Autism Spectrum Disorders

The fifth edition of *Autism Spectrum Disorders: Advancing Positive Practices in Education* provides readers with a comprehensive and accessible understanding of current research and evidence-based practices in autism spectrum disorders (ASD), linking research, theory, and practice. This new edition includes new chapters on trauma and co-morbidity, current trends in autism research, social media, neurodiversity, and aging in people with ASD. It features updated content, with added focus on culturally sustaining relevant practices. Aligned with DSM-5 diagnostic criteria, this text continues to be critical reading for students and researchers in special and inclusive education programs.

Angi Stone-MacDonald is Professor of Special Education and Department Chair at California State University, San Bernardino, USA.

David F. Cihak is Professor of Special Education and Associate Dean of Educator Preparation Programs at the University of Tennessee, Knoxville, USA.

Dianne Zager is Professor Emeritus at C.W. Post Campus/LIU and Pace University/NYC. Currently, she is a consultant and advocate for individuals with autism and their families.

Autism Spectrum Disorders

Advancing Positive Practices in Education

Fifth Edition

Edited by Angi Stone-MacDonald, David F. Cihak, and Dianne Zager, Founding Editor

Routledge
Taylor & Francis Group

NEW YORK AND LONDON

Designed cover image: © Getty Images

Fifth edition published 2023
by Routledge
605 Third Avenue, New York, NY 10158

and by Routledge
4 Park Square, Milton Park, Abingdon, Oxon, OX14 4RN

Routledge is an imprint of the Taylor & Francis Group, an informa business

First edition published by L. Erlbaum Associates 1992
Fourth edition published by Routledge 2017

ISBN: 9781032185637 (hbk)
ISBN: 9781032154176 (pbk)
ISBN: 9781003255147 (ebk)

DOI: 10.4324/9781003255147

Typeset in Sabon
by Newgen Publishing UK

We would like to dedicate this book to our students, friends, colleagues, and families who inspire us to keep learning, growing, and challenging our thinking. We hope this book will encourage our readers to further develop their own knowledge, skills, and understanding.

Contents

Contributors

Serra Acar, Ph.D., Assistant Professor of Early Childhood Education and Care, Department of Curriculum and Instruction, College of Education and Human Development, University of Massachusetts, Boston

Gabrielle Agnew, M.S., N.C.C., doctoral student in clinical psychology in the Graduate School of Biomedical Sciences, University of Texas Southwestern Medical Center

Megan M. Anderson, B.S., Graduate student in Healthcare Administration, Stonehill College, North Easton, Massachusetts

Kathryn Best, Ph.D., Director of Curriculum, Instruction, and Assessment at St. Michael's Episcopal School, Richmond, Virginia

Emily C. Bouck, Ph.D., Professor and Interim Associate Dean for Research at the College of Education, Michigan State University

Jonathan B. Bystrynski, Ph.D., Postdoctoral Fellow with the Department of Pediatrics and the MIND Institute, University of California, Davis

Irina Cain, Ph.D., Adjunct Instructor at the School of Education, Virginia Commonwealth University

Alice S. Carter, Ph.D., Professor in Clinical Psychology, College of Liberal Arts, University of Massachusetts, Boston

David F. Cihak, Ph.D., Professor of Special Education, Associate Dean of Professional Licensure, and Director of the Graduate School of Education, Department of Theory and Practice in Teacher Education, University of Tennessee, Knoxville

Debra L. Cote, Ph.D., Assistant Professor, Department of Special Education, College of Education, California State University, Fullerton

Christopher B. Denning, Ph.D., Associate Professor in the Department of Curriculum and Instruction and Associate Dean for Academic Affairs, College of Education and Human Development University of Massachusetts, Boston

Lindsay L. Diamond, Ph.D., Associate Professor in Special Education, College of Education, University of Nevada, Reno

E. Amanda DiGangi, Ph.D., BCBA-D, LBA, Clinical Associate Professor of Applied Behavior Analysis in the Mary Lou Fulton Teachers College, Arizona State University, Tempe, AZ

Samuel DiGangi, Ph.D., BCBA-D, Associate Professor of Special Education, Mary Lou Fulton Teachers College, Arizona State University, Tempe

Ben Edwards, Autistic and Disability Rights Activist, Research Aide at the Center on Developmental Disabilities, University of Kansas

Marc Ellison, Ed.D., Licensed Professional Counselor and Executive Director of the West Virginia Autism Training Center, Marshall University

Angel Fettig, Ph.D., Associate Professor and Special Education Doctoral Program Director, College of Education, University of Washington

Veronica P. Fleury, Ph.D., Associate Professor of Special Education, School of Teacher Education, Florida State University, Tallahassee

Deidre Gilley, M.S., Doctoral Candidate in Special Education, Florida State University

Ivy Giserman Kiss, Ph.D., Neurodevelopmental and Behavioral Phenotyping Service, National Institutes of Mental Health, Bethesda

Brenna Griffen, M.Ed., BCBA, Doctoral Student and Graduate Assistant CIED Doctoral Student, University of Arkansas Fayetteville

Monica Grillo, M.Ed., Doctoral candidate, Clinical Coach for Pre-Service Teachers at the University of Virginia, Adjunct Faculty Instructor, School of Education, Virginia Commonwealth University

Dedra Hafner, Ed.D., President of Innovations Now, Inc, LLC, Madison, Wisconsin

Shawna G. Harbin, Ph.D., Postdoctoral Scholar, College of Education, University of Washington, Seattle

Elizabeth A. Harkins Monaco, Ph.D., Assistant Professor, Department of Special Education, Professional Counseling, and Disability Studies, William Paterson University

Lindsey B. Hogue, Ph.D., College of Education at the University of Nevada, Reno

Kara Hume, Ph.D., Associate Professor and Faculty Fellow, Frank Porter Graham Child Development Institute Director, School of Education, University of North Carolina at Chapel Hill

Delia Kan, B.S., Doctoral student in the Applied Developmental Sciences and Special, School of Education, University of North Carolina at Chapel Hill

Dylan Kapit, M.A., GBTQ+ Outreach Coordinator at Barnard College and doctoral student at the School of Education, University of Pittsburgh

Mary Jo Krile, Ph.D., Assistant Professor of Special Education, Eastern Kentucky University

Holly Long, M.Ed., Graduate Student, College of Education, Michigan State University

Elizabeth R. Lorah, Ph.D., BCBA-D, Associate Professor of Special Education, Department of Curriculum and Instruction, University of Arkansas Fayetteville

Kayla Malone, M.Ed., Intervention Coach, graduate research assistant and doctoral student, School of Education, University of North Carolina at Chapel Hill

Melissa P. Maye, Ph.D., Assistant Scientist, Center for Health Policy and Health Services Research, Henry Ford Health System, Detroit

Meaghan M. McCollow, Ph.D., BCBA-D, Assistant Professor, Department of Educational Psychology, California State University East Bay

Celeste Michaud, Doctoral Student/Lecturer, College of Education and Health Professions, University of Arkansas, Fayetteville

Amelia K. Moody, Ph.D., Professor in the Watson College of Education, University of North Carolina, Wilmington

Michael C. Morrow, Doctoral Student in the Theory and Practice of Special Education, University of Tennessee, Knoxville

Nikki L. Murdick, Ph.D., Professor Emerita, School of Education, Saint Louis University, Saint Louis

Margaret O'Riordan, M.Ed., Doctoral Student, Department of Curriculum and Instruction, College of Education and Human Development, University of Massachusetts, Boston

Ozden Pinar Irmak, M.A., Doctoral Candidate and Graduate Assistant, Department of Curriculum and Instruction, University of Massachusetts, Boston

Jamie Prosser, Deputy Chief, Las Vegas Metropolitan Police Department

Orla Putnam, M.S., Doctoral Student in Speech and Hearing Sciences, University of North Carolina at Chapel Hill

Sheida K. Raley, Ph.D., Assistant Research Professor at the Center on Developmental Disabilities and Assistant Professor in the Department of Special Education, University of Kansas

Devon Ramey, PhD, Lecturer, School of Social Sciences, Education and Social Work, Queen's University Belfast, Ireland

Sarah Robison, M.Ed, BCBA, LBA, Doctoral Candidate in Disability and Psychoeducational Studies, University of Arizona, Tucson

Jenny R. Root, Ph.D., BCBA, Associate Professor of Special Education, School of Teacher Education, Florida State University

Jacquelin A. Sauer, B.S., Graduate Student in Healthcare Administration, Stonehill College

Peggy Schaefer Whitby, Ph.D., BCBA-D, Associate Professor, Department of Curriculum and Instruction, University of Arkansas, Fayetteville

LaRon A. Scott, Ph.D., Associate Professor and Developer and Executive Director of the Minority Educator Recruitment, Retention, and Equity Center, School of Education, Virginia Commonwealth University

Karrie A. Shogren, Ph.D., Director of the Center on Developmental Disabilities, Senior Scientist at the Schiefelbusch Life Span Institute, and Professor in the Department of Special Education, University of Kansas

Jordan Shurr, Ph.D., Associate Professor and Graduate Supervisor, Faculty of Education, Queen's University

Tom E.C. Smith, Ed.D., Professor of Special Education, Department of Curriculum and Instruction University of Arkansas, Fayetteville

Cate C. Smith, Ph.D., Clinical Associate Professor of Special Education, Department of Theory and Practice in Teacher Education, University of Tennessee, Knoxville

Shannon L. Sparks, Ph.D., Associate Professor and Special Education Program Coordinator, Department of Special Education, Rehabilitation & Counseling, California State University, San Bernardino

L. Lynn Stansberry Brusnahan, Ph.D., parent of a young adult with autism, Professor, University of St. Thomas

Angi Stone-MacDonald, Ph.D., Professor and Department Chair, Department of Special Education, Rehabilitation, and Counseling, California State University, San Bernardino

Kochy Tang, D.O. Medical Director at M Family Care, Henderson, Nevada

Colleen A. Thoma, Ph.D. Professor & Associate Dean of Academic Affairs and Graduate Studies, School of Education, Virginia Commonwealth University

Julie L. Thompson, Ph.D., BCBA, Assistant Professor of Special Education, Department of Educational Psychology, College of Education and Human Development, Texas A&M University

Danielle A. Waldron, Ph.D., Assistant Professor in Healthcare Administration at Stonehill College and Lecturer in the Department of Gerontology, McCormack Graduate School, University of Massachusetts, Boston

Michael L. Wehmeyer, Ph.D., Ross and Marianna Beach Distinguished Professor in Special Education, University of Kansas

Allison White, Ph.D., Licensed Behavior Analyst, Department of Counseling, Educational Psychology, and Special Education, Michigan State University

Andrew Wojcik, Ph.D., Assistant Professor and Assistant Coordinator, Counseling and Special Education, Virginia Commonwealth University

Amanda Wood, Ph.D., School Psychological Examiner at Wentzville R-IV School District, Wentzville, Missouri

A. Leah Wood, Ph.D., Associate Professor of Special Education, California Polytechnic University, San Luis Obispo

Jo Nell Wood, Ed.D., Associate Professor of Educational Leadership, School of Education, Saint Louis University, Saint Louis

Lexi Woods-Catterlin, M.S., CCC-SLP, Doctoral Student, University of Arkansas

Dianne Zager, Ph.D., Professor Emeritus, C.W. Post Campus/LIU and Pace University/NYC

Songtian Zeng, Ph.D., BCBA, Assistant Professor, Department of Curriculum and Instruction, University of Massachusetts, Boston

About the Editors

Angi Stone-MacDonald, Ph.D., is Professor and Department Chair of Special Education, Rehabilitation, and Counseling at California State University, San Bernardino. Dr. Stone-MacDonald has a Ph.D. in Special Education and has worked and researched inclusive and early childhood education for over 20 years, including in East Africa. Her areas of research include early intervention, international special education for children with developmental disabilities, and teacher preparation for early intervention. She has served on the board of the Division of Autism and Developmental Disabilities, a division of the Council for Exceptional Children in multiple capacities over the last 15 years. She is currently researching the experiences of families who speak languages other than English in the early intervention system.

David F. Cihak, Ph.D., is Associate Dean of Professional Educator Programs and Director of the Bailey Graduate School of Education in the College of Education, Health and Human Science at University of Tennessee. As a Professor of Special Education, he has published over 75 data-based research studies focused on remedying classroom-based problems associated with academic and social/behavioral problems of individuals with severe disabilities and autism resulting in greater competency, community access, and acceptance. His research interests include the use of effective instructional and behavioral strategies, specifically video, augmented, virtual, and AI technologies for improving educational, functional, and social/communicative outcomes for students in classroom and community settings. David is also currently examining instructional technologies to facilitate the acquisition, generalization, and maintenance of functional digital media skills to improve digital inclusion and independence.

Dianne Zager, Ph.D., has been a teacher, researcher, administrator, and national leader in education. She is internationally recognized as a pioneer in autism education, and has served as president of the International Council for Exceptional Children's Division on Autism and Developmental Disabilities, New York State Council for Exceptional Children, and Northeastern Educational Research Association. She has chaired the Special Education and Literacy Department at the C.W. Post Campus of Long Island University and the Special Education Department at Pace University's NYC campus, where she created and directed one of the nation's first college support programs for students with autism. Selected organizations from which she's received recognition and honors include the Autism Society of America, American Academy of Child and Adolescent Psychiatry, New York City Department of Education, and the International Council for Exceptional Children's Division on Autism and Developmental Disabilities.

Preface

The 5th edition of this text provides readers with a comprehensive and reliable source for the current research and evidence-based practices in autism spectrum disorder, as well as emerging directions in education and interventions. As editors, our goal is to continue to be responsive to the changing definitions and the broadening of the understanding of autism spectrum disorders, as well as the systematic implementation of evidence-based practices across the lifespan. In this edition, we provide readers with more knowledge about current evidence-based and research-based practices with individuals with ASD and strategies to support the implementation of those practices in their daily work as educators, therapists, clinicians, and other service providers working with people with ASD. Chapter authors examine historical perspectives, evidence-based best practices, strategies for inclusion, and emerging trends in the field. This edition also provides a more interactional context for readers through the inclusion of case studies and examples of application in each chapter. Furthermore, we wanted to include more voices and perspectives, including those of autistic people in this edition. In reading the book, it is noticeable that not all chapters are written from the same perspective about education or working with autistic people. We hope that the chapters provide a variety of perspectives that can encourage conversations and support a multitude of perspectives that will help us all to learn more and better understand those perspectives we are less familiar with.

Since the 4th edition was published in 2016, autism has continued to grow in prevalence and the field practitioners have continued to expand how they have supported autistic individuals and their families. While autism centers have sprung up across the nation, offering a wide range of services including assessment, academic, social, communication, vocational/career support, and counseling, students have also been more integrated into schools and inclusive classrooms. Furthermore, many college programs for students with autism have been established or expanded in the last five years, providing students with autism a more typical college experience. Families and clinicians are being inundated with information from conferences, webinars, journals, and newsletters. The number of undergraduate and graduate university courses on autism has increased. The field of autism continues to be ever-present in the media. Furthermore, in the last ten years, there has been a unifying advocacy by the autistic community such that autism is more often seen as a form of diversity and intersectionality is more salient within the autistic community.

In response to the dramatic increase in the prevalence of the diagnosis of ASD, diagnostic criteria in the recently published DSM-5 are different than they were in the DSM IV-R. Throughout the text, authors have utilized the new *2020 Evidence-based Practices Report* in their chapters to highlight the latest information on evidence-based practices in autism.

Education and intervention have become increasingly scientifically-based with clinical decisions more frequently grounded in research and data. In schools, special education teams are using evidence-based practices on a regular basis to support students and address their individualized goals. Interdisciplinary collaboration is common practice. While early intervention and preschool education remain critical areas of focus, greater attention is being devoted to preparing students with autism for transition to postsecondary education, employment and community living. In addition, it is important to recognize that much of the research being done on evidence-based practices is not being done by or with autistic scholars and their voices. Their participation in research needs to be included in the more holistic understanding of autism.

In this edition, we not only address autism in an international context through the updating of a dedicated chapter on autism in low- and middle-income countries, but we also are more inclusive and conscientious of the cultural and linguistic diversity of people with autism in the US and how that impacts the research on and use of evidence-based practices. While we have made an effort to diversify the authors in this edited volume, it is important to acknowledge that not all perspectives may be represented here and some information or perceptions may be missed without more authors from culturally and linguistically diverse backgrounds.

The structure, content, and format of the 5th edition have been revised as needed to reflect these changes in the field and to illuminate the current state of the art in the study of autism. Case studies and evidence-based practices have been integrated throughout the content of each chapter.

We have added seven additional chapters that are timely and reflect additional areas not covered in the previous editions and address cross-cutting themes regardless of the age of the individuals. We have added these chapters in a fourth section discussing neurodiversity, digital safety and media inclusion; current research trends; sexuality, LGBTQ+ considerations and intersectionality; and interaction with first responders and medical staff. Finally, to ensure that autistic individuals are included, the final chapter is on neurodiversity and the culture of autism. This chapter provides some perspectives from the autistic community on topics discussed in this book. It is important to recognize that chapter authors and the editors of this volume are not speaking as spokespeople or representing the autistic community, but creating an opportunity to share many voices and perspectives about autism and about education, intervention, and life for autistic people and their families.

We would like to thank the authors for their contribution to this new edition of *Autism Spectrum Disorders: Advancing Positive Practices in Education*.

Angi Stone-MacDonald, David Cihak, and Dianne Zager

The Study of Autism

Historical and Global Perspectives

Chapter 1

Definitions and Classification of Autism Spectrum Disorders

Melissa P. Maye,[1] Ivy Giserman Kiss,[2] and Alice S. Carter[3]

[1]Center for Health Policy and Health Services Research, Henry Ford Health System, Detroit
[2]Neurodevelopmental and Behavioral Phenotyping Service, National Institutes of Mental Health, Bethesda
[3]Department of Clinical Psychology, University of Massachusetts, Boston

Autism spectrum disorder (ASD), a new diagnosis in the fifth edition of the Diagnostic and Statistical Manual (DSM-5), was developed to classify individuals with impairments due to difficulties with social communication and social interaction, as well as the presence of restrictive and repetitive behaviors, interests, or activities (American Psychiatric Association, 2013). ASD replaces a set of diagnoses that were included in the fourth edition of the *Diagnostic and Statistical Manual* (DSM-IV), including Autistic Disorder, Pervasive Developmental Disorder – Not Otherwise Specified, and Asperger's Disorder (APA, 2000). These diagnoses were previously grouped together within a category labeled Pervasive Developmental Disorders. At present, it is estimated that 1 in 44 children (4.2 times more prevalent in boys than girls) have an ASD diagnosis (Maenner et al., 2021).

In this chapter, the ways in which the conceptualization of the construct *autism* has changed over the last century are explored, and modifications made to the diagnostic criteria in each edition of the DSM are described. Special emphasis is placed on the most recent changes, introduced in the DSM-5 in 2013. Symptom criteria that are used to diagnose autism spectrum disorder in the DSM-5 are described in detail.

Many different screening tools and diagnostic measures have been developed to aid clinicians and researchers in making earlier and more accurate diagnoses of earlier diagnostic classifiers included under the category, "Pervasive Developmental Disorders" and the current diagnostic classifier, ASD (Lord et al., 2012; Lord, Rutter, & Le Couteur, 1994; Luyster et al., 2009; Robins et al., 2014; Rutter, Bailey, Lord, Cianchetti, & Fancello, 2008; Schopler, Van Bourgondien, Wellman, & Love, 2010; Stone; Coonrod, & Turner, 2004; Stone, McMahon, & Henderson, 2008). In addition to reviewing historical shifts in diagnostic criteria and

DOI: 10.4324/9781003255147-2

conceptualizations, three diagnostic measures that are widely used in diagnostic assessment and have strong evidence bases to support their use are presented in the chapter. It is important to note, however, that while these diagnostic measures are extremely useful as aids in clinical decision-making, they are not considered diagnostic instruments. They are designed to be used to inform, rather than to replace, clinical judgment.

Historical Changes in Diagnosis and DSM Criteria

The conceptualization of ASD has changed over time to accommodate our evolving understanding of the disorder. In 1911, Eugen Bleuler, a Swiss psychiatrist, coined the terms *autism* and *autistic*, which he developed from the root Greek word *autos* meaning self. Bleuler used the term *autism* to describe a symptom of schizophrenia, in which individuals actively withdrew from the external world and into themselves, "rejecting reality" (Moskowitz & Heim, 2011). Regarding this *autistic* behavioral pattern, Bleuler (1951) wrote, "the most severe cases withdraw completely and live in a dream world; the milder cases withdraw to a lesser degree" (p. 399). Rather than referring to individuals now understood to have ASD, Bleuler intended for his term *autism* to refer to the "isolated self" observed in individuals with psychosis. Thus, in DSM-I, published in 1952, the term *autism* was used to describe psychotic reactions observed in children with childhood-onset schizophrenia (American Psychiatric Association, 1952). DSM-II (American Psychiatric Association, 1968) also mentioned autism only within the context of childhood schizophrenia.

Between the 1940s and 1960s the symptom of autism continued to be widely regarded as an early indicator of childhood schizophrenia (Baker, 2013). Moreover, causing significant stigma, pain, and suffering to families, this symptom was often erroneously attributed to distant parenting (Weintraub, 2011). During this time, Leo Kanner, an American psychiatrist, sought to distinguish autism as its own disorder, which was characterized by a unique set of behaviors, independent of childhood schizophrenia. Kanner's 1943 publication, entitled "Autistic Disturbances of Affective Contact," presented 11 comprehensive case histories of children with characteristics similar to those by which ASD is defined today. Their shared symptoms included social withdrawal, echolalia, need for sameness/resistance to change, atypical sensory responses, and repetitive behaviors such as spinning and rocking. Eventually, Kanner rejected the commonly held belief that autism was a product of "cold" child-rearing environments, and instead came to believe that autism was congenital in nature (Baker, 2013; Kanner, 1943). Kanner's documentation of the common behavioral profiles of this group of patients broadened the definition and understanding of autism as a behavioral disorder.

Interestingly, at the same time that Kanner was completing his work in the United States, Hans Asperger, an Austrian pediatrician, used the term *autistic* to describe a group of four boys who had traits similar to Kanner's cohort of patients but who were higher-functioning in terms of cognitive capacities. In his classic "Autistic Psychopathology" article published in 1944, Asperger described deficits that were slightly more social in nature in the four boys who he characterized as "little professors," a term that was often applied to describe children who met criteria for the later defined Asperger's Syndrome, which was included in the DSM-IV, but removed from DSM-5. The symptoms of Asperger's Syndrome are considered within ASD in DSM-5.

Kanner and Asperger's work, as well as a book published in 1964 by Bernard Rimland, an American psychologist, suggested that autism was based in biology and not caused by distant or cold parenting. These early writings laid the groundwork for the emergence of infantile autism as its own disorder in the DSM-III in 1980. Infantile autism in the DSM-III, consisted of the following three major symptom clusters, each of which had to emerge before 30 months of age: lack of responsiveness to others, severe impairments in language development, and "bizarre responses" to aspects of the environment. Additionally, to distinguish infantile autism from childhood schizophrenia, the authors of the DSM-III included a requirement of an absence of delusions and hallucinations. DSM-III applied a monothetic approach (i.e., an individual had to meet all three diagnostic criteria) and therefore focused on what might now be considered "classic autism," as manifested in more severely affected individuals.

The conceptualization of the disorder changed significantly from DSM-III to DSM-III-R (APA, 1987), when a more developmental emphasis and polythetic criteria (i.e., an individual had to meet a certain minimal number of defining characteristics, but not all symptoms of the diagnostic criteria) was introduced in which individuals had to meet only eight of 16 defined criteria. In addition, the requirement for an age of onset prior to 30 months was removed. The descriptions of the 16 possible symptoms in the DSM-III-R reflected an attempt to enhance diagnostic precision based on the prevailing understandings of the disorder, which were rooted in both the extant research and clinical practice. To meet criteria for the diagnosis, an individual needed to show at least two of five symptoms that reflected evidence of impaired reciprocal social interaction, one of six symptoms that reflected evidence of impaired verbal and nonverbal communication, and one of five symptoms that reflected the presence of restricted and/or repetitive behavior. Furthermore, the authors of the DSM-III-R created an additional category called Pervasive Developmental Disorder – Not Otherwise Specified (PDD-NOS), for children who displayed some of these symptoms, but did not meet full criteria for a diagnosis of autistic disorder. While the given list of symptoms provided a more structured organization of the criteria for the disorder, the addition of PDD-NOS increased the overall flexibility of the application of the diagnosis and increased the number of individuals who met criteria for these disorders (Hansen, Schendel, & Parner, 2015).

While DSM-III-R included the addition of PDD-NOS, it was not until the 1990s that Lorna Wing, an English psychiatrist, and Uta Frith, an English psychologist, popularized the term *Asperger's Syndrome*. The work of Wing and Frith contributed to another shift in the conceptualization of autism when Asperger's Syndrome was officially recognized as a distinct subtype of the disorder in the publication of DSM-IV in 1994. The diagnostic criteria for Asperger's Syndrome were similar to that of autistic disorder, but required typical language development, average cognitive abilities, and average adaptive behavior abilities (other than in social interaction). At this point, clinicians and researchers began to conceptualize autism along a broad continuum or spectrum of functioning levels and abilities (Baker, 2013).

Similar to DSM-III-R, DSM-IV relied on a polythetic approach, such that a diagnosis of autistic disorder required at least six of 12 listed criteria. To receive the diagnosis, an individual was required to evidence at least two of four symptoms of "qualitatively" impaired social interaction, one of four symptoms of "qualitatively" impaired communication, and one of four restricted or repetitive behaviors or interests. Moreover, the age of onset criteria was reinstated: at least one of the behaviors needed to be evident prior to three years of age. The criteria for autistic disorder, PDD-NOS and Asperger's Syndrome did not change in DSM-IV-TR, published in 2000.

The publication of the DSM-5 (APA, 2013) sparked a great deal of controversy among individuals who had been diagnosed with Asperger's syndrome, family members, clinicians, and researchers, and captured the attention of the general public because marked changes were made to the criteria and manner in which disorders would be classified. Specifically, in a major change from the manner in which disorders were grouped in DSM-IV, multiple disorders are now subsumed under a single autism spectrum disorder classification. In addition, where appropriate, in DSM-5 clinicians are required to provide a qualifier to the ASD diagnosis, which is quantified along a continuum of severity. The qualifier is used to designate the degree of support the individual with ASD requires, spanning from individuals who require minimal support to those who require very substantial support. Additionally, the qualifier helps to describe an individual's current symptomatology with the recognition that severity may vary by context. The revision committee eliminated the subtypes of Asperger's Syndrome and PDD-NOS as well as the overarching category of Pervasive Developmental Disorders, replacing these classifications with a single classification termed autism spectrum disorder (Ozonoff, 2012).

This decision created a powerful discourse regarding the loss of an entire group's identity. For example, Giles (2013) discussed how a culture developed around the diagnosis of Asperger's Syndrome, and thus meeting criteria for this disorder shaped a "blueprint for social identity." The committee justified their decision of creating a single "autism spectrum disorder" (ASD) diagnosis based on a body of evidence supporting that differentiation of ASD from typical development and other childhood disorders was done reliably and validly, while the distinction between the three subtypes was found to be inconsistent and varied across research sites (Gibbs, 2012).

Moreover, in DSM-5 the traditional triad of symptom domains (i.e., social, communication, and atypical/repetitive behaviors) was reduced to a dyad of symptoms by combining social and communication symptoms into a single domain (social communication deficits) to emphasize the social nature of communication symptoms relevant in ASD. In addition, sensory abnormalities were added to the second domain of restricted, repetitive behaviors, interests, or activities (RRBIs). Sensory abnormalities were not included in the DSM-IV-TR RRBI criteria. In contrast to the polythetic criteria in the third and fourth editions of the manual, the DSM-5 re-adopted a mixed monothetic and polythetic approach that requires meeting all of the listed social-communicative criteria (i.e., monothetic) that is contrasted with a polythetic approach for RRBI criteria, for which only two of the four defined symptoms must be present to assign a diagnosis. Finally, the specific age of onset was removed so that symptoms of the disorder must be present in infancy or early childhood, recognizing that the full disorder may become apparent in later years as the social demands of interpersonal relations increase.

The development of the new DSM-5 diagnosis of ASD leaves some questions unanswered. Although the majority of individuals who would have met DSM-IV criteria are likely to also meet DSM-5 criteria, there will not be 100% concordance. It remains unclear who will gain and who will lose a diagnosis with the revised DSM-5 diagnostic criteria, and what the long-term effects will be on access to services. Revising the organization, criteria, and nomenclature for describing the children first identified by Kanner and Asperger as having a unique set of symptoms associated with impairment is not a new phenomenom. The conceptualization of ASD has undergone several shifts over time to accommodate new understandings of the etiology and developmental course of the disorder.

Symptoms

ASD is currently characterized by impairments in an individual's social communication as well as the presence of RRBIs. Both retrospective and prospective research has informed the current conceptualization of the diagnosis (Ozonoff, 2012). Below, the defining symptoms of ASD, as described in the DSM-5, are explained in detail. The symptoms are divided into two domains: (1) impaired social communication skills (including impaired social-emotional reciprocity, impaired nonverbal communication, and atypical social relationships) and (2) restrictive and repetitive behaviors and interests. See Table 1.1 for DSM-5 descriptions of social communication and social interaction symptoms and restricted, repetitive patterns of behavior, interests, or activities symptoms (APA, 2013).

A. Impaired Social Communication Domain

1. Impaired social-emotional reciprocity. Starting from a very early age, children with ASD show abnormal social-emotional responses (De Giacomo & Fombonne, 1998; Gillberg et al., 1999; Guinchat et al., 2012; Osterling & Dawson, 1994; Webb & Jones, 2009; Werner, Dawson, Osterling, & Dinno, 2000; Wimpory, Hobson, Williams, & Nash, 2000; Young, Brewer, & Pattison, 2003), including the presence of some or all of the following symptoms: lack of and/or abnormal eye contact or gaze, decreased frequency of looking at others' faces, lack of interest in playing with other children, preference for playing alone, absence of pointing, giving, and showing objects, and lack of response to social stimuli such as the child's own name being called. Such impaired social-emotional responses have been documented as early as within the first six months of life (Maestro et al., 2002). However, prospective studies of high-risk infants (infant-siblings of older children diagnosed with ASD) have revealed that most infants who go on to later receive an ASD diagnosis do not show significant differences in social-emotional responses until the second year of life (Ozonoff et al., 2010). By 12 months of age, some infants later diagnosed with ASD can be differentiated from those who remain unaffected by the absence of social-communication competencies and/or atypical social-communication behaviors, including limited or unusual eye contact (Zwaigenbaum et al., 2005) and failure to orient to name call (Frohna, 2007). However, other children become symptomatic and do not meet diagnostic criteria until 18, 24, 30 or even 36 months of age (Ozonoff et al., 2010). In preschool and older-aged children, adolescents, and adults impaired social-emotional reciprocity can also include a limited ability to engage in a back-and-forth conversation, reduced sharing of interests and emotions, and an absence of initiation of/ response to social interactions.

2. Impaired nonverbal communication. Nonverbal communication includes facial expressions, body postures, and gestures, and is used to communicate needs, wants, and desires directly (e.g., pointing to direct attention, reaching to be picked up, shrugging shoulders to indicate lack of knowledge). Nonverbal communication may also be used to add nuance or punctuation to verbal communication (e.g., winking during or following a statement, nodding the head and/or using hand gestures

Table 1.1 Autism Spectrum Disorder DSM-5 Criteria for Social Communication and Restricted and Repetitive Patterns of Behavior, Interests, or Activities

A. Persistent deficits in social communication and social interaction across multiple contexts, as manifested by the following, currently or by history (examples are illustrative, not exhaustive; see text):

1. Deficits in social-emotional reciprocity	**Examples:** abnormal social approach and failure of normal back-and-forth conversation, reduced sharing of interests, emotions, or affect, failure to initiate or respond to social interactions
2. Deficits in nonverbal communicative behaviors used for social interaction	**Examples:** poorly integrated verbal and nonverbal communication, abnormalities in eye contact and body language or deficits in understanding and use of gestures, a lack of facial expressions and nonverbal communication
3. Deficits in developing, maintaining, and understanding relationships	**Examples:** difficulties adjusting behavior to suit various social contexts, difficulties in sharing imaginative play or in making friends, absence of interest in peers

A. Restricted, repetitive patterns of behavior, interests, or activities, as manifested by at least two of the following, currently or by history (examples are illustrative, not exhaustive; see text):

1. Stereotyped or repetitive motor movements, use of objects, or speech	**Examples:** simple motor stereotypies, lining up toys or flipping objects, echolalia, idiosyncratic phrases
2. Insistence on sameness, inflexible adherence to routines, or ritualized patterns or verbal nonverbal behavior	**Examples:** extreme distress at small changes, difficulties with transitions, rigid thinking patterns, greeting rituals, need to take same route or eat food every day
3. Highly restricted, fixated interests that are abnormal in intensity or focus	**Examples:** strong attachment to or preoccupation with unusual objects, excessively circumscribed or perseverative interest
4. Hyper- or hyporeactivity to sensory input or unusual interests in sensory aspects of the environment	**Examples:** apparent indifference to pain/temperature, adverse response to specific sounds or textures, excessive smelling or touching of objects, visual fascination with lights or movement

while speaking) and supplements language to help engage and connect with listeners and emphasize messages. Children and adults with ASD show deficits in nonverbal communication that is used for social purposes. It is common for individuals with ASD to demonstrate a lack of or atypical use of eye contact, facial expressions, and body language, as well as a reduced use and understanding of gestures. Additionally, children and adults with ASD oftentimes show atypical prosody, or changes in intonation and rhythm in speech. Instead of modulating his or her tone of voice, a child or adult with ASD will babble or speak in an abnormal or flat/monotonous tone that lacks appropriate stress or emphasis (Jones, Gliga, Bedford, Charman, & Johnson, 2014).

3. Atypical social relationships. Across the lifespan, individuals with ASD have difficulties relating to others. In early childhood, infants and toddlers with ASD often demonstrate a reduced interest in people and show a decreased frequency of looking at faces as well as a lack of interest in playing with other children. Children with ASD have difficulty initiating and sharing in imaginative play; they tend to struggle to engage in pretend play, especially with regard to the frequency, complexity, spontaneity, and playfulness of the activity (Porter, 2012). As they grow older, children with ASD continue to have difficulty maintaining and understanding social relationships. For example, children with the disorder frequently show a limited ability to pick up social cues to appropriately adjust their behavior to various social contexts (Jing & Fang, 2014).

B. Repetitive and Restricted Behaviors and Interests Domain

1. Stereotyped or Repetitive Motor and Vocal Mannerisms. Because repetitive motor mannerisms are commonly seen in typical development, some of the behaviors that are characteristic of older children with ASD may be hard to distinguish from typical behaviors (Jones et al., 2014). However, well-documented stereotypes in young children include repetitive hand and body movements, lining up toys, repeating idiosyncratic words or phrases, and spinning, rotating, and/or exploring objects visually in an unusual manner sometimes described as peering (Ozonoff et al., 2008). A recent review of stereotypic behavior in ASD (DiGennaro Reed, Hirst, & Hyman, 2012) found that commonly reported forms of stereotypic behaviors in ASD included body/head rocking/swaying, unrecognizable vocalizations, and hand flapping/waving, along with 25 additional categories of stereotypies.

2. Inflexible adherence to routines or rituals. Starting in toddlerhood, individuals with ASD frequently begin to show a desire for, or insistence on sameness (Leekam et al., 2007), which can also manifest as distress when rituals and/or routines are disrupted. Across childhood, this desire can take the form of the following behaviors: extreme distress at small changes, challenges with transitions, or the need to follow the same routine every day (American Psychiatric Association, 2013). Additionally, rigid thinking patterns and cognitive inflexibility often emerge as children with ASD grow older, frequently leading to behavioral and social impairments (Memari, 2013).

3. Preoccupations and restricted interests. Children and adults with ASD often have highly narrow interests. The term *restricted interest* is frequently interchanged with the terms *circumscribed interest* and *special interest*. Examples of restricted interests for children with ASD are particular machines, train schedules, and dinosaurs (Porter, 2012). The intensive and extensive knowledge gained about a restricted interest may or may not have any utility (e.g., an interest in train schedules for a specific city in another country or in the past, or a preoccupation with memorizing and updating the map of the NYC subway). Individuals with ASD may become hyper focused on or preoccupied with restricted interests, and therefore may become cognitively "stuck" (Charman, 2008). Early intervention services for children with ASD often focus on the ability to be redirected and the skill of flexibility.

4. Sensory behaviors. Many children and adults with ASD respond differently than individuals with typical development to sensory stimuli. Prior to the DSM-5, sensory behaviors were not included in the diagnostic criteria for the disorder. A review by Hazen, Stornelli, O'Rourke, Koesterer, and McDougle (2014) describes the three most common categories of impaired sensory modulation. The first category is *sensory overresponsivity*, where an individual experiences distress or a strong negative reaction to sensory input, often leading to avoidance (e.g., a child having an intense negative reaction to the noise of sirens, leading her to cover her ears or run away from police cars and fire trucks). The second category is *sensory underresponsivity*, in which an individual may seem to be unaware of, or display a delayed reaction to, a sensory stimulus that would normally lead to a response (e.g., a toddler repeatedly banging his or her head on the bottom of a table as if nothing happened, a teenager not reacting when he puts his hand on a hot stove). The final category of impaired sensory modulation is sensory-seeking behavior, also referred to as *craving*, in which an individual demonstrates a preoccupation with certain sensory experiences (e.g., a child repetitively staring at things that move or emit light, or a child licking walls or the floor).

Current Assessment Tools for Diagnosis

Researchers have completed extensive research over the last several decades to define the construct of autism and to identify those at risk for an ASD. At present, autism screening and diagnostic research have made it possible to identify children at high risk for ASD based on elevated ASD symptoms and to diagnose ASD in children as young as 12 months of age (Luyster et al., 2009; Osterling, Dawson, & Munson, 2002; Ozonoff et al., 2008; Ozonoff et al., 2010; Zwaigenbaum et al., 2005) with relative stability in diagnosis starting at about 14 months of age (Pierce et al., 2019).

Screening tools, many described below, have been created to help professionals identify children who are in need of a more thorough ASD evaluation in research and clinical settings (e.g., pediatric offices). The majority of empirically validated screening tools developed in the United States and/or European countries have been translated to, or adapted for, various other languages and cultures. We highlight the Modified Checklist for Autism in Toddlers – Revised, with Follow-Up interview (M-CHAT-R/F) as it has been the most extensively validated in international adaptations and translations. However, clinicians and researchers should still proceed with caution when using *any* translated and/or adapted screening tool given the limited research that has been completed for each measure/assessment in any one specific culture or language (Maskari et al., 2018; Soto et al., 2014).

These measures include brief screening instruments such as the extensively tested, M-CHAT-R/F, a written screener that has been adapted, translated, and validated in many countries and cultures (written screener, age range: 16-to-30-months) (Guo et al., 2019; Robins et al., 2014; Soto et al., 2015; Tsai et al., 2019). New since the last edition, the Developmental Check-In (DCI) is a brief picture-based ASD screener that was created with, and developed for, a racially, ethnically, and socioeconomically diverse population in the United States (available in English and Spanish, age range: 24-to-60-months) (Harris et al., 2021; Janvier, 2019). The DCI demonstrated strong discriminative power (area under the curve = 0.80) and performed well across all age groups, genders, levels of maternal education, primary language, and ethnic and racial groups in the initial validation study.

Longer ASD screening questionnaires can capture variability in normative and atypical expressions of symptoms such as the Social Communication Questionnaire (48-months-of-age and older) (Rutter, Bailey, Lord et al., 2007), while observational, play-based assessments can supplement screening questionnaires or be used independently for screening. The following are examples of validated play-based screening assessments: Screening Tool for Autism in Toddlers and Young Children (18-to-36-months-of-age) (Stone, Coonrod, & Turner, 2004; Stone, McMahon, & Henderson, 2008); Autism Observation Scale for Infants (6-to-18-months-of-age) (Bryson, Zwaigenbaum, McDermott, Rombough, & Brian, 2008); and Communication and Symbolic Behavior Scales – Developmental Profile (9-to-24-months-of-age) (Wetherby & Prizant, 2002).

Original, adapted, and translated ASD screening tools are used in a number of community settings, including pediatric primary care offices. The M-CHAT-R/F has been the most extensively implemented and evaluated in this setting – both nationally and internationally (Carbone et al., 2020; Guthrie et al., 2019; Monteiro et al., 2019; Stenberg et al., 2014; Toh, et al., 2018). Researchers found that the M-CHAT-R/F worked less well in real-world pediatric primary care settings than in controlled research studies (Carbone et al., 2020; Guthrie et al., 2019; Monteiro et al., 2019; Stenberg et al., 2014; Toh, et al., 2018). Moreover, disparities among historically marginalized groups were detected in several of the studies (Carbone et al., 2020; Guthrie et al., 2019). Although the American Academy of Pediatrics continues to recommend that all toddlers be screened for ASD at 18-and 24-months of age, debate on the effectiveness of universal screening persists as a result of numerous studies identifying implementation and/or measurement inadequacies identified in real-world universal screening studies (Carbone et al., 2020; Guthrie et al., 2019; Monteiro et al., 2019; Stenberg et al., 2014; Toh et al., 2018). Continued research and quality improvement in universal screening for ASD are necessary in order to ensure that children with ASD symptoms can be detected and further evaluated to determine a diagnosis and to connect individuals with early intervention and/or other community supports (Zwaigenbaum & Maguire, 2019). Regardless of the universal screening debate, if a child screens positive on a validated ASD screening tool, pediatricians should consider and discuss the results with parents and, when clinically appropriate, make appropriate referrals to a psychologist, psychiatrist, or developmental pediatrician for developmental and diagnostic evaluations.

Once referred, children suspected to be at risk of having ASD should ideally receive an evidence-based assessment of their current behaviors and interactions. Numerous assessments and interviews, discussed below, have been developed to aid clinicians in making accurate diagnoses. Most of these measures have been translated to or adapted for various languages and cultures. However, to our knowledge, no systematic reviews have been completed examining the rigor of translation and adaptation of these measures. As such, clinicians should proceed with extreme caution and review all published research when considering an adaptation or translation of any diagnostic assessment for ASD.

The Autism Diagnostic Observation Schedule – Second Edition (ADOS-2, Lord et al., 2012) is considered the gold standard empirically validated observational assessment of ASD and is widely used clinically and in research to assess individuals with suspected and known ASD. A second empirically validated tool is the Childhood Autism Rating Scales, Second Edition (CARS2: Schopler, Van Bourgondien, Wellman, & Love, 2010). These two empirically validated observational measures allow clinicians to directly assess an individual's behaviors and interactions. Both the ADOS-2 and CARS2 are appropriate for very young children through adulthood; the CARS2 is recommended for children 24-months-of-age and older and the ADOS-2 has a specific Toddler Module (Luyster et al., 2009) that is appropriate for children as young as 12-months-of-age – the ADOS-2 has slightly more range.

The *Autism Diagnostic Interview – Revised* (ADI-R: Lord, Rutter, & Le Couteur, 1994) is an empirically validated semi-structured caregiver interview that provides information about the identified individual's social, communication, and restricted and repetitive behaviors. The ADI-R allows comprehensive data to be gathered regarding both the individual's current and past functioning and is suitable for use in children 3.5-years-old and older. In the following sections, each measure is described in relation to the population for which it was designed, how the measure is administered, and what psychometric data are available; including where appropriate, internal consistency, sensitivity, and specificity. These measures can be used in combination in clinical diagnostic practice.

The *Autism Diagnostic Observation Schedule-2* (ADOS-2; Lord et al., 2012) is an observational assessment that trained clinicians can use as one part of their diagnostic battery to assess for presence of ASD. The ADOS-2 takes approximately 45 minutes to 1 hour to complete and consists of five modules, which are appropriate for individuals across the lifespan and across different levels of linguistic and developmental functioning. The newest module, the Toddler Module, is appropriate for young children between 12 and 30 months of age, who have not yet obtained phrase speech but have a nonverbal mental age of at least 12 months, and are walking independently (Luyster, et al., 2009). A sixth module, the Adapted ADOS, is currently in development for older populations who are minimally verbal and are seeking an ASD evaluation (Bal, et al., 2020). Initial validation of the Adapted ADOS is considered promising with acceptable sensitivity, specificity, and internal consistency.

An administration of the ADOS-2 consists of a series of semi-structured play-based tasks that elicit social communication behaviors and skills that are rated on a variety of dimensions to acquire a score in the Social Affective Domain (SA Domain), as well as ratings of observed restricted interests, repetitive behaviors, and sensory interests in the Restrictive Repetitive Behavior domain (RRB domain). Throughout the administration the clinician takes detailed observational notes regarding the participant's verbalizations and behaviors in the SA, and RRB domains.

The Toddler Module is comprised of 11 semi-structured tasks that elicit behaviors that are used to assess a toddler's social communication abilities as well as the presence or absence of sensory interests and RRBIs. Some of these tasks include: a free play interaction, a bubble play task where the examiner blows bubbles without explicitly calling the toddler's attention to them and then pauses to see whether or how the child requests more bubbles, a bath time routine with a doll to assess the presence or quality of functional and pretend play, and anticipatory social routines where the examiner engages the toddler in an interaction and observes his or her responses.

During these different tasks, the examiner observes how the toddler responds and notes behaviors and verbalizations relevant for considering social communication skills and presence of RRBI. For example, during the bubble blowing task the examiner notes the toddler's reaction to the bubbles being blown around the room. We might expect a typical toddler to look up, make eye contact with the examiner and smile. The toddler also might notice the bubbles and direct his or her caregiver's attention to them by pointing at the bubbles, smiling, using eye contact, and looking back-and-forth between the bubbles and his or her caregiver. However, it is likely that toddlers with an ASD would use few of these joint attention strategies when noticing the bubbles. Additionally, sensory interests and RRBIs may be noted during this task. For example, a child may explore the bubble toy in a sensory seeking manner by visually inspecting the toy bubble blower while looking at it and watching the propellers spin out of the corner of his/her eyes. Or, the toddler may demonstrate a restricted interest in colors by labeling all of the colors on the toy bubble blower as well as most of the colors of other objects throughout the assessment.

Modules 1 and 2 of the ADOS-2 are for individuals older than 30 months of age who have not yet attained fluent speech. Module 1 is appropriate for individuals who are either non-verbal or use single words only and is comprised of 10 semi-structured tasks. Module 2 is appropriate for individuals who are using phrase speech and is comprised of 14 semi-structured tasks, with many tasks overlapping from Module 1.

Modules 1 and 2 both have tasks that overlap with the Toddler Module such as a free play interaction, a task testing the child's response to his name, a task assessing the child's response to joint attention, and anticipation of a social routine with the examiner. Different from Module 1, Module 2 includes tasks that require a higher level of language ability. For example, Module 2 includes tasks, such as making up a story using a picture book that has few words, having a simple conversation with the examiner, and demonstrating make-believe play using a variety of toys and figures.

A birthday party routine task is present in both Modules 1 and 2. The birthday party interaction follows a simple script where children are given multiple opportunities to imitate play, expand on the prompts the examiner provides, and create their own make believe play interaction. During this interaction examiners can note any relevant social communication skills, sensory interests or RRBIs. However, this task specifically tries to draw out functional play and creative behaviors, as well as social reciprocity in observing how the child responds to the social interaction with the examiner.

Modules 3 and 4 of the ADOS-2 are designed for individuals with fluent speech. This is estimated at approximately a 4-year-old's expressive language level and includes presence of complex sentences. Module 3 is comprised of 14 different semi-structured tasks and is appropriate for children and adolescents with adequate language. Module 4 is comprised of 15 semi-structured tasks and is appropriate for individuals over the age of 16 who have a higher level of responsibility. Modules 3 and 4 include tasks similar to Module 2 such as a puzzle making task, a make-believe task, and a story-telling task with a book that is primarily pictures. However, Modules 3 and 4 also include activities that require fluent speech and a higher level of social communication development. For instance, there are a series of questions that explore topics, such as social difficulties, friends, and relationships that require the individual to reflect on his/her experiences and describe those to the examiner. During these tasks the examiner is able to observe social communication behaviors such as reciprocal conversation, sharing of interests with others, and sharing of emotions or affect and presence of, friendships or romantic relationships.

At the end of the assessment, the behaviors and verbalizations that the examiner noted are coded using a standardized protocol and algorithm scores for both the SA and RRB domains are calculated. Examiners can then use these scores as a tool to determine whether an individual is at risk for an ASD (i.e., the Toddler Module only assesses risk) or has met the cut-off for a classification of ASD on the ADOS-2 (Modules 1–4). These scores are used in determining a clinical diagnosis of ASD but should not be used as an independent determination of diagnosis; all diagnostic measures are limited by their individual psychometric properties of sensitivity (e.g., the probability of a positive test among people with ASD) and specificity (e.g., the probability of a negative test among people without ASD).

The ADOS-2, Modules 1–4 and the Toddler Module demonstrate strong psychometric properties. All five modules of the ADOS-2 demonstrate strong internal consistency within the SA domain. However, internal consistency is reduced for the RRB domain across all five modules (Gotham, Risi, Pickles, & Lord, 2007; Luyster et al., 2009). The variability within the RRB domain was expected due to the heterogeneous nature of the symptoms within this category and is a limitation of the measure.

Sensitivity and specificity ratings exceed 85% for almost all individuals studied across the five modules (Gotham, Risi, Pickles, & Lord, 2007; Luyster et al., 2009). However, for nonverbal toddlers between

21–30 months of age on the Toddler Module and for individuals with nonverbal mental ages less than 15 months on Modules 1–4 specificity, but not sensitivity, is reduced (Gotham, Risi, Pickles, & Lord, 2007; Gotham et al., 2008; Lord et al., 2000; Luyster et al., 2009). Despite this one shortcoming, as a whole the ADOS-2 provides clinicians with an excellent tool to use as part of a comprehensive evaluation.

The *Autism Diagnostic Interview – Revised* (ADI-R; Lord et al., 1994) is a standardized interview that trained interviewers can use as one part of a diagnostic battery to assess for ASD. The ADI-R is administered to caregivers of individuals with ASD and is appropriate for individuals who are at least 3.5-years-old and have a mental age of at least 2-years-old, through adulthood. Caregivers are asked questions based on their child's age and verbal abilities. For example, caregivers of individuals without spoken language are not asked questions regarding their child's ability to carry a conversation and caregivers of individuals who are 3 years old are not asked questions about the period of time between their child's fourth and fifth birthday (a series of questions focus on this time period).

Interview questions primarily focus on social communication and the presence of restricted interests and repetitive behaviors. Throughout the administration, the interviewer codes caregiver responses based on their report of the individual's behavior as opposed to asking caregivers to choose a rating. When the interview is complete, the interviewer calculates a total score using one of three algorithms based on the child's age, nonverbal and verbal mental age, and reported language abilities. The ADI-R adjusts for expressive language levels with different algorithms and total score cutoffs available for children who use daily, functional, use of language (i.e., three-word phrases that sometimes include a verb) and those with very limited language abilities (i.e., mostly single words, or no words at all).

The ADI-R takes approximately 1.5 hours to complete for caregivers who are reporting on a child approximately 3.5–4 years old. However, the interview could take substantially longer for an older child. Though the interview is lengthy, Lord et al. (1994) report that parents found the interview to be relatively comfortable and felt as though the interviewers cared about their perspective of their child and were able to gain more information about their child than they would in an observational assessment.

The ADI-R has shown strong psychometric properties for individuals regardless of chronological or mental age. The ADI-R demonstrates strong internal consistency for the social domain and good internal consistency for the RRB domain (Lord et al., 1994). Further, sensitivity for all individuals studied was over 90%. Specificity was over 85% for all verbal groups. Specificity for non-verbal groups was measured as 79% (Lord et al., 1997). Overall, the ADI-R complements the ADOS-2 in terms of gathering information for a clinical diagnosis. However, it is rarely used in clinical settings due to the length of time the interview takes to complete.

The Childhood Autism Rating Scale, Second Edition (CARS2; Schopler et al., 2010) consists of three forms: the Childhood Autism Rating Scale, Second Edition-Standard Version (CARS2-ST), the Childhood Autism Rating Scale, Second Edition-High Functioning Version (CARS2-HF), and the Childhood Autism Rating Scale, Second Edition-Questionnaire for Parents or Caregivers (CARS2-QPC).

Trained examiners in a variety of settings including psychologists, psychiatrists, pediatricians, and special educators may administer the CARS2-ST and CARS2-HF. Different from the ADOS-2, there are no specific prompts, tasks, or interactions that examiners employ when making their ratings of the child. In contrast to the semi-structured standardized activities included in the ADOS modules, the CARS2-HF and CARS2-ST are flexible, in that examiners can make observations in any way that is convenient for the individual and their support system so long as adequate observational data are collected.

Prior to beginning the assessment, examiners complete a language sample to determine the most appropriate version of the CARS2. Individuals who are verbally fluent with full-scale IQ scores over 80 are administered the CARS2-HF and those who are not fluent with full-scale IQ scores below 80 are administered the CARS2-ST. Children under 6 years of age are administered the CARS2-ST regardless of cognitive ability and verbal fluency. These measures evaluate individuals who have been referred for an ASD evaluation and should not be used within the general population. The CARS2-ST and CARS2-HF were developed to provide quantitative data obtained through a comprehensive evaluation within a referred population.

During an administration of the CARS2-ST and CARS2-HF examiners take detailed notes on behaviors, verbalizations, and interactions and then use a standardized form to rate an individual across 15 different functional areas. Examiners should be very familiar with the 15 different functional areas and scoring system of the CARS2-ST and CARS-HF prior to rating an individual's behaviors. The CARS2-HF has been adapted to adjust for differences in cognitive development. Thus, while many of the functional areas are similar across both the CARS2-ST and the CARS2-HF, there are key differences of which examiners should be aware.

For example, relating to people is a functional area on both the CARS2-ST and the CARS2-HF. Both functional areas require the examiner to assess the individual's behavior in a variety of situations while interacting with other people. However, the expectations for level of social complexity are higher for individuals receiving the CARS2-HF. Additionally, though the functional areas are similar in definition, and both are scored on a four point scale, the CARS-ST and CARS-HF have different scoring criteria.

The CARS2-QPC is an optional parent interview that can be used in conjunction with the CARS2-ST or CARS2-HF to supplement information that was not collected during the observational period. The CARS2-QPC collects data from each of the 15 areas of the CARS2-ST/CARS2-HF. It was organized in a way that is most meaningful for caregivers and thus does not directly map onto the rating form for the CARS-ST or CARS2-HF. Following the data collection period (i.e., the CARS2-ST, CARS2-HF, and possibly the CARS2-QPC), a trained clinician codes the data across the 15 different categories and generates a total score that is used to assess the likelihood that an individual meets criteria for ASD. It is suggested that the CARS2-QPC be administered after the CARS2-ST/ CARS2-HF and used as supplementary data to fill in gaps that may have been overlooked during the observational data collection period.

The CARS and CARS2 demonstrate strong psychometric properties. Several studies have reported strong total score internal consistency reliability for the CARS and CARS2 (Chlebowski, Green, Barton, & Fein, 2010; Schopler, Reichler, DeVellis, & Daly, 1980; Schopler, Van Bourgondien, Wellman, & Love, 2010). Further, the CARS and CARS2 have consistently demonstrated excellent sensitivity and specificity, with percentages over 85% for each (Chlebowski et al., 2010; Perry, Caondillac, Freeman, Dunn-Geir, & Belair, 2005; Schopler, Van Bourgondien, Wellman, & Love, 2010).

The ADOS-2, ADI-R, and CARS2 are three diagnostic measures that are clinically useful and have strong psychometric properties. Individually, they can stand alone as good measures to aid clinical judgment in making an ASD diagnosis with all three demonstrating strong levels of sensitivity and specificity (Chlebowski, Green, Barton, & Fein, 2010; Gotham et al., 2008; Gotham, Risi, Pickles, & Lord, 2007; Lord et al., 1997; Lord et al., 2000; Lord et al., 2012; Lord, Rutter, & Le Couteur, 1994; Luyster et al., 2009; Perry, Caondillac, Freeman, Dunn-Geir, & Belair, 2005; Schopler, Reichler, DeVellis, & Dally, 1980; Schopler, Van Bourgondien, Wellman, & Love, 2010).

The use of several diagnostic measures increases the likelihood of making an accurate diagnosis. For example, it has been well documented that using both the ADOS-2 and ADI-R together in a comprehensive ASD assessment increases the likelihood that an accurate diagnosis is made (de Bildt et al., 2004; Kim & Lord, 2012; Le Couteur, Haden, Hammeal, McConachie, 2008; Risi et al., 2006). Though administering at least two diagnostic measures is time-consuming, each measure brings unique, as well as overlapping, information about the individual, providing a more comprehensive assessment (Kim & Lord, 2012). For example, the ADI-R asks about both past and current skills and behaviors whereas all versions of the ADOS-2 only consider current skills and behaviors. The CARS has not been considered in terms of increased sensitivity or specificity when combined with other instruments. Researchers have demonstrated a high degree of diagnostic agreement (85%) between the CARS and the ADI-R (Pilowsky, Yirmiya, Shulman, & Dovers, 1998). The authors hypothesized that the disagreement between the two measures was related, in part, to the method in which data were collected – observational (CARS) versus an interview comprised of both past and present information (ADI-R).

In summary, the ADOS-2, ADI-R, and CARS2 consistently provide diagnoses high in specificity and sensitivity when administered individually. Additional diagnostic certainty can be obtained by administering at least two diagnostic measures, preferably a direct observational measure (i.e., ADOS-2 or CARS2) and a caregiver interview (i.e., ADI-R, CARS-QPC) or one of the more thorough parent/caregiver screeners such as the SCQ (Rutter, Bailey, Lord et al., 2007 or the SRS (Constantino et al., 2003).

Summary and Conclusions

The construct of *autism,* which was coined over 100 years ago, has been evolving as scientists work towards understanding and refining a diagnostic entity that reflects a constellation of social communication, RRBIs, and sensory interest symptoms. At present, we have moved towards a spectrum approach to understanding and studying autism (ASD) and have broken away from categorical diagnoses (i.e., Autistic Disorder, Asperger's disorder, and PDD-NOS). While we continue to make progress in understanding how to best conceptualize the disorder, deficits in social communication and presence of RRBIs have been anchors of this diagnosis since DSM-III was published in 1980.

At this time, many screening tools and diagnostic measures have been developed to identify autism (Bryson, Zwaigenbaum, McDermott, Rombough, & Brian, 2007; Harris et al., 2021; Lord et al., 2012; Lord et al., 1994; Robins et al., 2014; Rutter, Bailey, Lord et al., 2007; Schopler et al., 1980; Schopler, Van Bourgondien, Wellman, & Love, 2010; Stone; Coonrod, & Turner; 2004; Stone, McMahon, & Henderson, 2008; Wetherby & Prizant, 2002). These measures focus on the core symptoms of ASD: social communication difficulties and presence of RRBIs and sensory interests and have enabled examiners to make earlier and more accurate diagnoses (Zwaigenbaum et al., 2009). In particular, the diagnostic measures discussed in this chapter boast high levels of sensitivity and specificity for most individuals (Chlebowski et al., 2010; Gotham, Risi, Pickles, & Lord, 2007; Gotham et al., 2008; Lord et al., 1997; Lord et al., 2000; Luyster et al., 2009; Perry, Caondillac, Freeman,

Dunn-Geir, & Belair, 2005; Schopler, Van Bourgondien, Wellman, & Love, 2010).

Diagnosticians are still limited in their ability to make accurate and reliable diagnoses for individuals who are minimally verbal and have very low cognitive abilities but research is advancing, as evidenced by the development of new diagnostic tools specifically for this population such as the Adapted ADOS. Continued research in refining our understanding of the presentation of symptoms of ASD among cognitively lower functioning individuals needs to be continued to provide earlier and accurate diagnoses among individuals of varying cognitive abilities.

Author Note

We have no known conflict of interest to disclose.

References

American Psychiatric Association. (1952). *Diagnostic and statistical manual of mental disorders* (1st ed.). Washington, DC: Author.

American Psychiatric Association. (1968). *Diagnostic and statistical manual of mental disorders* (2nd ed.). Washington, DC: Author.

American Psychiatric Association. (2013). *Diagnostic and statistical manual of mental disorders* (5thed.). Washington, DC: Author.

Asperger, H. (1944) Die 'AutistichenPsychopathen' imKindesalter. *Archivfür Psychiatrie und Nervenkrankheiten*117: 76–136.

Baker, J. P. (2013). Autism at 70—Redrawing the boundaries. *The New England Journal of Medicine, 369*(12), 1089–1091. doi:10.1056/NEJMp1306380

Bal, V. H., Maye, M., Salzman, E., Huerta, M., Pepa, L., Risi, S., & Lord, C. (2020). The adapted ADOS: A new module set for the assessment of minimally verbal adolescents and adults. *Journal of Autism and Developmental Disorders, 50*(3), 719–729. https://doi.org/10.1007/s10803-019-04302-8

Bleuler, E. (1951). Autistic thinking. In, *Organization and pathology of thought: Selected sources* (pp. 399–437). New York, NY US: Columbia University Press. doi:10.1037/10584-020

Bryson, S. E., Zwaigenbaum, L., McDermott, C., Rombough, V., & Brian, J. (2008). The Autism Observation Scale for Infants: Scale development and reliability data. *Journal of Autism and Developmental Disorders, 38*(4), 731–738. https://doi.org/10.1007/s10803-007-0440-y

Carbone, P. S., Campbell, K., Wilkes, J., Stoddard, G. J., Huynh, K., Young, P. C., & Gabrielsen, T. P. (2020). Primary care autism screening and later autism diagnosis. *Pediatrics, 146*(2). doi: https://doi.org/10.1542/peds.2019-2314

Charman, T. (2008). Autism spectrum disorders. *Psychiatry, 7*(8). 331–334.

Chlebowski, C., Green, J. A., Barton, M. L., & Fein, D. (2010). Using the childhood autism rating scale to diagnose autism spectrum disorders. *Journal of Autism and Developmental Disorders, 40*(7), 787–799. doi: 10.1007/s10803-009-0926-x

Constantino, J. N., Davis, S. A., Todd, R. D., Schindler, M. K., Gross, M. M., Brophy, S. L., ... & Reich, W. (2003). Validation of a brief quantitative measure of autistic traits: Comparison of the social responsiveness scale with the autism diagnostic interview-revised. *Journal of Autism and Developmental Disorders*, *33*(4), 427–433. doi:10.1023/A:1025014929212

De Bildt, A., Sytema, S., Ketelaars, C., Kraijer, D., Mulder, E., Volkmar, F., & Minderaa, R. (2004). Interrelationship between autism diagnostic observation schedule-generic (ADOS-G), autism diagnostic interview-revised (ADI-R), and the diagnostic and statistical manual of mental disorders (DSM-IV-TR) classification in children and adolescents with mental retardation. *Journal of Autism and Developmental Disorders*, *34*(2), 129–137. doi: 0162-3257/04/ 0400-0129/0

De Giacomo, A. A., & Fombonne, E. E. (1998). Parental recognition of developmental abnormalities in autism. *European Child & Adolescent Psychiatry*, *7*(3), 131–136. doi:10.1007/s007870050058

DiGennaro Reed, F. D., Hirst, J. M., & Hyman, S. R. (2012). Assessment and treatment of stereotypic behavior in children with autism and other developmental disabilities: A thirty year review. *Research in Autism Spectrum Disorders*, *6*(1), 422–430. doi:10.1016/j.rasd.2011.07.003

Frohna, J. G. (2007). Failure to respond to name is indicator of possible autism spectrum disorder. *The Journal of Pediatrics*, *151*(3), 327–328. doi:10.1016/ j.jpeds.2007.07.023

Gibbs, V., Aldridge, F., Chandler, F., Witzlsperger, E., & Smith, K. (2012). An exploratory study comparing diagnostic outcomes for autism spectrum disorders under DSM-IV-TR with the proposed DSM-5 revision. *Journal of Autism and Developmental Disorders*, *42*(8), 1750–1756. doi:10.1007/ s10803-012-1560-6

Giles, D. C. (2013). 'DSM-V is taking away our identity': The reaction of the online community to the proposed changes in the diagnosis of Asperger's disorder. *Health* (London), *0*(0) 1–13.

Gillberg, C., Ehlers, S., Schaumann, H., Jakobsson, G., Dalgren, S. O., Lindblom, R., Bagenholm, A., Tjuus, T., & Blidner, E. (1999). Autism under 3 years: A clinical study of 28 cases referred for autism symptoms in infancy. *Journal of Child Psychology and Psychiatry*, *31*(6), 921–934.

Gotham, K., Risi, S., Pickles, A., & Lord, C. (2007). The Autism diagnostic observation schedule: Revised algorithms for improved diagnostic validity. *Journal of Autism and Developmental Disorders*, *37*(4), 613–627. doi: 10.1007/ s10803-006-0280-1

Gotham, K., Risi, S., Dawson, G., Tager-Flusberg, H., Joseph, R., Carter, A., ... & Lord, C. (2008). A replication of the Autism diagnostic observation schedule (ADOS) revised algorithms. *Journal of the American Academy of Child & Adolescent Psychiatry*, *47*(6), 642–651. doi:10.1097/CHI.0b013e31816bffb7

Guinchat, V., Chamak, B., Bonniau, B., Bodeau, N., Perisse, D., Cohen, D., & Danion, A. (2012). Very early signs of autism reported by parents include many concerns not specific to autism criteria. *Research in Autism Spectrum Disorders*, *6*(2), 589–601. doi:10.1016/j.rasd.2011.10.005

Guo, C., Luo, M., Wang, X., Huang, S., Meng, Z., Shao, J., ... & Jing, J. (2019). Reliability and validity of the Chinese version of modified checklist for autism in toddlers, revised, with follow-up (M-CHAT-R/F). *Journal of Autism and*

Developmental Disorders, 49(1), 185–196. https://doi.org/10.1007/s10 803-018-3682-y

Guthrie, W., Wallis, K., Bennett, A., Brooks, E., Dudley, J., Gerdes, M., ... & Miller, J. S. (2019). Accuracy of autism screening in a large pediatric network. *Pediatrics*, 144(4). DOI: https://doi.org/10.1542/peds.2018-3963

Hansen, S. N., Schendel, D. E., & Parner, E. T. (2015). Explaining the increase in the prevalence of autism spectrum disorders: The proportion attributable to changes in reporting practices. *JAMA Pediatrics*, 169(1), 56–62. doi:10.1001/jamapediatrics.2014.1893

Harris, J. F., Coffield, C. N., Janvier, Y. M., Mandell, D., & Cidav, Z. (2021). Validation of the developmental check-in tool for low-literacy autism screening. *Pediatrics*, 147(1). DOI: https://doi.org/10.1542/peds.2019-3659

Hazen, E. P., Stornelli, J. L., O'Rourke, J. A., Koesterer, K., & McDougle, C. J. (2014). Sensory symptoms in autism spectrum disorders. *Harvard Review of Psychiatry*, 22(2), 112–124. doi:10.1097/01.HRP.0000445143.08773.58

Janvier, Y. M., Coffield, C. N., Harris, J. F., Mandell, D. S., & Cidav, Z. (2019). The Developmental Check-In: Development and initial testing of an autism screening tool targeting young children from underserved communities. *Autism*, 23(3), 689–698. https://doi.org/10.1177/1362361318770430

Jing, W., & Fang, J. (2014). Brief report: Do children with autism gather information from social contexts to aid their word learning? *Journal of Autism and Developmental Disorders*, 44(6), 1478–1482. doi:10.1007/s10803-013-1994-5

Jones, E. H., Gliga, T., Bedford, R., Charman, T., & Johnson, M. H. (2014). Developmental pathways to autism: A review of prospective studies of infants at risk. *Neuroscience and Biobehavioral Reviews*, 39 1–33. doi:10.1016/j.neubiorev.2013.12.001

Kanner, L. (1943). Autistic disturbances of affective contact. *The Nervous Child* 2: 217–250.

Kim, S. H., & Lord, C. (2012). Combining information from multiple sources for the diagnosis of autism spectrum disorders for toddlers and young preschoolers from 12 to 47 months of age. *Journal of Child Psychology and Psychiatry*, 53(2), 143–151. doi: 10.1111/j.1469-7610.2011.02458.x

Leekam, S., Tandos, J., McConachie, H., Meins, E., Parkinson, K., Wright, C., & ... Le Couteur, A. (2007). Repetitive behaviours in typically developing 2-year-olds. *Journal of Child Psychology and Psychiatry*, 48(11), 1131–1138. doi:10.1111/j.1469-7610.2007.01778.x

Lord, C., Pickles, A., McLennan, J., Rutter, M., Bregman, J., Folstein, S., ... & Minshew, N. (1997). Diagnosing autism: Analyses of data from the Autism Diagnostic Interview. *Journal of Autism and Developmental Disorders*, 27(5), 501–517. doi: 10.1023/A:1025873925661

Lord, C., Risi, S., Lambrecht, L., Cook Jr, E. H., Leventhal, B. L., DiLavore, P. C., ... & Rutter, M. (2000). The Autism Diagnostic Observation Schedule—Generic: A standard measure of social and communication deficits associated with the spectrum of autism. *Journal of Autism and Developmental Disorders*, 30(3), 205–223. doi: 10.1023/A:1005592401947

Lord, C., Rutter, M., DiLavore, P. C., Risi, S., Gotham, K., & Bishop, S. (2012). *Autism diagnostic observation schedule: ADOS-2*. Los Angeles, CA: Western Psychological Services.

Lord, C., Rutter, M., & Le Couteur, A. (1994). Autism Diagnostic Interview-Revised: A revised version of a diagnostic interview for caregivers of individuals with possible pervasive developmental disorders. *Journal of Autism and Developmental Disorders*, 24(5), 659–685. doi:0162-3257/94/1000-0659507.00/0

Luyster, R., Gotham, K., Guthrie, W., Coffing, M., Petrak, R., Pierce, K., ... & Lord, C. (2009). The Autism Diagnostic Observation Schedule—Toddler Module: A new module of a standardized diagnostic measure for autism spectrum disorders. *Journal of Autism and Developmental Disorders*, 39(9), 1305–1320. doi: 10.1007/s10803-009-0746-z

Maenner, M. J., Shaw, K. A., Bakian, A. V., Bilder, D. A., Durkin, M. S., Esler, A., ... & Cogswell, M. E. (2021). Prevalence and Characteristics of Autism Spectrum Disorder Among Children Aged 8 Years—Autism and Developmental Disabilities Monitoring Network, 11 Sites, United States, 2018. *MMWR Surveillance Summaries*, 70(11), 1.

Maestro, S., Muratori, F., Cavallaro, M., Pei, F., Stern, D., Golse, B., & Palacio-Espasa, F. (2002). Attentional skills during the first 6 months of age in autism spectrum disorder. *Journal of the American Academy of Child & Adolescent Psychiatry*, 41(10), 1239–1245. doi:10.1097/00004583-200210000-00014

Al Maskari, T. S., Melville, C. A., & Willis, D. S. (2018). Systematic review: Cultural adaptation and feasibility of screening for autism in non-English speaking countries. *International Journal of Mental Health Systems*, 12(1), 1–19. DOI: https://doi.org/10.1186/s13033-018-0200-8

Memari, A. H., Ziaee, V., Shayestehfar, M., Ghanouni, P., Mansournia, M. A., & Moshayedi, P. (2013). Cognitive flexibility impairments in children with autism spectrum disorders: Links to age, gender and child outcomes. *Research in Developmental Disabilities*, 34(10), 3218–3225. doi:10.1016/j.ridd.2013.06.033

Monteiro, S. A., Dempsey, J., Berry, L. N., Voigt, R. G., & Goin-Kochel, R. P. (2019). Screening and referral practices for autism spectrum disorder in primary pediatric care. *Pediatrics*, 144(4).

Moskowitz, A. & Heim, G. (2011). Eugen Bleuler's dementia praecox or the group of schizophrenias (1911): A centenary appreciation and reconsideration. *Schizophrenia Bulletin*, 37(3), 471–479. doi:10.1093/schbul/sbr016

Osterling, J., & Dawson, G. (1994). Early recognition of children with autism: A study of first birthday home videotapes. *Journal of Autism and Developmental Disorders*, 24(3), 247–257. doi:10.1007/BF02172225

Osterling, J. A., Dawson, G., & Munson, J. A. (2002). Early recognition of 1-year-old infants with autism spectrum disorder versus mental retardation. *Development and Psychopathology*, 14(02), 239–251. doi:10.1017/S0954579402002031

Ozonoff, S. (2012). Editorial perspective: Autism spectrum disorders in DSM-5—An historical perspective and the need for change. *Journal of Child Psychology And Psychiatry*, 53(10), 1092–1094. doi:10.1111/j.1469-7610.2012.02614.x

Ozonoff, S., Iosif, A.-M., Baguio, F., Cook, I. C., Hill, M. M., Hutman, T., ... Sigman, M. (2010). A prospective study of the emergence of early behavioral signs of autism. *Journal of the American Academy of Child & Adolescent Psychiatry*, 49(3), 256–266.

Ozonoff, S., Macari, S., Young, G. S., Goldring, S., Thompson, M., & Rogers, S. J. (2008). Atypical object exploration at 12 months of age is associated with autism in a prospective sample. *Autism*, *12*(5), 457–472. doi: 10.1177/1362361308096402

Perry, A., Condillac, R. A., Freeman, N. L., Dunn-Geier, J., & Belair, J. (2005). Multi-site study of the Childhood Autism Rating Scale (CARS) in five clinical groups of young children. *Journal of Autism and Developmental Disorders*, *35*(5), 625–634. doi: 10.1007/s10803-005-0006-9

Pierce, K., Gazestani, V. H., Bacon, E., Barnes, C. C., Cha, D., Nalabolu, S., ... & Courchesne, E. (2019). Evaluation of the diagnostic stability of the early autism spectrum disorder phenotype in the general population starting at 12 months. *JAMA pediatrics*, *173*(6), 578–587. doi:10.1001/jamapediatrics.2019.0624

Pilowsky, T., Yirmiya, N., Shulman, C., & Dover, R. (1998). The Autism Diagnostic Interview-Revised and the Childhood Autism Rating Scale: Differences between diagnostic systems and comparison between genders. *Journal of Autism and Developmental Disorders*, *28*(2), 143–151. doi: 0162-3257/98/0400-0143$15.00/0

Porter, N. (2012). Promotion of pretend play for children with high-functioning autism through the use of circumscribed interests. *Early Childhood Education Journal*, *40*(3), 161–167. doi:10.1007/s10643-012-0505-1

Risi, S., Lord, C., Gotham, K., Corsello, C., Chrysler, C., Szatmari, P., ... & Pickles, A. (2006). Combining information from multiple sources in the diagnosis of autism spectrum disorders. *Journal of the American Academy of Child & Adolescent Psychiatry*, *45*(9), 1094–1103. doi: 10.1007/s10803-006-0280-1

Robins, D. L., Casagrande, K., Barton, M., Chen, C. M. A., Dumont-Mathieu, T., & Fein, D. (2014). Validation of the modified checklist for autism in toddlers, revised with follow-up (M-CHAT-R/F). *Pediatrics*, *133*(1), 37–45. doi: 10.1542/peds.2013-1813

Rutter, M., Bailey, A., Lord, C., Cianchetti, C., & Fancello, G. S. (2007). *SCQ: Social Communication Questionnaire: manuale*. Giunti OS.

Schopler, E., Reichler, R. J., DeVellis, R. F., & Daly, K. (1980). Toward objective classification of childhood autism: Childhood Autism Rating Scale (CARS). *Journal of Autism and Developmental Disorders*, *10*(1), 91–103. doi: 0162-3257/80/0300-0091$03.00/0

Schopler, E., Van Bourgondien, M. E., Wellman, J., & Love, S. (2010). *Childhood autism rating scale-second edition (CARS2): manual*. Los Angeles: Western Psychological Services.

Soto, S., Linas, K., Jacobstein, D., Biel, M., Migdal, T., & Anthony, B. J. (2015). A review of cultural adaptations of screening tools for autism spectrum disorders. *Autism*, *19*(6), 646–661. doi: https://doi.org/10.1177/1362361314541012

Stenberg, N., Bresnahan, M., Gunnes, N., Hirtz, D., Hornig, M., Lie, K. K., ... & Stoltenberg, C. (2014). Identifying children with autism spectrum disorder at 18 months in a general population sample. *Paediatric and Perinatal Epidemiology*, *28*(3), 255–262. doi: https://doi.org/10.1111/ppe.12114

Stone, W. L., Coonrod, E. E., Turner, L. M., & Pozdol, S. L. (2004). Psychometric properties of the STAT for early autism screening. *Journal of Autism and Developmental Disorders*, *34*(6), 691–701. doi:10.1007/s10803-004-5289-8

Stone, W. L., McMahon, C. R., & Henderson, L. M. (2008). Use of the Screening Tool for Autism in Two-Year-Olds (STAT) for children under 24 months: An exploratory study. *Autism, 12*(5), 557–573. doi:10.1177/1362361308096403

Toh, T. H., Tan, V. W. Y., Lau, P. S. T., & Kiyu, A. (2018). Accuracy of Modified Checklist for Autism in Toddlers (M-CHAT) in detecting autism and other developmental disorders in community clinics. *Journal of Autism and Developmental Disorders, 48*(1), 28–35. doi: https://doi.org/10.1007/s10803-017-3287-x

Tsai, J. M., Lu, L., Jeng, S. F., Cheong, P. L., Gau, S. S. F., Huang, Y. H., & Wu, Y. T. (2019). Validation of the modified checklist for autism in toddlers, revised with follow-up in Taiwanese toddlers. *Research in Developmental Disabilities, 85*, 205–216. https://doi.org/10.1016/j.ridd.2018.11.011

Webb, S., & Jones, E. H. (2009). Early identification of autism: Early characteristics, onset of symptoms, and diagnostic stability. *Infants & Young Children, 22*(2), 100–118. doi:10.1097/IYC.0b013e3181a02f7f

Weintraub, K. (2011). Autism counts. *Nature, 479*(7371), 22–24. doi:10.1038/479022a

Werner, E., Dawson, G., Osterling, J., & Dinno, N. (2000). Brief report: Recognition of autism spectrum disorder before one year of age: A retrospective study based on home videotapes. *Journal of Autism and Developmental Disorders, 30*(2), 157–162. doi:10.1023/A:1005463707029

Wetherby, A. M., & Prizant, B. M. (2002). *Communication and symbolic behavior scales: Developmental profile.* Baltimore, MD: Paul H Brookes Publishing Co.

Wimpory, D. C., Hobson, R., Williams, J. G., & Nash, S. (2000). Are infants with autism socially engaged? A study of recent retrospective parental reports. *Journal of Autism and Developmental Disorders, 30*(6), 525–536. doi:10.1023/A:1005683209438

Zwaigenbaum, L., Bryson, S., Carter, A. S., Lord, C., Rogers, S., Chawarska, K., Constantino, J., Dawson, G., Dobkins, K., Fein, D., Iverson, J., Klin, A., Landa, R., Sigman, M., Messinger, D., Ozonoff, S., Stone, W. & Yirmiya, N. (2009). Clinical assessment and management of toddlers with suspected ASD: Insights from studies of high-risk infants. *Pediatrics, 123*, 1383–1391. doi: 10.1542/peds.2008-1606

Zwaigenbaum, L., Bryson, S., Rogers, T., Roberts, W., Brian, J., & Szatmari, P. (2005). Behavioral manifestations of autism in the first year of life. *International Journal of Developmental Neuroscience, 23*, 143–152. doi: 10.1016/j.ijdevneu.2004.05.001

Zwaigenbaum, L., & Maguire, J. (2019). Autism screening: Where do we go from here?. *Pediatrics, 144*(4). doi: https://doi.org/10.1542/peds.2019-0925

Chapter 2

Historical Overview of Autism Spectrum Disorder

Peggy Schaefer Whitby,[1] *Tom E.C. Smith,*[1] *and Celeste Michaud*[2]

[1]Department of Curriculum and Instruction, University of Arkansas, Fayetteville
[2]College of Education and Health Professions, University of Arkansas, Fayetteville

One might ask, why study the history of how individuals with autism spectrum disorder (ASD) have been educated and treated. The American Historical Association states that we should study history to "gain access to the laboratory of human experience." The organization goes on to say that through the study of history "we emerge with an enhanced capacity for informed citizenship, critical thinking, and simple awareness" (American Historical Association, 2021). Studying the history of the education and treatment of persons with ASD can provide us with an informed view of what has been accomplished as well as help us identify where we need to go in the future.

Autism spectrum disorder is used to describe individuals with a variety of characteristics primarily affecting social communication with the display of restricted, repetitive behaviors or interests. The deficits are pervasive, sustained, and affect social functioning (American Psychiatric Association, 2013; Goldstein, Naglieri, & Ozonoff, 2009). Myths surrounding individuals with ASD are fueled by history, culture, and psychosocial influences across time. By reviewing the history of ASD, teachers, professionals, and families will develop an improved paradigm as it is appreciated in its current practice.

The purpose of this chapter is to discuss the history of ASD in society, the criteria for diagnosis of ASD, and the changing prevalence and policy that impacts individuals with ASD. The key points for this chapter are:

1. Clinical cases of individuals with autism have been documented since the late 1700s.
2. Autism definitions and diagnostic criteria have evolved.
3. Autism identification, interventions, and treatments have improved over time and are historically based upon psychosocial culture across time.
4. The evolution of services available for individuals identified with autism has been driven by advocacy efforts, litigation, and subsequent legislation.

DOI: 10.4324/9781003255147-3

History of Autism Spectrum Disorder

In 1798, prior to the conceptualization of ASD, Dr. Jean Itard, a French physician, adopted and educated Victor, a 12-year-old feral boy. Itard's clinical descriptions of Victor describe the characteristics of autistic disorder as classified in modern times. It is unknown whether Victor was abandoned in the woods due to his disability or if developmental delay resulted from the absence of stimulation needed to acquire language and social development. Regardless, while Victor made progress under Itard's care, including the acquisition of several words and the development of simple attachment behaviors, he continued to display indications of developmental disability (Goldstein et al., 2009; Malson, 1972; Wolff, 2004).

Additional accounts of suspected ASD have been documented in the psychiatric literature, as well as in cultural accounts of fictional and non-fictional characters throughout history. Uta Frith identified a Scottish landowner named Hugh Blair who in the late 1700s displayed numerous characteristics currently associated with ASD, including echolalia and processing delays; repetitive behaviors; insistence on sameness; collecting unusual objects; difficulty with social interactions; and insensitive, tactless interactions (Wolff, 2004). In 1867, Henry Maudsley, a leading author in the field of psychiatry in England, authored a text titled *The Physiology and Pathology of the Mind (1867)* in which he described the characteristics of insanity as manifested in children, including sensory-motor responses to environmental stimuli, ineffective communication skills, aggressive outbursts, and rigid movements or actions. Maudsley's accounts appear to be consistent with modern-day descriptions of ASD (Goldstein et al., 2009; Wolffe, 2004). In 1809 Haslam described cases of "insane children" in which one case describes a child with a possible ASD (Wolff, 2004). Through extensive record reviews, researchers have identified many early cases and have ascertained that the authors are describing an ASD as we conceptualize it in modern times (Frith, 2000; Frith, 2003; Wing, 1976).

Theodore Heller, a pioneer in special education from Vienna, documented a regressive pattern of behavior in children after two years of age in 1908. Heller described a loss of skills in the areas of language and social interaction, as well as adaptive behaviors, following a period of typical development. In addition, these children displayed rigid patterns of behavior, with repetitive, stereotypical interests. The loss of skills was noted to be pervasive and severe (Westphal, Schelinski, Volkmar, & Pelphrey, 2013). This disorder, initially coined "Heller syndrome" and later referred to as dementia infantilis or childhood psychosis, was aligned with initial theories that autism was a psychotic disorder. In 1904 this regressive pattern was identified as childhood disintegrative disorder (American Psychiatric Association, 1994). Regressive patterns of skill loss in children with ASD are still reported today.

In 1911, the term translated as "autism" was introduced by Eugene Bleuler, a Swiss psychiatrist known for his work in the area of schizophrenic disorders (Fitzgerald, 2014). The origin of the term coined by Bleuler, *autismus*, is derived from two Greek terms translated as *self* (*autos*) with the suffix (*ismos*) translated as an action or state. When introducing the term, *autismus*, Blueler was referring to a condition of schizophrenic disorder manifesting as difficulty in interpersonal relations due to detachment or affective incongruence. As a result, autism was originally more closely aligned with schizophrenia. It was not until 1980 that autism was introduced as a developmental disorder classified outside of schizophrenia (American Psychological Association, 1980; Baker, 2013).

In the 1940s, two pioneers in the field published research findings documenting the characteristics of ASD. In 1943, Leo Kanner described children with deficits in language development and use, social interaction, and communication, as well as the display of repetitive behaviors/restricted interests. Kanner's extensive body of work suggested an emotional disorder with biological etiology and implications of genetic predisposition with symptoms present since birth that he termed *Autistic Disturbances of Affective Contact*.

Around the same time as Kanner's initial research, a German psychiatrist named Hans Asperger was studying similar children. These children were very similar to the children Kanner described, although no cognitive delay was noted and the children displayed typical patterns of language development in the early years. He described these children as "Little Professors." As a German scholar, Asperger's work was overlooked until the 1980s (Wolff, 2004).

The theory of poor parenting as a cause of autism was promoted in the 1960s by Freudian psychologists, including Bettleheim who coined the term "refrigerator mothers". During this period, children with autism were placed in therapeutic hospitals to address the attachment to their mother issues. Therapeutic interventions included holding the children to a woman's chest, extensive psychoanalysis, and explicit instruction in language development and use.

During the same era, Bernard Rimland, a psychiatrist, had a son who was diagnosed with infantile autism. In 1964 he published *Infantile Autism: The Syndrome and its Implications for a Neural Theory of Behavior* which suggested autism was a neurodevelopmental disability with genetic predispositions similar to Kanner's original ideas on the neurological basis for autism (Wolff, 2004). In 1965, Rimland organized families and started the Autism Society of America, which is still an active organization today.

During the 1960s rapid research development in the area of ASD was beginning and continues in present day. In 1966, Rett's syndrome was identified, in 1968, Rutter validated the characteristics of Asperger, and in 1971, Kolvin distinguished autism from schizophrenia. Historical events related to ASD across the years are outline in Figure 2.1.

In the 1970s and 1980s, Drs. Lorna Wing and Judy Gould extensively explored the work of both Kanner and Asperger in Great Britain. They found similarities in the early cases of ASD across Kanner's and Asperger's work, including impairments in social interaction, communication, and restricted interests/repetitive behaviors. They coined these three areas as the "triad of impairments" and suggested that Asperger syndrome was a form of high-functioning autism (Wolff, 2004). Wing later referred to her original work discussing Asperger's clinical discussions as opening *Pandora's box*. She understood the controversy surrounding the issue of Asperger syndrome as high-functioning autism would unfold.

In the 1990s, Uta Frith translated the writings of Asperger's, initiating the debate regarding the differentiation of Asperger syndrome as a distinct disorder, apart from Autistic Disorder. Asperger believed it was a separate disorder. In 1987, Asperger syndrome was included as a separate diagnostic criterium under the umbrella of pervasive developmental disorder (American Psychiatry Association, 1987).

Also in the 1990s, the term "neurodiversity" was introduced by Judy Singer, an Australian sociologist (Singer, 1999). She used the term to describe the natural variations in neurological functioning and compared it to the biodiversity of living things. Neurodiversity is now commonly referred to as variations in neurocognitive function (Jaarsma & Welin, 2012). When a person is considered neurodivergent, they have neurocognitive functions that deviate from the most common patterns of the general population and creates natural variation in the human species.

New understandings of genetic and neurological origins of ASD resulted in increasing advocacy for individuals with this disorder. At first, parents and family members were the primary advocates. Later, self-advocates made use of the internet and began to organize with a new platform (Ortega, 2009). The term "neurodiversity" was adopted by advocacy groups; these groups initiated the rights movement of the neurodivergent population to ensure autonomy and inclusion in light of perceived neurotypical privilege (Jaarisma & Weilm, 2012). The movement advocates for the social model, which focuses on the subjective quality of life and does not focus on a cure or the reduction of harmless behaviors as represented by medicalized perspective of disability (Kapp et al., 2013).

Controversy in the field continued in 1998 when Wakefield published a study suggesting that vaccinations were the cause of ASD. This theory was believable at the time as the prevalence of ASD appeared to be increasing and parents were reporting typical developing children until around the age of immunization. However, when Thermosal, the

	Timeline	
Case Description of Hugh Blair 1737	1700s	1798 Itard Case Description of Victor
Haslam *Cases of Insane Children* 1809	1800s	1879 Maudsley *Insanity in Early Life*
Heller describes Dementia Infantilis 1908	1900s	1911 Blueler coins the word *"autism"*
Kanner describes Children with Autistic 1943 Disturbances of Affective Contact. Rett's Syndrome discovered 1966		1965 Rimland started the Autism Society of America 1967 Bettlehiem coins the term *"refrigerator mothers"* 1971 Kolvin distinguishes Autism from Schizophrenia
Rutter's validates Aspergers as a syndrome 1968 PDD Category Added to the DSM III. 1980 Infantile Autism is included Neurodiversity Movement Begins 1990 Defeat Autism Now! 1995 *Hartmann v. Loudoun County Board of Education* 1997 Wakefield publishes article suggesting 1998 immunizations cause ASD		1981 Wing and Gould reintroduce Asperger Syndrome 1993 *Delaware IU v. Martin K.* 1994 DSM IV Diagnosis expanded and included Asperger Syndrome 1995 Cure Autism Now! Campaign 199$ Frith and Happe introduce Cognitive Theories of ASD 1999 Zoghbi discovers genetic mutation for Rett Syndrome
Gill ex rel. Gill v. Columbia 93 School District 2000 CDC announces prevalence of 1:150 2000 IDEA requires the use of evidence-based practices 2004 Autism Speaks 2005 CDC reports prevalence of 1:110 2006 States begin mandating insurance coverage 2006 NAC publishes the first evidence-based practice guide 2008 CDC reports prevalence of 1:68 *2010* Defeat Autism Now! Discontinued 2011 *CDC reports prevalence of 1:69 2012* *Autism Collaboration, Accountability, Research, 2014 Education and Support Act* Autism Speaks removes *cure from their mission.* 2015 CDC reports a prevalence of 1:44 2021	2000s	2000 *Children's Health Act* 2004 CDC reports prevalence of 1:125 2004 Immunization Theory Debunked and Wakefield is barred from practicing medicine 2006 Formal Establishment of the Autism Self Advocacy Network 2006 *Combatting Autism Act* 2008 CDC reports prevalence of 1:88 2009 NPDC publishes an evidence-based practice guide *2011 Combating Autism Reauthorization Act* 2013 DSM V moves to Autism Spectrum Disorder Category Rett's Removed from the DSM-V 2014 CDC reports a prevalence of 1:59 2016 CDC reports a prevalence of 1:54 2018 Endrew F. v. Douglas County

Figure 2.1 Overview of Significant Events in the History of Autism: Prevalence, Diagnosis, Clinical Features, Legislation, and Litigation.

component in vaccines believed to cause ASD was removed from vaccinations the prevalence remained consistent. Later, it was determined that Wakefield was fraudulent and barred from practicing medicine. Other environmental triggers have been suggested to cause ASD but none have been verified as causes.

The evidence-based practice (EBP) movement in special education and in ASD services emerged in the 2000s and aligned with the mandate of the use of EBP's in IDEA 2004. Evidence-based practices in special education are identified by organizations that review quality studies using criteria to identify effective practices. This in turn may help to narrow the research-to-practice gap by identifying practices supported by quality research and making them available to educators. The purpose for the use of EBPs is to improve the possibilities of attaining desired outcomes when implemented with fidelity. Because EBPs are identified through quality research to work with most but not all students (Cook & Odom, 2013), implementation and measurement are necessary to determine if the selected practice results in the acquisition of desired skills for a particular population. In 2009, the National Autism Center published the first ASD EBP guide (NAC, 2009) followed in 2010 by the second ASD specific EBP guide published by the National Professional Development Center on Autism (Odom et al., 2010).

History of Diagnosis

The Diagnostic and Statistical Manual of Mental Health Disorders, 3rd Edition, included the first categorical diagnostic criteria for pervasive developmental disorders (PDD) (1980). It was under this new class that infantile autism made an entry separate from schizophrenia (Volkmar, Bregman, Cohen, & Cicchetti, 1988). In addition to infantile autism, additional related disorders included in this class were childhood-onset pervasive developmental disorder, residual infantile autism, and residual childhood-onset pervasive developmental disorder. The criteria for infantile autism were based on the work of Kanner and Rutter and included onset prior to 30 months of age, pervasive lack of social relationships, deficits of language/communication, and the absence of delusions or hallucinations. A developmental approach was emphasized and the term infantile was removed to capture both the developmental and age-related variables.

Asperger syndrome was officially added as a category under the classification of PDD in the fourth revision of the DSM, published in 1994 (American Psychiatric Association, 1994). The DSM-IV identified five potential categorical placements within the classification of PDD, including autistic disorder, PDD-NOS, Asperger disorder, Rett's Syndrome, and childhood disintegrative disorder. The DSM-IV-TR

(2000) continued the placement of autism under the category of PDD. There were three possible classifications of autism identified under the category of PDD: autistic disorder, pervasive developmental delay – not otherwise specified (PDD-NOS), and Asperger's syndrome. Autistic disorder required the identification of six characteristics, including two from the area of social interaction, one from the area of communication, and one from the area of restricted behaviors or activities (American Psychiatric Association, 1994, 2000).

Asperger syndrome was maintained on the spectrum of disorders, with distinct differences from autistic disorder. A key difference between the two was the diagnosis of Asperger syndrome was not reliant on identification prior to age 2, no requirement of characteristics identified within the area of communication, and no differences in cognitive impairment (Gibbs, Aldridge, Chandler, Witzlsperger & Smith 2012).

In the DSM-V (2013), the organization was restructured to reflect a focus on the dimensional aspects of mental health, maintaining a categorical approach but also reflecting the continuum and commonality between disorders. The philosophy behind this reorganization reflects a representation of developmental issues, advances in genetics and neuroimaging, neuroscience, and neuropsychology, a streamlined classification of disorders, and the conceptualization of personality disorders. The DSM-V replaces the previous category of Pervasive Development Disorders, used in DSM-IV, with the broad continuum of Autism Spectrum Disorders which is then specified by severity level, accompanying intellectual disability, language impairment, known medical or genetic conditions, environmental factors, and neurodevelopmental, mental, or behavior disorders.

Within this category, specific classes were eliminated, including the differentiation between autistic disorder, Asperger syndrome, and PDD-NOS. Viewing autism as a multifaceted spectrum with varying dimensions allows for clarification when diagnosing, identifying resources, and completing research. The specific nuances between the various labels are dismissed, allowing for the focus to remain on identifying the impact of the disorder on overall functioning (Szatmari, 2011).

History of the Prevalence

In modern media, the increasing prevalence of ASD has been described as an epidemic. However, the history of ASD in relation to prevalence suggests otherwise. Indeed, the prevalence has increased significantly over time. In the 1960s, researchers suggested the prevalence of ASD was 1:2500 children. In 2000, the Centers for Disease Control established the Autism Diagnostic Monitoring Network to monitor the prevalence of ASD. At this time, the CDC (2021) suggested 1:150 children would be diagnosed with ASD by the age of eight and in 2021 the number increased to 1:44 children (see Figure 2.1). Researchers have suggested three reasons for the increased prevalence: diagnostic substitution, broadening of the diagnostic criteria over time, and increase awareness.

Diagnostic substitution refers to children who had been earlier diagnosed with cognitive disabilities or emotional behavior disorders and were switched to a diagnosis of ASD as the diagnostic criteria changed. Furthermore, with the increased awareness of diagnosticians, children who in the past may have been diagnosed with cognitive or behavioral disorders are now given the appropriate diagnosis of ASD. As a result of diagnostic substitution, the prevalence of cognitive disabilities and behavioral disorders for certain demographic groups decreased as the prevalence of ASD increased.

When reviewing the changes in the educational and diagnostic criteria over time, it is clear that the criteria were broadened which resulted in increased prevalence of the disorder. In 1990, IDEA included autism as one of the specific service categories eligible for special education. This resulted in IEP teams identifying children under the autism category which increased the number of children given the educational label of autism. In 1994, Asperger's Syndrome was included in the DSM-IV capturing those individuals who in the past may not have met criteria for an autism type disorder.

As the public became more aware of ASD, more families sought ASD screenings, assessments, and services. Given the increased need for childhood screenings and early intervention, the American Pediatrics Association changed its policy and began recommending childhood screening for ASD by the age of two (2006). This increased awareness led to more children receiving the appropriate diagnosis as they children are routinely screened.

Advocacy and Litigation

In 1965 Rimland started the *Autism Society of America*, which was followed by the founding of many additional advocacy groups. The type and mission of the advocacy group tend to align with the social norms across time. For example, the *Defeat Autism Now* (DAN) network (1995) offered alternative treatments to parents who were seeking to cure autism. In the wake of the evidence-based practice movement and advocacy movement, DAN came under great scrutiny and was discontinued in 2011. The self-advocacy movement started in the 1990s but was formally organized in 2006 when the Autism Self Advocacy Network, a volunteer organization, became a powerful advocacy group. Autism Speaks promoted a *Cure Autism Now* campaign and came under great scrutiny from the neurodiversity self-advocacy movement. Subsequently, Autism

Speaks has changed its mission and moved away from curing ASD to supporting families and individuals with ASD. These examples illustrate the evolution of the concept of ASD and neurodiversity across time.

The importance of advocacy and its direct link to litigation and legislation cannot be underestimated. Indeed, as a result of the development of advocacy organizations and the push from families for ASD services, numerous court cases have focused on this group of individuals and resulted in significant opportunities. The number of due process hearings and court cases related to students with ASD has been increasing parallel to the number of students identified as having ASD (Hill, Martin, & Nelson-Head, 2011). Issues in these cases have ranged from the right to education, educational placement, applied behavior analysis, and employment. Gorn (1999) noted that the majority of court cases dealing with students with ASD have focused on educational methodology, the quantum of benefit, or generalization. The following provides an overview of several court cases dealing with students with autism:

Delaware IU v. Martin K. (1993). The parents of a 3-year-old boy with pervasive developmental disabilities requested reimbursement from the school district for their use of a private Lovaas instructor. The school had told the parents that they would develop an IEP for the student in November but did not produce the IEP until January, at which time they were proposing using the TEACCH method. The court ruled in favor of the parents based on procedural errors in developing the IEP, and for not providing educational programming that would result in an educational benefit.

Gill ex rel. Gill v. Columbia 93 School District (2000). In this case, parents were requesting the school pay for private Lovaas services for their 7-year-old child with autism. The Eighth Circuit, U.S. Court Appeals, ruled in favor of the district. The court found that the intervention techniques used by the district were sufficient and that decisions regarding methodology should be left to experts in the schools (Hulett, 2009).

Hartmann v. Loudoun County Board of Education (1997). In this case, the parents of an 11-year-old boy diagnosed with autism wanted the student to remain in the general education classroom with an aide. The district wanted to move the student to a more restricted setting because he was not making academic progress in the general classroom and was disruptive to other students. The U.S. Court of Appeals, Fourth Circuit, ruled in favor of the school, noting that including students in general classroom settings is not required when the student would not receive educational benefit, the student is disruptive, and any benefits of inclusion would be outweighed by benefits received in a more restrictive setting (Hill & Hill, 2012).

Endrew F. v. Douglas County (2018). In this case, Endrew demonstrated significant interfering behavior that impacted progress on the

Individual Education Program (IEP). His parents withdrew him from public school and enrolled him in a private school for students with autism where he made significant progress. His parents ask the district to pay for his tuition because they believed the district had not provided Endrew with a free and appropriate public education (FAPE) (Decker & Hurwitz, 2017). The lower courts in this case agreed with the school district. However, the parents' attorney found cases in other circuits in which judges ruled that students needed to make more than minimal progress on their IEPs. As a result of the inconsistency, the parents' attorney appealed to the U.S. Supreme Court. Endrew's guardians asserted the district committed both procedural and substantive violations of the Individual with Disabilities Education Act (IDEA) (Yell & Bateman, 2017). The result was the Supreme Court unanimously ruled, "A school must offer an IEP reasonably calculated to enable a child to make progress appropriate in light of the child's circumstances" (*Endrew,* 2017, p. 15). The Supreme Court stated, "goals may differ, but every child should have the chance to meet challenging objectives" (*Endrew,* 2017, p. 1,000). The Supreme Court ruled the promise of some educational benefit no longer meets the requirements of IDEA (Endrew F. v. Douglas County, 2018). This decision went further than the previous U.S. Supreme court case, *Rowley v. Board of Education* in 1984 that seemed to establish a minimum educational benefit as the acceptance of "appropriate".

While the courts have routinely ruled that educational methodology should be the decision of the school district, many parents have prevailed in court cases dealing with the Lovaas method by portraying it as an alternative to programs provided by the schools that were not producing educational benefit, the hallmark of the *Rowley* case in determining FAPE. Yell and Drasgow (2000) reviewed 45 cases dealing with students with autism and the Lovaas method and found that parents prevailed in 34 of the cases or 76 percent of the time. In the majority of these decisions, schools lost by either violating procedural safeguards or not showing that their programs provided meaningful benefit to the student.

History of Legislation

For the most part, early legislation focused on the general population of individuals with disabilities but was also applied to individuals with ASD. These include the Individuals with Disabilities Education Act (IDEA), Section 504 of the Rehabilitation Act of 1973, and the Americans with Disabilities Act (ADA). There are, however, in addition to these general acts, several specific pieces of legislation directly related to individuals with ASD. An overview of the ASD specific legislation is presented below followed by critical legislation for people with all disabilities.

In 2000, Congress passed the *Children's Health Act*. This legislation authorized the establishment of Centers of Excellence to encourage research into autism. The act called for the Centers for Disease Control (CDC) and the National Institutes of Health (NIH) to monitor the etiology, diagnosis, early detection, prevention, and treatment of autism.

The *Combatting Autism Act* was signed into law by President George W. Bush on December 19, 2006. This act focused on addressing the growing number of individuals with autism through research, screening, intervention, and education. The *Combating Autism Act* authorized approximately $950 million over a five-year period to address autism issues. The Act provided money for the Centers for Disease Control (CDC) to conduct programs to determine the prevalence of autism spectrum disorders, and to coordinate with the Department of Health and Human Services and the National Institutes of Health (NIH).

In 2011, Congress passed the *Combating Autism Reauthorization Act*. This act authorized $231 million per year for five years to continue the provisions of the original act. On August 8, 2014, President Obama, reauthorized the act a second time by signing the *Autism Collaboration, Accountability, Research, Education and Support Act* (CARES). This act dedicated $1.3 billion in federal funding for autism over five years, primarily focused on research, and continued prevalence monitoring, training medical professionals in the identification of ASD, and efforts to develop treatments of medical conditions associated with ASD. An important component of CARES required the federal government to review services for adults with ASD. With many children identified with ASD becoming adults, this addition to the act came at a critical time.

One area related to ASD and legislation deals with insurance coverage. In 2012, the National Conference of State Legislatures reported that 37 states and the District of Columbia had passed legislation related to autism and insurance coverage (2012). In 2021, all states and the District of Columbia had passed some type of legislation addressing autism insurance coverage. Most state legislation related to coverage for individuals with ASD was passed in 2007.

In addition to federal legislation specifically targeting individuals with ASD, there are three laws mandating services and protections for a wide variety of individuals with disabilities, including those with autism. The law that has had the greatest impact on the education of students with autism spectrum disorders is the Individuals with Disabilities Education Act (IDEA). Originally passed in 1975 as Public Law 94-142, the law requires schools to provide a free, appropriate public education (FAPE) for all school-age children, in the least restrictive environment (Smith, et al., 2020). Originally, ASD was not included as a specific disability covered, meaning that for students with ASD to be eligible for services they had to be identified as having one of the approved disability categories. The result was that some children with ASD were identified as having intellectual disabilities or emotional and behavioral disorders to be eligible for services (Smith, et al., 2020).

The 1990 reauthorization of IDEA included autism as one of the specific disabilities resulting in eligibility for IDEA services. Therefore, since 1990, children with ASD who need special education have been eligible for IDEA services under the distinct category of autism. IDEA is a very comprehensive, very prescriptive law that requires schools to provide students with disabilities a free appropriate public education.

Section 504 of the Rehabilitation Act of 1973, which is civil rights legislation for persons with disabilities, prohibits discrimination against any *otherwise qualified* individual with a disability in entities that receive federal funds. Unlike IDEA, Section 504 does not provide a list of disabilities for eligibility purposes; rather it requires that a student have a physical or mental impairment. It also does not require that an individual need special education, but that the physical or mental impairment substantially limits a major life activity (Smith, & Patton, 2016). Because autism is considered a mental impairment and is likely to substantially limit a major life activity, individuals with ASD are most often eligible for services and protections under Section 504.

The Americans with Disabilities Act (ADA), passed in 1990, is also a civil rights act for individuals with disabilities. The reason the ADA was passed, after Section 504 had already been in place for 17 years, was that Section 504 only applies to entities that receive federal funds while the ADA applies to many more entities, including department stores, entertainment venues, hotels, restaurants, and many other establishments that do not receive federal funds. The result is that individuals with disabilities, including those with ASD, cannot be discriminated against in hotels, restaurants, and other public accommodations, or by government entities. Since 504 and the ADA are civil rights laws, the focus of interventions in the prevention of discrimination. Therefore, as long as individuals with autism have equal opportunities to be successful as individuals without disabilities, the intent of these laws is achieved. This could require schools and employers to provide accommodations and modifications.

Future Considerations

The Ramifications of Endrew. A letter issued by the U.S. Department of Education emphasized that the *Endrew* decision requires schools to provide an IEP "reasonably calculated to enable a child to make progress appropriate in light of the child's circumstances" and thus rejects the "merely more than de minimis (i.e. more than trivial) standard applied by the Tenth Circuit" (U.S. Department of Education, 2017, p.3). The higher standard has resulted in substantial implications in how students with ASD are served. Yell and Bateman (2017) note that in order to meet the higher standard set by the *Endrew* case IEP teams must "(a) assess and analyze all of a student's unique educational needs; (b) develop ambitious, meaningful, and measurable annual goals; (c) rely on research-based special education procedures; and (d) collect actual data and make instructional decisions based on the data" (p. 290). This legislation will continue to impact how schools provide services to students with ASD, push the use of EBP to facilitate progress, and require students make reasonable progress.

The Promise of Intervention Outcomes. ASD intervention and the related outcomes have advanced significantly. However, the outcomes continue to vary widely across individuals (Eldevik, Berg Titlestad, Aarli, & Tønnesen, 2019). Research studies report approximately 30 percent of children with ASD that receive intensive early intervention are considered rapid learners and have outcome similar to their neurotypical peers (Eldevik, Hastings, Jahr, & Hughes, 2012; Sallows & Graupner, 2005). Others who have received intensive ASD interventions make progress but do not achieve the same level as neurotypical peers have been described as *moderate learners* (Sallows & Graupner, 2005). Some learners show little or no improvement (Eldevik et al., 2019) and some learners fail to acquire speech even with intensive intervention (e.g., Koegel, Shirotova, & Koegel, 2009). Varied outcomes suggests that a *one size fits all model of intervention* is not appropriate and practitioners should individualize treatment (Koegel, Shirotova, & Koegel, 2009). It is important to note that there is no cure for ASD and even with learning or optimal outcomes, the individual is still neurodiverse and should be respected as such. The goal should not be to cure ASD as individuals with ASD have much to offer society but to provide interventions to increase quality of life.

The Promise of Genetics. Identification of a specific genetic cause for ASD has not yet been found. However, researchers have suggested ASD is a genetic disorder and many different genetic profiles can contribute to an individual having an ASD (Jeste & Gerschwind, 2014). As researchers discover the genetic markers for disorders such as Rett's Disorder and Fragile X they are moved out of the category of mental disorder and can be diagnosed via a blood test. Given the complexity of the current genetic research the possibility of using genetic testing for diagnosis and access to early intervention is unlikely in the very near future but may be on the horizon for diagnosing different types or variants of ASD. Great ethical care and consideration needs to be taken should a genetic profile or marker be confirmed. The use of genetics for diagnosis and access to intervention could make the process objective but remains controversial and will lead to discussions on the ethics of genetic testing to ameliorate variants of ASD.

Advocacy and Acceptance. Fortunately, the civil rights movement provided the structure for which the neurodiverse community can and does advocate for their needs and acceptance in society. Individuals with ASD across history have made great contributions to society. It has been said that Albert Einstein, Bill Gates, Charles Darwin, Emily Dickinson and many other famous people in history had characteristics of ASD. Without the contribution of individuals with ASD society would be at a great loss. The neurodiverse community pushes society to move beyond awareness, rejects the idea that individuals with ASD need to conform to the neurotypical norms of society, and promote the education of both neurotypical and neurodiverse population to increase the quality of life for all. This community, along with other advocates for other disabilities, views disability as natural and a normal part of human diversity.

Conclusion

Despite historical references to the specific characteristics of ASD dating back to the 1700s, focused research did not begin until the 1940s with the work of Kanner and Asperger. In the time since the classification of ASD and intervention strategies have undergone significant change. Once thought of as a manifestation of early-onset schizophrenia, autism is now identified as a neurodevelopmental disorder with genetic and environmental factors influencing manifestation. There are still many unknown variables in the cause of the disorder; however, research continues to identify factors influencing symptoms and response to treatment. The most recent research indicates the manifestation of ASD falls on a continuum with a range of severity levels and comorbid conditions. Primary predictors for improvement include the level of language impairment and intellectual ability. In the community and school settings, advancements have been fueled by litigation and legislation, leading to improved educational opportunities, improved opportunities for inclusion in society, and more importantly, improved outcomes in treatment and management of the symptoms related to autism spectrum disorders.

Discussion Questions

1. Name two historical cases in which it was believed a child had ASD. What characteristics did the child present with that made people believe it could have been a case of ASD?
2. Describe how the diagnostic profile of autism has changed over time. How was this influenced by the psychosocial culture of the time?
3. Discuss the legislation that drives ASD services. Who has had the greatest influence on legislation and why do you think it is important for teachers, professionals, and researchers to understand the influences on legislation?
4. Discuss the evolution of evidence-based practices. How has the psychosocial culture of the times influenced treatment? Why is it important to focus on evidence-based practices?

Author Note

We have no known conflict of interest to disclose.

References

American Historical Society. Why study history? Retrieved December 12, 2021. from www.historians.org/teaching-and-learing/why-study-history

American Psychiatric Association. (1980). *Diagnostic and statistical manual of mental disorders*. Washington, DC: American Psychiatric Association.

American Psychiatric Association. (1987). *Diagnostic and statistical manual of mental disorders: DSM-III-R*. Washington, DC: American Psychiatric Association.

American Psychiatric Association. (1994). *Diagnostic and statistical manual of mental diseases: DSM-IV. 4th ed*. Washington, DC: American Psychiatric Association.

American Psychiatric Association. (2000). *Diagnostic and statistical manual of mental disorders, text revision (DSM-IV-TR)*. Washington, DC: American Psychiatric Association.

American Psychiatric Association. (2013). *Diagnostic and statistical manual of mental disorders (DSM-5®)*. American Psychiatric Pub.

Cook, B. G., & Odom, S. L. (2013). Evidence-based practices and implementation science in special education. *Exceptional children, 79*(2), 135–144.

Eldevik, S., Hastings, R. P., Jahr, E., & Hughes, J. C. (2012). Outcomes of behavioral intervention for children with autism in mainstream pre-school settings. *Journal of Autism and Developmental Disorders, 42*(2), 210–220. https://doi.org/10.1007/s10803-011-1234-9

Eldevik, S., Titlestad, K. B., Aarlie, H., & Tønnesen, R. (2019). Community implementation of early behavioral intervention: Higher intensity gives better outcome. *European Journal of Behavior Analysis*. https://doi.org/10.1080/15021149.2019.1629781

Frith, C.D. (2000). The role of dorsolateral prefrontal cortex in the selection of action as revealed by functional imaging. *Control of cognitive processes, 18*, 544–565.

Frith, C.D. (2003, January). What do imaging studies tell us about the neural basis of autism. In *Novartis Found Symp* Vol. 251, pp. 149–166.

Goldstein, S., Naglieri, J.A., & Ozonoff, S. (2009). *Assessment of Autism Spectrum Disorders*. New York, NY, US: Guilford Press.

Gorn, D. (1999). *What Do I Do When.... The Answer Book On Special Education Law*. Horsham, PA: LRP Publications.

Hill, D.A., Martin, E.D., & Nelson-Head, C. (2011). Examination of case law (2007–2008) regarding autism spectrum disorder and violations of the Individuals with Disabilities Education Act. *Preventing School Failure, 55*, 214–225.

Hill, D.A., & Hill, S.J. (2012). Autism spectrum disorder, Individuals with Disabilities Education Act, and case law: Who really wins? *Preventing School Failure, 56*, 157–164.

Hulett, K.E. (2009). *Legal Aspects of Special Education*. Upper Saddle River, NJ: Pearson.

Jeste, S.S., & Gerschwin, D.H. (2014). Disentangling the heterogeneity of autism spectrum disorder through genetic findings. *Nature, 10*, 74–81.

Kapp, S. K., Gillespie-Lynch, K., Sherman, L. E., & Hutman, T. (2013). Deficit, difference, or both? Autism and neurodiversity. *Developmental psychology, 49*(1), 59.

Koegel, R. L., Shirotova, L., & Koegel, L. K. (2009). Antecedent stimulus control: using orienting cues to facilitate first-word acquisition for nonresponders with autism. *The Behavior Analyst, 32*(2), 281–284.

Malson, L. (1972). *Wolf Children and the Problem of Human Nature*; and *Jean Itard The Wild Boy of Aveyron* (trsl by E. Fawcett, P. Ayton and J. White). NLB, London.

Maudsley, H. (1867). *The Physiology and Pathology of the Mind*. New York: Appleton.

National Autism Center (2009). National Standards Project-Addressing the need for evidence-based practice guidelines for autism spectrum disorders. Randolph, MA: National Autism Center.

National Conference of State Legislatures (2012). *Insurance coverage for autism*. www.ncsl.org/research/health/autism-and-insurance-coverage-state-laws.aspx. Downloaded 4/1/2015

Ortega, F. (2009). The cerebral subject and the challenge of neurodiversity. *BioSocieties, 4*(4), 425–445.

Sallows, G. O., & Graupner, T. D. (2005). Intensive behavioral treatment for children with autism: Four-year outcome and predictors. *American journal on mental retardation, 110*(6), 417–438.

Smith, T.E.C., Polloway, E.A., Doughty, T.A., Patton, J.R., & Dowdy, C.A. (2020). *Teaching Students With Special Needs in Inclusive Settings*, 8th ed. Austin: Pro-Ed.

Singer, J. (1999). Why can't you be normal for once in your life? From a 'problem with no name' to the emergence of a new category of difference. In M. Corker & S. French (Eds.), Disability discourse (pp. 59–67). London, England: Open University Press.

Szatmari, P. (2011). New recommendations on autism spectrum disorder. *BMJ, 342*.

U. S. Department of Education. Dec. 7, 2017 Questions and Answers on Supreme Court Case Decision Endrew F., v. Douglas County School District Re-1

Volkmar, F.R., Bregman, J., Cohen, D.J., & Cicchetti, D.V. (1988). DSM-III and DSM-III-R diagnoses of autism. *The American Journal of Psychiatry, 145*(11), 1404–1408.

Westphal, A., Schelinski, S., Volkmar, F., & Pelphrey, K. (2013). Revisiting regression in autism: Heller's dementia infantilis. *Journal of Autism and Developmental Disorders, 43*(2), 265–271.

Wing, J.K. (1976) Kanner's syndrome: a historical introduction. In L. Wing (Ed.), *Early Childhood Autism: Clinical, educational and social aspects (2nd ed.)*. Oxford: Pergamon.

Wolff, S. (2004). The history of autism. *European child & adolescent psychiatry, 13*(4), 201–208.

Yell, M.L., Bateman, D.F. (2017). Endrew F. v. Douglas County School District (2017): FAPE and the U.S. Supreme Court. *TEACHING Exceptional Children*, 50(1), 7–15.

Yell, M.L., & Drasgow, E. (2000). Litigating a free appropriate public education: The Lovaas hearing and cases. *The Journal or Special Education*, 33, 205–214.

Zager, D. (Ed.). (2004). *Autism Spectrum Disorders: Identification, Education, and Treatment*. Mahwah, NJ: Lawrence Erlbaum Publishers.

Chapter 3

Legislation, Evidence Based Practices, and State Implementation

Nikki L. Murdick,[1] *Jo Nell Wood,*[1] *and Amanda Wood*[2]
[1]School of Education, St. Louis University, St. Louis
[1]St. Louis University, St. Louis, Missori
[2]Wentzville R-IV School District, Wentzville, Missouri

> Public education reflects the society it serves. In the past half century, the United States has transitioned, evolved, and morphed in ways that brought concurrent schoolhouse changes: from desegregation to transgender bathrooms, from Title I and the War on Poverty to Title IX and the battle for gender equality, from No Child Left Behind (NCLB) to the Every Student Succeeds Act (ESSA), from prayer out of schools to lockdown drills in the schools. Public education is not the master of its destiny but rather the mirror through which society reflects.
>
> (Claypool & McLaughlin, 2017, p. 1)

While public schooling may be seen as a monolith, a one size for all, which looks correct when looking at the overall schooling, then one is looking at the forest and not the trees. However, if one focuses on the trees and not the forest, one sees "that decades of efforts in response to changes in society are there among the branches and the leaves" (Claypool & McLaughlin, 2017, p. 11). Although autism was recognized and identified in the early 1960s, education and treatment programs at that time were scarce. Nevertheless, parents were organizing and initiating programs for their children with autism. The history of autism legislation reflects the same confusion education and health professionals encountered when trying to provide services to children with autism and their families. Unarguably, the most important legislation for children and youth with disabilities was IDEA (Individuals with Disabilities Education Act). However, bowing to political demands, autism was not listed as a category under IDEA until 1990. Still, individuals with autism were eligible for some services under other disability legislation that burst into the public consciousness through personal accounts from movies, books, advocacy groups, and changes in legislation, program development, and service delivery that expanded at the same time. This chapter

DOI: 10.4324/9781003255147-4

provides information on legislation that helped define the programs and services designed to meet the growing need, evidence-based practices used to assist individuals with autism, and an outline of state-by-state and international efforts focused on supporting individuals with autism.

Legislation Impacting Individuals with Autism

Over the decades, information concerning autism spectrum disorder (ASD) has expanded. As a result, the "growing prevalence of ASD is shaping current law and policy relating to all disabilities and will have a profound impact on children with disability, particularly concerning special education" (Dicker & Bennet, 2011, p. 416). Table 3.1 lists key legislation related to education and Table 3.2 lists key legislation related to ASD.

Autism originally was known as a low incidence category, inferring that the number of children with this type of disability were few. As

Table 3.1 General Legislation Related to Education and Disability

Achieving a Better Life Experience Act (ABLE) of 2014. Public Law 113-297, 26 U.S.C. § 529

Affordable Care Act of 2010. Public Law 111-148

Children's Health Act of 2000, Public Law 106-301, 42 U.S.C. 201 *et seq.*

Developmental Disabilities Assistance and Bill of Rights Act of 2000, Public Law 106-402, 42 U.S.C. § 6000 *et seq.*

Education for All Handicapped Children Act of 1975. Public Law 94-142, 20 U.S.C. § 1471 *et seq.*

Education of the Handicapped Act of 1970, Public Law 91-230, 20 U.S.C. § 1401 *et seq.*

Education of the Handicapped Act of 1974, Public Law 93-380, 20 U.S.C. § 1232 *et seq.*

Elementary and Secondary Education Act (ESEA) of 1965, Public Law 89—10, 20 U.S.C. § 16301 *et seq.*

Elementary and Secondary Education Act, amended by Public Law 89-750, 20 U.S.C. § 1401 *et seq.*

Every Student Succeeds Act of 2015, 20 U.S.C. § 6301

Handicapped Children's Protection Act of 1986, Public Law 99-372, 20 U.S.C. § 1401 *et seq.*

Higher Education Opportunity Act of 2008, Public Law 110-315, 20 U.S.C. § 1001 *et seq.*

Individuals with Disabilities Education Act of 1990, Public Law 101-476, 20 U.S.C. § 1400 *et seq.*

Individuals with Disabilities Education Act Amendments of 1997, Public Law 105-17, 20 U.S.C. § 1400 *et seq.*

Individuals with Disabilities Education Act of 2001, Public Law 107-110, 20 U.S.C. 70 § 6301 *et seq.*

No Child Left Behind Act of 2001, Public Law 107-110, 20 U.S.C. 70 § 6301 *et seq.*

Patient Protection and Affordable Care Act of 2010, Public Law 111-148, 42 U.S.C. § 1801 *et seq.*

Rehabilitation Act of 1973, Section 504, Public Law 93-112, 39 U.S.C. §794 *et seq*

Table 3.2 Autism Specific Legislation

Autism CARES Act of 2014, Public Law 113-156, 42 U.S.C. 201 et seq.
Autism CARES Act of 2019, Public Law 116-60, 42 U.S.C. 201 et seq.
Combatting Autism Act of 2006, Public Law 109-416, 42 U.S.C. 201 et seq.
Combatting Autism Reauthorization Act of 2011, Public Law 112-32, 42 U.S.C. 201 et seq.

a result, prior to 1975, children with autism were routinely excluded from attending schools because of the belief they could not learn or they would interfere with the learning of other students in the class (Dicker & Bennett, 2011; Hass, 2008). Thus, many children who would now be considered as having autism were labeled under the category of mental retardation or emotional disturbance, spending most their lives in an institutional setting. As a result, much of the pre-1990 legislation did not include autism specifically as a category of disability. A brief description of legislation that was important in the provision of services for children with autism and other disabilities follows.

Rehabilitation Act (Section 504) (Public Law 93-112; Public Law 114-95)

Public Law 93-112, known as the Rehabilitation Act, was enacted in 1973. It was an expansion of several earlier acts beginning in the early 1900s with the Soldier's Rehabilitation Act (1918). One part of the Act, Section 504, is the part of this legislation that focuses on nondiscrimination of individuals with a disability. Specific categories of disability are not included in the Rehabilitation Act as it used a functional definition focusing entirely on the existence of a disability and its impact on the individual's chance for success. The Rehabilitation Act is basically civil rights legislation for persons with disabilities and, as such, is more inclusive in its outlook than other education-focused pieces of legislation, such as the Individuals with Disabilities Education Act. In 1998 the Rehabilitation Act was reauthorized and included amendments to Section 508 that focused on accessibility of electronic and information technology for persons with disabilities. The latest reauthorization was in 2015 as P.L. 114-95. At this time the Act replaced the Vocational Rehabilitation Act, extended the authorization of grants to states for vocational rehabilitation services, created a linkage between state vocational rehabilitation programs and workforce investment activities and established special responsibilities with respect to individuals with disabilities within and across programs administered by the federal government (Institute for Disability Research, Policy and Practice, 2021; U.S. Department of Education, 2017).

Developmental Disabilities Assistance and Bill of Rights Act (Public Law 106-402)

There has been ongoing controversy over the classification of persons with mental retardation and other disabilities and how they should be identified. As a result of this moral question, in 1975 a new more global category was invented – developmental disabilities (Eyal et al., 2010). This piece of legislation was an amendment of a 1963 act known as the Mental Health Centers Construction Act. The act included a variety of changes including a functional, as opposed to a categorical, definition of disability, i.e., developmental disabilities (DD), and an expansion of state involvement through state plans, state grants, and State Developmental Disabilities Councils.

In addition, it included a Bill of Rights for Persons with Disabilities. Because it includes a functional definition, autism was not named specifically, although individuals could be served under the eligibility rubric of DD. This piece of legislation was most recently reauthorized in 2000 to continue its focus on programs for individuals with developmental disabilities (Title I), family support (Title II), and programs for direct support workers who assist individuals with developmental disabilities (Title III).

Education for All Handicapped Children Act (Public Law 94-142)

In 1975, a piece of legislation considered to be the most important in the last century for persons with disabilities was enacted. The Education for All Handicapped Children Act (EAHCA) essentially included a Bill of Rights for Children with Disabilities with the assurance that all children with disabilities receive a free, appropriate, public education, abbreviated as FAPE (Murdick et al., 2014). Thirteen specific categories of disability were listed and explicitly covered by this legislation. Autism was not included as one of these, as it still was considered to be a rare disability. As such, autism was subsumed within the disability category of *seriously emotionally disturbed (SED)* and later in 1981 moved to the *other health impaired (OHI)* category (Zager et al., 2012). The EAHCA was amended once more before the new decade began. The Education of the Handicapped Amendments (EHA) of 1986 included two new programs addressing the needs of infants and toddlers with disabilities and, also, pre-school children ages three to five years old. Although the law was expanded, still autism was not included as a separate category in the legislation.

As the country moved into the 1990s, autism finally was recognized as a separate category. It was believed by specifically naming autism as a category, more appropriate research, education, and legislation could be provided for individuals with autism and their families. Subsequently, during the past 25 years, the number of pieces of legislation that have included or focused on children with autism has increased, as has research on ASD.

Individuals with Disabilities Education Act and its Reauthorizations (Public Law 101-476, 105-17, and 108-446)

In 1990, a more extensive reauthorization of the EASHCA occurred including a name change to reflect the field's move to focus on people first language. Thus, the new law was entitled the Individuals with Disabilities Education Act (IDEA) of 1990. Additional changes included expansion of service delivery to students with disabilities ages 18-21 years old, inclusion of transition services and assistive technology as approved special education services, and rehabilitation counseling and social work services under the list of related service. But to the field of autism, the most important aspect was the inclusion of autism as a specific, free-standing category for the first time (Murdick et al., 2014). The law has been reauthorized and revised three more times since. The first reauthorization was in 1991, titled the Individuals with Disabilities Education Act Amendments (IDEAA) with changes in the Part H program for infants and toddlers and the inclusion of an Individualized Family Service Plan (IFSP) instead of an Individualized Education Plan (IEP) for children ages three to five. The second reauthorization of the law was in 1997, with changes focusing on school safety, parental participation, and finances.

In 2004, a major revision of IDEA was completed. This reauthorization known as the Individuals with Disabilities Education Improvement Act (IDEIA), included a definition of highly qualified special education teachers, a provision for reducing paperwork, appropriate education for homeless or migrant children, changes in procedural safeguards, and a revision of state performance goals and requirements to bring IDEIA into compliance with the reauthorization of the Elementary and Secondary Education Act (ESEA) of 1965. The ESEA was later reauthorized and renamed as the No Child Left Behind Act (NCLB) and then as the Every Student Succeeds Act (ESSA). In addition, this IDEA reauthorization addressed the programmatic needs of children with autism by calling for the development and expansion of programs to train teachers for this group of students (Dicker & Bennett, 2011) and to increase the use of research-based teaching methodologies (Zager et al., 2012). According to Murdick et al. (2014, p. 30), "the changes to IDEA may be seen as an attempt to reduce the conflict between IDEA and No Child Left Behind Act (NCLB) of 2001 (PL 107-110)," that is, the individual focus of IDEA and the group focus of NCLB have led to concerns over the appropriateness of programming and assessment of student progress. The NCLB was revised with the enactment of the Every Student Succeeds Act in 2015 with some sections addressing issues related to children with disabilities. The ESSA was scheduled for reauthorization at the end of the 2020-2021 school year.

Children's Health Act (Public Law 106-310)

The Children's Health Act of 2000 was signed by President Clinton to increase research and treatment in a variety of health issues including autism. There are five sections of the law that focus on the issues related to autism. Section 101 focuses on the "expansion, intensification, and coordination of activities of National Institutes of Health with respect to research on autism" (U.S. GPO, 2000). Section 102 focuses on developmental disabilities surveillance and research programs for individuals with autism, including the National Autism and Pervasive Development Disabilities Surveillance Program, the Centers of Excellence in Autism and Pervasive Developmental Disabilities Epidemiology, and a Clearinghouse at the CDC for storage of data generated under this section. Section 103 expands and implements a program to provide information and education to professionals and the general public about the field of autism. Section 104 of this law mandates the establishment of a group to oversee and coordinate research in the field of autism known as the Interagency Autism Coordinating Committee (IACC). The IACC's mission is to "facilitate the effective and efficient exchange of information on autism activities among the member agencies and to coordinate autism-related activities" (U.S. Department of Health and Human Services, 2003). And the final section, 105, requires a yearly report to Congress on the progress of these sections of the legislation.

As a result of this act, the National Child Study was instituted in what was called its Vanguard or "pilot" phase in which the feasibility and cost of a longitudinal study was to be considered to address the need for research on autism. During this phase about 5000 children in 40 countries were enrolled with enrollment ending in 2013. At that time, an expert review committee reviewed the information collected during the pilot phase and based on the results advised the director of the NIH that the main study should not be completed. They believed additional research was currently not the best way "to add to the understanding of how environmental and genetic factors influence child health and development". The result was the National Children's Study was closed as of December 2014 (Children's Health Act, 2020). All data collected to that time was to be made available to researchers as of 2015, but no additional research would be completed. Thus, the Children's Health Act was not reauthorized as it had addressed its original goals.

No Child Left Behind Act (Public Law 107-110)

The No Child Left Behind Act of 2001, or NCLB, was a reauthorization of the Elementary and Secondary Education Act (ESEA) and was considered to be one of the most sweeping pieces of legislation since IDEA was first enacted in 1975. According to the Office of the Under Secretary of the U.S. Department of Education (2002) "[t]his historic reform gives states and school districts unprecedented flexibility in how they spend their education dollars in return for setting standards for student achievement and holding students and educators accountable for results" (p. 3). Thus, the purpose of the act is to "close the achievement gap by holding states, local school districts, and schools accountable for improving the academic achievement of children" (Wright et al., 2004, p. 21). This focus on academic accountability using state-developed tests becomes one of the most controversial, as there are concerns that the focus on testing as the means to identify progress may impact negatively on students with disabilities and those from minority or poverty-stricken areas of the country.

Combatting Autism Act and Reauthorizations (Public Laws 109-416, 112-32, 113-57, and 116-60)

The Combatting Autism Act of 2006 (CAA, P.L. 109-416) was enacted in 2006 by President Bush "in recognition of the rapid growth in the number of children diagnosed with autism" (White et al., 2012, p. 8). This legislation was developed from previously included sections of the Child Health Act of 2000 (CHA) which addressed issues related to autism (Congressional Research Service, 2012). The CAA was enacted as a stand-alone piece of legislation because of a growing concern over the increasing rates of children being diagnosed with autism. Its goals were to increase existing autism research funding authorizations and to stimulate state-level coordination of health, education, and disability programs. It authorized funding for ASD surveillance, research, and education through four agencies: the Department of Health and Human Services (HHS), the Centers for Disease Control and Prevention (CDC), the Health Resources and Service Administration (HRSA), and the National Institutes of Health (NIH). The CAA was reauthorized by President Obama in 2011 as the Combating Autism Reauthorization Act of 2011 (CARA) to extend appropriations for programs established in the CAA of 2006 and to require the Secretary of Health and Human Services to submit a yearly progress report related to the implementation of the act.

As re-authorization of the CARA of 2011 was being debated in early 2014, ASAN (the Autistic Self Advocacy Network) and 14 other disability organizations submitted a letter to Congress urging changes to the act including a revision of the title of the Act which they believed was both hurtful and stigmatizing (Congressional Research Service, 2012). Later in 2014 CARA was reauthorized as the Autism Collaboration, Accountability, Research, Education, and Support Act of 2014 or Autism CARES Act of 2014 (P. L. 113-156). It reauthorized the Public Service Health Act to reauthorize research, surveillance, and education activities related to autism conducted by various agencies within the Department of Health and Human Services. This act was again reauthorized in 2019 (*Autism Cares Act* of 2019, P.L. 116–60) to ensure support for research, services, prevalence tracking, to increase the amount of federal spending on autism efforts, and to expand the focus of government activities to include the lifespan of people with autism (Autism Society, 2019; White House Blog, 2014).

Higher Education Opportunity Act (Public Law 110-315)

The Higher Education Opportunity Act of 2008 is usually considered to focus on students with intellectual disability. The Act was the latest of many reauthorizations of the Higher Education Act of 1965, enacted to improve access to college or career schools for students with intellectual disability (ID) (Center for Autism Research, 2014a; Lee, 2009). This Act provided increased access for these students to Pell grants and other financial aid opportunities for those students with intellectual disability who are "enrolled or accepted for enrollment in a comprehensive transition and postsecondary program at specific institution of higher education (IHE) and maintain satisfactory progress in the program" (Lee, 2009, p. 1). Although this act focused on students with intellectual disability (ID), there is increasing evidence that many students with ID also have autism. According to the Center for Disease Control's (CDC) later prevalence study of records since 2008, 10 percent of those individuals who primary diagnosis is ID also have a secondary diagnosis of Autism Spectrum Disorder (ASD), and 38 percent of those individuals whose primary diagnosis is ASD have a secondary diagnosis of ASD (Center for Autism Research, 2014b). As a result, professionals and parents addressing the programmatic needs and future plans for students with ASD should be cognizant of the provisions of this Act.

The Higher Education Act was to be reauthorized every five years, but no reauthorization has occurred since 2008. The Act has continued as the result of a series of temporary extensions with efforts in Congress each year to address its extension although none have gone past the committee stage (ACE, 2021). In 2019 the College Affordability Act (CAA) was introduced in the House of Representatives which was a substantial rewriting and revision of the HEA. The bill with revisions was stalled in the Senate as of 2021. According to the American Council on Education (ACE), this bill as written had concerns that prevented its support by the ACE. As they noted:

> The CAA is a dense, complicated piece of legislation, with a number of provisions that would be beneficial for students and institutions, such as significant increases in student aid and support for institutions that have historically been under resourced. However, these provisions are offset by intrusive, complicated, or burdensome requirements that will undercut the bill's primary goal to make higher education more affordable.
>
> (ACE, 2021)

Affordable Care Act (Public Law 111-148)

The Patient Protection and Affordable Care Act of 2010, commonly called the Affordable Care Act and signed by President Obama, includes a significant section for children with autism as individuals with ASD can face complex health needs throughout their lifespan (Autism Speaks, 2015a). For most families of children with autism, it is critical that they have some type of financial support to manage the variety of medical, behavioral, and development health services required for their child. According to Autism Speaks (2015a), this can require a complex navigation of multiple medical professionals and insurance reimbursement rules that may not cover all the needed services. As a result of this problem, many reported they had to pay much of the medical costs themselves. With the enactment of the Affordable Care Act, insurance companies are prohibited from denying coverage to children with pre-existing conditions that include autism. The Act also includes behavioral health treatments on its list of essential benefits. Even with this change, there continues to be concern that parents with fewer resources still will be unable to access appropriate services for their child with autism.

Achieving a Better Life Experience Act (Public Law 113-295)

As noted previously, many individuals with disabilities (and their families) have had difficulty paying for their disability related services (Autism Speaks, 2015b). To address part of this issue, the Achieving Better Life Experience Act, or the ABLE Act of 2014, an amendment to the Internal Revenue Code of 1986, was signed by President Obama. Its purpose was to:

Encourage and assist individuals and families in saving private funds for the purpose of supporting individuals with disabilities to maintain health, independence, and quality of life; and (2) provide secure funding for disability-related expenses of beneficiaries with disabilities that will supplement, but not supplant, benefits private insurance, Title XVI (Supplemental Security Income) and Title XIX (Medicaid) of the Social Security Act, the beneficiary's employment, and other sources to allow parents to set up a special tax-free savings account for disability-related expenses.

(Library of Congress, 2015)

According to the National Down Syndrome Society (2021) essential expenses include "medical and dental care, education, community-based supports, employment training, assistive technology, housing and transportation." With the enactment of this Act, individuals with disabilities now can have college savings accounts, health savings accounts and individual retirement accounts the same as any other individual.

Every Student Succeeds Act, 20 U.S.C. § 6301 (2015)

On December 10, 2015, the Every Student Succeeds Act of 2015 (ESSA) was signed by President Barack Obama and became the United States' current national education law. The ESSA was a long overdue reauthorization of the Elementary and Secondary Education Act of 1965 (ESEA) replacing both ESEA and NCLB. Unlike previous ESEA reauthorizations, the ESSA shifted much educational authority from the federal government to state and local education agencies (Sharp, 2016). "The law requires states to develop plans on how they plan to reduce bullying and harassment, restraint and seclusion, and suspensions and expulsions—all of which disproportionately affect students with disabilities" (Samuels, 2015, p. 1). While ESSA was set to be reauthorized by 2021, no new reauthorization has taken place. Although major changes and legislative support expanded the options for individuals with ASD, problems continue to arise. Most noteworthy is children with autism who are high functioning may not be eligible to receive needed special education and related services because of the way the regulations are written. In addition, the NCLB's focus on alternative testing for those with a disability may hamper the educational future of these students because these tests may be unable to adequately measure ability. Also, legislation is occurring across the states, which holds promise for children with autism and their families but leaves concern that consistency of education programming will not occur since all states could pass legislation with differing requirements.

Standards Project, Evidence-based Practices, and State and International Efforts Supporting Individuals with Autism

Flowing from the legislative background supporting individuals with autism was the next important area, the standards projects. These projects were designed to identify the various evidence-based practices that were supported by research as being effective. In addition, they were to identify state initiatives in place to support individuals with autism. On the national arena, one can access the National Standards Project Report (Wilczynski, 2009; National Autism Center, 2015) for information about effective practices. According to the National Autism Center (2015), *The National Standards Report* answers the question of how to effectively treat individuals with autism spectrum disorder (ASD). This project was begun in 2005 by the National Autism Center in collaboration with an expert panel of scholars, researchers, and other national leaders. It is the most comprehensive analysis of evidence-based interventions targeted toward children, adolescents, and young adults with autism. Phase 2 provided an updated examination for this age group and extended the research base to adults over age 22.

The National Standards Research Project

According to the National Autism Center (2015), the National Research Project is an expansion of a 2001 report by the National Research Council (NRC). That report identified effective practices such as early intervention, instructional programming, parent involvement, utilization of deliberate teaching, small group or one-to-one instruction, and a communication-rich environment (NRC, 2001). Even with the publication of that report, families, educators, and service providers were still confused with the myriad and sometimes conflicting information about available treatments. Thus, the 2015 report was seen as a much-needed step in "helping to reduce the resulting turmoil and uncertainty by addressing the need for evidence-based practice standards and providing guidelines for how to make choices about interventions" (National Autism Center, 2015, p. 2). The 2017 analysis provided the most comprehensive list of research-based effective practices to that date.

Services for persons with autism have developed quickly, but through research data educators and medical professionals learned some important principles. First, early interventions lead to better outcomes. Parent involvement is not only important, but it leads to better outcomes for both the child and the family. Autism spans all ages, but its impact differs according to the age of the person with autism. Thus, services must develop a lifespan approach. Finally, the National Standards Project report identified effective practices such as early intervention, instructional programming, parent involvement, utilization of a deliberate teaching, small group or one-to-one instruction, and a communication-rich environment as a result of a thorough examination of research data.

Evidence-based Practices

In efforts to have a positive impact on the life trajectory of individuals with autism, teachers and practitioners working in clinics, early intervention centers and schools, as well as other human service programs search for effective intervention strategies when working with children and youth with autism (IRIS Center, n.d.). "The increased prevalence of autism has intensified the demand for effective educational and therapeutic services, and intervention science is providing mounting evidence about practices that positively impact outcomes" (Steinbrenner et al., 2020, p. 7). The current focus on evidence-based practices (EBPs) for children and youth with autism was first outlined in Cochrane's (1972) report concerning how health and medical services be based on "empirical, scientific evidence of its efficacy" (Hume et al., 2021, para. 3). A contribution of the evidence-based medicine movement was "identification and verification of evidence-based practice *is just the first step*" (Hume et al., 2021, para. 3). The selection and application of scientifically based practices depends on the skills and knowledge of the implementer in selecting appropriate practices for the autistic individual and applying them with fidelity. Hume et al. (2021) indicated:

> This multi-step process of blending information about scientifically identified, efficacious practices with practitioners' knowledge and skill has been adopted in the evidence-based movements in education (Davies, 1999; Odom et al., 2005), psychology (American Psychological Association, 2006) and other human services.
>
> (American Speech and Hearing Association, 2004, para 3)

From the work of the National Standards Project, examples of research-based practices (EBPs) for individuals with autism were outlined as the preferred methods of supporting development for these individuals. While not all of these EBPs are preferred or agreed upon methods in the eyes of practitioners the research does support each of the following as an EBP. For more information on EBPs, see Steinbrenner et al., 2020.

State by State Efforts to Assist Individuals with Autism

In every state and territory, programs authorized by the Developmental Disabilities Assistance and Bill of Rights Act (DD

Act) empower individuals with developmental disabilities and their families to help shape policies that impact them. DD Act programs conduct important research and test innovative new service delivery models. They work to bring the latest knowledge and resources to those who can put it to the best use, including self-advocates, families, service providers, and policymakers.

(Administration for Community Living, n.d., para. 3)

Most states began their work on autism with a task force charged by the governor or legislature to develop strategy to address the needs of individuals with autism within their state. Many states now have departments or offices to oversee implementation of the task force recommendations (Easter Seals, 2016). Some states have developed their own guides to assist the members of the multidisciplinary team in selecting appropriate evidenced-based practices for use with children with autism. For state examples, review Virginia's *Models of Best Practice* (2011), Ohio's *Autism Reaching for a Brighter Future* (2011), and Missouri's *Autism Spectrum Disorders: A Guide to Evidence-Based Interventions* (2012). Utilizing the Easter Seals (2016) website, all states with initiatives were investigated to identify what, if any, initiatives had been or were developed. See Table 3.3 for this information. All but seven states (Georgia, Hawaii, Louisiana, Maine, Oklahoma, South Dakota, and Wyoming) had some type of task force actively in place to assist with this effort with one state (Missouri) providing no information.

International Efforts to Support Individuals with Autism

While the road to recognition and awareness of autism and the rights of individuals with autism has been a long and winding one, there continues to be a continuing need to ensure the human rights of people with autism, such as the right to inclusive education and health needs. Individuals with autism should be given the opportunity to develop their full potential so they can flourish within a school setting so they can lead life as autonomously and interdependently as possible. Internationally, this road began in 1948 when the United Nations created the Universal Declaration of Human Rights (UDHR), which outlined the rights and freedoms of all human beings. It was adopted as a precursor to the human rights laws, which were later created. Thus, it led the way to future declarations by countries around the world (Roleska et al., 2018). Shortly afterward in 1959, the Declaration of the Rights of the Child was adopted by the United Nations. Principle 5 of the Declaration of the Rights of the Child posits if a child has special needs because of their mental or physical condition, appropriate treatment, education, and care should be provided (Roleska et al., 2018).

Table 3.3 State by State Autism Initiatives

State	Autism Initiatives
Alabama	• Alabama Interagency Autism Coordinating Council (AIACC) • Autism Spectrum Disorder Card • Autism Centers
Alaska	• Governor's Council on Disabilities and Special Education (GCDSE) • Alaska Autism Resource Center (AARC)
Arizona	• Autism Spectrum Disorder (ASD) Advisory Committee
Arkansas	• Arkansas Legislative Task Force on Autism • Arkansas Autism Partnership, a Medicaid waiver program
California	• Senate Select Committee on Autism and Related Disorders • Autism Therapy as a Medi-Cal Benefit • Superintendent's Autism Advisory Committee (SAAC) • Autism Pilot Program – Regional Center Excellence in Community Autism Partnerships (RE CAP) program
Colorado	• The Colorado Autism Commission • Colorado Home and Community-Based Services Waiver – Children with Autism Waiver
Connecticut	• Autism Spectrum Disorder Advisory Council • Connecticut Task Force on the Issues for the Education of Children with Autism • Guidelines for the Identification and Education of Children and Youth with Autism
Delaware	• Delaware Autism Adults Service Needs Task Force • Delaware Autism Program • Autism Surveillance and Registration
District of Columbia	• The District of Columbia does not have an active task force on autism at this time. • Governor's Task Force on Autism Spectrum Disorders
Florida	• Florida Regional Autism Centers • Florida Autism Center of Excellence
Georgia	• The State of Georgia does not have an active statewide task force on autism at this time.
Hawaii	• Hawaii does not have an active task force on autism at this time.
Illinois	• Illinois Autism Task Force • ISBE-Autism Peer Buddy Program • The Autism Program of Illinois • Autism Spectrum Disorder Wallet Card
Indiana	• Indiana Commission on Autism • Autism Training for Law Enforcement • Autism Training for Emergency Responders • Indiana Resource Center for Autism
Iowa	• Iowa Autism Council • The Autism Support Program • Regional Autism Assistance Program (RAP)
Kansas	• Kansas Autism Task Force • Kansas Home and Community-Based Services Waiver: KS Autism • TASN Autism and Tertiary Behavior Support

(continued)

Table 3.3 Cont.

State	Autism Initiatives
Kentucky	• Kentucky Commission on Autism Spectrum Disorders • The Office of Autism housed at the University of Kentucky and the University of Louisville • Kentucky Advisory Council on Autism Spectrum Disorders • Kentucky Autism Training Center
Louisiana	• Louisiana has no active Autism Task Force at this time
Maine	• Maine does not have an active task force on autism at this time
Maryland	• Maryland Commission on Autism • Task Force to Study an Online Assisting Students with Autism • Maryland Home and Community-Based Services Waiver:Easter Seals Serving • DC | MD |VA Waivers for Children w/Autism Spectrum Disorder (Autism Waiver) • Early Childhood Autism Workgroup • The Autism "Portal" Project • Maryland Autism and Developmental Disabilities
Massachusetts	• Monitoring Project Massachusetts • Towson University Hussman Center for Adults with Autism • Autism Commission • Massachusetts Home and Community-Based Services Waiver: MA Children's Autism Spectrum Disorder
Michigan	• Autism Council • The Michigan Autism Program • Michigan Medicaid and MIChild Autism Benefit • The Autism Coverage Fund
Minnesota	• Autism Spectrum Disorder Task Force • Minnesota Autism Project and Network
Mississippi	• Autism Advisory Committee • Autism Pilot Program
Missouri	• No information was provided on this website
Montana	• Montana Autism Task Force • Autism Services in Traditional Medicaid • Montana Autism Center
Nebraska	• The State of Nebraska does not have an active task force on autism at this time. • Nebraska Home and Community-Based Services Waiver: NE Autism • Nebraska Autism Spectrum Disorder (ASD) Network
Nevada	• The Nevada Commission on Autism Spectrum Disorders • Autism Assistance Treatment Program
New Hampshire	• New Hampshire Council on Autism Spectrum Disorders
New Jersey	• New Jersey Adults with Autism Task Force • New Jersey Governor's Council on Medical Research and Treatment for Autism • First Responders Training • Autism Registry • New Jersey Autism Website • Autism Programs Fund

Table 3.3 Cont.

State	Autism Initiatives
New Mexico	• The State of New Mexico does not have an active task force on autism at this time. • Voluntary Autism Registry
North Carolina	• No information was provided on this website
North Dakota	• Joint Committee on Autism Spectrum Disorder, Law Enforcement, Public Safety, and First Responders • Autism Spectrum Disorders Program • Treatment and Education of Autistic and Related Communication-handicapped Children (TEACCH) • Autism Alert • A task force on autism spectrum disorders • North Dakota Home and Community-Based Services Waiver: ND Autism Spectrum Disorder Birth Through Four • Autism Voucher Program • Autism Spectrum Disorder Database
Ohio	• Ohio Autism Task Force • Ohio Interagency Workgroup on Autism • Autism Scholarship Program • Ohio Center for Autism and Low Incidence • Ohio Autism Diagnosis Education Pilot Project
Oklahoma	• The State of Oklahoma does not have an active task force on autism at this time
Oregon	• Oregon Commission on Autism Spectrum Disorders • Oregon Regional Programs & Oregon Program Autism Training Sites and Supports (OrPATS)
Pennsylvania	• Bureau of Autism Services • Pennsylvania Home and Community-Based Services • Waiver: Adult Autism • The ASERT Collaborative (Autism Services, Education, Resources and Training) • Adult Community Autism Program (ACAP) • Law Enforcement Training
Rhode Island	• Joint Commission to Study Autism in the State of Rhode Island • Autism Support Center • Rhode Island Evaluation and Treatment Act
South Carolina	• The State of South Carolina does not have an active autism task force at this time. • South Carolina Department of Disabilities and Special Needs – Autism Division • Carolina Autism Resource and Evaluation (CARE) Center
South Dakota	• The State of South Dakota does not have an active task force on autism at this time.
Tennessee	• Autism Spectrum Disorder Task Force
Texas	• Texas Council on Autism and Pervasive Developmental Disorders • Texas Autism Research and Resource Center (TARRC) • Texas Legislature Approves Program for Autism

(continued)

Table 3.3 Cont.

State	Autism Initiatives
Utah	• Utah Registry of Autism and Developmental Disabilities (URADD) • Utah Home and Community-Based Services Waiver: UT Autism
Vermont	• Vermont Autism Planning Committee • Autism Advisory Council • Autism Tuition Assistance Grant Program • Autism Priority Project – Training & Technical Assistance Center
Virginia	• Virginia Commonwealth University Autism Center for Excellence (VCU-ACE) • Autism Study
Washington	• The Caring for Washington Individuals with Autism Task Force • Autism Outreach Project
West Virginia	• The State of West Virginia does not have an active task force on autism at this time. • The West Virginia Autism Training Center • Autism Trust Funds
Wisconsin	• Governor's Task Force on Autism • Autism Advisory Council • Autism Services as a Statewide Medicaid Benefit: ForwardHealth
Wyoming	• The State of Wyoming does not have an active task force on autism at this time. • ATTAIN: New Horizons in Autism

Easter Seals website https://www.easterseals.com/explore-resources/living-with-autism/state-autism-profiles.html.

In 1971, the Declaration on the Rights of Mentally Retarded Persons was instituted focusing on the fact that all people should have equal rights and the right to education with the aim to fully develop the potential of those with a disability. However, since it was not specific as to the meaning of disability, in 1975 the Declaration on the Rights of Disabled Persons was signed which expanded disability to include all people with disabilities including autism (Roleska et al., 2018). While these declarations touch on the right to education nothing is explicitly spelled out. As a result of these documents, countries were obligated to take into consideration the needs of persons with disabilities, including autism, when creating their legislation and these documents influenced most policies developed by the European Union (EU). In 1992, the Charter for Persons with Autism was created by Autism-Europe (Roleska et al., 2018).

In 2000, these documents were collected into one, legally binding document – the Charter of Fundamental Rights of the European Union. In the preamble, the rights were highlighted by creating the charter intended to enhance protection and assist in creating a closer union based on common values. Following these declarations in 2006, the Convention on the

Rights of People with Disabilities (CRPD) was held which resulted in articles outlining the rights to be protected by EU Countries. And in 2010, the European Commission adopted the European Disability Strategy 2010–2020 highlighting inclusive education of children with disabilities focusing on its important and beneficial aspects of development. While individuals with autism were not specifically mentioned, disability was treated as a unified concept (Roleska et al., 2018).

In addition, the World Health Organization (WHO) has recognized that people with autism have the right "to enjoyment of the highest attainable standard of physical and mental health" (WHO, 2021, section 5). To support this statement, the WHO adopted a resolution on autism spectrum disorders (WHA67.8) in May of 2014 at the Sixty-seventh World Health Assembly. More than 60 countries supported the resolution of "comprehensive and coordinated efforts for the management of autism spectrum disorders (ASD)" (WHO, 2021, section 6). This resolution was an effort to collaborate with member states and agencies to strengthen national capacities to address ASD by focusing efforts on:

- increasing the commitment of governments to taking action to improve the quality of life of people with autism;
- providing guidance on policies and action plans that address autism within the broader framework of health, mental health and disabilities;
- contributing to strengthening the ability of caregivers and the health workforce to provide appropriate and effective care for people with autism; and
- promoting inclusive and enabling environments for people with autism and other developmental disabilities.

(WHO, 2021, Section 7)

In 2015, the Written Declaration on Autism was adopted and co-signed by 418 Members of the European Parliament (Roleska et al., 2018). This Declaration outlined the importance of early diagnosis to provide support and education for individuals with autism. It also called upon the European countries to create a European Autism Strategy for ensuring the needs of people with autism are met as well as to expand autism research and prevalence studies (Roleska et al., 2018).

International organizations and countries continue to focus on how to support individuals with autism and the United Nations continues to maintain a focus on efforts as well. As a result of this focus April 2, 2021 was recognized as World Autism Awareness Day (Autism Europe, 2021a). The foregoing declarations and the continuing focus on autism assists countries internationally in providing the support needed by individuals with autism.

Where Do We Go From Here?

As the number of new cases of autism continues to rise, families and professionals agree there are questions that need answers. These questions are mainly focused in two areas – political issues and health issues. The issues of legislation and litigation concerning individuals with autism as well as ways to address their health issues throughout the life span continue to be of concern both in the U.S. and internationally.

Politically, the focus on research on autism has been slipping and no new legislative action has occurred. Thus there is a need for parents and professionals to advocate both nationally and internationally for future legislation and additional declarations concerning the rights of individuals with autism. In the U.S., the Every Student Succeeds Act was to be reauthorized in 2021, but as yet has not been introduced to the House of Representatives. Internationally, no legislation concerning individuals with autism has been introduced since 2019 when the European Accessibility Act was enacted (Autism Europe, 2021b).

In terms of health issues, there is a need for continued research both in the U.S. and internationally to address universal understanding of issues surrounding the health of individuals with autism. It is essential that a focus on research concerning autism, it causes, and its interventions continues. The CDC released its report in advance of April's World Autism Month and World Autism Awareness Day (April 2, 2021), which was dedicated to increasing global understanding and acceptance of people with autism. Key findings in the CDC report (2021) include:

- One in 54 children had a diagnosis of ASD by age 8 in 2016, a nearly 10 percent increase over 2014 when the estimate was 1 in 59.
- While the CDC found no difference in prevalence rates between black and white children, a gap remains in prevalence among Hispanic children, indicating a need to expand screening and intervention among this group. Further, black and Hispanic children identified with autism received evaluations at older ages than similar white children, again indicating that more needs to be done in this area.
- The number of children who had a developmental screening by age 3 increased from 74 percent to 84 percent, a sign of potential progress toward earlier and more consistent screening by healthcare providers.
- Boys are four times as likely to be diagnosed as girls, holding steady from previous reports. This indicates the need for more research to understand the gap in prevalence and ensure girls on the spectrum are receiving the care they need.
- Significant differences remain in the frequency of autism diagnosis between the CDC's monitoring sites. These range from a low of 1 in

76 in Colorado to a high of 1 in 32 in New Jersey. This may be due to how autism is diagnosed and documented in different communities.

As national and international legislation and health research indicates, there is a need for continued research in the field of autism. Additional questions have arisen as to what should be the focus of future research and what legislation should be enacted to support individuals with autism and their families? Some of the questions that continue to be asked are: What are the underlying causes of autism? What evidence-based interventions are the most appropriate? Which educational and behavioral programs are the most effective in addressing the needs of individuals with autism throughout their lifespans? What type of future educational service delivery options is most appropriate? How can parents and family members be more involved with their children with autism as they transition into adulthood? What types of legislation should be enacted to support individuals with autism throughout their lifespans? We know that research and legislation continues to address many of these questions. But we also know that the journey that began in the early 1960s with the search for how to address these intense, diverse, and sometimes overwhelming needs of the individual with autism is not over yet. The following chapters provide information to guide the provision of services from birth to adulthood, ending with the need for collaboration and teamwork.

References

Administration for Community Living. (n.d.). The Developmental Disabilities Assistance and Bill of Rights Act of 2000. https://acl.gov/about-acl/authoriz ing-statutes/developmental-disabilities-assistance-and-bill-rights-act-2000

American Council on Education. (2021). Renewing the Higher Education Act. www.acenet.edu/Policy-Advocacy/Pages/HEA-ED/Renewing-the-Higher-Education-Act.aspx

Autism Europe. (2021a). *World autism awareness day.* www.autismeurope.org/what-we-do/world-autism-awareness-day/

Autism Europe. (2021b). *European Accessibility Act.* www.autismeurope.org/what-we-do/rights-promotion/european-accessibility-act/

Autism Society. (2019). *Detailed summary of the Autism CARES Act of 2019.* www.autism-society.org/wp-content/uploads/2019/10/Detailed-Summary-of-the-Autism-CARES-Act-of-2019.pdf

Autism Speaks. (2015a). *The Affordable Care Act and autism.* http://autismspe aks.org

Autism Speaks. (2015b). Federal initiatives. http://autismspeaks.org

Center for Autism Research. (2014a). Higher Education Opportunity Act of 2008. *The Children's Hospital of Philadelphia Research Institute.* http://carau tismroadmap.org/

Center for Autism Research. (2014b). Intellectual disability and ASD. *The Children's Hospital of Philadelphia Research Institute.* http://carautismroad map.org/

Claypool, M. K., & McLaughlin, J. M. (2017). *How autism is reshaping special education.* Rowman & Littlefield.

Cochrane, A. L. (1972). Effectiveness and efficiency: random reflections on health services. London: Nuffield Provincial Hospitals Trust. Retrieved from https:// repository.library.georgetown.edu/handle/10822/764041

Congressional Research Service. (2012). *The Combatting Autism Act: Overview and funding.* https://20121227_R42369_c9f6f9ac27a216e6ca1b3edc22e65 0f7ab4f8cd4.pdf

Dicker, S., & Bennett, E. (2011). Engulfed by the spectrum: The impact of autism spectrum disorders on law and policy. *Valparaiso University Law Review, 45*(2), 415–455.

Easter Seals. (2016). *Annual update of the state autism profiles.* www.easterseals. com/explore-resources/living-with-autism/executive-summary-state.pdf

Eyal, G., Hart, B., Onculer, E., Oren, N., & Rossi, N. (2010). *The autism matrix: The social origins of the autism epidemic.* Polity.

Hass, T. (2008). School-based services. In G. R. Buckendorf (Ed.), *Autism: A guide for educators, clinicians, and parents* (pp. 139–152). Thinking Publications.

Hume, K., Steinbrenner, J. R., Odom, S. L., Morin, K. L., Nowell, S. W., Tomaszewski, B., Szendrey, S., McIntyre, N. S., Yucesoy-Ozkan, & S., Savage, M. N. (2021). Evidence-based practices for children, youth, and young adults with autism: Third generation review. *Journal of Autism and Developmental Disorders. 51*(11), 4013–4032.

Institute for Disability Research, Policy, and Practice. (2021). United States Laws: The Rehabilitation Act of 1973 (Sections 504 and 508). *WebAIM.* https:// webaim.org/articles/laws/usa/rehab#:~:text=The%20Reauthorized%20Reh abilitation%20Act%20of,accessible%20to%20those%20with%20disab ilities.

Iris Center. (n.d.). *What do educators need to know about EBPs for children with autism?* https://iris.peabody.vanderbilt.edu/module/asd2/cresource/q1/ p01/#content

Lee, S. S. (2009). Overview of the Federal Higher Education Opportunity Act Reauthorization. *Insight, 1.* www.thinkcollege.net

Library of Congress. (2015). *Summary: H.R. 647-ABLE Act of 2014.* http:// congress.gov.

Murdick, N., Gartin, B. C., & Fowler, G. (2014). *Special education law* (3rd ed.). Pearson.

National Autism Center. (2015). *The national standards report.* https://nationala utismcenter.org/national-standards-project/

National Down Syndrome Society. (2021). Achieving A Better Life Experience (ABLE) Act overview. www.ndss.org/ableact/

National Research Council. (2001). *Educating children with autism.* National Academy Press.

Roleska, M., Roman-Urrestarazu, A., Griffiths, S., Rulgrok, A. N. V., Holt, R., van Kessel, R., McColl, K., Sherlaw, W., Brayne, C., & Czabanowska, K. (2018). Autism and the right to education inthe EU: Policy mapping and scoping review of the United Kingdom, France, Poland and Spain. *PLoS One*, *13*(8), e0202336. www.ncbi.nlm.nih.gov/pmc/articles/PMC6116926/#pone.0202336.ref014

Samuels, C. (2015). ESSA and the disability community. *Education Week*. www.autismpolicyblog.com/2015/12/essa-and-disability-community.htm

Sharp, L. A. (2016). ESEA reauthorization: An overview of the Every Student Succeeds Act. *Texas Journal of Literacy Education*, *4*(1), 9–13.

Steinbrenner, J. R., Hume, K., Odom, S. L., Morin, K. L., Nowell, S. W., Tomaszewski, B., Szendrey, S., McIntyre, N. S., Yucesoy-Ozkan, S., & Savage, M. N. (2020). *Evidence-based practices for children, youth, and young adults with autism spectrum disorder*. The University of North Carolina at Chapel Hill, Frank Porter Graham Child Development Institute, National Clearinghouse on Autism Evidence and Practice Review Team. https://ncaep.fpg.unc.edu/sites/ncaep.fcg.unc.educ/files/imce/documents/EBP%20Report%202020.pdf

U. S. Department of Education. (2017). The Rehabilitation Act of 1973. *About ED*. www2.ed.gov/policy/speced/reg/narrative.html

U. S. Department of Health and Human Services, Interagency. (2003). *Report to congress on autism activities under the Children's Health Act of 2000 (Fiscal year 2002)*. http://iacc.hhs.gov.

U. S. Government Printing Office. (2000). *Public Law 106-310*. http://gpo.gov

White, M. L., Smith, T. E. C., & Stodden, R. (2012). Autism spectrum disorders: Historical, legislative, and current perspectives. In D. Zager, M. L. Wehmeyer, & R. L. Simpson (Eds.), *Educating students with autism spectrum disorders: Research-based principles and practices* (pp. 3–12). Routledge.

White House Blog. (2014, Aug. 11). President Obama signs bill to support the needs of people with autism. http://whitehouse.gov

Wilczynski, S., Green, G., Ricciardi, J., Boyd, B., Hume, A., Ladd, M., & Rue, H. (2009). National standards report: The national standards project: Addressing the need for evidence-based practice guidelines for autism spectrum disorders. *National Autism Center, Randolph (MA)*.

World Health Organization. (2021). Autism spectrum disorders. www.who.int/news-room/fact-sheets/detail/autism-spectrum-disorders

Wright, P. W. D., Wright, P. D., & Heath, S. W. (2004). *No Child Left Behind*. Harbor House Law Press.

Zager, D., Wehmeyer, M. L., & Simpson, R. L. (2012). *Educating students with autism spectrum disorders: Research-based principles and practices*. Routledge.

Chapter 4

Global Perspectives
Autism Education and Interventions in Low- and Middle-Income Nations

Angi Stone-MacDonald,[1] *Serra Acar,*[2]
Songtian Zeng,[2] *and Ozden Pinar Irmak*[2]
[1]Department of Special Education, Rehabilitation, and Counseling, California State University, San Bernardino
[2]Department of Curriculum and Instruction, University of Massachusetts, Boston

While autism was first written about in Europe in the 1940s, there have been stories of suspected cases of autism documented as early as 1724 (Feinstein, 2010). Autism exists all over the world. On World Autism Awareness Day in 2013, UN Secretary General Ki-Moon stated, "Autism is not limited to a single region or country; it is a worldwide challenge that requires global action. This international attention is essential to address stigma, lack of awareness and inadequate support structures" (Smith, 2014). Autism exists in all cultures, but the neurobiological expression of autism spectrum disorder (ASD) can look different in different cultures. Autism is truly a spectrum disorder, not just in the level of severity, but also in the symptoms that are most commonly observed in different cultures. Until recently, the importance of culture was generally ignored in relation to autism, both in diagnosis and treatment, and it has been viewed narrowly from a lens of specific racial or ethnic groups that are often discussed in the United States (Daley, 2002; La Roche, Bush, & D'Angelo, 2018). At the same time, there was a misconception in some countries outside of North America and Europe that autism was the result of modernization, and it did not exist outside of "Western" countries (Daley & Sigman, 2002; Hudec, 2012). This belief is still present amongst some people in various countries with low levels of knowledge about ASD and disability. The general diagnosis of ASD around the world is based on whether behavior deviates from what is considered typical in that culture, but there is less consensus among research where the line between behavior differences lie and diagnosis of an autism spectrum disorder (Freeth, Milne, Sheppard, & Ramachandran, 2014; Grinker, 2008).

In Chapter 1 of this volume, Maye et al. discussed the formal DSM definition and the characteristics and symptoms of autism used to identify and diagnose autism. In low- and middle-income countries, it is more

DOI: 10.4324/9781003255147-5

common for doctors and rehabilitation staff to have traditionally used the WHO definition. According to the World Health Organization, ASD comprises a group of complex, lifelong, neurodevelopmental disorders usually noticeable prior to 3 years of age. The conditions are characterized by qualitative impairments in reciprocal social interaction, impairments in verbal and nonverbal communication skills, and a restricted pattern of interest or behavior (World Health Organization, 1992; American Psychiatric Association, 2013). More recently, the International Classification of Functioning, Disability and Health Core Set for Autism has been developed for capturing functional information in clinical practice, but this core set is a complete set of categories and sub-sets to help describe behaviors and functioning for individuals with ASD within various age brackets and types of challenges such as mental functioning or reception of language (Schiariti, et al., 2018). Unfortunately, this tool is not user friendly and still very deficit-focused. ASD is found in every race, ethnic group, and socioeconomic class. Despite the universality, relatively less research and resources have been used to address people with ASD in low- and middle-income countries. Dyches et al. (2004) found that "students with multicultural backgrounds and autism are challenged on at least four dimensions: communication, social skills, behavioral repertoires, and culture. The professional literature continues to address the first three; it is imperative to now consider the third: multicultural issues" (p. 221).

While the DSM and WHO have clear definitions based on characteristics and symptomology, often children in countries without standardized assessment protocols are diagnosed with autism because they meet the core criteria of autism, but their presentation of symptoms look different from some more classic cases of autism in the US. For example, in studies in Sub-Saharan African countries hand flapping is a very rare symptom and is rarely reported (Bakare & Munir, 2011). In Sub-Saharan African countries, spinning, hand flapping and object spinning were less common than in a US sample, whereas more children with ASD were non-verbal and possessed poor non-verbal communication skills as well (Bello-Mojeed et al., 2014). In addition, some behaviors assessed by standardized screening and assessment tools such as the M-CHAT and ADOS, may not be viewed as deviant in certain cultures, so they are not seen as concerns for autism by parents and caregivers (Daly, 2004; Freeth, Milne, Sheppard, & Ramachandran, 2014). For example, in some Asian countries, eye contact with adults is not normal, so it is not considered deviant to not make eye contact with parents and caregivers. Behaviors exhibited by children with autism may look different in different cultures. In studies in several Sub-Saharan African countries, over half of children diagnosed with autism were also non-verbal in one study and over 70 percent were non-verbal in the other study, but it is not clear if they were truly non-verbal or did not meet the clinical threshold to be counted as verbal (Belhadj, Mrad, & Halayem, 2006; Mankoski et al., 2006). In addition, over 60 percent of children also were diagnosed with intellectual disability, despite not having cultural normed tools to assess concepts necessary to make this determination (Bakare & Munir, 2011). Observational measures and functional skill assessments are most commonly used in low- and middle-income countries, because there are not culturally validated or normed measures and/or health care workers do not have training in standardized assessments, and more importantly, the measures are often not available or normed in the language spoken in the home. There is a complex relationship between culture and all developmental disabilities, including autism that needs to be addressed through more research. In India, Daley (2004) found that some pediatricians and psychiatrists used the terms autism, autistic traits, and PDD interchangeably and did not use standardize tools or a systematic process for diagnosis.

In working with families and conducting research on autism, it is critical to focus assessment and intervention for the child or adult with autism's ability to function in society and community within the culture and not use American or Eurocentric models of assessment and diagnosis, because it introduces systematic bias (Freeth, Milne, Sheppard, & Ramachandran, 2014). That is not to say that certain assessment tools cannot be used as a guide, but we need to assess their validity within the language and cultural context before they are used as a standardized method of assessment and make the necessary adjustments for language and culture. For example, the M-CHAT autism screening tool has been modified and culturally validated in many countries and languages including Mali, China, Moroccan Arabic, and Northern Sotho in South Africa. Furthermore, there are more culturally and linguistically validated tools that are now available in different languages, but it is important for practitioners and researchers to verify that they are culturally validated. In a scoping review of the translation and cultural adaptation of the Ages and Stages Questionnaire (ASQ), a very common screening tool used in early childhood education and early childhood special education, Rousseau et al. (2021) found that of the 37 cultural adaptations representing 29 languages and 27 countries, few made cultural modifications and those that did were minor. The cultural modifications were more likely to help the translation stick closer to the original content than to adapt the content to an appropriate cultural context. Practitioners and educators working with families should focus on helping supporting children and adults with ASD to increase their ability to gain skills and knowledge most relevant to their community and build towards successful community membership and participation (Stone-MacDonald, 2014).

Labels and Stigma Around ASD and Developmental Disabilities

Diagnosing someone with ASD can be a daunting task, both because it can be difficult for health care professionals and educators to determine if a person has ASD based on diagnostic criteria due to lack of training, lack of standardized assessment tools, and cultural differences in the expression of symptoms in different countries. In addition, a diagnosis does not always lead to services or an understanding by caregivers about the implications of the diagnosis and how that will impact the child and family's life. In India, parents are often not given the specific diagnosis of autism because the label itself does not provide additional services. Children need a label of intellectual disability to receive additional mental health and educational services (Daley 2004). In South Korea, mothers often reject any label because of the intense stigma associated with the label and the desire to continue to see their child as normal (Grinker & Cho, 2013). In Vietnam, the prevalence of ASD remains below 1 percent and is seen as primarily a psychological or mental health disorder (Ha & Whittaker, 2022). South Korean mothers referred to their children as "border children," where they viewed their children as living with a temporary deficit in the single domain of social impairment (Grinker & Cho, p. 46). Furthermore, if children were able to attend a typical primary school school and do well in some school subjects, then the label was incompatible with their child having a pervasive developmental disorder such as ASD.

Labels can also be linked to beliefs about the causes of the disability. Cultural factors influence acceptance and understanding of intervention strategies (Mandell & Novak, 2005). In several Sub-Saharan African countries, people hold both biological and spiritual beliefs about the causes of disability (Ampetee & Chiyito, 2009; Stone-MacDonald & Butera, 2012). Mankoski et al. (2006) found that it was believed that severe cases of malaria or a Vitamin D deficiency in the first two years of life caused ASD. In Tanzania, while it is recognized that children with disabilities, especially children with developmental disabilities such as ASD or ID, should be cared for and families should meet their needs, it is not necessary to educate children with disabilities and some people do not believe that these children can learn and participate in society (Stone-MacDonald, 2014). Historically, children with disabilities were hidden due to stigma (Bello-Mojeed et al., 2014; Butera & Stone-MacDonald, 2012). These attitudes are slowly changing, and children are given educational opportunities, but often in Sub-Saharan African countries, children with autism are taught in separate classrooms or separate schools that can provide more intensive interventions.

In African and Middle Eastern countries, stigma is attached to labels of disability (Bello-Mojeed et al., 2014). Families experience shame because often they feel that a family member or family member's action is to blame for the disability (Holroyd, 2003). Samadi, McConkey, and Kelly (2013) found in Iran that there was a great deal of stigma for the family of an individual with ID or ASD. "Having a child who has a disability is considered by many religious Iranians to be a result of a sin and hence disability is a source of shame for the broader family, with negative effects on the marriage prospects of siblings, for example" (p. 4). In Chinese culture, mental health conditions and disabilities attract social shame, and denial may be preferable to seeking advice (Mak & Kwok, 2010). Often families also still feel stigma over having a child with autism, because there is still a belief that a family member (often the mother) did something wrong to cause the disability (Holroyd, 2003). McCabe (2007) interviewed 38 families about their perceptions on having a child with autism and found a high level of concern amongst caregivers about stigma and discrimination:

> caregivers' perceptions of the existence of beliefs and practices that discriminate against individuals with disabilities and their families, due to a low awareness and acceptance of disability and difference. Almost every family interviewed for this study mentioned their fear of being discriminated against if others found out that their child had autism (or was in some way "different" from typically developing children). This meant that it was often difficult for them to take the steps necessary to seek assistance.
>
> (p. 43)

Several studies have reported that because ASD is often seen as an "invisible" disability, families feel more stigma from friends, family, and the community, especially when their child exhibits challenging behaviors (Cohen & Miguel, 2018; Holloway et al., 2018). While parents in several studies conducted by McCabe sought support and interventions, parents talked of others they knew with children with autism or other developmental disabilities who did not seek support out of a fear of stigma from friends and family (McCabe, 2007).

Assessment, Education, and Parental Perspectives Around the World

In this chapter, we have chosen to focus on issues around identification and awareness about autism, assessment and education of individuals with autism, and parental perspectives using four countries or regions as examples. Because we cannot talk about all countries in this short chapter, we wanted to focus on low- and middle-income countries where less research is done and disseminated worldwide. We will focus on the following areas: 1) Sub-Saharan African Countries; 2) China; 3) Turkey; and 4) the Middle East. We chose these areas because they represent both low- and middle-income countries and the literature available was in English. We were unable to include research on Central or South America because most of the research is published in Spanish. To begin, we will look at overall prevalence and identification in each region/country.

Prevalence and Identification

Sub-Saharan African Countries

Although there has been extensive research on the assessment and diagnosis of ASD in North America, Europe, and Asia, people in many low and middle-income regions, such as many Sub-Saharan African countries, still do not have access to ASD assessment and diagnostic services (Elsabbagh et al., 2012). But three published meta-analyses found that there are no population-based studies or reports on the specific prevalence of ASD or PDD in Sub-Saharan African countries and more research is needed (Ametepee & Chiyito, 2009; Bakare & Munir, 2011; Elsabbagh et al., 2012). Nevertheless, studies have documented the existence of autism in Sub-Saharan African countries since 1978 (Lotter, 1978; Ampetee & Chiyito, 2009). A higher male-to-female ratio was consistent across studies in Sub-Saharan African Countries and consistent with studies from the United States and Europe. (Khan & Hombarume, 1996; Lotter, 1978; Mankoski et al., 2006). Studies also showed an over representation of higher socioeconomic background and higher frequency of cases co-morbid with intellectual difficulties. Most children who were identified as having both ID and autism were nonverbal.

In the last 10 years, more assessment and screening tools are being validated in other languages and countries, including work on the M-CHAT-R in Mali conducted in French (Sangare et al., 2019) and multiple languages in South Africa (Vorster et al., 2021). Prevalence in Sub-Saharan African countries is difficult to establish due to the lack of research and lack of healthcare or educational professionals with knowledge and expertise to identify ASD in children. At present there are no ASD diagnostic instruments validated for use in Swahili, a language that is spoken by millions of people in Kenya, Tanzania, and Uganda. There are other tools to assess more general characteristics of developmental disabilities or specific skills for individuals with disabilities or delays (e.g. Bitta et al., 2021; Stone-MacDonald & Fettig, 2019). In other Sub-Saharan African countries, there are also no validated measures for use in the local language. Furthermore, there remain noteworthy disparities in the age of onset and identification of ASD with a prominent problem of late identification among children in Africa diagnosed with ASD (Mandell et al., 2007; Bello-Mojeed et al., 2011; Bakare and Munir, 2011a).

In South Africa, there are an estimated 135,000 children with autism (*The Global Challenge of Autism*, 2014). At the same time, a recent database study by Pillay et al. (2017) found that ASD was under identified in South Africa, and the created long waiting lists for assessment and identification, further exacerbated by the lack of qualified professionals available to assess students. Furthermore, there are no legal mandates in South Africa that require students with ASD to receive any services, so even with a diagnosis, it is hard to find and access services (Viljoen et al., 2019).

Among healthcare workers in Nigeria, Bakare et al. (2008, 2009) and Igwe et al. (2011) found a low level of knowledge and awareness about ASD among healthcare workers with the highest level observed among those in working psychiatric facilities in Nigeria. Amongst the general population, they found a very low level of knowledge and understanding about ASD. Furthermore, psychiatrists, who often diagnose children with autism are rare in many Sub-Saharan African Countries. In Nigeria and Ghana, each country has only one psychiatrist to serve over one million people in each country, respectively, and Liberia has one psychiatrist for over 3.4 million people (*The Global Challenge of Autism*, 2014).

China

In China, national estimates of the autism prevalence are not available based on data collection, but instead were estimated utilizing the school-age children data. Regardless, the autism spectrum disorder (ASD) prevalence in China has been reported to be lower than the United States or European countries. For example, a recent report on the prevalence of ASD in China suggested that the observed prevalence rate was 0.29 percent (95% CI: 0.26%–0.32%) for the 6–12-year-old children population (Zhou et al., 2020). This is likely due to at least two reasons: (1) most studies in China only included the special school population, overlooking the mainstream school population; and (2) most studies in China have not used contemporary screening and diagnostic methods. Another study utilizing both mainstream and special school data revealed a similar prevalence of autism in China, about 1 percent (108 per 10,000 in Jilin City for example). Similarly, the prevalence rate among 18–36-month-old children are estimated to be 27.5 per 10,000 (Huang et al., 2014). In short, the prevalence estimates could be varied depending on the source of data and the inclusion policy for children with ASD.

Several challenges may contribute to the under diagnosis in mainland China. First, similar to many other countries, there are regular physical and developmental checkups at local clinics (e.g., local community hospitals as well as health care centers for women and children) in mainland China. Unfortunately, ASD and neurodevelopmental screenings are not part of standard practice in pediatric primary care settings. Physicians and pediatricians at this level are often not trained to perform these types of screenings and are often unfamiliar with the symptoms of ASD (Duan et al., 2015; Huang et al., 2013). As a result, early detection of ASD relies mostly on parents' awareness of symptoms and persistence in obtaining the appropriate services. It has been reported that parent's education level is significantly related to the early detection of ASD in mainland China (Zhou et al., 2014). If parents fail to report behavioral difficulties associated with ASD, their children are typically overlooked by professionals.

Second, diagnostic evaluations are inconsistently conducted because of the training level of professionals and availability of assessment tools and resources. In mainland China, it has been proposed that the diagnostic procedures should include the following three steps: 1) interviews with caregivers to clarify the developmental history and symptoms of concern; 2) structured observations and multicomponent behavioral assessments; and 3) an official diagnosis based on ASD-specific instruments and standardized diagnostic criteria (Huang et al., 2014). In practice, however, not all of these steps are followed. It has been reported that in China, the diagnostic assessment is typically conducted in 15–30 min, and the diagnosis is typically given by physicians based on medical history and parent interviews (Huang et al., 2013). Objective assessments and observations are not always utilized to support the diagnosis. When these assessments are performed, the instruments used are typically Chinese-translated versions of popular screening tools developed in the US or Europe that have potential cultural biases (details in the assessment instruments session). Systematic observations across multiple settings (e.g., school, home, or community) are not commonly conducted, and evaluations by a multi-disciplinary team (i.e., including pediatricians, child psychiatrists, psychologists, or other related professionals) are very rare (Sun et al., 2013).

Turkey

The current prevalence of children with ASD in Turkey is unknown, however a local study in Istanbul, Turkey found an estimate of 1 in 117 children with ASD (Oner & Munir, 2020). The Public Health Agency of Turkey recommends evaluating children between 18 and 36 months of age at least once with a focus on ASD (Turkish Ministry of Health, 2015). In Turkey, pediatricians and child and adolescent psychiatry professionals are known as the first professionals who evaluate children with

ASD symptoms (e.g., difficulties in social interaction and communication, and unusually repetitive and restricted behaviors and interests). In general, comprehensive assessments and standardized diagnostic evaluations are done in child psychiatry departments. The final diagnosis and the referral to special education centers are made by child and adolescent psychiatry professionals. However, Çitil and colleagues (2021) revealed that the knowledge of pediatricians and pediatric residents about diagnostic criteria regarding ASD was insufficient and some of them had misconceptions and out of date dated knowledge about the etiology, intervention, and prognosis regarding ASD.

The Middle East

In the Middle East and North Africa, there are various prevalence estimates for several countries, but it is still suspected that autism is under-diagnosed and under-reported for the same reasons as in other low- and middle-income countries, namely lack of qualified personal and resources and lack of knowledge and awareness about ASD. It has been estimated that 1.4 per 10,000 children of Omani children (aged 0–14 years) have ASD (Al-Farsi et al., 2011), 4.3 per 10,000 in Bahrain (Al-Ansari & Ahmed, 2013), 6.3 cases per 10,000 in Iran (Samadi et al., 2012), 29 per 10,000 in the United Arab Emirates (Eapen et al., 2007) and 59 per 10,000 in Saudi Arabia (Aljarallah et al., 2006). Seif Eldin et al. (2008) reported the prevalence of ASD to be 11.5–33.6 percent among children with developmental disabilities in Tunisia and Egypt, respectively. The low prevalence rate in Oman, Bahrain and Iran does not prove that ASD is less prevalent in those countries, but rather reflects under-diagnosis, and under-reporting of cases based on limited access to educational and medical services (Al-Farsi et al., 2011; Taha & Hussein, 2014). The difference in prevalence rate might also be due to cultural attitudes such as stigma and no national studies estimating the prevalence of ASD (Taha & Hussein, 2014).

In Lebanon, Chaaya et al. (2016) conducted the Modified Checklist for Autism in Toddlers (M-CHAT) for examining the prevalence rate of ASD. Similarly, in a study of ASD among children with developmental disabilities, Seif Eldin et al. (2008) used the M-CHAT to screen for young children with ASD in a multinational Arab population in Tunisia and Egypt, two Northern African Countries. A study by Alsaedi (2020) used the Bruininks-Oseretsky Test of Motor Proficiency, Second Edition (BOT-2) standardized test to determine the prevalence, severity and nature of the motor abnormalities in children with ASD between the age of 6–12 in Bahrain, Saudi Arabia, and the UAE. The results showed that the majority of children with ASD fell outside the normal range in terms of motor performance. In Qatar, ASD was added as a disability category after 2012 (Ministry of Development Planning and Statistics, 2016) and most of the centers use the ADI-R or ADOS as diagnostic tools with DSM-4 and DSM-5 criteria for diagnosis (Alshaban et al., 2017). In Iran, preschool children with ASD are usually diagnosed by medical doctors privately or at a non-profit clinic prior to starting school. In Oman, clinical information was collected and validated, Arabic childhood autism rating scale (CARS) was administered for diagnosis in multiple studies (Al-Shomari & Al-Saratwai, 2002; Al Farsi et al., 2011). More Middle Eastern countries are using standardized assessments that have been validated in Arabic and align with the DSM-V criteria for ASD. Seif Eldin et al. (2008) studied the use of the M-CHAT as an early screening tool for autism in nine Arabic speaking countries using an Arabic version. The team felt this was a good screening tool because you did not need to be a trained medical professional to use it, but could be easily trained in the tool. The team argued for expanded usage to gather additional clinical data about children and their families.

Education and Intervention

Sub-Saharan African Countries

In many Sub-Saharan African countries, children with ASD attend special schools or are in segregated classes, if they have the opportunity to attend school. Provision of special education and rehabilitation services are impeded in sub-Saharan Africa by several factors including lack of resources, teachers, and teacher training facilities. Kalabula (2000) pinpoints a number of these factors: including wide gaps between knowledge and expectations of national education officials and classroom teachers close to the problem; a lack of understanding of specific needs of individual children with ASD and other disabilities by administrators of education system at different levels of service delivery; negative attitudes of regular education teachers, other children, and other school staff toward the services and children with special educational needs; and lack of advocacy. In a recent study by Soni et al. (2021), they found that in sub-Saharan African countries the key factors that predicted if a child transitioned to an early childhood setting or primary school were health; bullying and discriminatory experiences; parents' beliefs about the benefits and education and the ability of the school to meet their child's needs; perceptions of disability, perceptions of education (based on type of setting); and teachers' knowledge, experience, and confidence. In Tanzania, society has given very little attention to the needs of children with ASD and their families. Most educational efforts for children with ASD exist within non-governmental organizations and children with autism are often turned away from public primary schools and sent to special schools when parents can afford that resource (Stone-MacDonald, 2014; Stone-MacDonald & Fettig, 2019). The government has put little effort into establishing schools or services for children with ASD and other developmental disabilities. In Mbwilo, Smide, & Aarts (2010), many families expressed concerns that their children were not benefiting from schooling, because the children were not receiving the specialized instruction they needed and often received very little attention in the crowded classroom. More recently, Soni et al. (2021) also found similar results and noted that families were concerned about the costs of school to the family, the lack of resources for their children who needed specialized supports, and the travel required to go to school, which usually required a parent or adult escort.

In Ghana, those children attending school (86%) were in private school settings (Dixon, et al., 2015). Children received group educational instruction, speech therapy, behavioral therapy, and recreation. The majority of children had a paraprofessional to help them work throughout the day on individual goals. Interviewees were asked to list the services that are needed to help their children with autism. The most frequently reported service needs were speech therapy (36%), teacher education (36%), parent/family training (32%), and behavior management (28%) (Dixon et al.). This list is fairly typical for Sub-Saharan African countries. With the exception of South Africa, many countries have only a few or no speech therapists. In the literature published after 2015, scholars called for more behavior interventions targeted at both parent education and behavioral interventions that parents could implement at home to fill in some of the gaps in service (Harrison et al., 2016; Viljoen et al., 2019).

Specifically, Ghana is an exception where there are a larger number of inclusion programs. In Ghana, the majority of children with disabilities are schooled in general education classrooms rather than segregated special education classrooms solely for children with disabilities (Dixon, Badoe, & Owusu, 2015). At the same time, the results suggested that children with ASD did not have access to needed special education services and they experienced ostracism and discrimination resulting from the social stigma of having an ASD. Research from Zimbabwe expressed similar frustrations with the lack of progress over time to include children with ASD in inclusion early childhood settings and the failure to provide the necessary pedagogical and curriculum supports (Majoko, 2017). Unfortunately, many educators and health care professionals still do not have a strong knowledge of autism themselves, which makes it difficult to advise and support children with ASD and their families (Fewster et al., 2020; Odunsi et al., 2017; Sampson & Sandra, 2018).

China

China has made significant progress on inclusion education for children with disabilities. At the level of national policies, the Chinese government has taken initiatives to support inclusion (Zhao & Zhang, 2018). Effective from May 1, 2017, the revised 1994 Regulations for Educating Students with Disabilities mandate inclusion and necessary accommodations as well as mandating that teachers be prepared to work with students who have disabilities and provide supports for pre-service and in-service teachers. This complements the lack of mandate in China's Compulsory Education Law to accommodate the needs of students with disabilities (Zhang & Spencer, 2015). In the new five-year (2021–2025) protection and development plan for people with disabilities issued in July 2021, the Chinese government mandates the continuous improvement of the education system for people with disabilities at all educational levels (i.e., from early childhood education to graduate programs). However, education in China is clearly complicated when it comes to serving the needs of children with ASD. Studies have reported misunderstandings, confusion, prejudice, and discrimination against disabled students in mainstream schools in China (Xu et al., 2018). In addition, not only does the quality of services for children with autism vary, but there is also variation in the level of knowledge about autism among healthcare and educational professionals (Liu et al., 2016). Despite what appears to be a welcoming trend regarding increased awareness of autism, for the most part, teachers' knowledge of autism is quite basic. According to researchers, teachers often report having heard the term "autism," but beyond that, they lack the knowledge and expertise that are important to provide effective classroom instruction.

Although public awareness and professional knowledge of autism has increased substantially over time (Fan, 2018; Wang et al., 2018), children with ASD are still at risk for not receiving evidence-based services. Fan found that only 37% of the 47 organizations studied that were providing autism treatment were using interventions that would be considered "well established" or "evidence-based." Most support services are for children with ASD younger than six years old, both private and government owned. Intervention is provided primarily by private centers and a smaller number of public centers in China (McCabe, 2013; Sun et al., 2013a). Less than one-third of children with ASD receive intervention services in public medical institutions, and most receive interventions services in high-cost private rehabilitation centers (Zou et al., 2020). The majority of preschool and kindergarten teachers lack knowledge and skills to work with ASD populations (Liu et al., 2016). Wang et al. revealed that in China a child is usually referred by preschool teachers for further ASD assessment and diagnosis due to the lack of a developmental surveillance in most Chinese cities.

Data published in 2016 in the *Report on the Development of Autistic Children in China* show that there were 1,345 autism rehabilitation institutions registered with the China Disabled Persons' Federation. Recently, Wang et al. (2018) found 1,600 such institutions in a database of the China Association of Persons with Psychiatric Disability and their Relatives (CAPPDR), which is reportedly the largest national autism association in China and is responsible for all autism services in the country. Although promising, research has clearly shown that there are too few treatment options for families whether they live in urban areas or rural regions of the country (e.g., Li et al., 2011). However, families in rural China are far worse off as there are few, if any, services within hundreds of miles from people's homes. The same is true about families accessing an education for their child. Options for schooling are extremely limited, or non-existent for children with ASD in rural areas. Although most families cannot afford the cost of travel to ensure their child can attend school, many will make tremendous sacrifices to ensure that their child has the opportunity to have an education (Feuerberg, 2013).

After seven years old, children with normal IQ will attend typical schools, and those diagnosed with different disabilities will usually attend special schools, including children with ASD. However, children with ASD and normal IQ usually attend typical schools, though there are rarely any services for them. Children with ASD and low IQ sometimes attend typical schools depending on the available services in the schools in China. Schools however, also face pressure from parents of typically developing students to dedicate their full effort to provide instruction for the majority, and not spend time helping students with special needs (Xiong et al., 2011).

Turkey

Turkey is increasingly investing in resources to address the educational needs of children with ASD; however, the dosage and quality of support are debatable. In Turkey, public education funded interventions comprise weekly two-hour individualized and one-hour group education sessions for individuals with ASD (Kilincaslan et al., 2019). Depending on the school's decision to accept a child with ASD in their program, children with ASD can attend mainstream schools, and/or special schools with classes for children with ASD only.

According to the Turkish Ministry of National Education (Milli Eğitim Bakanlığı, 2018), children with disabilities can have access to compulsory early childhood education by 36 months old. After early childhood education, children with ASD can attend 12 years of compulsory schooling.

Children who can function with ASD and meet the benchmarks of the national Turkish curriculum, can enroll in special classrooms within mainstream public schools. It should be noted that the national Turkish curriculum is developed for children who do not have disabilities and/or delays. The Turkish Ministry of National Education also provides Special Education and Application Centers, which is mostly preferred for children who have difficulties with following the national curriculum. In these centers, children receive an individualized education program with a one-to-one teaching approach. They follow a curriculum for children with ASD focusing on self-care skills, daily routine development, and functional academic skills. Lastly, the Turkish Ministry of National Education provides home schooling and education, and healthcare options are available for children with ASD.

It should be noted that there is a shortage of teachers who could support inclusive classrooms. While exploring the intervention and opportunities for children with ASD, it is important to consider the teacher education/personnel preparation programs in Turkey. Currently, there is not a personnel preparation program specifically for autism available for pre-service teachers (Yazici & McKenzie, 2020). There is an increasing need to support teachers who work with children with ASD.

In addition to supporting pre- and in-service teachers' professional development in inclusive settings, there is growing evidence to suggest that school-wide social-emotional interventions are needed. Recent literature indicated that children with ASD are at greater risk of bullying victimization than their peers who are developing typically in Turkey. Children with ASD experienced both verbal and emotional bullying victimization, in the forms of nicknaming, exclusion, and being threatened (Eroglu & Kilic, 2020). Teachers and related education personnel play a critical role to prevent peer bullying and support positive social-emotional development. This means more attention needs to be paid to the well-being of children with or without disabilities.

The Middle East

In several Middle Eastern countries, the systems addressing children with disabilities and delays are rudimentary (Eapen et al., 2007; Profanter 2009). As a result, the family caring for a child with a disability must take the initiative (Read & Schofield, 2010). In the Middle East, educational services vary significantly for children in both general and special education. For example, in Oman, the government has invested a lot of money in improving the education and healthcare systems. In Jordan, special education schools and centers are more common options for children with ASD, but the educational system is moving towards inclusion of students in general education settings (Al-Rossan, 2012). In a study of perceptions of teachers in Jordan about inclusion, young teachers with bachelor's degrees had a more favorable view of inclusion for children with autism because the philosophy of inclusion was taught in pre-service education and demonstrated a willingness to differentiate and support children with ASD in classrooms (Abu-Hamour & Muhaidat, 2013). Because there are no standard educational options or settings for children with ASD, children tend to end up in a variety of settings based on parental input and resources (Seif Eldin et al., 2008). This often results in parents resorting to 'doctor shopping' where parents with more means and more flexible employment options are able to secure more services for their child (Al Farsi et al., 2013; Chakrabarti, 2009).

A study by Taresh et al. (2020) revealed that many preschool teachers in Yemen have misconceptions about ASD and believe that religious healers could treat children with ASD.

In Egypt, autism care is usually home-based (Gobrial, 2018). Fewer than 2 percent of Egyptian children with disabilities are enrolled in school and children with ASD receive little to no education and have limited access to disability support services and child healthcare facilities (Gobrial, 2018). Rehabilitation and social care services are generally available in the capital and big cities and the services are mostly provided by private clinics (Gobrial, 2018; Okasha, 2005; Omar, 2014; Taha & Hussein, 2014). Often, the parents of children with ASD cannot afford the rare and expensive private facilities and most children with ASD in Egypt remain uneducated at home for an indefinite period (Gobrial et al., 2019).

One of the key societal responses to children with developmental disabilities, such as those with ASD is to provide special education services. Oman has led the region in advocating for the integration of children with special needs (Al-Lamki & Ohlin, 1992). Initially, the modern Omani education system focused on increasing literacy rates and this effort has been successful (Al-Adawi, 2006). However, education and the services for children with special needs have been lagging behind other developments in the country. It is still unclear what the impact is for children and families who are trying to access relevant intervention, rehabilitation and special education services in the country (Al Farsi et al., 2013).

In Iran, state-funded special schools are part of the Iranian public school system, but many parents choose to enroll their children in private schools or engage private therapists for their children with ASD. Children with severe and multiple disabilities can participate in state-funded day treatment programs. However, these services are available only in larger cities and often only for more affluent families (Samadi, McConkey, & Kelly, 2013). More formalized services are available to families who can afford private settings and private therapists, but there is limited evidence that children who use the public systems are receiving specific services for children with ASD. In the literature from Middle Eastern countries, the focus is on general services that are available and assessment, but studies were not available on the effectiveness of specific interventions for children with ASD. This is an area in need of future research.

Parental Perspectives

In low and middle income countries, three common themes arose after reviewing the literature from the selected areas for families with a child with ASD: 1) having a child can cause emotional and financial stress on the family due to lack of resources and information and the effort required to find and utilize educational opportunities and services; 2) parents generally want to care for their children, but can face considerable discrimination from people in their countries due to a lack of information about ASD and characteristics and capabilities of an individual with ASD; and 3) families wanted and needed benefits from the comradery of support groups, parent-to-parent groups, and professional support, but these resources were hard to find and maintain based cost, distance, and time constraints.

Sub-Saharan African Countries

In Sub-Saharan African countries, support services for rehabilitation or to support families of children with ASD or other developmental disabilities are often rare and run by local non-governmental organizations (NGOs). While several countries on the continent have implemented disability policies and inclusive school policies, children with ASD and other developmental disabilities are often still turned away from public schools because typical primary and secondary teachers do not have any training in working with children with disabilities and have little or no knowledge of autism (African Decade of Disabled Persons, 2009; Fakolade, & Adeniyi, 2009; Stone-MacDonald, 2014; Stone-MacDonald & Fettig, 2019). While various summits and meetings have occurred amongst researchers, the work on the ground to provide support to parents and interventions is slow, with most research done in South Africa and Nigeria (*Africa Regional International Meeting for Autism Research, 2017*; Franz et al., 2017; *The Global Challenge of Autism, 2014*). Miles and Kaplan (2005) found that in Africa, children with disabilities may belong to any number of marginalized groups and "tend to be disproportionately represented in the out-of-school population" (p. 78).

In a Ghanaian study, parents stated that they wanted training, support groups, and behavior management training and support for their child with ASD. In addition, parents wanted their children's healthcare workers and educators to have more training and support to work with their child and their unique needs based on the ASD diagnosis areas

(Dixon, Badoe, & Owusu, 2015). In Tanzania, parents wanted and needed more education and interventions to support their child, but the limited number of child psychologists and psychiatrists made it difficult to effectively deliver this information (Harrison et al., 2016). At the same time, there is a strong argument that educators using a train-the trainer model could train many parents about evidence-based interventions that have been culturally adapted with the support of a autism specialist. This method would not only increase the knowledge and skills of more educators and parents, but empower educators and parents and contribute to much needed capacity building. Parent education and support services are needed across the continent.

In Tanzania, two studies found similar results to the Ghanaian study discussed above. McNally and Meenan (2013) found that the parents also experienced financial burdens and emotional stress, but most critically a lack of money for daily living supplies. Parents were positive about their children and used coping mechanisms such as spirituality and support from the community and neighbors. In a study by Gona et al. (2016), researchers found very similar results in Kenya, but also found that parents focused on diet management and respite care.

Although the demands of care are high, parents do not feel burdened or overwhelmed by their children. The parents do not see the child as the problem. It is the inability to provide for the child that creates the most stress and the lack of support within the systems within the society that adds more stress (Gona et al.). Carers have a clear idea of what they need in the present and the future to care for their child. Parents do not doubt their parenting abilities (McNally & Meenan). Mbwilo, Smide, & Aarts (2010), came to similar conclusions, but parents focused more on the hardships faced and the lack of educational supports and the financial burdens of caring for a child with a disability. In reviewing the literature from Sub-Saharan African countries, the concerns have not changed in the last ten years, but the research has become more focused to state that these are challenges and coping strategies specifically for families of children with ASD, not just developmental disabilities or disabilities in general.

China

Raising a child with ASD can be challenging. Providing care for a child with ASD can be challenging for the family and cause stress (Zeng et al., 2020). In China, current federal policies have not yet authorized formal family support programs. Informal social support to families of children with ASD is usually provided in three ways: counseling services and information support from the registered parent support organizations; professional support on parenting skills from special education schools; and emotional support and information sharing from self-organized parent-to-parent support groups (Zeng et al.). Family support is critical in promoting family quality of life (FQOL) and helps to buffer the negative effect of stress deriving from raising a child with ASD. Family support had a direct effect on parental FQOL. Family support is critical in promoting FQOL, consistent with research done in the United States (Davis & Gavidia-Payne, 2009), and applies in the Chinese context. Moreover, there is a significant mediating effect of family support on parental stress and FQOL. Although previous studies suggest raising a child with ASD can be stressful for parents and can negatively impact their FQOL, if robust family support is available to meet the demands associated with parenting a child with ASD, the stress can be mediated (Abidin, 1990).

Given the limited resources, it is important to empower parents with evidence-based practices. Parents with lower education levels tended to report more behavioral issues in their children (Tsai et al., 2017). It is important to establish a parent training system to reach families with limited professional resources due to financial hardship. Since a significant portion of the people in mainland China rely on the internet and social media (such as WeChat, a platform similar to Facebook) to obtain information, it is also critical to launch educational programs through these channels. Health professionals in the field can be invited to directly train parents and disseminate data-driven, unbiased information because they are more aware of the divergence between the clinical reality and the social perception. Educational websites, online forums, and professional accounts on WeChat can be created to provide resources for diagnosis and intervention, explain medical insurance policies, and recommend information about special education services in an interactive manner. Through these programs, we hope that more training resources and accurate information of ASD can be delivered to parents and the caregivers (Tang & Bie, 2016). The parenting stress and self-blame can be reduced, further enhancing parents and caregivers' confidence and willingness to seek professional help. In addition, school educators would have more knowledge and resources to work with students with disabilities and be more willing to work with parents and clinicians to support these families.

Turkey

In Turkish culture, parents/main caregivers of children with autism take on excessive responsibilities, which may include medical, educational issues and daily routine activities. Bozkurt and colleagues (2019) studied the caregiver burden and stress coping styles of parents of children with ASD and the associated factors. Their study indicated the caregiver burden was significantly higher ($p < 0.05$) for parents of one child as compared to parents with more children, and parents with daughters compared to parents with sons. The mothers were found to have higher scores of submissive approach and seeking social support than fathers. In another study, Yildiz and colleagues (2019) conducted an exploratory digital ethnography study to learn from the discussions of parents of children with ASD on an online platform (i.e., Facebook group). Their findings revealed that parents develop individual ways to cope with the disability and re-define autism, empower each other, and share daily life strategies from their own experiences under a dominant medical discourse around autism in Turkish culture.

Arslan and Diken (2020) examined the relationship between Turkish fathers' interactional behaviors and the engagement of their children with ASD. The results showed that fathers had a moderate to low level of interactional behaviors while playing with their children with ASD. Fathers' sensitivity-responsivity and emotional expressiveness were positively correlated with child's engagement. However, when fathers used achievement-oriented, directive or teaching-oriented interactional behaviors, child engagement decreased.

The Middle East

Parents in the Middle East experience many of the same joys and concerns as parents in the other regions. According to Hassan (2019), attitudes on autism in Arab countries are slowly changing and it is not uncommon for parents to hide their children with ASD from the society due to the feelings of shame.

Religious belief and spirituality are still used as coping mechanisms among parents and the literature is limited on health, educational and social services for children with ASD in Arab countries (Khaateb et al., 2019). Studies from this region focused heavily on the impact that lack of knowledge by parents and caregivers had on the families and family functioning. In Iran, Samadi, Mahmoodizadeh, and McConkey (2012) surveyed Iranian parents about their knowledge of ASD and the impact it had on their lives. Families faced stress and health problems similar to those of parents in other countries, with a tendency to rely on emotionally focused coping and experienced more difficulties in family functioning. However, many families lacked accurate information about ASD and its causes and they had few opportunities to gather information, advice and support for themselves as parents, either informally or from professional services (Dunst, Trivette, & Hamby, 2007).

Families with children with ASD face several challenges such as lack of information and financial burdens that contribute to their stress and anxiety (Zarafshan et al., 2019). In Egypt, autism care is typically home-based but parents lack awareness and resources, which causes dramatic and adverse effects on the family's life (Gobrial et al., 2019). Limited options to support their children with ASD can also lead to family isolation and frustration (Taha & Hussein, 2014). One significant benefit of increased knowledge about ASD and its causes is that families were more able to counter the stigma they experienced from others, including professionals (Farrugia, 2009), which in itself can be another source of stress for parents (Mak & Kwok, 2010).

In the Middle East, religion played a large role in parents' perception and positive feelings about their child. Their religion urged them to maintain a positive attitude and to do everything they could to help their child. Muslim families believed that they had been chosen to care for their child with autism and this child was special and given to the family as a gift from Allah; their child was part of their fate (Jegatheesan, Miller & Fowler, 2010), because Allah wants to test that particular family to see if they can care for that child (Taresh et al., 2020). Religious and spiritual traditions also influence ASD treatment and parent's attitudes. For instance, most Yemeni parents struggle with finding the right help for ASD since they believe that ASD is a scourge from Allah or the curse of the evil eye (Taresh et al., 2020).

Internationally, there is a clear need for families of children with ASD to be better informed about this disorder and to be supported to cope with the stresses that most experience in raising their children. However, in low and middle income countries where access to service by experts and professionals is limited, greater reliance will need to be placed on individual families and training will need to be adapted to the cultural context and sensitivities. Moreover, establishing the feasibility and effectiveness of these culturally relevant, methodologically sound interventions should encourage their implementation (Samadi, McConkey, & Kelly, 2013).

Discussion and Future Research

Each of these regions face many of the same challenges: resources; lack of awareness and education of service providers, doctors, and educators; lack of knowledge of parents; stigma and discrimination; and lack of culturally relevant and validated assessment tools and interventions. While many of these countries are moving toward inclusive policies in their education systems for children with ASD, the implementation of those inclusive practices is still fragmented. At the same time, individuals with ASD are also not receiving the intensive and specialized interventions that they may need to support their development and to grow into productive members of their communities.

In countries like Costa Rica, China, and Tanzania, the concept of inclusion naturally reflects the collective attitudes of society and natural tendencies to care for children with disabilities. In Costa Rica, this relationship between societal attitudes and inclusion seems to have advanced inclusion's development. However, in China and Tanzania, other factors such as a lack of resources, a competitive educational system, and a huge number of children to serve seem to have overshadowed the positive societal attitudes toward inclusion and have hindered the progress toward inclusion for children with autism and other disabilities (Hippensteel, 2008).

When determining research priorities, it is important to look at issues that will improve the lives of individuals with autism and their families. Vitally important, research and interventions should be "rigorous, empirical, family-centered, culturally grounded, and methodologically sound" (Freeth, Milne, Sheppard, & Ramachandran, 2014, p. 999). There are several areas of future research that need to be addressed. Certainly, more work needs to be done in creating and implementing culturally responsive, but also valid measures of assessment of ASD in many different languages. Interventions need to be adapted and researched in the local context. In many of these countries, parents do not receive definitive diagnoses, but still need education and support for the needs of their child, regardless of the child's specific diagnosis. In countries where the general population has lower levels of knowledge about ASD, it would be advantageous to start with interventions designed to provide knowledge to parents of children with ASD to create a base of advocacy and support (Harrison et al., 2016). In the higher income countries, the world of ASD and special education can involve many acronyms, jargon, and complex terminology that needs to be broken down and demystified for both providers and families. Furthermore, in low- and middle-income countries, biological parents may not be the primary caregivers or the daily caregivers. Primary caregivers could be other relatives such as grandparents or aunts or neighbors or friends. Providers need to respect and work with the family unit presented to them with the child. While interventions, assessments, and educational systems from the United States and Europe can inform policy and practice for children and families with ASD in other countries, those policies and practices should not be used without adaptation and cultural understanding/reciprocity. Most critically, researchers, providers, and policy makers need to remember the important role of cultural and local context in every step of diagnosis, intervention, education, and research to support families in ways that are meaningful and create systems that can be sustainable in the local context because they are built on local values, knowledge, and buy-in. While ASD is a worldwide phenomenon, the sustainable programs to help children and families participate actively in their communities will need to be based in those local context and cultures.

A Case Study to Consider

Given space constraints, it is not possible to provide case studies for all countries, but we hope these experiences from Turkey can give readers an idea of the nature of educational services in low- and middle-income countries.

Ayse is six years old and diagnosed with autism spectrum disorder. She lives in a two-bedroom apartment with her two older brothers, mother, father, and grandmother from her father's side in Turkey. Children share their room with their grandparents and parents share a room, they also have a living room, formal dining room, one kitchen where they have their meals together, and one and half bathrooms. Ayse started public preschool when she turned five and her teacher noticed that she showed little interest in social interactions, daily routine activities, had difficulty initiating social interactions with her peers, maintaining daily conversations, and also she had some trouble with appropriate communication such as adjusting her volume/tone of speech. When her preschool teacher shared her observations and concerns after Ayse's first month in preschool, Ayse's mother didn't think that these behaviors would be considered as early indicators of autism, because she thought Ayse learned lots of things from her two older brothers and simply copied them.

According to the Special Education Law, services in Turkey are planned and applied throughout the country by the Special Education Guiding and Consulting Services Head Office under the Ministry of Education. With the help of the school counselor, Ayse was referred to a Guidance and Research Center (GRC) for evaluation. In Turkey, educational evaluations and identifications of individuals with disabilities are done by GRCs. These centers operate under the Ministry of National Education with responsibilities of designing and providing both educational and psychological services for individuals with disabilities, their parents, and their teachers (Karasu, 2014). Moreover, GRC service providers make all decisions for the individual with disability regarding the type and degree of the disability, developmental characteristics, current performance, and educational placement. GRC also decides on the individual's present levels of performance, and educational and supportive opportunities that are available in proximity.

Then, following the educational evaluation, the GRCs' Special Education Evaluation Board prepares a report for the individual who is going to benefit from special education. These reports are prepared by considering the principle of the least restrictive environment. These GRC reports are usually issued on a one-year basis, with rare exceptions of six-month or two-years. Following the evaluation process, the individual with disability might be directed to an inclusive general education classroom, a special education classroom in a general education school, a special education school, homeschooling, or hospital school (Ministry of National Education, 2018). An individual with disability could also be directed to a private Special

Education and Rehabilitation Center (SERC) as another option, or an additional option to their educational placement based on the family's decision. In Ayse's case, GRC decided Ayse should attend the same preschool classroom and receive two hours of communication support through the GRC.

Ayse's mother brought her to the center every week for two hours and she didn't miss one single week. Ayse's mother waited in the waiting room with other parents, while Ayse was working 1:1 with the GRC service provider on her communication skills. They used naturalistic language strategies and social narratives. GRC service providers worked with Ayse about one year to support her communication skills and expressive language, starting with responding to her name, however they couldn't make any significant difference in her communication skills. In fact, she didn't respond to her name at all. Her preschool teacher was also concerned because next year all of her peers will continue with first grade and she was worried Ayse may not be able to reach her goals before the next academic year. When GRC service providers systematically talk to her mother and discuss their activities, they always hear the same feedback from her mother, their routine is the same, Ayse plays with her brothers, she is a happy child.

For the end of year celebration, Ayse's preschool teacher organized a potluck and invited all the parents. Ayse's mother went to the potluck with burek with feta filling (traditional Turkish pastry) which is Ayse's favorite food. However, Ayse's teacher noticed that she called Ayse, "Elif" which is a very common Turkish name for girls. Ayse's teacher puzzled for a second, because she knew that Ayse didn't have a middle name or a nickname. She asked her mother why she was using Elif, and the mother explained that they took Ayse to a *hodja*, known as a religious community leader, to heal her autism and communication issues. Hodja recommended the family to go to their family cemetery before the sun rises and ask the first person they see to rename their child. Hodja said Ayse is a "heavy name" for the child and needs to be changed in order to heal her soul and communication issues in time. Ayse's parents followed hodja's guidance and changed her name and started to call her Elif.

Discussion Questions

1. As you read through the case story, were there points at which you were surprised? Please use these "surprising moments" to reflect on which of your own values, beliefs, education experiences made you reach this way.

2. At points in the process would you have suggested something different and why? How does that fit in with the cultural norms and values?

References

Abidin, R. R. (1990). Parenting Stress Index, 3rd Edition: Test Manual. Charlottesville, VA: Pediatric Psychology Press.

Abu-Hamour, B., & Muhaidat, M. (2013). Special education teachers' attitudes towards inclusion of students with autism in Jordan. *Journal of the International Association of Special Education, 14*(1), 34–40.

African Decade of Disabled Persons. (2009). Declaration of the African decade. Retrieved March 25, 2009, from www.africa-union.org/africandecade/declaration.htm.

Africa Regional International Meeting for Autism Research 2017. Spectrum. (2017, September 12). Retrieved March 14, 2022, from www.spectrumnews.org/conference-news/africa-regional-international-meeting-autism-research-2017/

Al-Adawi, S. (2006). Adolescence in Oman. In J. J. Arnett (Ed.), International encyclopedia of adolescence: A historical and cultural survey of young people around the world. New York: Routledge.

Al-Ansari, A. M., & Ahmed, M. M. (2013). Epidemiology of autistic disorder in Bahrain: prevalence and obstetric and familial characteristics. *Eastern Mediterranean Health Journal, 19*(9).

Al-Farsi, Y. M., Al-Sharbati, M. M., Al-Farsi, O. A., Al-Shafaee, M. S., Brooks, D. R., & Waly, M. I. (2011). Brief report: Prevalence of autistic spectrum disorders in the Sultanate of Oman. *Journal of Autism and Developmental Disorders, 41*(6), 821–825.

Al-Farsi, Y. M., Al-Sharbati, M. M., Al-Farsi, O. A., Al-Shafaee, M. S., Brooks, D. R., & Waly, M. I. (2011). Brief report: Prevalence of autistic spectrum disorders in the Sultanate of Oman. *Journal of Autism and Developmental Disorders*. https://doi.org/10.1007/s10803-010-1094.

Al-Farsi, Y. M., Waly, M. I., Al-Sharbati, M. M., Al-Shafaee, M., Al-Farsi, O., Al-Fahdi, S., ... & Al-Adawi, S. (2013). Variation in socio-economic burden for caring of children with autism spectrum disorder in Oman: caregiver perspectives. *Journal of Autism and Developmental Disorders, 43*(5), 1214–1221.

Al Khateeb, J. M., Kaczmarek, L., & Al Hadidi, M. S. (2019). Parents' perceptions of raising children with autism spectrum disorders in the United States and Arab countries: A comparative review. *Autism, 23*(7), 1645–1654.

Al-Lamki, Z., & Ohlin, C. (1992). A Community-based study of childhood handicap in Oman. *Journal of Tropical Pediatrics, 38*(6), 314–316.

Al-Shomari, T., & Al-Saratwai, Z. (2002). The Saudi and Kuwaiti standards of childhood autism rating scale (CARS): Standardization and validation. *Journal of Special Education Academy, 1*, 1–39.

Al-Rossan, F. (2012). Introduction to special education. *Amman: Dar Al-fker*.

Aljarallah, A., Alwaznah, T., Alnasari, S., & Alhazmi, M. (2006). A study of autism and developmental disorders in Saudi children. *Report, King Abdulaziz City for Science and Technology, Kingdom of Saudi Arabia*, 1–10.

Alsaedi, R. H. (2020). An assessment of the motor performance skills of children with autism spectrum disorder in the Gulf Region. *Brain Sciences, 10*(9), 607.

Alshaban, F., Aldosari, M., El Sayed, Z., Tolefat, M., El Hag, S., Al Shammari, H., ... & Fombonne, E. (2017). Autism spectrum disorder in Qatar: Profiles and correlates of a large clinical sample. *Autism & Developmental Language Impairments*, 2, 2396941517699215.

American Psychiatric Association [APA]. (2013). Diagnostic and statistical manual of mental disorders (5th ed.). Washington, DC: Author.

Ametepee, L. K., & Chitiyo, M. (2009). What we know about autism in Africa: A brief research synthesis. *The Journal of the International Association of Special Education, 10*(1), 11–13.

Bakare, M. O., Ebigbo, P. O., Agomoh, A. O., Eaton, J., Onyeama, G. M.,Okonkwo, K. O., . . . Aguocha, C. M. (2009). Knowledge about childhood autism and opinion among healthcare workers on availability of facilities and law caring for the needs and rights of children with childhood autism and other developmental disorders in Nigeria. *BMC Pediatrics*, 9(1), 1.

Bakare, M. O., Ebigbo, P. O., Agomoh, A. O., & Menkiti, N. C. (2008). Knowledge about childhood autism among health workers (KCAHW) questionnaire: Description, reliability and internal consistency. *Clinical Practice and Epidemiology in Mental Health*, 4(1), 17.

Bakare, M. O., & Munir, K. M. (2011). Autism spectrum disorders (ASD) in Africa: a perspective. *African Journal of Psychiatry*, 14(3), 208–210.

Belhadj, A., Mrad, R., & Halayem, M. B. (2006). A clinic and a paraclinic study of Tunisian population of children with autism. About 63 cases. *La Tunisie Medicale*, 84(12), 763–767.

Bello-Mojeed, M. A., Bakare, M. O., & Munir, K. (2014). Identification of autism spectrum disorders (ASD) in Africa: Need for shifting research and public health focus. In Comprehensive Guide to Autism (pp. 2437–2453). New York: Springer.

Bello-Mojeed, M. A., Ogun, O. C., Omigbodun, O. O., Adewuya, A. O., & Ladapo, H. T. O. (2011). Late identification of autistic disorder in Nigeria: An illustration with 2 case reports. *Nigerian Journal of Psychiatry*, 9(2).

Bitta, M. A., Kipkemoi, P., Kariuki, S. M., Abubakar, A., Gona, J., Philips-Owen, J., & Newton, C. R. (2021). Validity and reliability of the Neurodevelopmental Screening Tool (NDST) in screening for neurodevelopmental disorders in children living in rural Kenyan coast. *Wellcome Open Research*, 6.

Bozkurt, G., Uysal, G., & Düzkaya, D. S. (2019). Examination of care burden and stress coping styles of parents of children with autism spectrum disorder. *Journal of Pediatric Nursing*, 47, 142–147.

Chaaya, M., Saab, D., Maalouf, F. T., & Boustany, R. M. (2016). Prevalence of autism spectrum disorder in nurseries in Lebanon: a cross sectional study. *Journal of Autism and Developmental Disorders*, 46(2), 514–522.

Chakrabarti, S. (2009). Early identification of autism. *Indian Pediatrics*, 46(5).

Çitil, G., Çöp, E., Açıkel, S. B., Sarı, E., Karacan, C. D., & Şenel, S. (2021). Assessment of the knowledge and awareness of pediatric residents and pediatricians about autism spectrum disorder at a single center in Turkey. *Journal of Community Psychology*, 49(7), 2264–2275.

Daley, T. C. (2004). From symptom recognition to diagnosis: children with autism in urban India. *Social Science & Medicine*, 58(7), 1323–1335.

Daley, B. J. (2002). Context: Implications for learning in professional practices. In M.V. Alfred (ed.), Learning and sociocultural contexts: Implications for adults, community, and workplace education (pp. 79–88). San Francisco: Jossey Bass. (New Directions for Adult and Continuing Education, No. 96).

Daley, T. C., & Sigman, M. D. (2002). Diagnostic conceptualization of autism among Indian psychiatrists, psychologists, and pediatricians. *Journal of Autism and Developmental Disorders*, 32,12–23.

Daly, M. (2004) Families and family life in Ireland. Challenges for the future, report of public consultation for a. Department of Social & Family Affairs. Retrieved from www.welfare.ie/en/downloads/iyf2004.pdf. Accessed June 2, 2015.

Davis, K., & Gavidia-Payne, S. (2009). The impact of child, family, and professional support characteristics on the quality of life in families of young children with disabilities. *Journal of Intellectual and Developmental Disability*, 34(2), 153–162.

Dixon, P., Badoe, E. V., & Owusu, N. A. V. (2015). Family perspectives of autism spectrum disorders in urban Ghana. *JICNA*, 1(1).

Dyches, T. T., Wilder, L. K., Sudweeks, R. R., Obiakor, F. E., & Algozzine, B. (2004). Multicultural issues in autism. *Journal of Autism and Developmental Disorders*, 34(2), 211–222.

Duan, G., Chen, J., Zhang, W., Yu, B., Jin, Y., Wang, Y., ... Yao, M. (2015). Child abuse & neglect physical maltreatment of children with autism in Henan province in China: A cross-sectional study. *Child Abuse & Neglect*, 48, 140–147. http://dx.doi.org/10.1016/j.chiabu.2015.03.018.

Dunst, C. J., Trivette, C. M., & Hamby, D. W. (2007). Meta-analysis of family-centered helpgiving practices research. *Mental Retardation and Developmental Disabilities Research Reviews*, 13(4), 370–378.

Eapen, V., Mabrouk, A. A., Zoubeidi, T., & Yunis,F. (2007). Prevalence of pervasive developmental disorders in preschool children in the UAE. *Journal of Tropical Pediatrics*. https://doi.org/10.1093/tropej/fml091.

Elsabbagh, M., Divan, G., Koh, Y. J., Kim, Y. S., Kauchali, S., Marcín, C., . . . Yasamy, M. T. (2012). Global prevalence of autism and other pervasive developmental disorders. *Autism Research*, 5(3), 160–179.

Eroglu, M., & Kilic, B. G. (2020). Peer bullying among children with autism spectrum disorder in formal education settings: Data from Turkey. *Research in Autism Spectrum Disorders*, 75, 101572.

Fakolade, O. A., & Adeniyi, S. O. (2009). Attitude of teachers toward the inclusion of children with special needs in the general education classroom: The case of teachers in selected schools in Nigeria. *The Journal of the International Association of Special Education*, 10(1), 60–64.

Fan, Y. (2018). *The current state and outlook of autism in Mainland China*. Presentation at the annual conference of the International Society for Autism Research, Rotterdam, Amsterdam.

Farrugia, D. (2009). Exploring stigma: Medical knowledge and the stigmatisation of parents of children diagnosed with autism spectrum disorder. *Sociology of Health & Illness*, 31(7), 1011–1027.

Feinstein, M. M. (2010). Holocaust survivors in postwar Germany, 1945–1957. Cambridge: Cambridge University Press.

Feuerberg, G. (2013, July 13). Children with disabilities excluded in China. Epoch Times. Retrieved from www.theepochtimes.com/children-with-disabilitiesexcluded-in-china_218365.html

Fewster, D. L., Uys, C., & Govender, P. (2020). Interventions for Primary Caregivers of Children with Autism Spectrum Disorder: A cross-sectional study of current practices of stakeholders in South Africa. *South African Journal of Occupational Therapy*, *50*(1), 41–48.

Franz, L., Chambers, N., von Isenburg, M., & de Vries, P. J. (2017). Autism spectrum disorder in sub-saharan africa: A comprehensive scoping review. *Autism Research*, *10*(5), 723–749.

Freeth, M., Milne, E., Sheppard, E., & Ramachandran, R. (2014). Autism across cultures: Perspectives from non-Western cultures and implications for research. Handbook of Autism and Pervasive Developmental Disorders, Fourth Edition.

Grinker, R. R. (2008). Unstrange minds: Remapping the world of autism. Cambridge, MA: Da Capo Press.

Grinker, R. R., & Cho, K. (2013). Border children: Interpreting autism spectrum disorder in South Korea. *Ethos*, *41*(1), 46–74.

Gobrial, E. (2018). The lived experiences of mothers of children with the autism spectrum disorders in Egypt. *Social Sciences*, *7*(8), 133.

Gobrial, E., McAnelly, S., & Shannon, P. (2019). Education of children and young people with autistic spectrum disorders in Egypt. *British Journal of Learning Disabilities*, *47*(1), 29–34.

Gona, J. K., Newton, C. R., Rimba, K. K., Mapenzi, R., Kihara, M., Vijver, F. V., & Abubakar, A. (2016). Challenges and coping strategies of parents of children with autism on the Kenyan coast. *Rural and remote health*, *16*(2), 3517.

Ha, V. S. & Whittaker, A. (2022): "Pray to all four directions": a qualitative study of syncretic care seeking by Vietnamese families for their children with autism spectrum disorder, Disability and Rehabilitation, DOI: 10.1080/09638288.2022.2040613

Harrison, A. J., Long, K. A., Manji, K. P., & Blane, K. K. (2016). Development of a brief intervention to improve knowledge of autism and behavioral strategies among parents in Tanzania. *Intellectual and Developmental Disabilities*, *54*(3), 187–201.

Hippensteel, L. F. (2008). Comparative study: Educating a student with autism in Tanzania and the United States. University of Tennessee Honors Thesis Projects. Retrieved from http://trace.tennessee.edu/utk_chanhonoproj/1192. Accessed March 12, 2015.

Hudec, T. (2012). The attitudes of social workers in Kerala to complementary and alternative interventions for children with autism spectrum disorders (Doctoral dissertation, Doctoral thesis). Masarkova University, Czech Republic. Retrieved from http://is.muni.cz/th/365957/fss_m/Attitudes-Kerala.pdf). Accessed March 12, 2015.

Holloway, S. D., Cohen, S. R., & Dominguez-Pareto, I. (2018). Culture, stigma, and intersectionality: Towards equitable parent-educator relationships in early childhood special education. In M. Siller & L. Morgan (eds.), Handbook of Parent-Implemented Interventions for Very Young Children with Autism (pp. 93–106). New York: Springer.

Holroyd, R. A. (2003). Fields of experience: Young people's constructions of embodied identities. Unpublished dissertation, Loughborough University, Loughborough.

Hassan, A. (2019). Arab views on autism. *Encyclopedia of Autism Spectrum Disorders*. New York, NY. Springer. doi, *10*, 978–1.

Huang, A. X., Jia, M., & Wheeler, J. J. (2013). Children with autism in the People's Republic of China: Diagnosis, legal issues, and educational services. *Journal of Autism and Developmental Disorders, 43*(9), 1991–2001.

Huang, J. P., Cui, S. S., Yu, H. A. N., Hertz-Picciotto, I. R. V. A., Qi, L. H., & Zhang, X. (2014). Prevalence and early signs of autism spectrum disorder (ASD) among 18–36 month old children in Tianjin of China. *Biomedical and Environmental Sciences, 27*(6), 453–461.

Igwe, M. N., Ahanotu, A. C., Bakare, M. O., Achor, J. U., & Igwe, C. (2011). Assessment of knowledge about childhood autism among paediatric and psychiatric nurses in Ebonyi state, Nigeria. *Child & Adolescent Psychiatry & Mental Health, 5*, 1–8.

Jegatheesan, B., Fowler, S., & Miller, P. J. (2010). From symptom recognition to services: How South Asian Muslim immigrant families navigate autism. *Disability & Society, 25*(7), 797–811.

Kalabula, M. D. (2000). Inclusive education in Africa: A myth or reality? A Zambian case. Retrieved May 1, 2005, from www.isec2000.org.uk/abstra cts/papers_k/ kkalabula_1.htm.

Karasu, N. (2014). Guidance and research centers of Turkey: From the perspective of parents. *European Journal of Special Needs Education, 29*(3), 358–369.

Kilincaslan, A., Kocas, S., Bozkurt, S., Kaya, I., Derin, S., & Aydin, R. (2019). Daily living skills in children with autism spectrum disorder and intellectual disability: A comparative study from Turkey. *Research in Developmental Disabilities, 85*, 187–196.

Khan, N., & Hombarume, J. (1996). Levels of autistic behaviour among the mentally handicapped children in Zimbabwe. *The Central African Journal of Medicine, 42*(2), 36–39.

La Roche, M. J., Bush, H. H., & D'Angelo, E. (2018). The assessment and treatment of autism spectrum disorder: A cultural examination. *Practice Innovations, 3*(2), 107.

Li, N., Chen, G., Song, X., Du, W., & Zheng, X. (2011). Prevalence of autism-caused disability among Chinese children: A national population-based survey. *Epilepsy & Behavior, 22*, 786–789. doi:10.1016/j.yebeh.2011.10.002

Liu, X., Liu, J., Xiong, X., Yang, T., Hou, N., Liang, X., ... & Li, T. (2016). Correlation between nutrition and symptoms: nutritional survey of children with autism spectrum disorder in Chongqing, China. *Nutrients, 8*(5), 294.

Lotter, V. (1978). Childhood autism in Africa. *Journal of Child Psychology and Psychiatry, 19*(3), 231–244.

Mandell, D. S., Ittenbach, R. F., Levy, S. E., & Pinto-Martin, J. A. (2007). Disparities in diagnoses received prior to a diagnosis of autism spectrum disorder. *Journal of autism and developmental disorders, 37*(9), 1795-1802.

Mbwilo, G., Smide, B., & Aarts, C. (2010). Family perceptions in caring for children and adolescents with mental disabilities: A qualitative study from Tanzania. *Tanzania Journal of Health Research, 12*(2), 129–137.

McCabe, H. (2007). Parent advocacy in the face of adversity autism and families in the People's Republic of China. *Focus on Autism and Other Developmental Disabilities, 22*(1), 39–50.

McCabe, H. (2013). Bamboo shoots after the rain: Development and challenges of autism intervention in China. *Autism*, *17*(5), 510–526.

McNally, A., & Mannan, H. (2013). Perceptions of caring for children with disabilities: Experiences from Moshi, Tanzania. *African Journal of Disability*, *2*(1), 1–10.

Majoko, T. (2017). Practices that support the inclusion of children with autism spectrum disorder in mainstream early childhood education in Zimbabwe. *SAGE Open*, *7*(3), 2158244017730387.

Mak, W. W., & Kwok, Y. T. (2010). Internalization of stigma for parents of children with autism spectrum disorder in Hong Kong. *Social Science & Medicine*, *70*(12), 2045–2051.

Mankoski, R. E., Collins, M., Ndosi, N. K., Mgalla, E. H., Sarwatt, V. V., & Folstein, S. E. (2006). Etiologies of autism in a case-series from Tanzania. *Journal of Autism and Developmental Disorders*, *36*(8), 1039–1051.

Mandell, D. S., & Novak, M. (2005). The role of culture in families' treatment decisions for children with autism spectrum disorders. *Mental Retardation and Developmental Disabilities Research Reviews*, *11*(2), 110–115.

Miles, S., & Kaplan, I. (2005). Using images to promote reflection: An action research study in Zambia and Tanzania. *Journal of Research in Special Educational Needs*, *5*(2), 77–83.

Milli Eğitim Bakanlığı (2018). *Özel Eğitim Hizmetleri Yönetmeliği*. Retrieved from http://orgm.meb.gov.tr/meb_iys_dosyalar/2018_07/09101900_ozel_egitim_hizmetleri_yonetmeligi_07072018.pdf

Ministry of Development Planning and Statistics. (2016). *Statistics*. Retrieved from www.psa.gov.qa/en/pages/default.aspx

Odunsi, R., Preece, D., & Garner, P. (2017). Nigerian teachers' understanding of autism spectrum disorder: A comparative study of teachers from urban and rural areas of Lagos State. *Disability, CBR & Inclusive Development*, *28*(3), 98–114.

Okasha, A. (2005). Mental health in Egypt. *Journal of Psychiatry and Related Sciences*, *42*(2), 116–125.

Omar, M. (2014). Early intervention services as perceived by parents of children with autism in Egypt and Saudi Arabia. *International Interdisciplinary Journal of Education*, *3*(2), 238–249. http://doi.org/10.12816/0003002.

Oner, O., & Munir, K. M. (2020). Modified checklist for autism in toddlers revised (MCHAT-R/F) in an urban metropolitan sample of young children in Turkey. *Journal of Autism and Developmental Disorders*, *50*, 3312–3319.

Pillay, S., Duncan, M., & De Vries, P. J. (2017). A systematic database search for known cases of ASD in the Western Cape Province. In *Poster presentation at the University of Cape Town. Conference: Regional IMFAR SA-ACAPAP 2017At: Cape Town, South Africa*.

Profanter, A. (2009). Facing the challenges of children and youth with special abilities and needs on the fringes of Omani society. *Children and Youth Services Review*, *31*(1), 8–15.

Read, N., & Schofield, A. (2010). Autism: are mental health services failing children and parents? Recent research suggests that many CAMHS need to improve. *Journal of Family Health Care*, *20*(4), 120–125.

Rousseau, M., Dionne, C., Savard, R. T., Schonhaut, L., & Londono, M. (2021). Translation and Cultural Adaptation of the Ages and Stages Questionnaires

(ASQ) Worldwide: A Scoping Review. *Journal of Developmental & Behavioral Pediatrics*, 42(6), 490–501.

Samadi, S. A., Mahmoodizadeh, A., & McConkey, R. (2012). A national study of the prevalence of autism among five-year-old children in Iran. *Autism*, 16(1), 5–14.

Samadi, S. A., McConkey, R., & Kelly, G. (2013). Enhancing parental well-being and coping through a family-centred short course for Iranian parents of children with an autism spectrum disorder. *Autism*, 17(1), 27–43.

Sampson, W. G., & Sandra, A. E. (2018). Comparative study on knowledge about autism spectrum disorder among paediatric and psychiatric nurses in Public Hospitals in Kumasi, Ghana. *Clinical Practice and Epidemiology in Mental Health: CP & EMH*, 14, 99.

Sangare, M., Toure, H. B., Toure, A., Karembe, A., Dolo, H., Coulibaly, Y. I., Kouyate, M., Traore, K., Diakité, S. A., Coulibaly, S., Togora, A., Guinto, C. O., Awandare, G. A., Doumbia, S., Diakite, M., & Geschwind, D. H. (2019). Validation of two parent-reported autism spectrum disorders screening tools M-CHAT-R and SCQ in Bamako, Mali. *eNeurologicalSci*, 15, 100188. https://doi.org/10.1016/j.ensci.2019.100188.

Schiariti, Verónica, et al. "International Classification of Functioning, Disability and Health Core Sets for Cerebral Palsy, Autism Spectrum Disorder, and Attention-deficit-hyperactivity Disorder." *Developmental Medicine and Child Neurology*, vol. 60, no. 9, 2018, pp. 933–941.

Seif Eldin, A., Habib, D., Noufal, A., Farrag, S., Bazaid, K., Al-Sharbati, M., ... & Gaddour, N. (2008). Use of M-CHAT for a multinational screening of young children with autism in the Arab countries. *International Review of Psychiatry*, 20(3), 281–289.

Smith, C. (2014). The global challenge of autism. *House Hearing of the Subcommittee on Africa, Global Health, Global Human Rights and International Organizations*. Retrieved from http://chrissmith.house.gov/uploadedfiles 2014-07-23_global_autism_hearing.pdf. Accessed June 2, 2015.

Soni, A., Reyes Soto, M., & Lynch, P. (2021). A review of the factors affecting children with disabilities successful transition to early childhood care and primary education in sub-Saharan Africa. *Journal of Early Childhood Research*, 1476718X211035428.

Stone-MacDonald, A. (2014). Community-based education for students with developmental disabilities in Tanzania. Dordrecht, Netherlands: Springer.

Stone-MacDonald, A., & Butera, G. (2012). Cultural beliefs and attitudes about disability in Sub-Saharan Africa. *Review of Disability Studies*, 8, 62–77.

Stone-MacDonald, A. & Fettig, A. (2019). Culturally Relevant Assessment and Support of Grade 1 Students with Mild Disabilities in Tanzania: An Exploratory Study. *International Journal for Disability, Development and Education*, 66, 374–388. doi: 10.1080/1034912X.2019.1591616.

Sun, X., Allison, C., Auyeung, B., Matthews, F. E., Baron-Cohen, S., & Brayne, C. (2013). Service provision for autism in mainland China: Preliminary mapping of service pathways. *Social Science & Medicine*, 98, 87–94.

Taha, G. R., & Hussein, H. (2014). Autism Spectrum Disorders in Developing Countries: Lessons from the Arab World. In V. B. Patel (Ed.), Comprehensive Guide to Autism (pp. 2509–2531). New York, NY: Springer.

Tang, L., & Bie, B. (2016). The stigma of autism in china: an analysis of newspaper portrayals of autism between 2003 and 2012. *Health Communication*, *31*(4), 445–452.

Taresh, S. M., Ahmad, N. A., Roslan, S., & Ma'rof, A. M. (2020). Preschool Teachers' Beliefs towards Children with Autism Spectrum Disorder (ASD) in Yemen. *Children*, *7*(10), 170.

Tsai, H. W. J., Cebula, K., & Fletcher-Watson, S. (2017). The role of the broader autism phenotype and environmental stressors in the adjustment of siblings of children with autism spectrum disorders in Taiwan and the United Kingdom. *Journal of Autism and Developmental Disorders*, *47*(8), 2363–2377.

Turkish Ministry of Health. (2015). *Recommended periodic health examinations and screening tests in family medicine practice*. Ministry of Health, Republic of Turkey.

Viljoen, M., Mahdi, S., Griessel, D., Bölte, S., & de Vries, P. J. (2019). Parent/caregiver perspectives of functioning in autism spectrum disorders: A comparative study in Sweden and South Africa. *Autism*, *23*(8), 2112–2130.

Vorster, C., Kritzinger, A., Coetser, L. E., & Linde, J. V. D. (2021). Preliminary reliability of South African adaptation and Northern Sotho translation of the Modified Checklist for Autism in Toddlers, Revised with Follow-Up. *South African Journal of Communication Disorders*, *68*(1), 1–7.

Wang, K., Wang, C., Guo, D., van Wijngaarden, M., & Begeer, S. (2018). Children with autism spectrum disorder from China and the Netherlands: Age of diagnosis, gender, and comorbidities. *Research in Autism Spectrum Disorders*, *54*, 76–82. https://doi:10.1016/j.rasd.2018.07.004.

World Health Organization (1992), ICD-10 Classification of mental and behavioral disorders, clinical description and diagnostic guidelines. Geneva: World Health Organization.

Xiong, N., Yang, L., Yu, Y., Hou, J., Li, J., Li, Y., ... & Jiao, Z. (2011). Investigation of raising burden of children with autism, physical disability and mental disability in China. *Research in developmental disabilities*, *32*(1), 306–311.

Xu, Y., Yang, J., Yao, J., Chen, J., Zhuang, X., Wang, W., ... & Lee, G. T. (2018). A pilot study of a culturally adapted early intervention for young children with autism spectrum disorders in China. *Journal of Early Intervention*, *40*(1), 52–68.

Yazici, M. S., & McKenzie, B. (2020). Strategies used to develop sociocommunicative skills among children with autism in a Turkish special education school and implications for development of Practice. *International Journal of Disability, Development and Education*, *67*(5), 515–535.

Yildiz, Gatos, D., Subasi, Ö., Yantac, A. E., & Kuscu, K. (2019). Examining online practices of an autism parent community in Turkey: Goals, needs, and opportunities. *Proceedings of the 2019 on Designing Interactive Systems Conference*, 373–384. https://doi.org/10.1145/3322276.3322344

Zarafshan, H., Mohammadi, M. R., Abolhassani, F., Motevalian, S. A., Sepasi, N., & Sharifi, V. (2019). Current status of health and social services for children with autism in Iran: Parents' perspectives. *Iranian Journal of Psychiatry*, *14*(1), 76.

Zeng, S., Hu, X., Zhao, H., & Stone-MacDonald, A. (2020). Examining the relationships of parental stress, family support and family quality of life: A structural equation modeling Approach. *Research in Developmental Disabilities*, *96*, 1–9. doi: https://doi.org/10.1016/j.ridd.2019.103523.

Zhang, D., & Spencer, V. G. (2015). Addressing the needs of students with autism and other disabilities in China: Perspectives from the field. *International Journal of Disability, Development, and Education*, *62* (2), 168–181. https://doi:10.1080/1034912X.2014.998175.

Zhao, X., & Zhang, C. (2018). From isolated fence to inclusive society: The transformational disability policy in China. *Disability & Society*, *33*(1), 132–137. https://doi.org/10.1080/09687599.2017.1375246.

Zhou, W. Z., Ye, A. Y., Sun, Z. K., Tian, H. H., Pu, T. Z., Wu, Y. Y., ... & Wei, L. (2014). Statistical analysis of twenty years (1993 to 2012) of data from mainland China's first intervention center for children with autism spectrum disorder. *Molecular Autism*, *5*(1), 1–14.

Zhou, H., Xu, X., Yan, W., Zou, X., Wu, L., Luo, X., ... & Wang, Y. (2020). Prevalence of autism spectrum disorder in China: a nationwide multi-center population-based study among children aged 6 to 12 years. *Neuroscience Bulletin*, *36*(9), 961–971.

Section II

Education and Intervention in the Early Years

Chapter 5

Early Intervention Services for Children with Autism

*Shawna G. Harbin[1], Angel Fettig,[1]
and Veronica P. Fleury[2]*
[1] University of Washington, Seattle
[2] Florida State University, Tallahassee

Introduction

The rising prevalence of Autism Spectrum Disorder (ASD) has increasingly become an important public health concern with significant impact on Early Intervention (EI) systems, schools, and communities. Children's caregivers and other close family members often notice some early behavioral indicators associated with ASD before the age of two years, although the child may not receive a medical diagnosis until later. National efforts by government and private organizations are working towards improving public awareness of early indicators to facilitate accurate and earlier diagnosis, which enables children to access critical EI services. It is well documented that early intervention services play a critical role in maximizing outcomes and reducing debilitating impacts for children with ASD (Hume et al., 2005; National Research Council, 2001; Rogers, 1999; Woods & Wetherby, 2003). This chapter aims to provide an overview of the purpose of EI services, specific interventions available for children with ASD, and issues and factors to consider when examining early intervention services for children with ASD.

Purpose of Early Intervention

Early intervention services for infants and toddlers with special needs from birth to age 3 have been a part of the Individuals with Disabilities Education Act (IDEA) since 1986. This section of the law is commonly known as Part C of IDEA. Early intervention focuses on providing family-centered services for children from birth to age 3 who have disabilities or are at risk for developmental delays, and their families. Eligibility for these services is determined by evaluating the child to see if a delay in

DOI: 10.4324/9781003255147-7

one or more domains of development or a disability exists. Children who meet these criteria, and their families, can receive early intervention services from the child's birth through their third birthday, and sometimes beyond in certain states through age five. Sometimes caregivers and professionals know from the moment a child is born that early intervention services will be essential in helping the child's growth and development. This is often the case for children who are diagnosed at birth with a specific condition, or who experience significant prematurity, very low birth weight, illness, or surgery soon after being born. Even before heading home from the hospital, this child's parents may be given a referral to their local early intervention agency to facilitate the start of early intervention services. Some children, like those with ASD, have a relatively routine entry into the world at birth, but may develop more slowly in certain domains than others, experience setbacks, or be diagnosed with a specific disability in the first few years of their lives. For these children, a visit with a developmental pediatrician and a thorough evaluation may lead to an early intervention referral and potentially a diagnosis of ASD.

IDEA provides states with federal grants to institute early intervention programs. Any child younger than age three who is experiencing significant delays in their development or has a physical or mental condition likely to result in a developmental delay, is eligible to receive early intervention services through these programs. Early intervention services can vary by state and region. However, services should address the child's unique, individualized needs and should not be limited to what is currently available or customary in the region where the child is being served. Following a comprehensive evaluation by a team of developmental experts, an Individual Family Service Program (IFSP) is created, which documents the child's needs, and the goals and services that will be provided to the child and their family. Additional information about legislation and service delivery is covered in an earlier chapter in this text (see Chapter 3).

Early Detection of ASD

Our knowledge regarding early behavioral manifestations of ASD has grown tremendously over the past two decades. Many symptoms and characteristics can be detected in children as young as 18 months of age, especially for children with less advanced language and adaptive skills (Zwaigenbaum et al., 2015). Although experienced professionals can provide reliable diagnoses by the age of 2, many children do not receive a final diagnosis until they are much older. This is due to a number of factors, particularly community settings with limited access to high quality healthcare providers who are knowledgeable about ASD (Daniels & Mandell, 2014) and a prevailing stigma associated with pursuing a diagnosis in some cultural groups (Lord et al., 2006). Also, research suggests racially minoritized children may be found to receive a later diagnosis compared to White children (Fombonne & Zuckerman, 2021; Mandell et al., 2009). National public efforts by the American Academy of Pediatrics (AAP, 2007) in concert with professional organizations such as the Center for Disease Control's "Learn the Signs. Act Early" program, have improved both procedures for detection and public awareness about early behaviors that may indicate a risk for ASD. These early behaviors, oftentimes referred to as "red flags," reflect the core difficulties that are characteristic of ASD, namely problems with social interaction, communication, and the presence of repetitive behaviors and mannerisms. Refer to Table 5.1 for a description of "red flags." Caregivers of infants who show two or more of these behaviors are encouraged to talk to their child's pediatric healthcare provider (AAP, 2006; Wetherby et al., 2004; Zwaigenbaum et al., 2015).

Table 5.1 Early "Red Flags" for ASD

Behavior of Concern	Description
Impairment in Social Interaction	
Lack of appropriate eye gaze	Child does not consistently make eye contact or look at items when directed
Limited facial expression	No big smiles or other warm, joyful expressions by 6 months or later
Lack of response to name	Child does not consistently look or attend when his/her name is called
Impairment in Communication	
Limited use of gestures	No back-and forth gestures such as pointing, showing, reaching, or waving by 12 months
Lack of coordination of nonverbal communication	No back and forth sharing of enjoyment. Non-verbal communicative attempts are not well integrated (i.e., child may point to an object, but does not pair it with eye contact)
Limited babbling or lack of words	No babbling at 12 months of age; no words at 16 months of age; no meaningful 2-word phrases by 24 months of age (does not include imitated or repeated phrases)
Unusual prosody of verbal language	Child's cries/speech has little variation in pitch, odd intonation, irregular rhythm, and/or unusual voice quality
Regression of skills	Any loss of speech, babbling or social skills at any age
Repetitive behaviors and restricted interests	
Repetitive movements of objects	Child plays with objects the same way repeatedly
Repetitive body movements	Repetitive movements or posturing of body, arms, hands, or fingers
Unusual play	Lack of pretend play; intense visual or tactile interaction with toys

Wetherby et al., 2004; AAP, 2006; Zwaigenbaum et al., 2015.

Table 5.2 Autism Screening Tools

Screening Tool	Description	Admin Time	Who Completes
Autism Behavior Checklist (ABC) (Krug et al., 1980)	ABC is used to assess behaviors and symptoms of autism in the categories of sensory, relating, body and object use, language, and social and self-help for children 3 and older.	10–20 mins	Parents or teachers; scored by professionals
Ages & Stages Questionnaire: Social- Emotional (ASQ-SE 2) (Squires et al., 2009)	ASQ-SE focuses on identifying social emotional behavior for children ages 1– 72 months.	10–15 mins	Parents and caregivers
Brief Infant Toddler Social Emotional Assessment (BITSEA) (Briggs-Gowen, J. & Carter, A., 2007)	BITSEA is a brief comprehensive screening instrument to evaluate social and emotional behavior for children ages 12-36 months.	7–10 mins	Parents and childcare providers
Communication and Symbolic Behavior Scales Developmental Profile Infant/ Toddler Checklist (CSBS-DP) (Wetherby & Prizant, 2002)	CSBS-DP is a screening tool used to identify children ages 6-24 months in need of further evaluation for autism and other developmental delays.	5–10 mins	Parents and caregivers
Modified Checklist for Autism in Toddlers, Revised, with Follow- Up (M-CHAT-R/F) (Robins et al., 2009)	M-CHAT-R/F is designed for children 16-30 months of age that assesses risk for autism spectrum disorder.	5–10 mins	Parents and caregivers
Screening Tool for Autism in Two-Year- Olds (STAT) (Stone et al., 2008)	STAT is designed to screen for autism in children between 24 and 36 months of age.	20 mins	Service providers and clinicians

The AAP recommends that pediatricians screen all children specifically for ASD during the 18-month and 24-month regular well-child visits in addition to general developmental surveillance and screening during regular well-child visits. Many subjective screening instruments rely solely on parents' responses to a questionnaire, while others involve a combination of parent report and direct observation. Screening tools are designed to be quick to administer and enable practitioners to focus on key "red flags" of ASD to guide their decision whether further evaluation is needed. In addition to subjective measures screening for "red flags," researchers are innovating objective measures, such as eye tracking (Kong et al., 2017) and brain-imaging tools, to detect ASD at an early age, even before the child's second birthday. A list of ASD-specific screening tools used by parents/caregivers and pediatricians is outlined in Table 5.2. By having procedures to identify children at risk for ASD combined with overall improved awareness of "red flags" means that children are being diagnosed at earlier ages, which ultimately translates to earlier opportunities to access important intervention.

Young children with ASD often have difficulty participating in appropriate play, meeting developmental milestones, communicating effectively with others, developing friendships, and conforming to expected behavioral norms. It is important that children with ASD start receiving services to address these concerns as soon as ASD is suspected. The effectiveness of early intervention has been clearly demonstrated by research (National Research Council, 2001). The question is no longer *Does early intervention work?* but rather, *How early can we intervene?* Some researchers believe that treatment will be most effective if intervention services begin before a child's second birthday (Dawson, 2008; Dawson et al., 2012; Sullivan et al., 2014; Zwaigenbaum et al., 2015). Accordingly, many professionals advocate for treatment to begin as soon as any early behavioral "red flags" are detected rather than waiting for a formal clinical diagnosis. The rationale behind this thinking is that the early behavioral characteristics of ASD prevent a young child from interacting with people and materials in their environment in meaningful ways that are believed to promote healthy development. Interventions that enable young children at risk for ASD to become more socially engaged and interactive can change a child's developmental trajectory, and even prevent these early symptoms from exacerbating to a point where they would no longer reach the clinical threshold for ASD (Dawson, 2008; Dawson et al., 2012). The following vignette describes the experience of one family as they seek support for their young child, Samuel:

> Samuel is two years old and lives with his mother, father, grandmother, and two older siblings. Samuel's parents are fluent in English, but their preferred language is Vietnamese, and Samuel's grandmother speaks Vietnamese primarily. Samuel himself is learning both Vietnamese and English in the home. At his two-year well child exam, Samuel's caregivers talk to their pediatrician about a few concerns they had been having about Samuel's behaviors. For instance, Samuel would sometimes scream unconsolably during daily routines, such as family meals or getting in the car. He also didn't seem as interested in playing with other children as his siblings or family

friends did. His mother explained to the pediatrician that they did not experience this with their first two children. The family pediatrician listened to their concerns and talked to them about red flags for Autism. She referred them to a neurodevelopmental pediatrician who could provide more support and answer their questions about Samuel's recent behaviors.

Approaches to Intervention

Over the years, interventions have been developed for children with ASD to address the core symptoms associated with ASD – social-communication and behavioral differences; however, children with ASD may also benefit from additional services to address any broader developmental needs. Children with ASD receive early intervention services to address global developmental delays as well as symptoms specific to ASD. Early intervention services are designed to meet the specific needs of children with ASD and their families by adopting a family-centered approach. As such, service providers need to individualize services to meet the needs of both the child and the family. Services focus on the family's priorities and strengths as well as their cultural, linguistic, and lifestyle practices (Dunst et al., 1991; Espe-Sherwindt, 2008). These services should occur in children's natural environments, that is, settings that are typical for children. During early childhood, these settings can include but are not limited to the family's home, childcare programs, and other community settings. Accordingly, early intervention services for children with ASD vary depending on a child's individual needs and may include, but are not limited to, early intensive behavioral intervention, speech and language therapy, occupational therapy, and physical therapy. In this section, we will first describe common services that children with ASD may receive as part of their early intervention programming. Although each of these services may differ in their focus, service providers should incorporate instructional strategies (referred to as *Focused Intervention Strategies*) that have strong evidentiary support as the basis for their instruction. Recommended focused intervention strategies for children with ASD will be discussed later in this section.

Early Intensive Behavioral Intervention (EIBI). Some families of children with ASD may choose to participate in EIBI programming in an effort to improve overall developmental outcomes for their child. Sometimes referred to as *comprehensive program models* (previously identified as Comprehensive Treatment Models but modified to avoid potentially ableist language) (Hume et al., 2021), these programs consist of a set of practices designed to achieve a broad learning or developmental impact on the core deficits of ASD (CTM; Odom et al., 2010; Wong et al., 2015). Specific instructional approaches vary across programming as do the amount of time children spend receiving services (range: 12–40 hours per week). The National Academy of Science Committee on Educational Interventions for Children with Autism (National Research Council, 2001) identified 10 comprehensive program models. Examples include the UCLA Young Autism Program by Lovaas and colleagues (Smith et al., 2000), the TEACCH program developed by Schopler and colleagues (Marcus et al., 2000), the LEAP model (Strain & Hoyson, 2000), and the Denver model designed by Rogers and colleagues (Rogers et al., 2000). It should be noted, however, that most of the research that has been conducted with these models focus on preschool-age children or older.

Speech and Language Therapy. Children with ASD vary widely in their speech and communication needs. Some children never develop functional speech and will learn to communicate using augmentative and alternative communication (AAC). Licensed speech language pathologists (SLP) can work with young children and their families to teach children an effective means of communicating. Options range from low-technology systems, such as sign language or using pictures to communicate (i.e., Picture Exchange Communication System; Bondy & Frost, 2001) to high-technology systems that include voice-output devices once children are older (Steinbrenner et al., 2020). Children with ASD who develop speech may continue to exhibit differences with pragmatics of language, or the social application of using speech. SLP services in early intervention can support children's language development by coaching parents and caregivers to embed language and communication strategies throughout daily routine activities in the language(s) preferred by the family (American Speech Language Hearing Association; n.d.).

Occupational therapy (OT). OT focuses on helping children be as independent as possible with participating in purposeful and meaningful daily activities and routines in their homes and communities (Clark et al., 2017). According to The Therapy Association (2010) for young children with ASD, the scope of OT services generally focuses on self-management skills (e.g., dressing, feeding, hygiene, and sleep), regulation of emotional and behavioral responses, processing of sensory information to ensure participation in natural settings, and development of social and interpersonal skills and peer relationships.

Physical Therapy (PT). Children with ASD often have challenges with developing motor skills such as sitting, walking, running, or jumping. PT focuses on supporting children's motor skill development by improving muscle tone, balance, and coordination. This reduces their developmental and functional obstacles, thereby increasing children's participation in natural routines and environments. Based on updated competencies, physical therapists practicing in early intervention settings are expected to demonstrate specific knowledge reflecting early intervention contexts, such as family systems theory, coordinated care, assessment, and intervention programs (Chiarello & Effgen, 2006).

> *Samuel's family put their name on a waitlist for an appointment with a developmental pediatrician and were expected to see the new doctor in several months. Their family pediatrician also referred Samuel and his caregivers to a local EI center, where a team of practitioners including an Educator, a Speech-Language Pathologist, and an Occupational Therapist conducted an evaluation with Samuel and his caregivers to determine if he qualified for EI services. Each of the practitioners spoke English as their primary language, and the Occupational Therapist also spoke Spanish. A Vietnamese language interpreter was present for the evaluation to ensure the family and practitioners could share important information with each other. Based on the practitioners' observations and the reports of Samuel's mother, father, and grandmother, the practitioners recommended Education and Speech services for Samuel and his family. With the family, they scheduled a time for the team (including Samuel's family) to participate in an Individualized Family Service Plan (IFSP) meeting the following week to talk about the family's strengths, their concerns, and their goals for Samuel's development.*

Focused-Intervention Strategies

The intervention literature for children with ASD has grown dramatically over the past decade. Practitioners and parents are often bombarded with conflicting information regarding treatment options, some of which may be ineffective or potentially harmful. Fortunately, there are resources that are publicly available to assist practitioners and parents in selecting strategies that are supported by research. Researchers with the National Clearinghouse for Autism Evidence and Practice (NCAEP) published a technical report in which they summarize the results of a systematic review of the intervention research for individuals with ASD from birth to age 21 (Steinbrenner et al., 2020). In this review, researchers identified 28 evidence-based practices (EBPs) that address a number of different outcomes for individuals with ASD. Of the 545 studies included in this review, 82 studies included children younger than three years old and 16 included this age group exclusively. Because these reviews only included research that targeted individuals who were identified as having ASD, this small number of studies is not surprising given that the average age of diagnosis is age three or later (Lord et al., 2006). There is, however, clearly a need to continue to conduct research to identify and validate strategies that are effective for infants and toddlers at risk for ASD.

Parent-Implemented Interventions. In nearly half of all of the studies targeting young children with ASD in the NCAEP report, parents were trained to deliver interventions with their toddler. As mentioned earlier, family-centered practices are the cornerstones of early intervention services. One of the key missions of early intervention is to build on and support the families and caregivers' confidence and competence as they support their children's development (Workgroup on Principles and Practices in Natural Environments, 2008). The family-centered approach highlights that family context and experiences are critical to a child's development and early intervention service providers must recognize that the family is the constant unit in the child's life and development (Bruder, 2000). Families know their children best and can provide an important source of information to ensure that early intervention services are meeting the needs of the child and their families. Early interventionists focus on preparing families and caregivers with skills they need to support the use of intervention skills in their daily lives. Involving families and caregivers in implementing intervention strategies allows the maximization of intervention provided in early intervention practices because families and caregivers can continue to support their child in using the learned skills throughout their daily routines.

In parent-implemented intervention (PII) programs, a toddler's caregiver is responsible for carrying out some or all of the components of the intervention. Caregivers are typically trained by the professional or member of the research team in either their homes or in community settings. The methods used to train caregivers vary across programs, but often will include didactic instruction, discussion, modeling, coaching, and feedback about the parent's or caregiver's performance (Schultz, 2013). Common toddler behaviors that are targeted in these programs also vary, but typically focus on improving communication, play, and self-help skills and/or decreasing challenging behavior (Steinbrenner et al., 2020). A major benefit of PII programs is that parents and caregivers are empowered to interact with their children in a meaningful way that can have major benefits in the child's development, as well as improve overall family functioning. A sample of PII research that highlighted infants and toddlers that was included in the NCAEP review can be found in Table 5.3.

Naturalistic interventions. Evidence suggests naturalistic interventions support young children from birth to three with reducing challenging behavior, while promoting prosocial behavior, communication, and social skills. Naturalistic interventions occur within typical settings (i.e., home, childcare), activities, and routines in which toddlers participate. Naturalistic interventions may include a variety of practices such as environmental arrangements, techniques to facilitate parent-child interactions, and other strategies based on applied behavior analysis. The

Table 5.3 Parent Implemented Interventions that Included Toddlers with ASD

Study	Intervention	Outcomes
Aldred et al. (2004)	Parents were trained to use adapted communication tailored to their child's individual competencies.	Significant improvements made in children's total ADOS scores, particularly in the areas of social interaction, expressive language, social initiations, and parent-child interactions.
Chiang et al. (2016)	Similar to Kasari et al. (2010), parents participated in an 8-week, 20 session Joint Engagement (JE) training. It also incorporated "creative movement play." Module topics included following and imitating their child, establishing and developing a play routine, finding a balance between imitation and demonstration, flexible play (toy and movement), sharing communication, supporting initiating communication for the child, management of the child's emotional regulation, and generalization.	The intervention could enhance joint engagement: child-initiated supportive and coordinated joint engagement was greater for the JE intervention group.
Green et al. (2010)	Preschool Autism Communication Trial [PACT]. Parents were taught to increase their sensitivity and responsiveness to children's communicative attempts.	Improvements in children's overall autism severity as measured by the ADOS, parent-child interaction, expressive language skills, and adaptive skills.
Hardan et al. (2015)	Parents were taught behavioral techniques to facilitate their child's language development as part of a Pivotal Response Therapy Group (PRTG).	Parents were able to successfully learn in a PRTG format. Children in the PRTG showed increased improvement in frequency of utterances and adaptive communication skills.
Kasari et al. (2010)	8-week intervention that used developmental procedures of responsive and facilitative interaction methods as well as aspects of applied behavior analysis. Parents were taught the following skills: following the child's lead and interest in activities, imitating child actions, talking about what the child was doing, repeating back what the child said, expanding on what the child said, giving corrective feedback, sitting close to the child and making eye-contact, and making environmental adjustments to engage the child.	Improvements in joint engagement, responsiveness to joint attention, and diversity of functional play acts.

Table 5.3 Cont.

Study	Intervention	Outcomes
Kasari et al. (2015)	Parents participated in JASPER (joint attention, symbolic play, engagement and regulation) for ten weeks.	Children experienced improvements in the primary outcome of joint engagement.
Stahmer & Gist (2001)	Assessed the effectiveness of a parent education support group in addition to an accelerated parent-education program.	Parents who participated in the parent education support group showed increased learning of teaching techniques, which led to improvement in children's language skills.
Najdowski et al. (2010)	Mothers were trained to implement differential reinforcement of alternative behavior (DRA) combined with non-removal of the spoon and demand fading for the treatment of their children's food selectivity.	Improvements in children's tolerance to different foods.
Reagon & Higbee (2009)	Three mothers of children with autism were taught to create, implement, and systematically fade scripts to promote vocal initiations during play.	Parents successfully implemented script-fading procedures in their homes and these procedures were effective in increasing children's vocal initiations during play.
Rocha et al. (2007)	Parents were trained to increase their joint attention bids using behavior analytic techniques to facilitate appropriate responding.	As parent joint attention bids increased, children's responses increased. Children's joint attention initiations also increased, even though this was not a direct target of the intervention.
Rollins et al. (2015)	Pathways Early Autism Intervention was investigated. Interventionists worked with caregivers weekly in the home. Each session included a 10-minute video of parent–child interaction.	Improvements were made in the measures of eye contact, social engagement, and verbal reciprocity.
Schertz & Odom (2007)	Parents were taught to promote joint attention in their children. The intervention consisted of four phases: focusing on faces, turn-taking, responding to joint attention, and initiating joint attention.	All children showed improvements in engagement and joint attention.
Kaiser et al. (2000)	Parents were trained to use a naturalistic teaching strategy, called Enhanced Milieu Teaching (EMT), to improve children's social-communication skills.	Positive effects were observed on the use of communication targets for all children and on the complexity and diversity of productive language for most children.

(continued)

Table 5.3 Cont.

Study	Intervention	Outcomes
Turner-Brown et al. (2019)	Parents were trained in Family Implemented TEACCH for Toddlers (FITT), which included 90-minute in-home sessions and parent group sessions.	Families in the FITT group showed decreased stress and improved well-being over time.
Wetherby et al. (2014)	Parents participated in one of two nine-month interventions within the Early Social Interaction (ESI) project. Each intervention taught parents how to embed strategies to support their child's social communication throughout everyday activities.	Children who had parents that received the intervention individually in their home 2-3 times each week developed social communication skills at a faster rate and greater improvements in receptive language.

Data extracted from Steinbrenner, J. R., Hume, K., Odom, S. L., Morin, K. L., Nowell, S. W., Tomaszewski, B., Szendrey, S., McIntyre, N. S., Yücesoy-Özkan, S., & Savage, M. N. (2020). Evidence-based practices for children, youth, and young adults with Autism. The University of North Carolina at Chapel Hill, Frank Porter Graham Child Development Institute, National Clearinghouse on Autism Evidence and Practice Review Team.

adult capitalizes on the toddler's interests and uses these strategies to naturally promote, support, and encourage the complexity of the skills, while relying on naturally reinforcing contingencies to maintain the behavior.

Pivotal Response Training (PRT) is a type of naturalistic intervention based on principles of applied behavior analysis that is particularly effective in improving communication, play, and social behaviors in young children. PRT specifically targets behaviors that are believed to be "pivotal learning variables," specifically, motivation, responding to multiple cues, and initiating social interactions. These are believed to be pivotal skills for toddlers because they provide a foundation upon which toddlers can make generalized improvements in other areas of development (see Table 5.4).

Other Focused Intervention Approaches Used with Toddlers. Interventions implemented by parents are the most commonly researched intervention practice for children under the age of three; however, researchers have begun to explore the use of other strategies to improve social-communication skills and reduce challenging behaviors for toddlers with ASD. These *focused intervention strategies* can be used by practitioners to create an eclectic intervention program for young children that can be individualized to align with child and family goals. We stress that the following list of intervention strategies did not have sufficient

Table 5.4 Naturalistic Interventions that Included Toddlers with ASD

Study	Intervention	Outcomes
Rollins et al. (2016)	Pathways Early Autism Intervention was the focus of this intervention. Interventionists conducted weekly home visits with caregivers to target child skills.	The intervention was effective for supporting children's eye contact, social engagement, and verbal reciprocity.
Harrop et al. (2016)	The Joint Attention, Symbolic Play, Engagement, and Regulation (JASPER) intervention targeted social-communication and restricted and repetitive behaviors of toddlers with ASD and caregivers' responses to behaviors.	Caregivers who received one-on-one coaching in the intervention group had more successful responses to their child's behaviors.
Vernon et al. (2012)	Parents were taught to deliver a social engagement intervention focusing on Pivotal Response Treatment (PRT) to their children with autism.	Children had increased eye contact, positive affect, and verbal initiations and parents demonstrated increased positive affect and synchronous engagement.
Ingersoll (2012)	Children with ASD in the treatment group received three hours per week of Reciprocal Imitation Training (RIT) targeting object and gesture imitation for ten weeks. During RIT sessions, therapists modeled specific actions for children to imitate.	Results of this randomized control trial showed that children in the intervention group achieved more gains in joint attention initiations and social-emotional functioning.
Schertz et al. (2013)	Parent and their toddlers with autism participated in Joint Attention Mediated Learning (JAML) during weekly visits with their intervention coordinators. JAML targeted toddlers' joint attention and early communication.	Toddlers in the JAML group showed improved preverbal social communication on select measures as well as improvement on standardized language measures.
Chiang et al. (2016)	Young children with ASD and their caregivers participated twenty 60-minute sessions occurring twice each week. Intervention sessions incorporated a caregiver-mediated joint engagement intervention program combined with movement play.	The intervention group toddlers showed greater joint attention compared to the control group at the three-month follow-up.

(continued)

Table 5.4 Cont.

Study	Intervention	Outcomes
Casenhiser et al. (2015)	Families in the treatment group spent two hours of therapy per week to learn how to facilitate social interaction and social communication with their child. Caregivers also met with the therapy team every eight weeks.	Children in the treatment group demonstrated greater gains than the community treatment group in mean length of utterances, number of utterances produced, and various speech act categories.
Shire et al. (2017)	In this randomized control trial, 113 children with ASD participated in the JASPER intervention or a waitlist group for ten weeks. Intervention was delivered by teaching assistants in public early intervention.	Young children receiving the JASPER intervention showed significant gains over the control group in joint engagement, joint attention, and play skills.
Landa et al. (2011)	Fifty-six toddlers with ASD received either the Interpersonal Synchrony or Non-Interpersonal Synchrony interventions for ten hours each week in the classroom. Interpersonal Synchrony group targeted social outcomes.	Toddlers in the Interpersonal Synchrony group showed significant comparative gains in socially engaged imitation, joint attention, and shared positive affect.
Pickles et al. (2016)	Young children with autism and their parents were randomized to the Preschool Autism Communication Trial (PACT) intervention targeting social communication in center and home environments.	Children receiving the PACT intervention showed long-term reduction in autism symptoms across social communication and restricted and repetitive behaviors.
Turner-Brown et al. (2019)	Toddlers with ASD and their parents participated in a six-month Family Implemented TEACCH for Toddlers (FITT) intervention including both in-home sessions and parent group sessions.	Participants in the intervention group showed improvements in parent stress and well-being and children's social communication skills.
Ingersoll et al. (2005)	Young children with ASD engaged in a Development, social-pragmatic (DSP) intervention targeting interactions with therapists in center-based settings. Intervention also included generalization of skills to parents in the home.	After the intervention, children demonstrated increased use of spontaneous speech with their therapists and their parents (parents were not trained in the intervention).

Table 5.4 Cont.

Study	Intervention	Outcomes
Kaiser et al. (2000)	Parents were trained to use a naturalistic teaching strategy, called Enhanced Milieu Teaching (EMT), to improve social-communication skills for children with ASD.	Positive effects were observed on the use of communication targets for all children and on the complexity and diversity of productive language for most children.
Nefdt et al. (2010)	Parents in the treatment group took part in a self-directed learning program (SDLP) addressing the use of PRT to increase child motivation to engage in social communication.	Compared to control group results, participants in the treatment group showed greater parent language opportunities, child verbal utterances, and parent confidence.

Data extracted from Steinbrenner, J. R., Hume, K., Odom, S. L., Morin, K. L., Nowell, S. W., Tomaszewski, B., Szendrey, S., McIntyre, N. S., Yücesoy-Özkan, S., & Savage, M. N. (2020). Evidence-based practices for children, youth, and young adults with Autism. The University of North Carolina at Chapel Hill, Frank Porter Graham Child Development Institute, National Clearinghouse on Autism Evidence and Practice Review Team.

research to qualify as evidence-based practices for toddlers according to NCAEP criteria; however, they have some preliminary research that shows promise for promoting positive outcomes for children with ASD under the age of three. Examples of how these strategies may relate to toddlers is presented here and more information about these strategies can be found in Chapter 9 (unless otherwise noted):

- *Reinforcement.* The consequences that occur after a toddler engages in a desired behavior can increase the likelihood that the behavior will reoccur in the future. These consequences may be purposefully manipulated by an adult but can also occur naturally in the environment. Examples of positive reinforcement for the young child may include praise, tickles, or access to preferred toys. Negative reinforcement may involve the toddler taking off his coat, thereby removing the uncomfortable feeling of being too hot.
- *Prompting.* Prompts can take different forms depending on the skill being taught and the toddler's learning style. Common forms of prompting for toddlers include physical (i.e., hand-over-hand guidance), verbal (i.e., telling the child more information to demonstrate the behavior), visual (i.e., using picture cues), and gestural assistance (i.e., pointing).
- *Time Delay*: Time delay is useful for systematically fading prompts for toddlers and is always used in conjunction with prompting

procedures. With this practice, an adult may provide a child with an instruction and then include a brief delay before providing any additional instruction or prompts.

- *Modeling.* Modeling is a procedure that involves correctly performing a target behavior so that a young child may acquire the behavior. This strategy can support toddlers with learning a variety of skills, such as putting on clothing, using new words, or engaging in positive interactions.
- *Video Modeling.* Some research has used video technology to teach toddlers a new skill. An adult shows the toddler a video of someone performing the target behavior and the toddler is then given an opportunity to practice the skill they watched in the video.
- *Augmentative and Alternative Communication (AAC)*: These interventions teach children to use aided or unaided communication systems in lieu of verbal/vocal forms of communications. Sign language, Picture Exchange Communication System® (PECS®; Bondy & Frost, 2001), speech generating devices, and applications that allow other devices (i.e., tablets), are common choices for supporting toddlers' communication (more information about AAC is provided in Chapter 8).
- *Functional Behavior Assessment.* Challenging behaviors are believed to have a communicative function. Toddlers may engage in challenging behaviors in order to obtain something (i.e., parent's attention; access to a desired item) or escape undesired activities or parental demands. Functional Behavior Assessment (FBA) provides a systematic way for professionals to determine the underlying function of a challenging behavior, create a hypothesis about why the toddler engages in the challenging behavior, and develop an effective behavior intervention plan to decrease or eliminate the challenging behavior.
- *Antecedent-Based Interventions.* Antecedent-Based Interventions (ABI) involve an adult modifying environmental conditions that are believed to elicit a toddler's challenging behavior. The types of modifications used in ABI for toddlers may include incorporating choices in undesired activities, modifying the child's schedule, enriching the environment to provide additional cues for appropriate behavior (i.e., visual supports), or access to additional materials.

Challenges for Accessing Early Intervention Services

Prior to receiving early intervention services, children need to be diagnosed with a disability or identified as having a delay in one or more developmental domains. The American Academy of Pediatrics recommends that young children are screened twice for autism before the age of 24 months, at the 9–18 and 24–30 month well baby check visits

(Johnson & Myers, 2007). Researchers have documented children with ASD who may demonstrate developmental differences when compared to neurotypical children in the first year of life (Zwaigenbaum et al., 2013). Over the past two decades, researchers have made significant advances in developing reliable screening measures to detect ASD in children as young as 14 months (Deitz et al., 2006; Dumont-Mathieu & Fein, 2005; Stone et al., 2008). Yet, despite the greater availability of reliable ASD-specific and broader developmental delay screening measures, ASD diagnosis is often delayed until children are in preschool (Mandell et al., 2005; Shattuck et al., 2009; Wiggins, et al., 2006), though children's age of diagnosis is decreasing over time (Daniels & Mandell, 2014). Various studies have noted that parents' concerns about their children almost always arise before or around the second year of age (Chawarska et al., 2007; Hess & Landa, 2012) and are predictive of children later receiving a diagnosis (Ozonoff et al., 2009). Nonetheless, the gap between initial parental concern and receipt of diagnosis continues to be wide (Kozlowski et al., 2011; Zuckerman et al., 2015). Delay in diagnosis hinders young children from benefiting from critical opportunities for early intervention, which not only fosters optimal development, but also decreases lifelong care costs (Peters-Scheffer et al., 2012; Warren & Stone, 2011; Zwaigenbaum et al., 2015).

As methods for earlier detection become available, infants diagnosed with ASD or flagged at risk for ASD, and their parents, may likewise benefit from early intervention (Landa, 2018). Because of the complex etiology of ASD (multiple areas of developmental needs), intensive early intervention is recommended to ensure that children's development is maximized. While the need for intensive early intervention is documented, there is often a long wait for these interventions due to the demands of these services. These wait times vary from an average of nine months to three years, with younger children, and their families, enduring longer wait times (Dimian et al., 2021; Yingling et al., 2018). Some families might choose to pay out of pocket or seek insurance coverage for private services, which can be costly. While many families resort to waiting until services become available, many others choose to receive less intensive early intervention services until a diagnosis is made (Monteiro et al., 2016).

It is important to highlight the need for collaborative efforts when providing support for young children. As mentioned earlier in this chapter, children with ASD, and their families, often require services from a team of professionals, including speech and language therapists, occupational therapists, physical therapists, as well as early developmental pediatricians and psychologists. It is critical that service providers work together to create the best intervention approach for the young child and their family (Division for Early Childhood (DEC, 2014)). Though the importance of interdisciplinary intervention to ensure children with ASD are receiving services required, communications among the key contributors to the intervention plan is often lacking. Additionally, the field of early intervention needs to train their providers to be competent in serving families from diverse linguistic and cultural backgrounds (Lee et al., 2003). Early intervention providers who are culturally competent actively reflect on how individual families' backgrounds affect children's development and behavior as well as how their own values and beliefs impact their service delivery. To the extent possible, a "match" between the provider and a family should be targeted. This "match" in cultural and linguistic compatibility will support professionals in maximizing family strengths when identifying and delivering early intervention services.

One of the major challenges of early intervention services for children with ASD is the involvement of families and caregivers in the intervention services provided. While family-centered practices are the key to ensure successful and effective early intervention services (DEC, 2014), many barriers are present that make family-centered early intervention practices difficult. For instance, families may see the service delivery time as a respite time for them, thus removing themselves from fully participating in the intervention sessions. Additionally, families may carry the belief that the professionals know what is best for their children, thus minimizing the importance of their expertise in their children during service delivery. Likewise, practitioners may need to develop skills necessary to support families with participating in early intervention services in a meaningful way (Bradshaw, 2013). Early intervention professionals must acknowledge and support families' strengths and their critical role in these services and empower families to fully participate in all aspects of early intervention services for their children with ASD.

At the IFSP meeting, Samuel's caregivers talked about their strengths, their concerns for Samuel, and their hopes and dreams for his growth and development. Again, an interpreter was present to support the team. In their conversation with the practitioners, Samuel's caregivers chose outcomes for their family and to support Samuel's communication and play skills. Together, the team decided that the Educator and Speech Language Pathologist would make weekly visits to the family's home to support the family with working towards their chosen goals, such as supporting mealtimes and play with his siblings. The team discussed how visits would be conducted, with the practitioners spending most of their home visit time supporting the family members in their interactions with Samuel instead of working with him directly. They talked about using Naturalistic Interventions, which the family would be able to incorporate into their daily routines and activities based on Samuel's interests. They also discussed using Parent-Implemented Interventions, so Samuel's caregivers could choose which strategies they might like to learn to use during mealtimes between home visit sessions to help them enjoy this routine together as a family.

Conclusion

As the field of early intervention and early childhood special education advances in their techniques to enhance the screening practice and early identification of children with ASD, early intervention professionals are also tasked with the responsibility of providing intervention practices that are beneficial in supporting children's development and family outcomes. Early intervention professionals must capitalize on family strengths and professional collaboration to create an intervention plan that best meets the needs of the families and children with ASD.

Discussion Questions

1. What role might the family play in supporting their young child with ASD through the diagnosis process, selecting intervention approaches in EI, and implementing EI services?
2. Which evidence-based intervention strategies are most featured in research for supporting outcomes for children from birth to three-years-old with ASD? In what ways are these strategies well-suited for addressing the needs of young children?

References

Aldred, C., Green, J., & Adams, C. (2004). A new social communication intervention for children with autism: Pilot randomized controlled treatment study suggesting effectiveness. *Journal of Child Psychology and Psychiatry, 45*(8), 1420–1430.

American Academy of Pediatrics (2006). Understanding autism spectrum disorders. Elk Grove, IL: Author.

American Academy of Pediatrics (2007, October 29). New AAP reports help pediatricians identify and manage autism earlier. Retrieved from www.aap.org

American Occupational Therapy Association. (2010). The scope of occupational therapy services for individuals with an autism spectrum disorder across the life course. *American Journal of Occupational Therapy, 64*, 125–136.

American Speech-Language-Hearing Association (n.d.). Early Intervention. (Practice Portal). Retrieved November 05, 2021 from www.asha.org/Practice-Portal/Professional-Issues/Early-Intervention/.

Bondy, A., & Frost, L. (2001). The picture exchange communication system. *Behavior Modification, 25*(5), 725–744.

Bradshaw, W. (2013). A framework for providing culturally responsive early intervention services. *Young Exceptional Children*, 16(1), 3–15.

Briggs-Gowan, M. J., & Carter, A. S. (2007). Applying the infant-toddler social & emotional assessment (ITSEA) and brief-ITSEA in early intervention. *Infant Mental Health Journal*, 28(6), 564-583.

Bruder, M. B. (2000). Family-centered early intervention: Clarifying our values for the new millennium. *Topics in Early Childhood Special Education*, 20(2), 105–115.

Casenhiser, D. M., Binns, A., McGill, F., Morderer, O., & Shanker, S. G. (2015). Measuring and supporting language function for children with autism: Evidence from a randomized control trial of a social-interaction-based therapy. *Journal of Autism and Developmental Disorders*, 45(3), 846–857.

Chawarska, K., Paul, R., Klin, A., Hannigen, S., Dichtel, L., & Volkmar, F. (2007). Parental recognition of developmental problems in toddlers with autism spectrum disorders. *Journal of Autism and Developmental Disorders*, 37(1), 62–72.

Chiang, C. H., Chu, C. L., & Lee, T. C. (2016). Efficacy of caregiver-mediated joint engagement intervention for young children with autism spectrum disorders. *Autism*, 20(2), 172–182.

Chiarello, L., & Effgen, S. K. (2006). Updated competencies for physical therapists working in early intervention. *Pediatric Physical Therapy*, 18(2), 148–158.

Clark, G. F., Laverdure, P., Polichino, J., & Kannenberg, K. (2017). Guidelines for occupational therapy services in early intervention and schools. *AJOT: American Journal of Occupational Therapy*, 71(S2), 7112410010p1–7112410010p1.

Daniels, A. M., & Mandell, D. S. (2014). Explaining differences in age at autism spectrum disorder diagnosis: A critical review. *Autism*, 18(5), 583–597.

Dawson, G. (2008). Early behavioral intervention, brain plasticity, and the prevention of autism spectrum disorder. *Development and Psychopathology*, 20(03), 775–803.

Dawson, G., Jones, E. J., Merkle, K., Venema, K., Lowy, R., Faja, S., ... & Webb, S. J. (2012). Early behavioral intervention is associated with normalized brain activity in young children with autism. *Journal of the American Academy of Child & Adolescent Psychiatry*, 51(11), 1150–1159.

Dietz, C., Willemsen-Swinkels, S. H. N., van Daalen, E., van Engeland, H., & Buitelaar, J.K. (2006). Screening for Autistic Spectrum Disorder in children aged 14 to 15 Months. II: Population screening with the Early Screening of Autistic Traits (ESAT). Design and general findings. *Journal of Autism and Developmental Disorders*, 36, 713–722.

Dimian, A. F., Symons, F. J., & Wolff, J. J. (2021). Delay to early intensive behavioral intervention and educational outcomes for a Medicaid-enrolled cohort of children with autism. *Journal of Autism and Developmental Disorders*, 51(4), 1054–1066.

Division for Early Childhood. (2014). DEC RPs in early intervention/early childhood special education. Retrieved from www.dec-sped.org/recommendedpr actices

Dumont-Mathieu, T., & Fein, D. (2005). Screening for autism in young children: The modified checklist for Autism in toddlers (M-CHAT) and other measures. *Mental Retardation and Developmental Disabilities Research Reviews*, 11(3), 253–262.

Dunst, C. J., Johanson, C., Trivette, C. M., & Hamby, D. (1991). Family-oriented early intervention policies and practices: Family-centered or not?. *Exceptional children*, 58(2), 115–126.

Espe-Sherwindt, M. (2008). Family-centred practice: collaboration, competency and evidence. *Support for learning*, 23(3), 136–143.

Fombonne, E., & Zuckerman, K. E. (2021). Clinical profiles of Black and White children referred for autism diagnosis. *Journal of Autism and Developmental Disorders*, 1–11.

Green, J., Charman, T., McConachie, H., Aldred, C., Slonims, V., Howlin, P., … Pickles, A. (2010). Parent- mediated communication- focused treatment in children with autism (PACT): A randomized controlled trial. *The Lancet*, 375(9732), 2152–2160.

Hardan, A. Y., Gengoux, G. W., Berquist, K. L., Libove, R. A., Ardel, C. M., Phillips, J., Frazier, T. W., & Minjarez, M. B. (2015). A randomized controlled trial of Pivotal Response Treatment Group for parents of children with autism. *Journal of Child Psychology and Psychiatry and Allied Disciplines*, 56(8), 884–892. https://doi.org/10.1111/jcpp.12354

Harrop, C., Gulsrud, A., Shih, W., Hovsepyan, L., & Kasari, C. (2017). The impact of caregiver-mediated JASPER on child restricted and repetitive behaviors and caregiver responses. *Autism Research*, 10(5), 983–992.

Hess, C., & Landa, R. (2012). Predictive and concurrent validity of parent concern about young children at risk for autism. *Journal of Autism & Developmental Disorders*, 42(4), 575–584.

Hume, K., Bellini, S., & Pratt, C. (2005). The usage and perceived outcomes of early intervention and early childhood programs for young children with autism spectrum disorder. *Topics in Early Childhood Special Education*, 25(4), 195–207.

Hume, K., Steinbrenner, J. R., Odom, S. L., Morin, K. L., Nowell, S. W., Tomaszewski, B., … & Savage, M. N. (2021). Evidence-based practices for children, youth, and young adults with autism: Third generation review. *Journal of Autism and Developmental Disorders*, 1–20.

Ingersoll, B. (2012). Brief report: Effect of a focused imitation intervention on social functioning in children with autism. *Journal of Autism and Developmental Disorders*, 42(8), 1768–1773.

Ingersoll, B., Dvortcsak, A., Whalen, C., & Sikora, D. (2005). The effects of a developmental, social-pragmatic language intervention on rate of expressive language production in young children with autistic spectrum disorders. *Focus on Autism and Other Developmental Disabilities*, 20(4), 213–222.

Johnson, C. P., & Myers, S. M. (2007). Identification and evaluation of children with autism spectrum disorders. *Pediatrics*, 120(5), 1183–1215.

Kaiser, A. P., Hancock, T. B., & Nietfeld, J. P. (2000). The effects of parent- implemented enhanced milieu teaching on the social communication of children who have autism. *Early Education & Development*, 11(4), 423–446.

Kasari, C., Gulsrud, A., Paparella, T., Hellemann, G., & Berry, K. (2015). Randomized comparative efficacy study of parent-mediated interventions for toddlers with autism. *Journal of Consulting and Clinical Psychology, 83*(3), 554–563. https://doi.org/10.1037/a0039080

Kasari, C., Gulsrud, A. C., Wong, C., Kwon, S., & Locke, J. (2010). Randomized controlled caregiver mediated joint engagement intervention for toddlers with autism. *Journal of Autism and Developmental Disorders, 40*(9), 1045–1056.

Kong, H. K., Lee, J., & Karahalios, K. (2017). A comparative study of visualizations with different granularities of behavior for communicating about autism. *Proceedings of the ACM on Human-Computer Interaction, 1*(CSCW), 1–16.

Kozlowski, A. M., Matson, J. L., Horovitz, M., Worley, J. A., & Neal, D. (2011). Parents' first concerns of their child's development in toddlers with autism spectrum disorders. *Developmental Neurorehabilitation, 14*(2), 72–78.

Krug, D. A., Arick, J. R., & Almond, P. J. (1980). Behavior checklist for identifying severely handicapped individuals with high levels of autistic behavior. *Journal of Child Psychology and Psychiatry, 21*, 221–229.

Landa, R. J. (2018). Efficacy of early interventions for infants and young children with, and at risk for, autism spectrum disorders. *International Review of Psychiatry, 30*(1), 25–39.

Landa, R. J., Holman, K. C., O'Neill, A. H., & Stuart, E. A. (2011). Intervention targeting development of socially synchronous engagement in toddlers with autism spectrum disorder: A randomized controlled trial. *Journal of Child Psychology and Psychiatry, 52*(1), 13–21.

Lee, H., Ostrosky, M. M., Bennett, T., & Fowler, S. A. (2003). Perspectives of early intervention professionals about culturally-appropriate practices. *Journal of Early Intervention, 25*(4), 281–295.

Lord, C., Risi, S., DiLavore, P. S., Shulman, C., Thurm, A., & Pickles, A. (2006). Autism from 2 to 9 years of age. *Arch Gen Psychiatry, 63*(6), 694–701.

Mandell, D., Novak, M., & Zubritsky, C. (2005). Factors associated with age of diagnosis among children with autism spectrum disorders. *Pediatrics, 116*(6), 1480–1486.

Mandell, D. S., Wiggins, L. D., Carpenter, L. A., Daniels, J., DiGuiseppi, C., Durkin, M. S., ... & Kirby, R. S. (2009). Racial/ethnic disparities in the identification of children with autism spectrum disorders. *American Journal of Public Health, 99*(3), 493–498.

Marcus, L., Schopler, L., & Lord, C. (2000). TEACCH services for preschool children. In J. Handleman & S. Harris (Eds.), *Preschool education programs for children with autism* (2nd ed., pp. 215–232). Austin, TX: PRO-ED.

Monteiro, S. A., Dempsey, J., Broton, S., Berry, L., Goin-Kochel, R. P., & Voigt, R. G. (2016). Early intervention before autism diagnosis in children referred to a regional autism clinic. *Journal of Developmental & Behavioral Pediatrics, 37*(1), 15–19.

Najdowski, A. C., Wallace, M. D., Reagon, K., Penrod, B., Higbee, T. S., & Tarbox, J. (2010). Utilizing a home- based parent training approach in the treatment of food selectivity. *Behavioral Interventions, 25*(2), 89–107.

National Research Council. (2001). *Educating children with autism.* Committee on Educational Interventions for Children with Autism. C. Lord & J. P. McGee (Eds.). Washington DC: National Academy Press, Division of Behavioral and Social Sciences and Education.

Nefdt, N., Koegel, R., Singer, G., & Gerber, M. (2010). The use of a self-directed learning program to provide introductory training in pivotal response treatment to parents of children with autism. *Journal of Positive Behavior Interventions, 12*(1), 23–32.

Odom, S. L., Boyd, B., Hall, L., & Hume, K. (2010). Evaluation of comprehensive treatment models for individuals with autism spectrum disorders. *Journal of Autism and Developmental Disorders, 40,* 425–436.

Ozonoff, S., Young, G. S., Steinfeld, M., Hill, M. M., Cook, I., Hutman, T., & ... Sigman, M. (2009). How early do parent concerns predict later autism diagnosis?. *Journal of Developmental and Behavioral Pediatrics, 30*(5), 367–375.

Peters-Scheffer, N., Didden, R., Korzilius, H., & Matson, J. (2012). Cost comparison of early intensive behavioral intervention and treatment as usual for children with autism spectrum disorder in The Netherlands. *Research in Developmental Disabilities, 33*(6), 1763–1772.

Pickles, A., Le Couteur, A., Leadbitter, K., Salomone, E., Cole-Fletcher, R., Tobin, H., ... & Green, J. (2016). Parent-mediated social communication therapy for young children with autism (PACT): Long-term follow-up of a randomised controlled trial. *The Lancet, 388*(10059), 2501–2509.

Reagon, K. A., & Higbee, T. S. (2009). Parent- implemented script fading to promote play- based verbal initiations in children with autism. *Journal of Applied Behavior Analysis, 42*(3), 659–664.

Robins, D. L., Fein, D., & Barton, M. (2009). Modified Checklist for Autism in Toddlers, Revised, with Follow-Up (M-CHAT-R/F). Retrieved from www.autis mspeaks.org/sites/default/files/docs/sciencedocs/m-chat/m-chat-r_f.pdf?v=1

Rocha, M. L., Schreibman, L., & Stahmer, A. C. (2007). Effectiveness of training parents to teach joint attention in children with autism. *Journal of Early Intervention, 29*(2), 154–173.

Rogers, S. J. (1999). Intervention for Young Children with Autism: From Research to Practice. *Infants & Young Children, 12*(2), 1–16.

Rogers, S. J., Hall, T., Osaki, D., Reaven, J., & Herbison, J. (2000). The Denver Model: A comprehensive, integrated educational approach to young children with autism and their families. In J. Handleman & S. Harris (Eds.), *Preschool education programs for children with autism* (2nd ed., pp. 95–135). Austin, TX: PRO-ED.

Rollins, P. R., Campbell, M., Hoffman, R. T., & Self, K. (2016). A community-based early intervention program for toddlers with autism spectrum disorders. *Autism, 20*(2), 219–32. https://doi.org/10.1177/1362361315577217

Schertz, H. H., & Odom, S. L. (2007). Promoting joint attention in toddlers with autism: A parent- mediated developmental model. *Journal of Autism and Developmental Disorders, 37*(8), 1562–1575.

Schertz, H. H., Odom, S. L., Baggett, K. M., & Sideris, J. H. (2013). Effects of joint attention mediated learning for toddlers with autism spectrum disorders: An initial randomized controlled study. *Early Childhood Research Quarterly, 28*(2), 249–258.

Schultz, T. R. (2013). *Parent-implemented intervention (PII) fact sheet.* Chapel Hill: The University of North Carolina, Frank Porter Graham Child Development Institute, The National Professional Development Center on Autism Spectrum Disorders. Retrieved from http://autismpdc.fpg.unc.edu/ sites/autismpdc.fpg.unc.edu/files/Parent_Implemented_factsheet.pdf

Shattuck, P. T., Durkin, M., Maenner, M., Newschaffer, C., Mandell, D. S., Wiggins, L., & … Cuniff, C. (2009). Timing of identification among children with an autism spectrum disorder: Findings from a population-based surveillance study. *Journal of the American Academy of Child & Adolescent Psychiatry, 48*(5), 474–483.

Shire, S. Y., Chang, Y. C., Shih, W., Bracaglia, S., Kodjoe, M., & Kasari, C. (2017). Hybrid implementation model of community-partnered early intervention for toddlers with autism: A randomized trial. *Journal of Child Psychology and Psychiatry, 58*(5), 612–622.

Smith, T., Groen, A. D., & Wynn, J. W. (2000). Randomized trial of intensive early intervention for children with pervasive developmental disorders. *American Journal on Mental Retardation, 105,* 269–285.

Squires, J., Bricker, D. D., & Twombly, E. (2009). *Ages & stages questionnaires: A parent-completed child monitoring system.* Paul H. Brooks Publishing Company.

Stahmer, A. C., & Gist, K. (2001). The effects of an accelerated parent education program on technique mastery and child outcome. *Journal of Positive Behavior Interventions, 3*(2), 75.

Steinbrenner, J. R., Hume, K., Odom, S. L., Morin, K. L., Nowell, S. W., Tomaszewski, B., Szendrey, S., McIntyre, N. S., Yücesoy-Özkan, S., & Savage, M. N. (2020). Evidence-based practices for children, youth, and young adults with Autism. The University of North Carolina at Chapel Hill, Frank Porter Graham Child Development Institute, National Clearinghouse on Autism Evidence and Practice Review Team.

Stone, W. L., McMahon, C. R., & Henderson, L. M. (2008). Use of the screening tool for autism in two-year-olds (STAT) for children under 24 months: An exploratory study. *Autism, 12*(5), 557–573.

Strain, P. S., & Hoyson, M. (2000). On the need for longitudinal, intensive social skill intervention: LEAP follow-up outcomes for children with autism as a case-in-point. *Topics in Early Childhood Special Education, 20*(2), 116–122.

Sullivan, K., Stone, W. L., & Dawson, G. (2014). Potential neural mechanisms underlying the effectiveness of early intervention for children with autism spectrum disorder. *Research in Developmental Disabilities, 35*(11), 2921–2932.

Turner-Brown, L., Hume, K., Boyd, B. A., & Kainz, K. (2016). Preliminary efficacy of family implemented TEACCH for toddlers: Effects on parents and their toddlers with autism spectrum disorder. *Journal of Autism and Developmental Disorders, 49*(7), 2685–2698. https://doi.org/10.1007/ s10803-016-2812-7

Vernon, T. W., Koegel, R. L., Dauterman, H., & Stolen, K. (2012). An early social engagement intervention for young children with autism and their parents. *Journal of Autism and Developmental Disorders, 42*(12), 2702–2717.

Warren, Z., & Stone, W. L. (2011). Why is early intervention important in ASC?. In S. Bölte, J. Hallmayer (Eds.), *Autism spectrum conditions: FAQs on autism, Asperger syndrome, and atypical autism answered by international experts* (pp. 167–169). Cambridge, MA US: Hogrefe Publishing.

Wetherby, A. M., Guthrie, W., Woods, J., Schatschneider, C., Holland, R. D., Morgan, L., & Lord, C. (2014). Parent-implemented social intervention for toddlers with autism: An RCT. *Pediatrics, 134*(6), 1084–1093. https://doi.org/ 10.1542/peds.2014-0757

Wetherby, A. M., & Prizant, B. M. (2002). *Communication and symbolic behavior scales: Developmental profile.* Paul H Brookes Publishing.

Wetherby, A., Woods, J., Allen, L., Cleary, J., Dickinson, H., & Lord, C. (2004). Early indicators of autism spectrum disorders in the second year of life. *Journal of Autism and Developmental Disorders, 34,* 473–493. Based on research at the Florida State University FIRST WORDS® Project.

Wiggins, L. D., Baio, J., & Rice, C. (2006). Examination of the time between first evaluation and first autism spectrum diagnosis in a population-based sample. *Journal of Developmental and Behavioral Pediatrics, 27*(Suppl2), S79–S87.

Woods, J. J., & Wetherby, A. M. (2003). Early identification of and intervention for infants and toddlers who are at risk for autism spectrum disorder. *Language, Speech, and Hearing Services in Schools, 34*(3), 180–193.

Wong, C., Odom, S. L., Hume, K. A., Cox, A. W., Fettig, A., Kucharczyk, S., ... & Schultz, T. R. (2015). Evidence-based practices for children, youth, and young adults with autism spectrum disorder: A comprehensive review. *Journal of autism and developmental disorders, 45*(7), 1951–1966.

Workgroup on Principles and Practices in Natural Environments, OSEP TA Community of Practice: Part C Settings. (2008, March). *Agreed upon mission and key principles for providing early intervention services in natural environments.* Retrieved from http://ectacenter.org/~pdfs/topics/families/Finalmissionandprinciples3_11_08.pdf

Yingling, M. E., Hock, R. M., & Bell, B. A. (2018). Time-lag between diagnosis of autism spectrum disorder and onset of publicly-funded early intensive behavioral intervention: Do race–ethnicity and neighborhood matter?. *Journal of Autism and Developmental Disorders, 48*(2), 561–571.

Zuckerman, K. E., Lindly, O. J., & Sinche, B. K. (2015). Parental concerns, provider response, and timeliness of autism spectrum disorder diagnosis. *The Journal of Pediatrics, 166*(6), 1431–1439.

Zwaigenbaum, L., Bauman, M. L., Fein, D., Pierce, K., Buie, T., Davis, P. A., ... & Wagner, S. (2015). Early screening of autism spectrum disorder: recommendations for practice and research. *Pediatrics, 136*(Supplement 1), S41–S59.

Zwaigenbaum, L., Bryson, S., & Garon, N. (2013). Early identification of autism spectrum disorders. *Behavioural Brain Research, 251,* 133–146.

Additional Important Resources

1. Division for Early Childhood (DEC): www.dec-sped.org/

Chapter 6

Preschool Years

Christopher B. Denning,[1] Amelia K. Moody,[1]
and Margaret O'Riordan[1]
[1]University of Massachusetts Boston

Case Study

Students diagnosed with autism can be placed in many different learning environments and settings. In Ethan's case he was placed in a center-based sub-separate classroom. This is a classroom where there are nine students all on Individualized Education Plans with two teachers: one lead teacher and one paraprofessional. Ethan was involved in early intervention and then at the age of 2 years and 11 months was placed in this classroom setting in his public school district. He was in this setting until he aged out at five years old.

Like any child Ethan has his interests and specific preferred activities he likes to engage in. Ethan enjoys logos, especially movie logos like Fox, Pixar, Paramount, and Disney. He loves the movie, *Cars*. Ethan was diagnosed during early intervention with Autism Spectrum Disorder (ASD). When he is excited, he repetitively flaps his arms, makes limited eye contact, and focuses on a preferred item. Ethan has many strengths that include being able to identify all upper and lowercase letters, as well as identify and verbally name sight words. He is advanced for his age in math and literacy skills; however, he needs support in fine motor skills such as writing and utensils for eating.

His individualized education goals revolve mainly around self-regulation and readiness skills. In the classroom, structure and consistency are key for Ethan. He has a visual schedule to know what his day will look like, along with getting a five-minute and two-minute warning to the next transition. This is essential for Ethan because he may bolt from the classroom or flop on the floor when he is leaving a preferred activity. To help with behavior, Ethan receives six hours a week of ABA (Applied Behavior Analysis). He works with the ABA instructor to help find strategies to increase his positive behavior and decrease negative behavior. The strategies used in ABA are also used daily in the classroom when his ABA instructor is not there. For example, during rest time Ethan struggled to stay on his mat quietly, instead he tried to run from

DOI: 10.4324/9781003255147-8

the classroom, wandered the classroom, or repeated loud noises. One of Ethan's preferred items is drawing on the tablet. The teacher explained to Ethan that if he stays on his mat for two minutes (he can watch the timer) he will earn drawing on the iPad during rest time. Over time Ethan was able to increase his wait time to ten minutes, and he was able to sit quietly and patiently on his mat until the timer went off.

Knowing your student is incredibly important. By knowing Ethan's preferred activities his teacher was able to help him master a self-regulation skill he had been struggling with. Strategies and plans should be tailored to the student to help give them the motivation they need to achieve success.

Historical Perspective

Changes in the definition for ASD are affecting diagnosis and supports for young children with ASD. The most recent definition of autism by the American Psychological Association (APA, 2013) made changes that may have effects on the early childhood classroom. Evidence suggests that fewer individuals meet criteria using the newest definition for autism, especially infants and toddlers (e.g., Peters & Matson, 2020). Early childhood educators will need to closely examine these populations to ensure access to necessary supports and services.

Prevalence

Although autism was once viewed as a rare disorder, the incidence rate has increased dramatically over the past 20 years. The Center for Disease Control (Maenner et al., 2021) now estimates that 1 in 44 children have an autism spectrum disorder. This represents a current prevalence rate of over 2% in the general population and an increase of 150% from 2006 and 57% from 2012. Boys are 4.2 times more likely to be diagnosed with ASD than girls (Maenner et al., 2021). The median age of earliest known ASD diagnosis ranged from 36 months in California to 63 months in Minnesota (Maenner et al., 2021). This variation across states will impact early childhood educators. On average, 35.2% of children were assessed as having an intelligence quotient (IQ score) ≤ 70. Black (49.8%) children were more likely to be diagnosed with IQ scores ≤ 70 than Hispanic (33.1%) or White (29.7%) children (Maenner et al., 2021). It is important that research examines these variabilities to provide equitable access to assessments and services for young children.

Cultural Disparities in Identification

A recent report from the U.S. Center on Disease Control (CDC; Maenner et al., 2021) indicated that no differences were found between the number of Black and White children diagnosed with ASD. Notable differences were found for Hispanic children who were identified at a lower rate than their Black and White peers. Tek & Landa (2012) compared 84 toddlers (19 minority and 65 White) diagnosed with ASD. Results indicated that upper- and middle-class families were the largest groups regardless of ethnicity. The authors noted that cultural practices might influence communication during assessment. These findings suggest that socioeconomic status and culture should be considered when diagnosing young children with ASD (Waligórska et al., 2019). Individualized services are needed to ensure appropriate diagnosis and support are provided for families.

Services and Placement Decision Satisfaction

Early intervention services are key to addressing challenges associated with ASD. McDonald and colleagues (2019) examined special education services received by 89 children diagnosed with ASD and found that 56.2% of children with ASD received services under the autism classification. Most children received additional services, including 70.8% in speech therapy and 56.2% in occupational therapy. Only 15.7% were on behavior support plans, and 16.9% received social skills instruction. Although more young children with ASD are served in inclusive settings, the decisions vary greatly across districts and states (e.g., Kurth, 2014). Placement options should be decided by the IEP team and should occur in the least restrictive environment (LRE; IDEA, 2004).

In Ethan's case study he was diagnosed with ASD early before 2.8 years of age. When it came to start attending his district's public schools, he was assessed by the Early Intervention team and then along with his family they made the decision to enroll him in the district's sub-separate center based classroom. The decision was made based on Ethan's abilities, age, and what would be the best for Ethan's development while considering the least restrictive environment. Ethan was in this early education classroom for three years. Once he turned five, Ethan's team, including his teachers and family, met again for his Aging Out Meeting. This is a meeting where the team was able to meet again and decide what Kindergarten classroom would best meet his needs and support Ethan the best.

McIntyre & Zementic (2017) researched services and parent satisfaction in 60, 2–7-year-old children with ASD in the Northeast. Most families reported an average of 13 hours of therapy per week for older children and an average of three hours for children in birth to 3-year-old settings. Findings indicated that parents became more dissatisfied as children grew older. Inequities in services were also found because higher family income was correlated with receiving more hours of services.

Families of preschool age children should be aware that advocating for increased service hours and equitable treatment based on income is important.

Evidence-Based Practices

Evidence-Based Practices (EBPs) are instructional interventions that researchers have examined to ensure they are safe and effective for children with ASD (Wong, 2015). There are currently 27 practices that meet the criteria as an EBP and had demonstrated effects for preschool aged children with ASD (Steinbrenner et al., 2020). Table 6.1 lists each practice and the areas that have been identified as effective (e.g., academic, adaptive, behavioral, communication, play).

One must consider the child's age, range on the spectrum, and cultural needs to determine best practices. The goal is to offer teachers, service providers, and caregivers some guidance about which interventions will be most effective. EBPs can include environmental supports, behavioral supports, and instructional supports. We will highlight EBPs below that address the development in multiple areas such as social, communication, self-help, cognition, motor, and behavior/mental health and are commonly used in PreK classrooms.

Environmental Supports

The structure of a preschool environment can play an integral role in the participation of children with ASD in educational and social activities. Research indicates that children with disabilities participate less frequently in educational, social, and leisure activities than their typically developing peers (Rosenberg et al., 2013). This may be due to deficits in social and academic readiness skills. Khalifa and colleagues (2020) examined participation patterns in children with ASD and they determined that discrepancies in behavior and social skills can place children with ASD at risk for low participation.

In Ethan's classroom there were many visual aids in his classroom to help support his readiness goals. Examples of this include a visual aid to hang up his backpack and coat, a visual aid to wash his hands, and built up to a visual aid of approaching peers. Visual aids are wonderful but it is essential that teachers teach the students the visuals, it is a scaffolding tool that needs to first be learned by the student and then with consistency Ethan was able to independently follow the aids.

Classroom materials should be well organized and have picture and word labels to assist children in knowing where to find and put back materials. This promotes independence by providing visual support which can impact thinking, learning, and behavior (Hume & Turner-Brown, 2018).

Table 6.1 Evidence-Based Practices for Preschoolers with ASD

Environmental

Intervention	Positive Outcomes
Antecedent Behavior Interventions (ABI)	- Communication, social, and play - Academic readiness skills - Self-help and challenging behavior
Augmentative and Alternative Communication (AAC)	- Communication, social, joint attention, and self-help - Academic readiness skills - Challenging behavior
Naturalistic Intervention (NI)	- Communication, social, play, and joint attention skills - Cognitive and academic readiness skills - Self-help, challenging behaviors, and motor skills - Mental health
Sensory Integration (SI)	- Communication and social skills - Cognitive and academic readiness skills - Self-help, challenging behaviors, and motor skills
Visual Supports (VS)	- Communication, social, play, and joint attention skills - Academic readiness and cognitive skills - Self-help and challenging behaviors

Behavioral

Intervention	Positive Outcomes
Behavioral Momentum Intervention (BMI)	- Communication and social skills - Joint attention and play skills - Cognitive and academic readiness skills - Self-help and challenging behavior
Differential Reinforcement of Alternative, Incompatible, or Other Behavior (DR)	- Communication and social skills - Joint attention and play skills - Cognitive and academic readiness skills - Self-help, behavioral, and motor skills
Exercise and Movement (EXM)	- Communication, social, joint attention, and play skills - Cognitive and academic readiness skills - Self-help and challenging behavior - Motor skills
Extinction (EXT)	- Communication and social skills - Academic readiness skills - Self-help and challenging behaviors
Functional Behavioral Assessment (FBA)	- Academic readiness skills - Challenging behaviors
Functional Communication Training (FCT)	- Communication, social, and play skills - Academic readiness skills - Self-help and challenging behaviors
Reinforcement (R)	- Communication, social, play, and joint attention skills - Academic readiness skills - Self-help, challenging behaviors, and motor skills
Response Interruption/ Redirection (RIR)	- Communication, social, and play skills - Academic readiness skills - Self-help and challenging behaviors
Self-Management (SM)	- Cognitive skills - Academic readiness - Challenging behaviors

Table 6.1 Cont.

Environmental	
Intervention	Positive Outcomes

Instructional

Direct Instruction (DI)	- Communication, social, play, and joint attention skills - Academic readiness skills
Discrete Trial Training (DTT)	- Cognitive skills - Social, joint attention, and play skills - Self-help skills
Music-Mediated Intervention (MMI)	- Communication, social, and play skills - Academic readiness - Challenging behaviors and motor skills
Parent-Implemented Intervention (PII)	- Communication, social, play, and joint attention skills - Cognitive and academic readiness skills - Self-help, challenging behaviors, and motor skills - Mental health
Prompting (PP)	- Communication, social, play, and joint attention skills - Cognitive and academic readiness skills - Self-help, challenging behaviors, and motor skills
Social Narratives (SN)	- Communication, social, play, and joint attention skills - Academic readiness - Self-help and challenging behaviors
Social Skills Training (SST)	- Communication, social, and play skills - Cognitive - Challenging behaviors
Task Analysis (TA)	- Communication and joint attention - Self-help skills
Technology-Aided Instruction and Intervention (TAII)	- Communication, social, play, and joint attention skills - Cognitive and academic readiness skills - Self-help, challenging behaviors, and motor skills - Mental health
Time Delay (TD)	- Communication, social, play, and joint attention skills - Cognitive and academic readiness skills - Self-help, challenging behaviors, and motor skills
Video Modeling (VM)	- Communication, social, play, and joint attention skills - Academic readiness skills - Self-help, challenging behaviors, and motor skills
Modeling (MD)	- Communication, social, joint attention, and play skills - Academic readiness skills - Self-help, behavioral, and motor skills
Peer-Based Instruction and Interventions (PBII)	- Communication, social, play, and joint attention skills - Academic readiness skills

Antecedent-based Interventions (ABI)

ABIs are changes made to the environment that can change the learners' behaviors (Steinbrenner et al, 2020). These can include picture schedules, individual workspaces, preferred activities, choice, and sensory equipment. ABIs are used alongside other EBPs such as reinforcement and extinction and can assist with improving outcomes in communication, social, and play skills; school readiness and pre-academic skills; and self-help and challenging behaviors (Steinbrenner et al., 2020).

Augmentative and Alternative Communication (AAC)

AAC teaches the use of communication systems such as voice output devices, picture exchange, or the use of gestures so children who are nonverbal or developing verbal skills can communicate (Steinbrenner et al., 2020). For example, a teacher might ask yes/no questions to a child who has to respond by pressing a yes or no image on an iPad.

Naturalistic Interventions

Strategies employed in natural routines that promote the development of academic and behavioral skills (Steinbrenner et al., 2020) that are embedded in typical activities and/or routines in which the learner participates to naturally promote, support, and encourage target skills/behaviors. For example, a teacher might pass out playdough to two children but wait for the third child to ask for help before sharing playdough to promote communication.

Visual Supports

A support that is visual in nature and allows the learner to engage and learn new skills without additional prompts (Steinbrenner et al., 2020). One example would be the use of an activity schedule. Activity schedules can help children organize their day, plan for changes in their routine, support transitions, and complete tasks by augmenting expressive and receptive language abilities (e.g., Akers et al., 2016). Ethan had an activity schedule that helped him anticipate transitions. For students with ASD transitions can be a challenging time. Ethan was able to better transition after consistency with a visual schedule.

Schedules provide a visual warning prior to transitions and help students plan for the day's events. By letting students know what will happen in advance, teachers can help reduce anxiety and allow students time to prepare for an activity. These supports help to promote children's functional independence and decrease their disruptive behaviors (Kimball et al., 2003). For example, Dettmer and colleagues (2000) utilized a visual schedule, a sub schedule that consisted of a finished box routine, and a Time Timer™ to support appropriate behavior and work completion. The finished box was used during independent work sessions. It consisted of 3 x 5-inch note cards that described instructions and a coffee can with a slot in the top that was large enough for the card to slide through when the task was completed. Results indicated that transition times decreased, and the intervention reduced the need for physical and verbal prompts. The target child's mother also reported starting visual schedules at home after noting the success in school.

Behavioral Supports

Behavioral supports are designed to prevent or reduce disruptive or repetitive behaviors using EBPs. Challenging behaviors can serve as barriers to educational progress. It is important the educator, caregivers, and service providers understand how to address these behaviors to ensure progress. Understanding ways to support young learners is critical to ensure positive outcomes.

Behavioral Momentum Intervention

Behavioral Momentum Intervention is an effective antecedent strategy that increases compliant behavior by using a series of high probability requests to increase compliance with lower probability requests (Steinbrenner et al., 2020). A teacher might gain eye contact with a student and make a low demand request such as, "Please wash your hands". This is a simple request, so the student complies and gets positive feedback. Once a positive behavioral pattern is in place for easy tasks the teacher might ask for lower probability tasks such as, "Sit down because it is time for math". The child will be more likely to respond in a positive manner since he complied with easy tasks and got positive feedback.

Functional Communication Training (FCT)

This is a process that aims to replace difficult behaviors with more appropriate communication that can achieve the same outcome. This can be verbal or non-verbal (e.g., AAC). For example, a teacher might offer a goldfish to a child. The child may scream and throw the snack on the floor if he does not want it. If this is replaced with a yes/no card, the child can convey that he doesn't want the snack and the behavior will be eliminated.

Reinforcement

Positive reinforcement is an event or activity that occurs after the target behavior and increases the likelihood of the behavior occurring again in the future (Wong et al., 2015). Whether it is a positive comment, fist bump, or a tangible reward, it can assist children in understanding what they are doing right. For example, teachers and parents can state what a child is doing correctly and why. For example, "Nice sitting." Increasing the frequency of positive reinforcement can increase desirable behaviors.

Sensory Integration

This approach offers sensory experiences (visual, auditory, tactile, and vestibular) to assist children with sensory processing issues ways to respond using positive behavior Interventions that target a person's ability to integrate sensory information (visual, auditory, tactile, proprioceptive, and vestibular) from their body and environment to respond using organized and adaptive behavior.

Instructional Supports

Teachers face several challenges in educating young children with ASD. Strain et al. (2011) suggested that teachers need to be able to identify the instructional needs of students, develop plans to support identified needs, match interventions to instructional needs, evaluate progress, and adjust programs to ensure success. The last phase is crucial as it supports on-going needs and monitors progress. Potential areas to consider for change include ensuring that the intervention is implemented with fidelity, exploring varying types of reinforcement, adjusting the intensity of the intervention, or changing the intervention or strategy being used.

Choice

Choice can be highly motivating, increase the likelihood of task completion, and reduce disruptions for young children with ASD (Koegel et al., 2010). Koegel and colleagues (2010) utilized choice, embedding reinforcers within tasks, and interspersing maintenance tasks to increase motivation and assignment completion. Choice included materials (e.g., type of pen, color) and setting (i.e., where would you like to sit?). In our case study, Ethan preferred Fox, Pixar, Paramount, and Disney so these materials could be used to increase his engagement (e.g., a Pixar pen). Embedding reinforcement included having a child write about playing outside and then playing outside when the task was completed or completing math problems using Cheerios and then eating the Cheerios when the problems were completed. Results indicated decreases in latency to begin tasks, increases in task completion, and decreases in disruptive behavior. Choice has been used to increase language use. Choice has been used to support social interactions and can increase motivation to participate and support generalization of learned skills to other settings. Vitello et al. (2012) observed the use of choice and found children were more engaged in free choice activities when compared to teacher directed activities. Therefore, offering a balance of activities is important.

Common Interests

Common interests can build engagement by offering choice. Harrop et al. (2019) examined 246 articles on the use of special interests in improving outcomes for children with ASD. Thirty-one studies were eligible for inclusion. Common interests utilized were TV shows or movies (N = 21), popular characters (N = 18), computers/video games (N = 12) and transportation (N = 11). Results suggested that the inclusion of choice within interventions can lead to positive effects across several domains. In the case of Ethan, his teacher took the time to understand and talk with him about his interests. This allowed his teacher to build rapport and motivational activities for him.

Prompting

Prompts are defined as visual/pictorial, gestural, verbal, or physical supports provided to learners by an adult or peer before they attempt to perform the target behavior or skill to help them complete the skill successfully (Wong et al., 2015). Prompts are ordered from least to most intrusive. Teachers should focus on the least intrusive prompt to support a child in completing tasks. Visual prompts include picture cues that represent an action to be completed, such as eating. Gestural prompts involve pointing to or touching an object to indicate a child should perform a skill. Verbal prompts include an oral cue such as "Say, yes." Physical prompts range from full physical support where an adult uses hand over hand assistance to help a child complete an activity.

Ethan was scaffolded by both visual and verbal prompting regularly. When trying to engage with peers or other teachers, Ethan's teacher would prompt him with a consistent phrase. For example, if Ethan wanted to play with a train at Center time but another student was already using it, instead of Ethan trying to take it by force or flopping to the ground. His teacher would say "Say, can I have a turn please?". The teacher would also support the other student in his response as well as prepare Ethan for the response that came.

Modeling (MD)

Modeling is a useful intervention for teaching a variety of skills to individuals with autism who have imitation skills (Steinbrenner et al., 2020). This can be done in the classroom by using videos. For example, a child might watch a video about how to set the table and then imitate what they saw in the classroom.

Positive Reinforcement

Positive reinforcement is an event or activity that occurs after the target behavior and increases the likelihood of the behavior occurring again in the future (Wong et al., 2015). Whether it is a positive comment, fist bump, or a tangible reward, it can assist children in understanding what they are doing right. For example, teachers and parents can state what a child is doing correctly and why. For example, "Nice sitting." Increasing the frequency of positive reinforcement can increase desirable behaviors.

Priming

Priming helps prepare students for the day or for a specific activity. Priming reduces surprises and helps students plan for the day. Teachers or parents can prime children by providing background knowledge, preparing them for the expectations, and providing examples (Cihak et al., 2012). Strategies include providing access to visual material that discusses the day's topics, providing books on tape or in digital format for students to review at home, or briefly discussing the day's plan when the day starts. Koegel et al. (2003) used daily priming sessions that were implemented at home and were reported to last for one hour. Results indicated that priming appeared to positively impact academic responding and decreased problem behaviors.

Social Narratives (SN)

Social narratives describe social situations that describe what to do in a specific scenario or how to behave in a specific situation (Steinbrenner et al., 2020). For example, a child might get a social narrative on how to get a tissue and wipe her nose.

Assessment of Interventions

Evaluating the effectiveness of the interventions we use with children is an integral part of the instructional process. Goldstein et al. (2014) suggest that assessments should include analysis of specific behaviors and the tools used during the intervention. For example, if a student is using play-based therapy and interest items to learn joint attention it would be important to evaluate the effectiveness of the play-based intervention and the interest materials as well as the unique needs of the child for a comprehensive understanding of what the target behaviors are and how they are influenced by educational tools and interventions. This way we can discover what tools and interventions work well for each unique child with ASD.

Support for Generalization and Maintenance

Generalization and maintenance plans can assist in ensuring new skills can be utilized in a variety of settings over time. This is critical for children with ASD because they often have difficulties using new skills in novice settings (Bellini et al., 2007). Generalization is defined as the transfer of newly learned skills to new settings (Denning & Moody, 2018). Maintenance is one's ability to perform newly developed skills in natural settings over time (Gresham et al., 2001). Without proper maintenance, skills can be lost over time.

Cultural Factors

Children with diverse backgrounds can enter preschool with varying cultural differences that may play a role in a child's schooling. Lee (2011) explains that age, ethnicity, language, religion, gender, sexuality, and socioeconomic factors can all play a valuable role in the learning process. The way teachers and caregivers view behaviors, social interactions, and autism symptoms can vary widely. It is important to collect research on interventions and curricula being used with diverse populations of students so we can determine what works for various groups of students.

Content Rich, Culturally Grounded Curricula

Bateman and Wilson (2021) indicate that the number of culturally and linguistically diverse children diagnosed with ASD is on the rise. Culturally grounded curricula can assist in promoting equity and inclusion for diverse students diagnosed with ASD. It is important to offer instruction using a curriculum that appeals to families' cultures and perspectives while remaining evidence based. McDevitt et al. (2020) describe the need to adapt curricula while considering cultural and contextual influences. For example, when developing rules and expectations it is important to consider social norms in varying environments.

Comprehensive Team Approaches

Collaboration between schools, caregivers, and service providers is important for children with ASD, since they often get assistance in multiple settings, by a variety of specialists. The National Association for Special Education Teachers (2021) defines collaboration as interactions amongst a group of people working towards a common goal. Collaborations in the preschool classroom might include joint planning of IEP goals, service providers working together, or parents having monthly meetings with the IEP team.

Related Service Providers

It is common for preschool children diagnosed with ASD to require multiple service providers to address the comprehensive needs of children. This can include Board Certified Behavioral Analysts (BCBA), counselors/psychologists, early interventionists, occupational therapists, physical therapists, and speech language pathologists (see Table 6.2).

Each provider addressed challenges presented by the child. Designated providers are outlined in the IEP and the amount of time for each service is indicated. Finally, a start and end date of services is provided.

Classroom Placements

Legislation suggests that children with autism be included in classrooms with typically developing children. When deciding on when and how to include children in the special education classroom parents should consider time with peers. Hansen and colleagues (2014) conducted a systematic review of research between 2005–2012 and found that many interventions are available to support children with ASD in inclusive preschool settings including discrete trial training, behavioral momentum, modeling, and priming. When considering placements, Delmolino and Harris (2012) recommended that teams consider the following

Table 6.2 Service Providers Working in Early Intervention

Service Provider	What the Service Provider Does
Board Certified Behavioral Analyst (BCBA)	Conduct behavioral assessment and analyze results.
Counselor/Psychologist	Conduct evaluations, make recommendations and provider counseling and social skills training.
Early Interventionist	Provide services to children ages birth through three years. They coordinate services and provide interventions.
Occupational Therapist	Provide training in handwriting, cutting, motor skills, and the development of daily living skills.
Physical Therapist	Assist with large muscle groups and rebuild physical function.
Speech Language Pathologist	Treat communication and speech impairments., language skills, conversation skills, and social pragmatics.

Adapted from Association for Science (2022).

factors: setting, instructional variables, treatments, evaluation methods, and family involvement.

Designing Inclusive Environments

The classroom environment offers opportunities for students with ASD to learn, engage, socialize, and understand routines. Understanding environments may play an important role in children's learning experiences. Function, predictability, and comfort should be considered when designing inclusive preschool classrooms (e.g., McAllister & Barry, 2012). Children with autism can benefit from visual support in the classroom. For example, teachers who want to take attendance in the morning might provide a visual by a student's cubby to serve as a reminder to sign in each day. Using specific spaces for activities can also be helpful. For example, a child should not eat at the same table where they work because it can cause confusion. Gersten et al. (2007) promoted the use of classroom routines to increase familiarity in students and support learning. For example, teachers could offer a block of time for morning work and use a numbered bin system to promote self-regulation, completion, and enhance organization. These types of support can be easily embedded into a school day, encourage independence, and offer the teacher time to work with small groups.

An organized classroom can help students better understand how to move about the space, how to find materials, where to go to calm down, and can help minimize distractions (see Hurth et al., 1999). Supports that promote predictability include the arrangement of the physical environment, such as defining classroom boundaries (e.g., tape off areas, label items, create workstations), considering indoor and outdoor safety (e.g., add bell to door so you know when someone enters or leaves, create calming areas in the room to encourage children to stay), and creating a sensory area in the room (e.g., bean bags, weighted blankets, and fidgets). Activity length is important to consider based upon age, developmental levels, and maturity. Decreasing or increasing lesson times may increase engagement and minimize frustration especially for young children.

Educators should teach behavioral expectations using visuals that focus on positive behaviors and classroom boundaries to support behavioral and communication difficulties (see Arthur-Kelly et al., 2009). Task analyses offer supports to breakdown and teach components of tasks. For example, Meaden et al. (2011) supported the use of durable, portable, and age-appropriate visual tools as behavioral reminders to teach expectations.

Flexibility is an integral part of successfully including students with ASD into inclusive environments. Choice can be embedded into activities (e.g., love of trains) to promote engagement. Teachers can also vary activities by the level of challenge they provide. For example, The Premack Principle (Premack, 1959) suggests that less desirable activities should be introduced first and preferred activities later for students who have difficulties attending for long periods of time. This concept is also known as "First -> Then" or Grandma's Rule that you need to eat your vegetables before dessert. Behavioral momentum is a similar strategy that can also promote task completion (Nevin et al., 1983).

Parent Engagement

Effective communication between school and home is essential to keep structure and consistency for the student. Teachers should implement interventions to help students achieve self-regulation and readiness goals and include the family in plans so that they can continue implementing them at home. This way the student has consistency in an intervention and family and teachers can see if that strategy is having the desired effect. Having a child in the special education sector means that the family will be invited to participate in all team meetings about the student. Communication and notice to these meetings need to be communicated and teachers are the ones ensuring information gets to the intended person.

It is also important that you establish the best form of communication with the family. What works best for one family might not work for another. For example, one family may prefer communicating through emails, while another may prefer a logbook that goes back and forth from the school to the home in the student's backpack. Sending out a form/survey at the beginning of the school year asking parents for their preferred form of communication ensures that important information is being received and there is open communication to monitor progress and ask questions. In preschools, parents and teachers can also use apps to communicate and track behaviors. With technology advances many classroom teachers are using new apps to better communicate with families. Applications such as Class Dojo or Talking Points allow teachers to send both class announcements and individual family messages. Talking Points allows for communication to be translated into the family's home language. This is especially helpful when there is a language barrier between the teacher and family. Understanding the Home life behaviors and schedule allows the school to make informed decisions and that starts by creating a relationship with the family.

There needs to be open communication especially if a child has multiple behaviors where they could hurt themselves or their peers. Teachers should track behaviors and then update parents daily or weekly (depending on severity) of behaviors and progress. The relationship should go both ways. Some students with ASD struggle with morning routines and can come into school showing challenging behaviors. Families should feel comfortable enough to share with their student's teacher about how the morning routine went. Having that information allows the teacher to have all the information going into the day and allows the teacher to support students most effectively. Creating a valuable family-teacher relationship has also been proven to improve student behaviors. According to the National Research Council it is a best practice for parents to be involved (Zablotsky et al., 2012).

Understanding goals and preferences ensures growth success. In the case study of Ethan, he had items and activities that motivated him to stay on track to achieve his IEP goals. Ethan was able to stay on his mat during rest time and work on his self-regulation skills because teachers knew his preferred items. Families know what their child prefers. Whether it is specific like yellow Lamborghini cars or Disney movies. When students are comfortable, they are more willing to learn and make progress. Families are the key to making students feel more comfortable in the classroom. Preferences and preferred items also change, and families usually know first. Knowing how your student reacts at home can help identify behaviors as well as strategies to use in the classroom. Knowing the behaviors happening at home can be addressed in the classroom. Families have valuable information that teachers and support staff need to help the student make progress. Families are included in the special education process, and it is critical that they participate in the making of their student's goals.

When there is a strong relationship between school staff and families, families participate more effectively (Zablotsky et al., 2012). Teachers need to reach out to families and tell them that advocacy and participation in their child's education is necessary and wanted (Zablotsky et al., 2012). In the case of Ethan, his teacher reached out to the family before meetings as well as sent home reports before the meeting so that they could be fully prepared for the upcoming meeting for their child. They could then come in with questions and ideas. With the creation of this relationship by school staff and the family, the team was able to collaborate to best fit the needs of Ethan. If the family is willing, getting a report of how life at home is going adds a lot of weight to the overall assessment of well-being of the student. Hearing insights from the parent adds a perspective that school staff may not have. Listening to the family's perspective on educational, social-emotional, or behavioral goals may add strategies and goals. Their perspective holds value.

Transitions

Family collaborations are an essential component of the preschool experience because children continue to require a strong family support system as they develop independence. However, transitions are a high source of stress for families in the early years (Buescher et al., 2014). This may be due to the complexity of issues dealt with during transitions. Marsh and colleagues (2017) completed a review of transition research and found that children with ASD who struggle with social interactions often have challenges when transitioning. The implementation of school-based interventions can often assist children when starting school. Taking pictures of a new school and creating a social story, visiting the school, and meeting new teachers are all useful ways children can prepare for changes. Transitions are defining moments for young children, especially children with ASD who naturally struggle with changes in routines. The Early Learning Network (2020) recommends that teachers align PreK and kindergarten curricula and invest in culturally grounded curricula.

Emerging Trends in the Field

Multiple emerging trends continue as the field of early intervention seeks to improve support and access to services for families and young children with ASD. These include a continued focus to access and universal PreK and a strength-based approach to supporting children with ASD. Early intervention is one cost effective method for increasing future academic and social development for young children with ASD by providing children with interactional opportunities and a wealth of new experiences.

Autism and other disabilities are viewed almost exclusively from a deficit perspective focusing on what individuals can't do. This is neither fair nor helpful. Since limited consideration is given to the strengths that individuals with ASD may possess, we may be underestimating the overall ability and IQ levels of individuals with autism (e.g., Christensen et al., 2016). For example, Christensen and colleagues (2016) reported that 44% of individuals with ASD test at the average or above average level of intellectual ability. These findings may underestimate overall abilities. Many individuals with ASD have strengths that can help them in the classroom or could translate into future careers (e.g., Meilleur et al., 2015), such as relating to concrete ideas, and both understanding and working effectively with details (Bauminger-Zviely, 2013) and visual processing (e.g., Kaldy et al., 2016). An increased understanding of the mechanisms surrounding these strengths may inform decisions around targeted interventions and developmental outcomes (Kaldy et al., 2016).

In a worldwide examination of research Carmona-Serrano and colleagues (2020) found emerging topics in inclusion and diagnosis as well as transitions. There was also a new body of literature emerging from 2018–2019 surrounding mothers of children with ASD and the children themselves, specifically, through transitions. Additionally, research on girls with ASD is starting to garner attention. Technology supports for individuals with ASD have also been highlighted.

Discussion Questions

1. What factors should families consider when choosing a preschool program for their young children with ASD?
3. Discuss the similarities and differences between various forms of play therapies. What characteristics might guide a parent to the right individualized approach for his/her child?
4. How can preschool educators provide culturally competent instruction? What instructional considerations should they make?

References

Association for Sciences. (2022). Description of Service Providers retrieved from https://asatonline.org/for-parents/learn-more-about-specific-treatments/appl ied-behavior-analysis-aba/aba-techniques/description-of-service-providers/.

Akers, J., Higbee, T., Pollard, J., Pellegrino, A., Gerencser, K. (2016). An evaluation of photographic activity schedules to increase independent playground skills in young children with autism. *Journal of Applied Behavior, 49*(4). Doi: 10.1002/jaba.327

American Psychiatric Association (APA). (2013). Diagnostic and statistical manual of mental disorders (5th ed.). Washington, DC: American Psychiatric Association.

Arthur-Kelly, M., Sigafoos, J., Mathisen, B. & Arthur-Kelly, R. (2009). Issues in the use of visual supports to promote communication in individuals with autism spectrum disorder. *Disability Rehabilitation, 31*(18), 1474. doi: 10.1080/ 09638280802590629

Bateman, K. J., & Wilson, S. E. (2021). Supporting Diverse Learners with Autism Through a Culturally Responsive Visual Communication Intervention. *Intervention in School and Clinic, 56*(5), 301–307.

Bauminger-Zviely, N. (2013). *Social and academic abilities in children with high-functioning autism spectrum disorders.* New York, NY: The Guilford Press.

Bellini, S., Peters, J. K., Benner, L., & Hopf, A. (2007). A meta-analysis of school-based social skills interventions for children with autism spectrum disorders. *Remedial and Special Education, 28,* 153–162.

Buescher, A., Cidav, C., Knapp, M. & Madell, D. (2014). Costs of ASD Spectrum Disorders in the United Kingdom and the United States. *JAMA Pediatrics,* 168(8), 721–728-DOI: 10.1001.

Carmona-Serrano, N., López-Belmonte, J., López-Núñez, J., & Moreno-Guerrero, A. (2020). Review trends in autism research in the field of education in web of science: Abibliometric study. *Brain Sciences, 10,* 1018–1040.

Cihak, D. F., Smith, C. C., Cornett, A., & Coleman, M. (2012). The use of video modeling with the picture exchange communication system to increase independent communicative initiations in preschoolers with autism and developmental delays. *Focus on Autism and Other Developmental Disabilities*, 27(1), 3–11.

Christensen, D. L., Baio, J., Braun, K. V. N., Bilder, D., Charles, J., Constantino, J. N., … & Yeargin-Allsopp, M. (2016). Prevalence and characteristics of autism spectrum disorder among children aged 8 years—autism and developmental disabilities monitoring network, 11 sites, United States, 2012. *MMWR Surveillance Summaries*, 65(3), 1.

Delmolino, L. & Harris, S. (2012). Matching children on the autism spectrum to classrooms: a guide for parents and professionals. *Journal of Autism and Developmental Disorders*, 42(6), 1197–1204. doi: 10.1007/s10803-011-1298-6.

Denning, C. B. & Moody, A. (2018). Inclusion and autism spectrum disorder: Strategies to support students. New York: Routledge.

Dettmer, S., Simpson, R. L., Myles, B. S., & Ganz, J. B. (2000). The use of visual supports to facilitate transitions of students with autism. Focus on Autism and Other Developmental Disabilities, 15(3), 163–169.

Gersten, R., Baker, S. K., Shanahan, T., Linan-Thompson, S., Collins, P., & Scarcella, R. (2007). *Effective literacy and English language instruction for English learners in the elementary grades: A practice guide* (NCEE 2007-4011). Washington, DC: National Center for Education Evaluation and Regional Assistance, Institute of Education Sciences, U.S. Department of Education. Retrieved from http://ies.ed.gov/ncee/wwc/publications/practiceguides.

Goldstein, H., Lackey, K. C., & Schneider, N. J. (2014). A new framework for systematic reviews: Application to social skills interventions for preschoolers with autism. *Exceptional Children*, 80(3), 262–286.

Gresham, F. M., Sugai, G., & Horner, R. H. (2001). Outcomes of social skills training for students with high-incidence disabilities. *Teaching Exceptional Children*, 67, 331–344.

Hansen, S. G., Blakely, A. W., Dolata, J. K. et al. (2014). Children with autism in the inclusive preschool classroom: A systematic review of single-subject design interventions on social communication skills. *Review Journal of Autism and Developmental Disorders* 1, 192–206. https://doi.org/10.1007/s40489-014-002-y

Harrop, C., Amsbary, J., Towner-Wright, S., Reichow, B., & Boyd, B. (2019). That's what I like: The use of circumscribed interests within interventions for individuals with autism spectrum disorder. A systematic review. *Research in Autism Spectrum Disorders*, 57, 63–86. Doi.org/10.1016/j.rasd.2018.09.008.

Hume, K., & Turner-Brown, L. (2018). Family implemented TEACCH for toddlers. In *Handbook of parent-implemented interventions for very young children with autism* (pp. 321–337). Springer, Cham.

Hurth, J., Shaw, E., Izeman, S. G., Whaley, K., & Rogers, S. J. (1999). Areas of agreement about effective practices among programs serving young children with autism spectrum disorders. *Infants and Young Children*, 12(2), 17–26.

Individuals With Disabilities Education Act, 20 U.S.C. § 1400 (2004).

Kaldy, Z., Giserman, I., Carter, A. S., & Blaser, E. (2016). The mechanisms underlying the ASD advantage in visual search. *Journal of Autism and Developmental Disorders*, 46, 1513–1527.

Khalifa, G., Rosenbaum, P., Georgiades, K., Duku, E., & Di Rezze, B. (2020). Exploring the participation patterns and impact of environment in preschool children with ASD. International *Journal of Environmental Research and Public Health, 17*(17), 5677. doi: 10.3390/ijerph17165677

Kimball, J., Kinney, E., Taylor, B., & Stromer, R. (2003). Video enhanced activity schedules for children with autism: A promising package for teaching social skills. *Education and Treatment of Children, 27,* 280–298.

Koegel, L., Koegel, R. L., Frea, W., & Green-Hopkins, I. (2003b). Priming as a method of coordinating educational services for students with autism. *Language, Speech, and Hearing Services in Schools, 34*(3), 228–235. doi: 10.1044/0161-1461(2003/019)

Koegel, L. K., Singh, A. K., & Koegel, R. L. (2010). Improving motivation for academics in children with autism. *Journal of Autism and Developmental Disorders, 40,* 1057–1066. doi: 10.1007/s10803-010-0962-6

Kurth, J. A. (2014). Educational placement of students with autism: The impact of state of residence. *Focus on Autism and Other Developmental Disabilities, 30*(4), 249–256.

Lee, H. J. (2011). Cultural factors related to the hidden curriculum for students with autism and related disabilities. *Intervention in School and Clinic, 46*(3), 141–149. doi: 10.1177/1053451210378162

Maenner, M. J., Shaw, K. A., Bakian, A. V., Bilder, D. A., Durkin, M. S., Esler, A., ... & Cogswell, M. E. (2021). Prevalence and characteristics of autism spectrum disorder among children aged 8 years—autism and developmental disabilities monitoring network, 11 sites, United States, 2018. *MMWR Surveillance Summaries, 70*(11), 1.

Marsh, A., Spagnol, V., Grove, R., & Eapen, V. (2017). Transition to school for children with autism spectrum disorder: A systematic review. *World Journal of Psychiatry, 7*(3), 184.

McAllister, K. & Barry, B. (2012). A design model: the autism spectrum disorder classroom design kit. *British Journal of Special Education, 39*(4), 201–208.

McDevitt, S. E., Jiang, H., Xu, Y., & Pei, D. (2020). Culturally relevant special education curriculum for children with autism in China. *Childhood Education, 96*(3), 56–61.

McDonald, C. A., Donnelly, J. P., Feldman-Alguire, A. L., Rodgers, J. D., Lopata, C., & Thomeer, M. L. (2019). Special education service use by children with autism spectrum disorder. *Journal of Autism and Developmental Disorders, 49*(6), 2437–2446.

McIntyre, L. L., & Zemantic, P. K. (2017). Examining services for young children with autism spectrum disorder: Parent satisfaction and predictors of service utilization. *Early Childhood Education Journal, 45*(6), 727–734. doi: https://doi.org/10.1007/s10643-016-0821-y

Meadan, H., Ostrosky, M., Triplett, B., Michna, A., & Fettig, A. (2011). Using visual supports with young children with autism spectrum disorder. *Teaching Exceptional Children, 43,* 28–35.

Meilleur, A. A. S., Jelenic, P., & Mottron, L. (2015). Prevalence of clinically and empirically defined talents and strengths in autism. *Journal of Autism and Developmental Disorders, 45*(5), 1354–1367.

Peters, W. J., & Matson, J. L. (2020). Comparing rates of diagnosis using DSM-IV-TR versus DSM-5 criteria for autism spectrum disorder. *Journal of Autism and Developmental Disorders*, *50*(6), 1898–1906.

Premack, D. (1959). Toward empirical behavior laws: I. Positive reinforcement. *Psychological Review*, *66*, 219–233.

Rosenberg, L., Jarus, T., Bart, O., & Ratzon, N. (2013). Complementary contribution of parents and therapists in the assessment process of children. *Australian Occupational Therapy Journal*, *6*, 410–500. doi: 10.1111/1440-1630.12041

Strain, P. S., Schwartz, I. S., & Borton, E. E. (2011). Providing interventions for young children with autism spectrum disorders: What we still need to accomplish. *Journal of Early Intervention*, *33*, 321–332. doi: 10.1177/1053815111429970

Tek, S., & Landa, R. J. (2012). Differences in autism symptoms between minority and non-minority toddlers. *Journal of Autism and Developmental Disorders*, *42*(9), 1967–1973.

The Early Learning Network. (2020). https://earlylearningnetwork.unl.edu/wp-content/uploads/2020/11/201105-Policy-Brief-PreK-K-Transition.pdf

Vitiello, V., Booren, L., Downer, J., & Williford, A. (2012). Variation in children's classroom engagement throughout a day in preschool: Relations to classroom and child factors. *Early Childhood Research Quarterly*, *27*(2), 210–220. doi: 10.1016/j.ecresq.2011.08.005

Wong, C., Odom, S. L., Hume, K. A., Cox, C. W., Fettig, A., Kurcharczyk, S., et al. (2015). Evidence-based practices for children, youth, and young adults with autism spectrum disorder: A comprehensive review. *Journal of Autism and Developmental Disorders*. Advance online publication. doi: 10.1007/s10803-014-2351-z

Zablotsky, B., Boswell, K., & Smith, C. (2012). An evaluation of school involvement and satisfaction of parents of children with autism spectrum disorders. *American Journal on Intellectual and Developmental Disabilities*, *117*(4), 316–330.

Chapter 7

Teaching Communication to Individuals with Autism Spectrum Disorders

Brenna Griffen, Lexi Woods-Catterlin,
Elizabeth R. Lorah, and Peggy Schaefer Whitby
University of Arkansas Fayetteville

The ability to communicate is foundational to future learning across all developmental domains, is considered a quality-of-life indicator, and is essential to form social connections with those around us (Drmic et al., 2018; Prelock et al., 2011). Studies show that for individuals with autism spectrum disorder (ASD), early language skills are a predictor of successful communication, social functioning, and independence in adulthood (Ben-Itzchak & Zachor, 2020; Drmic et al., 2018; LeGrand et al., 2021). As social communication, including prelinguistic and non-vocal communication is a diagnostic category for ASD, focused interventions are often needed to teach such skills (American Psychiatric Association [APA], 2013; Drmic et al., 2018; Prelock et al., 2011). For the 30% of individuals with ASD who lack functional vocal output, educators need to provide and teach alternative systems of communication to supplement or replace vocal speech (LeGrand et al., 2021).

This chapter provides an overview of communication and language impairments associated with ASD, an introduction to assessments that drive communication interventions, evidence-based practices used during instruction, guidance for interdisciplinary teaming to enhance communication, and strategies to train communicative partners. In addition, this chapter discusses the use of augmentative and alternative communication (AAC) systems, including the use of picture exchange systems and handheld technology to provide a means of communication for individuals with limited vocal abilities. The key points are:

1. Children with ASD present with varying levels of social communication impairments.
2. Appropriate assessment to identify a child's current level is necessary to drive instruction.
3. Evidence-based interventions are critical for addressing the communication needs of children with ASD.
4. AAC systems, including picture exchange systems and speech-generating devices (SGD) can increase communicative abilities.

DOI: 10.4324/9781003255147-9

5. Coordinating communication interventions with other professionals improves outcomes for children with ASD.
6. Training communication partners can help children with ASD communicate in all environments.

Lucía is a 3-year-old Latina girl diagnosed with ASD-level three. She exhibits severe qualitative impairments in social interaction, communication, and repetitive behaviors. While Lucía produces sounds and some babbling, she does not imitate sounds or use any words. She is considered non-vocal. To communicate her needs, Lucía often demonstrates crying, screaming, and pulling hands to objects. Lucía has been recommended for an assessment to help drive instruction of early learner skills, including communication.

Communication and Language Issues in ASD

Communicative ability varies greatly across individuals with ASD, ranging from no functional vocal output to individuals with high levels of vocal ability who struggle with modifying speech to fit various social contexts (Prelock et al., 2011; Skinner et al., 2021). The ability to use conventional and socially appropriate vocal and non-vocal communication across contexts enables individuals with ASD to interact with and form meaningful relationships with those around them (Prelock et al., 2011). This requires the ability to change behavior based on factors in an environment and self-monitor behavior in relation to others. Social skills can have a tremendous impact on relationships with loved ones, peers, and acquaintances.

Early developmental milestones for communication include eye gaze, babbling, imitation, pointing, gestures, responding to requests, joint attention, using words, following directions, naming objects, articulation, and using pronouns and other language-based rules (Center for Disease Control and Prevention [CDC], 2015). However, not every child develops typically. The wide range of language abilities in children with ASD can make teaching communication and language skills difficult since instructors must be able to identify the specific areas of focus for each child. Areas of impairment may include expressive language (i.e., word imitation, labeling, and requesting), receptive language (i.e., responding to one's name, following directions, and identifying objects by name), articulation (i.e., specific sound pronunciation), and fluency (i.e., ability to speak without stuttering; LeGrand et al., 2021).

Additionally, children with ASD may have difficulty using language for a variety of communicative functions (LeGrand et al., 2021; Shumway & Wetherby, 2009). Language use may be restricted to expressing preferences, such as requesting preferred items and rejecting or protesting nonpreferred activities, instead of a wide range of social functions, such as commenting and sharing attention (LeGrand et al., 2021; Shumway & Wetherby, 2009). Many studies have illustrated that the development of functional language skills in early childhood is one of the best predictors of social behaviors and independence in adulthood (Ben-Itzchak & Zachor, 2020; Drmic et al., 2018).

Because many individuals with ASD are unable to acquire functional communicative abilities without direct instruction, early intervention using evidence-based strategies can be effective in developing these skills (Prelock et al., 2011). Understanding the strengths and weaknesses of the individual learner through assessment leads to the selection of evidence-based practices to systematically teach communication skills.

Assessment to Drive Instruction

The process of acquiring both speaker and listener repertoires can be lengthy, complex, and full of detours. Having an organized and clear understanding of both a learner's skill level and a future teaching pathway is vital to producing a language-rich future (Trembath et al., 2021). The purpose of assessments is to identify gaps in skills and compare an individual's performance to a set of predetermined criteria or performance standards. These standards represent what a person is expected to know or be able to do at a certain age, level of education, or developmental stage (Westby et al., 2013). Once developmental gaps are identified, instructors must identify what skills are needed to fill these gaps and identify evidence-based strategies to teach these skills. Instructors can collect data on skill acquisition and reassess skills periodically to ensure acquisition (Vietze & Lax, 2020).

There are a variety of assessments, including the *Verbal Behavior Milestones and Placement Program* (VB-MAPP; Sundberg, 2014), the *Assessment of Basic Language and Learning Skills—Revised* (ABLLS-R; Partington, 2015), and other speech-language evaluations, that can be used to drive instructional programs. The first two examples are derived from a behavior analytic approach to teaching and learning. Table 7.2 highlights those assessments derived from a speech/language pathology perspective. These assessments have many similarities and differences and will be discussed in the context of the information they provide and the implications of the information they do not offer.

Verbal Behavior Milestones and Placement Program

The VB-MAPP is based on the analysis of verbal behavior as conceptualized by B.F. Skinner in his work *Verbal Behavior* (1957). The VB-MAPP (Sundberg, 2014) uses the same terminology as Skinner in its differentiation of the distinct repertoires of speaker and listener, as well as in the terminology of speaker behavior. Skinner (1957) categorized verbal behavior according to the function, or contingency that maintains that behavior. Within this framework, it is not the topography (e.g., vocal output, sign language, etc.), but rather the function of the behavior that is of interest. A behavior that requests an item or action from someone else is called a mand. A tact is a label of something in the environment. More complex communication, such as back-and-forth conversation, questions, and songs are referred to as intraverbals. The term echoic refers to instances when a response is repeated or echoed by another person. More in-depth information about verbal behaviors is discussed later in the chapter and provided in Table 7.5. Often, practitioners will begin by teaching manding, or requesting, skills because this allows learners to access preferred items and activities quickly and appropriately. This is called mand training.

In addition to verbal behavior, the VB-MAPP (Sundberg, 2014) includes learning and school readiness skills such as matching-to-sample, imitation, reading, writing, and math. This assessment was developed by a team of interdisciplinary professionals and comprehensively provides assessment, curriculum planning, and skill monitoring (Sundberg, 2014).

The assessment and curriculum of the VB-MAPP are based on typical developmental milestones up to 48 months (Sundberg, 2014). It contains up to 900 skills that comprise 170 language and social milestones across three developmental levels. The individual items can serve as targets within goals for a learner's individualized education program and be used to track progress towards skill acquisition (Vietze & Lax, 2020). In addition to the assessment of current repertoires, the VB-MAPP's strength is its assessment of barriers to language acquisition. It is praised for providing an assessment of language according to the source of control of the language response, versus only the topography, i.e., what the response looks or sounds like (Esch et al., 2010). It is not only essential to know a learner's current language development, but possibly more important to understand the faulty sources of control, competing contingencies, or other variables in the environment or learner's history that affects acquisition challenges. For example, self-stimulatory behavior may compete with other items or activities during mand training, blocking other potential sources of motivating operation control and serving as a barrier to mand acquisition. Finally, the VB-MAPP also includes a self-care checklist of skills based on developmental milestones (Sundberg, 2014). See Table 7.1 for a list of the domains included in the VB-MAPP.

Lucía was assessed using the VB-MAPP. Upon initial assessment, Lucía presented as a level 1 learner. Lucía has no mand, tact, listener, or echoic repertoire. She has some level 1 visual perceptual skills and matching to sample. She engages in parallel play and is beginning to emit speech sounds.

Table 7.1 Comparison of Domains Between VB-MAPP and ABLLS-R

VB-MAPP Domains (Sundberg, 2014)	ABLLS-R Domains (Partington, 2015)
Basic verbal operants (e.g., echoic, mand, tact, intraverbal)	Cooperation & Reinforcer Effectiveness
Listener skills	Visual Performance
Vocal output	Receptive Language
Independent play	Imitation
Social skills and social play	Vocal Imitation
Visual perceptual skills and matching-to-sample	Requests (mands)
Grammatical and syntactical skills	Labeling (tacts)
Group and classroom skills	Intraverbals
Beginning academic skills	Spontaneous Vocalizations
	Syntax & Grammar
	Play & Leisure
	Social Interaction
	Group Instruction
	Classroom Routines
	Generalized Responding
	Reading
	Math

The Assessment of Basic Language and Living Skills – Revised

Similar to the VB-MAPP, the ABLLS-R provides assessment, curriculum guidance, and a method for skill tracking based on developmental milestones. However, it includes information on a slightly broader range of skill types, and domains are based on criterion references for children slightly older than with the VB-MAPP (kindergarten age vs. 48 months).

The ABLLS-R can assess and plan for 500 skills across language, social, motor, self-help, and academic domains (Partington, 2015). See Table 7.1 for a side-by-side comparison of skill domains between the VB-MAPP and ABLLS-R. Like the VB-MAPP, the ABLLS-R provides differentiation of expressive language according to Skinner's analysis of verbal behavior. For example, it assesses and tracks mands, tacts, intraverbals, etc. Notable skill targets also include other precursor skills to language, such as joint attention (Partington, 2015). The ABLLS-R does not provide an assessment of possible learning barriers but does provide guidance on goal creation for individualized education programs.

The main weakness of both assessments is that although they provide information about current skill levels and plans for teaching acquisition skills, they do not identify teaching procedures that may result in the most efficient acquisition of skill targets. Neither assessment provides methods for determining the types of specific prompting and error-correction procedures that work best for an individual, as an individual's prompting or error-correction history may influence skill acquisition (Coon & Miguel,

2012). Conducting an additional initial assessment to identify prompts and error-correction procedures that best suit an individual's needs and choosing an evidence-based intervention to implement the curriculum is advised. McGhan and Lerman (2013) identify and describe this type of assessment as applied to four boys with ASD.

Speech-Language Based Assessments

In addition to the behavior analytic assessments, there are specific assessments from the field of speech-language pathology that can provide additional information about a learner's skills. The appropriateness of an evaluation is determined based upon the child's need, age, cultural background, and communication disorder (DiStefano & Kasari, 2016). Formal and informal assessments focus on the understanding of subcomponents that make up receptive language, including pragmatics, phonology, semantics, syntax, and morphology (Muller & Brady, 2016). Pragmatics is understanding and demonstrating the social components of language (Miller & Thiemann-Bourque, 2016). Phonology involves understanding and demonstrating phonological awareness, which refers to sounds in language. The ability to understand and demonstrate vocabulary in language is referred to as semantics. Syntax is the ability to understand and generate grammatically correct sentences. The final subcomponent is morphology, which is the ability to understand the parts of words and their meaning (Gleason & Ratner, 2017).

Table 7.2 provides an overview of common assessments used by speech-language pathologists. These assessments target various skills, including receptive language, expressive language, pragmatics, articulation, and fluency. Assessments are used for identifying receptive and expressive language baseline skills in the classroom (Gaffney, 2020). The pragmatic assessments listed in Table 7.2 focus on assessing the child's current social skills and identifying which areas are more difficult to comprehend and demonstrate in various scenarios. Assessments of articulation focus on specific speech sounds made at word and sentence level. Fluency is commonly informally assessed; however when systematically assessed, the speech-language pathologist collects data to determine the impact and the frequency of the stuttering (Gaffney, 2020).

Receptive language is the ability or capacity to understand language. Typically, humans can comprehend language before they express it. Babies begin to understand when their parent says "no" with a loud tone and volume before they can say the word "no." Many adult second language learners can understand more than they can express (DiStefano & Kasari, 2016). Expressive language is the ability to use language to communicate meaning. This language can consist of gestures, sounds, words, phrases, sentences, and conversation. This process may look different for each child with ASD and may include the use of AAC systems (DiStefano & Kasari, 2016).

Table 7.2 Speech-Language Assessments to Drive Communication Instruction

Communicative Domain	Age Range (in years)
Language	
*Test of Language Development – Fifth Edition (Intermediate) (TOLD-I:5)	4–9
*Oral and Written Language Scales – 2nd Edition (OWLS II)	3–21
*Expressive Vocabulary Test (EVT)	2.5–90
*Test of Language Competence Expanded Edition (ToLCE)	1.5–10 (Level 1); 9–19 (Level 2)
*Test for Auditory Comprehension of Language – Fourth Edition (TACL-4)	3–10
*Test of Early Language Development 3 (TELD-3)	2–8
*Clinical Evaluation of Language Fundamentals Preschool – 5th Edition (CELF)	3–22
*Comprehensive Assessment of Spoken Language (CASL)	3–21
*Preschool language scales (PLS-5)	Birth -7 years
*Children's Communication Checklist – 2nd Edition (CCC-2) Manual/ Scoring Program	4-16
*Functional Communication Profile – needs to be associated with non-verbal intellectual quotient	3 -adulthood
Test of Nonverbal Intelligence (TONI-4)	
Pragmatics	
*Pragmatic Language Skills Inventory (PLSI)	5–12
*Social Skills Improvement System (SSIS)	3–18
*Social Language Development Test: Elementary – Adolescent (SLDT-A)	6–17
Speech Sound Disorders	
*Kaufman Speech Praxis Test for Children (KSPT)	3–5
Arizona-4 (AAPS-4; 2017)	1.5–21
*Goldman Fristoe 2 Test of Articulation	2–21
Clinical Assessment of Articulation and Phonology – 2nd Edition (CAAP-2; 2013)	2.5–11
Fluency/Voice	
Stuttering Severity Instrument- Fourth Edition (SSI-4; 2009)	2–10
Test of childhood stuttering (TOCS; 2009)	4–12

*Adapted from Gaffney, A. (2020). Speech Pathology Assessment Resource List. Indiana Resource Center for Autism. Retrieved from www.iidc.indiana.edu/irca/articles/speech-pathology-assessment-resource-list.html.

Teaching Communication and Language

Once the assessment is complete, teaching goals should be identified. Both the VB-MAPP and the ABLLS-R are designed to identify skills based on a continuum of typical development across multiple domains (i.e.,

manding or requesting, tacting or labeling, etc.). After scoring these assessments, practitioners can identify the skills missing at the lower levels
of each domain and develop interventions to target these skills before
progressing to skills at the higher levels (Partington et al., 2018; Vietze
& Lax, 2020).

> *Based upon Lucía's results on the VB-MAPP, the intervention team
> chose to initially target mands using an iPad-based SGD with the
> Proloquo2Go application. This device has a screen with icons that
> when pressed provide an audible speech output. This form of com-
> munication was chosen because Lucía demonstrated a relative
> strength in visual performance and matching to sample. Her team
> decided to focus heavily on teaching manding skills, as mands use
> natural reinforcers and are highly motivating for children, thereby
> increasing engagement in the activity.*

After teaching goals have been identified, it is critical that practitioners,
teachers, and families have access to evidence-based interventions to teach
these goals. Fortunately, the National Autism Center ([NAC]; 2015),
the National Professional Development Center on Autism (Wong et al.,
2014), and The National Clearinghouse on Autism Evidence and Practice
(Steinbrenner et al., 2020) have developed practitioner and family guides
on evidence-based practices for teaching children diagnosed with ASD.
The specific intervention used depends on which area of communication is being targeted. Table 7.3 provides an overview and definitions of
these practices. Table 7.4 displays resources for learning more about each
intervention.

The NAC Guide for Evidence-based Practices (NAC, 2015), the
National Professional Development Center National Standards Report
(Wong et al., 2014), and the National Clearinghouse on Autism Evidence
and Practice (Steinbrenner et al., 2020) recognize teaching strategies
based on principles of applied behavior analysis (ABA) as evidence based.
When these practices are embedded within a behavior-treatment package,
it can lead to gains across all developmental domains for individuals with
ASD (NAC, 2015).

ABA is the systematic application of interventions based on the principles of learning to improve socially significant behavior and demonstrate that the intervention was responsible for the behavior change (i.e.,
functional relationship; Baer, Wolfe, & Risley, 1968). It should be noted
that ABA is not one teaching strategy, such as Discrete Trial Training
(DTT), but a technology of interventions based on learning theory
(Ghezzi, 2007). DTT is one strategy for teaching and has a strong evidence base for teaching communication.

Table 7.3 Definitions of Evidence-Based Practices

Evidence-Based Practice	Definition
Antecedent-Based Interventions (ABI)	Arrangement of events or circumstances that precede an activity or demand in order to increase the occurrence of a behavior or lead to the reduction of the challenging/interfering behaviors.
Augmentative and Alternative Communication (AAC)	Interventions using and/or teaching the use of a system of communication that is not verbal/vocal which can be aided (e.g., device, communication book) or unaided (e.g., sign language).
Cognitive Behavioral/ Instructional Strategies (CBIS)	Instruction on management or control of cognitive processes that lead to changes in behavioral, social, or academic behavior.
Differential Reinforcement of Alternative, Incompatible, or Other Behavior (DR)	A systematic process that increases desirable behavior or the absence of an undesirable behavior by providing positive consequences for demonstration/ non-demonstration of such behavior. These consequences may be provided when the learner is: a) engaging in a specific desired behavior other than the undesirable behavior (DRA), b) engaging in a behavior that is physically impossible to do while exhibiting the undesirable behavior (DRI), or c) not engaging in the undesirable behavior (DRO).
Discrete Trial Training (DTT)	Instructional approach with massed or repeated trials with each trial consisting of the teacher's instruction/ presentation, the child's response, a carefully planned consequence, and a pause prior to presenting the next instruction.
Extinction (EXT)	The removal of reinforcing consequences of a challenging behavior in order to reduce the future occurrence of that behavior.
Functional Behavioral Assessment (FBA)	A systematic way of determining the underlying function or purpose of a behavior so that an effective intervention plan can be developed.
Functional Communication Training (FCT)	A set of practices that replace a challenging behavior that has a communication function with more appropriate and effective communication behaviors or skills.
Modeling (MD)	Demonstration of a desired target behavior that results in use of the behavior by the learner and that leads to the acquisition of the target behavior.
Naturalistic Intervention (NI)	A collection of techniques and strategies that are embedded in typical activities and/or routines in which the learner participates to naturally promote, support, and encourage target skills/behaviors.
Parent-Implemented Intervention (PII)	Parent delivery of an intervention to their child that promotes their social communication or other skills or decreases their challenging behavior.

(continued)

Table 7.3 Cont.

Evidence-Based Practice	Definition
Peer-Based Instruction and Intervention (PBII)	Intervention in which peers directly promote autistic children's social interactions and/or other individual learning goals, or the teacher/ other adult organizes the social context (e.g., playgroups, social network groups, recess) and when necessary, provides support (e.g., prompts, reinforcement) to the autistic children and their peer to engage in social interactions.
Prompting (PP)	Verbal, gestural, or physical assistance given to learners to support them in acquiring or engaging in a targeted behavior or skill.
Reinforcement (R)	The application of a consequence following a learner's use of a response or skill that increases the likelihood that the learner will use the response/skills in the future.
Social Narratives (SN)	Interventions that describe social situations in order to highlight relevant features of a target behavior or skill and offer examples of appropriate responding.
Task Analysis (TA)	A process in which an activity or behavior is divided into small, manageable steps in order to assess and teach the skill. Other practices, such as reinforcement, video modeling, or time delay, are often used to facilitate acquisition of the smaller steps.
Time Delay (TD)	A practice used to systematically fade the use of prompts during instructional activities by using a brief delay between the initial instruction and any additional instructions or prompts.
Video Modeling (VM)	A video-recorded demonstration of the targeted behavior or skill shown to the learner to assist learning in or engaging in a desired behavior or skill.
Visual Supports (VS)	A visual display that supports the learner engaging in a desired behavior or skills independent of additional prompts.

Note. Adapted from Steinbrenner, J. R., Hume, K., Odom, S. L., Morin, K. L., Nowell, S. W., Tomaszewski, B., Szendrey, S., McIntyre, N. S., Yücesoy-Özkan, S., & Savage, M. N. (2020). Evidence-based practices for children, youth, and young adults with Autism. The University of North Carolina at Chapel Hill, Frank Porter Graham Child Development Institute, National Clearinghouse on Autism Evidence and Practice Review Team.

DTT is appropriate for teaching communication skills for those who present with little or no vocal language (Burggraff & Anderson, 2011). The characteristics of ASD in the area of social communication and social interaction may influence the motivation of a child to interact with others. By using tangible motivators (positive reinforcers), the learning environment can be arranged to increase motivation for the learner. DTT

Table 7.4 Evidence Based Interventions for Teaching Communication

Evidence-Based Practice	Age Range	Resource(s)
Antecedent-Based Intervention (ABI)	0–22	*Antecedent Based Interventions* (Ohio Department of Education, 2020)
Augmentative and Alternative Communication (AAC)	0–18	"A Systematic Review of Tablet Based Computers and Portable Media Players as Speech Generating Deices for Individuals with Autism Spectrum Disorder" (Lorah et al., 2015) *A Picture's Worth: PECS and Other Visual Communication Strategies in Autism* (Bondy & Frost, 2011)
Cognitive Behavioral/ Instructional Strategies (CBIS)	6–14	*CBT for Children and Adolescents with High-Functioning Autism Spectrum Disorders* (Scarpa et al., 2016)
Differential Reinforcement (DR)	6–14	*Applied Behavior Analysis* (Cooper et al., 2020)
Discrete Trial Training (DTT)	0–14	*Individualized Autism Interventions for Young Children: Blending Discrete Trial and Naturalistic Strategies* (Thompson, 2011) *A Brief Explanation of Discrete Trial Training* (Buckmann, 2016)
Extinction (EXT)	0–18	*Extinction Procedures* (Cosgrave, 2021)
Functional Behavior Assessment (FBA)	0–22	*Basic FBA to BSP: Trainer's Manual* (Loman et al., 2019)
Functional Communication Training (FCT)	0–22	*Functional Communication Training for Problem Behavior* (Reichle & Wacker, 2017)
Modeling (MD) and Video Modeling (VM)	0–22	*Video Modeling for Young Children with Autism Spectrum Disorder: A Practical Guide for Parents and Professionals* (Murray & Nolan, 2013)
Naturalistic Interventions (NI)	0–14	*Naturalistic and Incidental Teaching* (Charlop, 2018) *The PRT Pocket Guide: Pivotal Response Treatment for Autism Spectrum Disorders* (Koegel & Koegel, 2012)
Parent-Implemented Intervention (PII)	0–18	*Teaching Social Communication to Children with Autism and Other Developmental Delays: The Project ImPACT Manual for Parents* (Ingersoll & Dvortcsak, 2019)
Peer-based Instruction and Intervention (PBII)	3–14	*Peer Networks and Peer Support Arrangements* (Human Development Institute, 2015)
Prompting (PP)	0–22	*Autism Focused Intervention Resources and Modules: Prompting* (Sam & AFIRM team, 2015a)
Reinforcement (R)		*Behavior Analysis for Lasting Change* (Mayer et al., 2018)
Social Narratives (SN)	3–14	*The New Social Story Book: Over 150 Social Stories that Teach Everyday Social Skills to Children and Adults with Autism and Their Peers* (Gray, 2015)

(continued)

Table 7.4 Cont.

Evidence-Based Practice	Age Range	Resource(s)
Task Analysis (TA)	3–22	*Autism Focused Intervention Resources and Modules: Task Analysis* (Sam & AFIRM team, 2015b)
Time Delay (TD)	0–22	*Progressive Time Delay* (Ledford et al., 2016)
Visual Supports (VS)	0–14	*Practical Communication Tools for Autism: Using Visual Strategies for Lifelong Success* (Hodgdon, 2019) *Teach Me With Pictures: 40 Fun Picture Scripts to Develop Play and Communication Skills in Children on the Autism Spectrum* (Hodgdon et al., 2017)

uses a *stimulus-response-consequence* teaching format (Ghezzi, 2007). In this teaching sequence, a stimulus is presented, the child responds or the response is prompted, and a consequence, such as positive reinforcement, is provided. Tangible reinforcers are always paired with naturally occurring social reinforcers. Skills to be taught are broken into small, attainable tasks so that the child can obtain success and receive reinforcement often. When a skill is reinforced, it is more likely to occur in the future. Many times, the reinforcer is related to the task (i.e., manding for a preferred item), but it does not have to be explicitly linked to the task (point to a picture and immediately receive a toy). Learners acquire skills quickly when they are highly motivated. Many times, children with ASD need the frequent repetition of the *stimulus-response-consequences* to learn a skill (Burgraff & Anderson, 2011). The format of DTT is fast-paced and highly reinforcing, allowing for high repetition and quick learning. Figure 7.1 provides a graphic overview of the DTT teaching sequence.

When teaching communication, behavior analytic instruction focuses on the functional units of communication (i.e., the verbal operant) versus the form of the verbal behavior or what the behavior looks like (i.e., picture based vs. vocal; Sundberg, 2014). Verbal behavior differs from other operant analyses in that verbal behavior operates across a four-term contingency in which behavior is mediated by a listener (Reichle et al., 2021). This sequence is illustrated in Figure 7.2 and an overview of Skinner's (1957) verbal operants are presented in Table 7.5.

Specific instruction is often needed for children with ASD to generalize, or apply, newly acquired skills to novel situations, environments, or instructors. Using naturalistic intervention (NI), also known as natural environment teaching, involves systematically arranging the environment to set up teaching opportunities across multiple contexts and can help alleviate the need for additional instruction (Cowen & Allen,

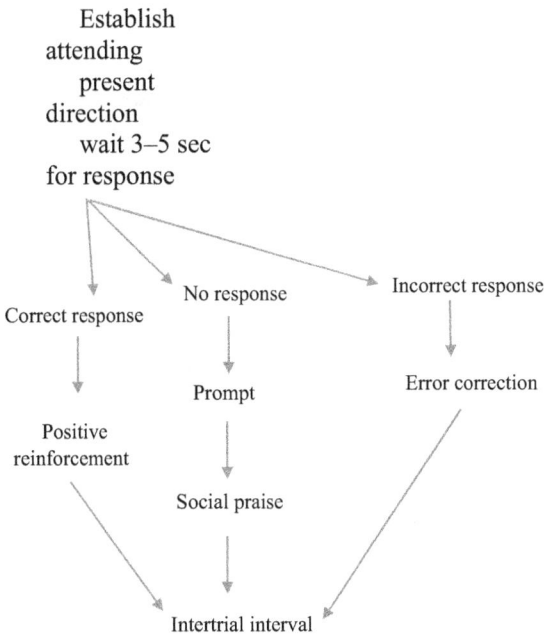

Figure 7.1 The Discrete Trial Instruction Sequence.

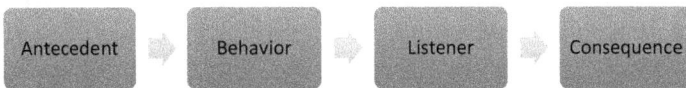

Figure 7.2 Verbal Behavior Four-Term Contingency.

2007). When teaching using NI, the same *stimulus-response-consequence* teaching pattern is followed, except it is embedded into daily activities and the learner's interests are used to guide the interventions (Cowen & Allen, 2007). NI was developed out of incidental teaching and milieu language intervention. Figure 7.3 displays a NI teaching sequence. Pivotal Response Training (PRT) is another evidence-based practice based on the same theoretical components of NI.

PRT emerged from the ABA field when researchers Koegel and Frea (1993) identified pivotal skills that differentiated successful learners from unsuccessful learners after receiving ABA therapy. When children learn these pivotal skills, other skills emerge without being explicitly taught.

Table 7.5 Skinner's Verbal Operants

Verbal Operant	Definition
Mand	Verbal operant that requests the "speaker" to do something. There is a unique relationship between the response and the reinforcement.
Tact	Verbal operant that elicits an evoked response and makes contact with the environment.
Echoic	Verbal operant that occasions a corresponding vocal verbal response and response is an exact replica of the original verbal stimulus.
Intraverbal	Verbal response occasioned by a verbal stimulus. It is not an exact replica of the original verbal stimulus (e.g. reciting the alphabet).
Textual	Verbal operant regulated by verbal stimuli that includes a correspondence between the stimulus and response.
Transcription	Verbal operant that includes a verbal stimulus that evokes a written response that includes a correspondence between the stimulus and response.

Note. Adapted from Skinner, B. F. (1957). *Verbal Behavior.* Copley Publishing Group.

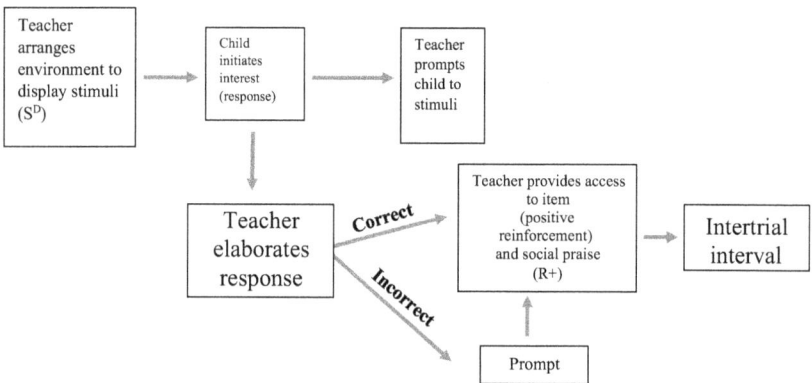

Figure 7.3 Naturalistic Intervention Teaching Sequence.

The pivotal skills include motivation, initiation, responsiveness to multiple cues, imitation, and joint attention (Reichle et al., 2021).

> *Several evidence-based practices were selected to teach Lucía to communicate. DTT was used to teach receptive labeling, picture discrimination, and motor imitation. NI was used to teach these basic skills within functional play activities. Each of these instructional methods included the use of additional evidence-based practices, such as reinforcement, prompting, and time delay procedures.*

Augmentative and Alternative Communication

Given the impairments demonstrated by individuals with ASD, coupled with individuals who struggle to develop vocal speech output capabilities, it is often necessary to incorporate the use of an AAC system when establishing verbal behavior for individuals with ASD (Schlosser, 2006). There are two broad categories of AAC systems: aided and unaided (Gevarter et al., 2013). Unaided systems do not require equipment and include systems such as manual sign language or gestures. Aided systems require equipment and include systems such as a picture-based system or SGD (also called vocal output communication systems).

Families are often hesitant to use AAC as a form of communication for their child as they want their child to "talk." To date, no studies suggest a decrease in vocal output based on the use of AAC. On the contrary, it has been suggested that AAC supplements vocal output, and in some cases, an increase in vocal output has been noted (Tincani et al., 2006). More research is needed in this area. However, the use of AAC as a functional communication system has been linked to a decrease in problem behaviors (Carr & Durand, 1985; Chezan et al., 2018; Durand & Carr, 1991).

Manual Sign

The use of gestures is, developmentally, one of the earliest forms of non-vocal communication (CDC, 2015). Neurotypical children generally develop gesturing before the development of functional vocal output. Procedures, such as time delay and differential reinforcement, can be incorporated into manual sign instruction and may increase vocal responses of children with ASD (Carbone et al., 2010; Schlosser & Wendt, 2008). However, recent studies have demonstrated that communication skills can be taught more effectively and efficiently with aided AAC systems (i.e., picture exchange and SGD) than with manual sign (Couper et al., 2014; Lorah et al., 2021; McLay et al., 2015). Additionally, participants in such research generally prefer aided AAC to unaided AAC (Lorah et al., 2015; Lorah et al., 2021). A final consideration for the use of manual sign is that it requires the communicative partner to understand the sign or gesture (Brodhead et al., 2020).

Picture Exchange

Picture exchange is the use of graphic symbols to teach communication skills (Gevarter et al., 2013). Some suggest that the use of pictures or graphic symbols may benefit the learner because the symbols are not transient and require less working memory (Ganz et al., 2012). Once a word is spoken it is gone, but a picture remains as long as the learner needs it. Picture exchange, icon-based communication systems, or the use of graphic symbols are different than Picture Exchange Communication Systems (PECS; Bondy & Frost, 1994; Gevarter et al., 2013), as they do not use the same teaching sequence as described by the creators and outlined below.

The Picture Exchange Communication System

PECS is a manualized intervention for teaching communication (Bondy & Frost, 1994). PECS uses picture symbols for the exchange in a six-phase teaching format. In phase one, learners are taught to exchange a picture for the desired item (mand training). Phase two involves teaching the learner to expand spontaneity and persistence to communicate, as the learner is required to exchange the picture with a communication partner across the room, using shaping and fading. Phase three requires the student to visually discriminate between two or more picture symbols, in a progressively complex field. Phase four begins teaching a sentence structure with manding ("I want …"). Phase five teaches the learner how to respond to direct questions ("What do you want?"). Finally, phase six teaches the learner to respond and spontaneously comment (Bondy & Frost, 1994). In their review of the literature, Ganz et al. (2012) found that only two studies showed participants advancing through all six phases of PECS with the majority showing participants advancing through only the first three phases. Since more complex language skills are targeted in phases four through six, there is limited evidence to support the use of PECS for more advanced communication. Some research suggests that after the first three phases are mastered, instruction begins to focus on vocal communication (Flippin et al., 2010).

Voice Output Technology

SGD are electronic devices that rely on the speaker's pressing of a picture, word, or symbol with sufficient force to evoke a digitized audio output, which typically occurs in the form of synthesized speech (Lorah et al., 2015). For example, if a child wants a "cookie," he or she can press the picture, word, or symbol that represents "cookie", and a digitized output of "cookie" will be produced by the device. AAC systems, including SGD, are considered an evidence-based practice and have empirical research to support its use (e.g., Lorah et al., 2015; Muharib & Alzrayer, 2017).

Access to relatively low-cost, handheld electronic devices has increased the use of technology as a tool for communication (Lorah, 2018). As the media report stories of people using technology to communicate, parents, as well as professionals, hope that technology is an answer for their children. It is important to understand that technology alone is not an intervention; it is simply the mechanism we use to teach the learner to use the device. Multiple evidence-based practices can be used in SGD instruction, such as time delay, prompting, reinforcement, task analysis, and discrete trial training that can lead to improved communication outcomes for children with ASD (Lorah et al., 2021).

SGD differ from other methods of aided AAC (such as picture-based communication) and unaided AAC (such as sign language), in several ways. First, because SGD generate intelligible audio output, the speaker is not first required to gain the attention of the listener, and the listener can interpret the speaker's message even if he or she is not looking at the speaker. Second, SGD produce audible speech more similar to natural speech production than picture-based communication systems or manual sign. Third, in using SGD, the speaker only needs to demonstrate one-response topography (i.e., pressing a button). This is not the case with manual sign, which requires multiple response topographies, or with picture-based communication, which commonly requires the speaker to remove and exchange a picture card with the listener. Finally, as a speaker acquires a larger vocabulary, the use of a picture-based communication system may become cumbersome in terms of storing and transporting picture cards. SGD, on the other hand, can store thousands of electronic "picture cards" in a compact manner (Lorah et al., 2015; Muharib & Alzrayer, 2017).

In the past, practitioners and caregivers faced exorbitant costs associated with SGD that possessed substantial technological capabilities, such as immediate customization options, which left few alternatives beyond low- to no-technology AAC. But given recent technological advances in the development of powerful, portable, off-the-shelf handheld devices, such as tablet computers (i.e., iPad®; Glaxay®), portable media players (i.e., iPod®), and applications such as Proloqu2Go™, stakeholders now have affordable alternatives. These devices have become increasingly more reliable and can be serviced at most electronic and department stores if necessary. Additionally, the use of tablets and/or portable multimedia players may be less stigmatizing than traditional SGD or picture-based communication since they can be used for additional functions, such as learning (Lorah & Parnell, 2014) or leisure activities (Lorah et al., 2015).

In terms of effectiveness, the use of SGD as an AAC has undergone more than 20 years of research on communication acquisition, teaching strategies, and comparisons to other methods (e.g., Beck et al., 2008; Dicarlo & Banajee, 2000; Lorah et al., 2021; Muharib & Alzrayer, 2017; Sigafoos et al., 2003; Thunberg et al., 2007). The results have been generally favorable, and the use of SGD for communication training is considered effective. Studies comparing SGD with picture-based communication have been largely inconclusive and/or have produced mixed results (Lorah et al., 2021). However, in studies that include a measure of participant preference, most participants demonstrated a preference for SGD over picture-based communication or manual sign (Lorah et al., 2021). Given that both methods of aided AAC may be a viable option for communication training, the preference of the learner should be taken into consideration.

Communication training with SGD can go beyond the basic mand (requesting) repertoire. For example, Lorah, Parnell, and Speight (2014) taught three preschool children with developmental disabilities to tact (label) environmental stimuli in complete sentences, such as "I see dog." Additionally, it has been shown that such devices can be used to teach children to accurately respond to questions such as, "What is it?" (Kagohara et al., 2012). Finally, it has been demonstrated that by using these devices educators can effectively teach children with ASD to respond accurately to questions about personal information such as, "What is your name?" (Strasberger & Ferreri, 2014).

When teaching communication with any form of AAC, practitioners must ensure they are using evidence-based teaching strategies and not simply providing the learner with the system and expecting communication acquisition. It is the AAC plus teaching that allows learners to acquire the ability to communicate (Lorah et al., 2021).

Functional Communication Training

Individuals with ASD often engage in higher levels of disruptive behavior, such as self-injury, aggression, and property destruction, in comparison to neurotypical peers due to a number of factors, including limited communication abilities and adaptive behavior skills, and environmental variables (Chezan et al., 2018). Functional communication training (FCT) is an evidence-based practice that can address these behaviors by teaching communication skills that allow the learner to gain access to preferred items or escape from aversive situations in socially appropriate ways (Carr & Durand, 1985; Chezan et al., 2018; Kurtz et al., 2011). The first step in FCT is conducting a Functional Behavior Assessment (FBA) to determine the underlying function of the challenging behavior. During an FBA, the interfering behavior is objectively defined and antecedent and consequent events that control the behavior are recorded or analyzed (Steinbrenner et al., 2020). The results generate a hypothesis for the function of the behavior as access to preferred materials, access to attention from others, escape from nonpreferred activities, automatic/ sensory stimulation, or a combination of these purposes (Chezan et al., 2018).

Once the function is determined, a replacement behavior is identified that is functionally equivalent (or produces the same outcome), requires less response effort, and is understood by communicative partners (Steinbrenner et al., 2020). The replacement behavior is then taught to the learner explicitly and in context. It is important that the challenging behavior be placed on extinction and the new replacement is reinforced. Differential reinforcement is an evidence-based practice commonly used in conjecture with FCT to provide positive consequences for the replacement behavior (Chezan et al., 2018). The replacement behavior may have to be prompted at first, but prompts should be faded as quickly as possible. Common replacement behaviors are the use of a break card, AAC, or requesting help by raising a hand. For many families of children with ASD, challenging behavior is a major concern. FCT can be utilized to decrease challenging behavior, thereby increasing the quality of life for the learner and family (Chezan et al., 2018). In training communication, it is essential that all the child's communicative partners, including family members, school staff, and therapy providers, actively participate in the growth of language (McLeskey et al., 2019).

> *Lucía's team decides to use an FBA to identify the function of her screaming behavior. After analyzing the results, they determine the function is escape from nonpreferred activities. Crying most commonly occurs when Lucía is presented with novel foods at mealtime. The team identifies pressing an "all done" icon on the SGD as an appropriate replacement behavior. When Lucía starts to whine and push the food away, she is prompted to press the "all done" icon. After pressing the "all done" icon, the food is removed from the table. The prompts are faded as Lucía's crying decreases and her independence increases.*

Interdisciplinary Teaming to Enhance Communication

Due to their complex needs, children with ASD often require specialized services across many disciplines. By working collaboratively, professionals can provide greater support to these individuals and their families (Gerenser & Koenig, 2019). Interdisciplinary teams may include occupational therapists, speech-language therapists, physical therapists, behavior analysts, teachers, caregivers, and other interventionalists (Shahidullah et al., 2020). Although highly beneficial for both the student and professionals involved, coordinating care between all members of a professional team can be challenging.

A barrier to effective collaboration is when professional scopes of practice overlap, causing ambiguous situations and unclear boundaries (Gerenser & Koenig, 2019). In addition, terminology and technical jargon can vary across professions, hindering communication abilities. Misconceptions and stereotypes about other professionals can lead to biases and judgments about other team members. Theoretical and historical differences can be an additional barrier to teamwork (Gerenser & Koenig, 2019; McClain et al., 2020).

One of the most important factors in overcoming these challenges is creating and maintaining open and honest communication with all team members (Shahidullah et al., 2020). This should happen early in the process, before the first meeting, by introducing yourself and establishing a preferred method of communication for the team (Gerenser & Koenig, 2019). Focusing on shared values and goals, such as student growth and progress, encourages everyone to remain respectful of one another (McClain et al., 2020). Meetings can be a time to share progress reports, create a joint plan to handle disruptive behaviors, and share functional communication phrases that the student is learning. Working as a member of a team presents many opportunities to learn from other professionals and other fields of discipline. Team members may share applicable research findings and updates that highlight the relevant strengths of other professions (Griffin, 2017; Spencer et al., 2021). If possible, team members should observe each other working with the student to learn from each other and offer support to one another (Griffin, 2017).

Among the many benefits of collaboration is an increase in service efficiency through reducing the unnecessary duplication of services (Gerenser & Koenig, 2019). By sharing knowledge and experience, professionals can spot problems and develop solutions more effectively while sharing in decision-making (McClain et al., 2020). Coordination of care can reduce parent confusion from receiving different or conflicting recommendations from professionals, increase parental involvement in services, and result in more consistent communication with families (Gerenser & Koenig, 2019). Despite its many challenges, interdisciplinary teaming can be beneficial for everyone involved since all communicative partners have an essential role in the learners' life.

Training Communicative Partners

For verbal behavior to be maintained or generalized, it must come in contact with reinforcement in the natural environment (Cooper et al., 2020). One way to facilitate generalization is to train communicative partners across a variety of contexts and settings. Researchers suggest that lack of training for communicative partners is a barrier to the successful use of AAC systems for communication (Donato et al., 2018; Sievers et al., 2018). This barrier can be overcome through systematic instruction in naturalistic contexts, including daily routines (Donato et al., 2018; Kent-Walsh et al., 2015; Shire et al., 2015). When teaching communication skills, it is essential for all communicative partners involved in the child's life to receive training (Meadan et al., 2012).

Therefore, the first step is to identify all communicative partners in the student's life. Training can begin by gathering these stakeholders and discussing the importance of communicative partners in the development of their loved ones' communication ability (Meaden et al., 2012). Stakeholders need to understand that 1) everyone has a right to communicate; 2) a communication system is the person's voice and it must always be available to the learner; 3) if a learner does not have a system to communicate, they may communicate with problem behavior; and 4) the communicative partners' behavior (setting up opportunities and responding to communicative attempts) will increase or decrease the likelihood of the learner's attempts to communicate.

Next, help stakeholders identify naturally occurring opportunities and daily routines in which communication takes place. Communication opportunities can be embedded within the naturally occurring activities and routines for the family (Akemoglu et al., 2020). This increases the likelihood that the interaction will occur as it is a meaningful activity for the child and partner and does not require the family to add anything to their day or change their routine. The next step is to set up the communication system and show the family how to use it (Donato et al., 2018). The system must be easy and efficient for both user and partner. Practice with the partner and learner in the natural environment while giving feedback to the partner to increase fidelity (Kent-Walsh et al., 2015). Once fidelity is achieved, instruct the partner and learner to continue to use the system during the identified routines and activities. Tell the partner and learner they can use the system in other activities. Collect data, provide feedback, and adjust the intervention according to the partner and learner feedback and skill acquisition.

Dialect

When evaluating and training communication, consideration should be given to the cultural background and communication history of each child. Not only is every child with ASD unique, but the communication styles, values, beliefs, and traditions of the family can vary greatly. Despite all these differences, many continuous patterns of articulation and dialect can be seen around certain ethnicities. Regional differences are common and sometimes mistaken as a speech disorder (Hendricks et al., 2021). Therefore, practitioners should research unfamiliar cultures and be aware of these differences. The common dialectical differences noted here are only a small sample of the diversity reflected across our expanding world (Hendricks et al., 2021).

African languages consist of more verbal than written communication. Practitioners have noted that children that speak African American English (AAE) have some patterns such as deleting consonants in clusters, (e.g. "hep" for help) due to African American tribal languages having limited consonant clusters. Another AAE language pattern is voiced and voiceless "th" being replaced by /f/ for /d/ such as "dis for this" (Velleman & Pearson, 2010). Also, use of double negatives, such as "I don't have no pencil" instead of "I don't have a pencil." They may articulate with the substitution of /ks/ for /sk/ for example, "ask" is articulated "aks" (Rickford & King, 2016; Stockman et al., 2016).

In our Spanish communities, there is an increase in children presenting as frontal lispers or pronouncing a "th" in place of a "s" sound. This means that the tongue protrudes past their teeth in articulation of fricatives /s/, /s/ -blends, and /z/. Spanish speakers often put the "eh" (as in egg) in front of the /s/ sounds, even when it is not spelled with the vowel in front. This vowel causes the tongue to start to automatically protrude before articulating the /s/. Therefore, when many of these speakers start to learn Spanish as a second language, the frontal tongue protrusion is already embedded and occurs naturally (Shi & Canizales, 2013).

Even across regions of the United States, there are differences in short /i/ and short /e/. In areas like Wisconsin, students may make the sound short /i/ and short /e/ sound differently. However, in areas such as Arkansas, the short /i/ and short /e/ may sound the same. For example, this can cause the name "Ben" to sound very similar to "bin" (Cristia et al., 2012).

There are up to 200 Native American languages that represent over 20 language families (Robinson-Zafiartu, 1996). This provides a rich ancestral language tradition that contains its own rules of pronunciation and grammar. These rules are produced by sound contrasts based on ancestral language, pronunciation that parallels sound inventories found in the local or regional dialects or combines principles from both sources to resemble standard English (Leap, 1993; Robinson-Zafiartu, 1996).

In addition to articulation and speech patterns, nasalance scores can vary across cultures. For example, southern Vietnamese speakers produce the higher nasalance scores on the vowel /a/, followed by /i/ and /u/. Nasalance scores also varied across stimuli with the falling and restricted tone producing significantly lower scores than those produced by other tones (Nguyen et al., 2021).

Many English as second language learners struggle with some consonants and vowels that are exclusive to the English language. For example, the H and R sounds are not present in Brazilian Portuguese. Many Asian languages do not have R or L sounds, and Arabic lacks a P and B sound, causing many of these individuals to struggle with English sound pronunciation (Wallace, 2015). These issues may be even more cumbersome for children with ASD. It is our responsibility as practitioners to be knowledgeable of these differences and be able to identify when communication difficulties can be attributed to the broader social communication impairments that characterize ASD.

Conclusion

Communication is essential to everyday life and builds connections and relationships with those around us (Prelock et al., 2011). Early language skills provide a basis for future learning across all developmental domains and may be a predictor of successful social and adaptive skills in adolescence and adulthood (Ben-Itzchak & Zachor, 2020; Drmic et al., 2018; LeGrand et al., 2021). In order to develop communication skills, individuals with ASD often require focused instruction that includes evidence-based practices, such as AAC, prompting, reinforcement, DTT, and NI. This chapter provided an overview of the language impairments associated with ASD, the assessments that drive instruction, and evidence-based practices used during instruction. Practical tips on working collaboratively with other professionals and important stakeholders were provided to guide practitioners.

After 6 months of intervention, at 9 hours per week, Lucía has moved from a level 1 learner to a level 2 learner in many areas. Lucía uses the SGD to independently communicate her basic needs. She is able to mand for at least 10 items without prompts, can tact at least ten items without echoic prompts, responds to her name, orients towards a speaker's voice, points to preferred items and is beginning to respond to simple one-step directions, such as "clap" and "wave.". Lucía continues to have strengths in visual performance and matching to sample. She has made great gains in play and social interaction. Lucía is able to participate in small group activities for up to 10 minutes with teacher support. Lucía has a limited echoic repertoire and continues to struggle with imitation and vocal response. Imitation is the ability to repeat what one hears. However, it should be noted that Lucía spontaneously uses vocal responses and has been heard using vocalizations in context such as "Mama, wow, I did it, stand up, fall down".

Discussion Questions

1. What resources can be used to choose evidence-based interventions for teaching communication to children with ASD?
2. How does the use of applied behavior analysis and speech language therapy fit within a communication training package?
3. What is verbal behavior?
4. What is functional communication training (FCT)? How do the aims of FCT differ from communication training?
5. What are some strategies for successful collaboration with other professionals? With caregivers and stakeholders?

References

Akemoglu, Y., Meadan, H., & Towson, J. (2020). Embedding naturalistic communication teaching strategies during shared interactive book reading for preschoolers with developmental delays: A guide for caregivers. *Early Childhood Education Journal*, 48, 759–766. doi: 10.1007/s10643-020-01038-4

American Psychiatric Association. (2013). *Diagnostic and statistical manual of mental disorders* (5th ed.). https://doi.org/10.1176/appi.books.978089 0425596

Baer, D.M., Wolf, M.M., & Risley, T.R. (1968). Some current dimensions of applied behavior analysis. *Journal of Applied Behavior Analysis*, 1, 91–97.

Beck, A.R., Stoner, J.B., Bock, S.J., & Parton, T. (2008). Comparison of PECS and the use of a VOCA: A replication. *Education and Training in Developmental Disabilities*, 43, 198–216.

Ben-Itzchak, E. & Zachor, D.A. (2020). Toddlers to teenagers: Long-term follow-up study of outcomes in autism spectrum disorder. *Autism*, 24(1), 41–50.

Bondy, A., & Frost, L. (1994). The picture exchange communication system. *Focus on Autistic Behavior*, 9(3), 1–19.

Bondy, A., & Frost, L. (2011). *A picture's worth: PECS and other visual communication strategies in autism.* Woodbine House.

Brodhead, M.T., Brouwers, L.F., Sipila-Thomas, E.S., & Rispoli, M.J. (2020). A comparison of manual sign and speech generating devices in the natural environment. *Journal of Developmental and Physical Disabilities*, 32, 785–800. doi: 10.1007/s10882-019-09720-1

Buckmann, S. (2016). *A brief explanation of discrete trial training.* Indiana Resource Center for Autism. www.iidc.indiana.edu/pages/A-Brief-Explanation-of-Discrete-Trial-Training

Burggraff, B., & Anderson, C.A. (2011) Discrete trial intervention for children with limited social and language skills and intellectual delays. In T. Thompson (Ed.), *Individualized Autism Intervention for Young Children* (pp. 73–98). Brookes Publishing.

Carbone, V.J., Sweeney-Kerwin, E.J., Attanasio, V., & Kasper, T. (2010). Increasing the vocal responses of children with autism and developmental disabilities using manual sign mand training and prompt delay. *Journal of Applied Behavior Analysis*, 43(4), 705–709.

Carr, E.G., & Durand, V.M. (1985). Reducing problem behavior through functional communication training. *Journal of Applied Behavior Analysis*, 18(2), 111–126.

Centers for Disease Control and Prevention (2015). *Developmental Disabilities Homepage.* www.cdc.gov/ncbddd/developmentaldisabilities/specificconditions. html

Charlop, M.H. (2018). *Naturalistic and incidental teaching* (2nd ed.). Pro-Ed Series.

Chezan, L.C., Wolfe, K., & Drasgow, E. (2018). A meta-analysis of functional communication training effects on problem behavior and alternative communicative responses. *Focus on Autism and Other Developmental Disabilities*, 33(4), 195–205. https://doi.org/10.1177/1088357617741294

Coon, J.T., & Miguel, C.F. (2012). The role of increased exposure to transfer-of-stimulus-control procedures on the acquisition of intraverbal behavior. *Journal of Applied Behavior Analysis, 45,* 657–666.

Cooper, J.O., Heron, T.E., & Heward, W.L. (2020). *Applied Behavior Analysis* (3rd ed.). Pearson Education Limited.

Cosgrave, G. (2021). *Extinction procedures.* Educate Autism. www.educateautism.com/applied-behaviour-analysis/extinction-procedure-aba.html

Couper, L., van der Meer, L., Schafer, M.C.M., McKenzie, E., McLay, L., O'Reilly, M.F., et al. (2014). Comparing acquisition of and preference for manual signs, picture exchange, and speech-generating devices in nine children with autism spectrum disorder. *Developmental Neurorehabilitation, 17*(2), 99–109.

Cowan, R.J., & Allen, K.D. (2007). Using naturalistic procedures to enhance learning in individuals with ASD: A focus on generalized teaching in the classroom setting, *Psychology in the Schools, 44*(7), 701–715.

Cristia, A., Seidl, A., Vaughn, C., Schmale, R., Bradlow, A., & Floccia, C. (2012). Linguistic processing of accented speech across the lifespan. *Frontiers in Psychology, 3,* 1–15. https://doi.org/10.3389/fpsyg.2012.00479

Dicarlo, C. F., & Banajee, M. (2000). Using voice output devices to increase initiations of young children with disabilities. *Journal of Early Intervention, 23,* 191–199.

DiStefano, C., & Kasari, C. (2016). The window to language is still open: Distinguishing between Preverbal and minimally verbal children with ASD. *Perspectives of the ASHA Special Interest Groups, 1*(1), 4–11. https://doi.org/10.1044/persp1.sig1.4

Donato, C., Spencer, E., & Arthur-Kelly, M. (2018). A critical synthesis of barriers and facilitators to the use of AAC by children with autism spectrum disorder and their communication partners. *Augmentative and Alternative Communication, 34*(3), 242–253. https://doi.org/10.1080/07434618.2018.1493141

Drmic, I.E., Szatmari, P., & Volkmar, F. (2018). Life course health development in Autism Spectrum Disorders. In N. Halfon, C.B. Forrest, R.M. Lerner, & E.M. Faustman (Eds.), *Handbook of life course health development* (pp. 237–274). Springer.

Durand, V.M., & Carr, E.G. (1991). Functional communication training to reduce challenging behavior: Maintenance and application in new settings. *Journal of Applied Behavior Analysis, 24,* 251–264.

Esch, B.E., LaLonde, K.B., & Esch, J.W. (2010). Speech and language assessment: A verbal behavior analysis. *The Journal of Speech and Language Pathology-Applied Behavior Analysis, 5*(2), 166–191.

Flippin, M., Reszka, S., & Watson, L.R. (2010). Effectiveness of the picture exchange communication system (PECS) on communication and speech of children with autism spectrum disorders: A meta-analysis. *American Journal of Speech-Language Pathology, 19,* 178–195.

Gaffney, A. (2020). *Speech Pathology Assessment Resource List.* Indiana Resource Center for Autism. www.iidc.indiana.edu/irca/articles/speech-pathology-assessment-resource-list.html

Ganz, J.B., Davis, J.L., Lund, E.M., Goodwyn, F.D., & Simpson, R.L. (2012). Meta-analysis of PECS with individuals with ASD: Investigation of targeted versus non-targeted outcomes, participant characteristics, and implementation phase. *Research in Developmental Disabilities*, *33*(2), 406–418. doi:10/1016/j.ridd.2011.09.023

Gerenser, J.E., & Koenig, M.A. (Eds.) (2019). *ABA for SLPs: Interprofessional collaboration for autism support teams*. Paul H. Brooks Publishing Co.

Gevarter, C., O'Reilly, M.F., Rojeski, L., Sammarco, N., Lang, R., Lancioni, G.E., & Sigafoos, J. (2013). Comparing communication systems for individuals with developmental disabilities: A review of single-case research studies. *Research in Developmental Disabilities*, *34*, 4415–4432.

Ghezzi, P. (2007). Discrete Trials Teaching. *Psychology in the Schools*, *44*(7), 667–679.

Gleason, J.B., & Ratner, N.B. (2017). *The development of language* (9th ed.). Pearson.

Gray, C. (2015). *The new social story book: Over 150 social stories that teach everyday social skills to children and adults with autism and their peers*. Future Horizons.

Griffin, R. (2017, May 17). *Ten collaboration tips for SLPs and behavior analysts treating students with autism*. ASHA Leader. https://leader.pubs.asha.org/do/10.1044/10-collaboration-tips-for-slps-and-behavior-analysts-treating-students-with-autism/full/

Hendricks, A.E., Watson-Wales, M., & Reed, P.E. (2021). Perceptions of African American English by students in speech-language pathology programs. *American Journal of Speech-Language Pathology*, *30*(5), 1962–1972. https://doi.org/10.1044/2021_ajslp-20-00339

Hodgdon, L., & Bryant, M. (2019). *Practical communication tools for autism: Using visual strategies for lifelong success*. QuirkRoberts Publishing.

Hodgdon, L., Harris, R., Griffin, S., & Butler, R. (2017). *Teach me with pictures: 40 fun picture scripts to develop play and communication skills in children on the autism spectrum* (2nd ed.). Jessica Kingsley Publishers.

Human Development Institute. (2015). *Peer networks and peer support arrangements*. Kentucky Peer Support Network Project. www.kypeersupport.org/

Ingersoll, B., & Dvortcsak, A. (2019). *Teaching social communication to children with autism and other developmental delays: The project ImPACT manual for parents* (2nd ed.). Guilford Press.

Kagohara, D.M., van der Meer, L., Achmadi, D., Green, V.A., O'Reilly, M.F., Lancioni, G.E., Sutherland, D., Lang, R., Marschik, P.B., & Sigafoos, J. (2012). Teaching picture naming to two adolescents with autism spectrum disorders using systematic instruction and speech-generating devices. *Research in Autism Spectrum Disorders*, *6*(3), 1224–1233.

Kent-Walsh, J., Murza, K.A., Malani, M.D., & Binger, C. (2015). Effects of communication partner instruction on the communication of individuals using AAC: A meta-analysis. *Augmentative and Alternative Communication*, *31*(4), 271–284. doi: 10.3109/07434618.2015.1052153

Koegel, R.L., & Frea, W.D. (1993). Treatment of social behavior in autism through the modification of pivotal social skills. *Journal of Applied Behavior Analysis*, *26*, 369–377.

Koegel, R.L., & Koegel, L.K. (2012). *The PRT pocket guide: Pivotal response treatment for autism spectrum disorders*. Brookes Publishing Company.

Kurtz, P.F., Boelter, E.W., Jarmolowicz, D.P., Chin, M.D., & Hagopian, L.P. (2011). An analysis of functional communication training as an empirically supported treatment for problem behavior displayed by individuals with intellectual disabilities. *Research in developmental disabilities*, 32(6), 2935–2942. https://doi.org/10.1016/j.ridd.2011.05.009

Leap, W.L. (1993). *American Indian English*. University of Utah Press.

Ledford, J.R., Chazin, K.T., & Maupin, T.N. (2016). *Progressive time delay*. Evidence-Based Instructional Practices for Young Children with Autism and Other Disabilities. http://ebip.vkcsites.org/progressive-time-delay

LeGrand, K.J., Weil, L.W., Lord, C., & Luyster, R.J. (2021). Identifying childhood expressive language features that best predict adult language and communication outcome in individuals with autism spectrum disorder. *Journal of Speech, Language, and Hearing Research*, 64, 1977–1991.

Loman, S., Strickland-Cohen, M.K., Borgmeier, C., & Horner, R. (2019). *Basic FBA to BSP: Trainer's manual*. U.S. Department of Education. www.pbis.org/resource/basic-fba-to-bsp-trainers-manual

Lorah, E.R. (2018). Evaluating the iPad Mini as a speech generating device in the acquisition of a discriminative mand repertoire for young children with autism. *Focus on Autism and Other Developmental Disabilities*, 33(1), 47–54. doi: 10.1177/1088357616673624

Lorah, E.R., Holyfield, C., Miller, J., Griffen, B., & Lindbloom, C. (2021). A systematic review of research comparing mobile technology speech-generating devices to other AAC modes with individuals with autism spectrum disorder. *Journal of Physical and Developmental Disabilities*, doi:10.1007/s10882-021-09803-y

Lorah, E.R., & Parnell, A. (2014). The acquisition of letter writing using portable multimedia players in young children with developmental disabilities. *Journal of Developmental and Physical Disabilities*, 26, 655–666. doi: 10.1007/s10882-014-9386-0

Lorah, E.R., Parnell, A., Schaefer-Whitby, P., & Hantula, D. (2015). A systematic review of tablet based computers and portable media players as speech generating devices for individuals with ASD spectrum disorder. *Journal of Autism and Developmental Disorders*, 45, 3792–3804. doi: 10.1007/s10803-014-2314-4

Lorah, E.R., Parnell, A., & Speight, D.R. (2014). Acquisition of sentence frame discrimination using the iPad as a speech generating device in young children with developmental disabilities. *Research in Autism Spectrum Disorders*, 8, 1734–1740.

Mayer, G.R., Sulzer-Azaroff, B., & Wallace, M. (2018). *Behavior analysis for lasting change* (4th ed.). Sloan Publishing.

McClain, M.B., Shahidullah, J.D., Mezher, K.R., Haverkamp, C.R., Benallie, K.J., & Schwartz, S.E. (2020). School-clinic care coordination for youth with ASD: A national survey of school psychologists. *Journal of Autism and Developmental Disorders*, 50, 3081–3091.

McGhan, A.C., & Lerman, D.C. (2013). An assessment of error correction procedures for learners with ASD. *Journal of Applied Behavior Analysis*, 46, 626–639.

McLay, L., van der Meer, L., Schafer, M.C., Couper, L., McKenzie, E., O'Reilly, M.F., Lancioni, G.E., Marschik, P.B., Green, V.A., Sigafoos, J., & Sutherland, D.

(2015). Comparing acquisition, generalization, maintenance, and preference across three AAC options in four children with autism spectrum disorder. *Journal of Developmental and Physical Disabilities*, 27(3), 323–339.

McLeskey, J., Maheady, L., Billingsley, B., Brownell, M., & Lewis, T. (2019). *High leverage practices for inclusive classrooms*. Routledge.

Meadan, H., Halle, J.W., & Kelly, S.M. (2012). Intentional communication of young children with autism spectrum disorder: Judgments of different communication partners. *Journal of Developmental and Physical Disabilities*, 24(5), 437–450. https://doi.org/10.1007/s10882-012-9281-5

Miller, T.M., & Thiemann-Bourque, K. (2016). Integrating written text and graphic cues into peer-mediated interventions: Effects on reciprocal social communication skills. *Perspectives of the ASHA Special Interest Groups*, 1(1), 20–28. https://doi.org/10.1044/persp1.sig1.20

Muharib, R., & Alzrayer, N.M. (2017). The use of high-tech speech-generating devices as an evidence-based practice for children with autism spectrum disorders: A meta-analysis. *Review Journal of Autism and Developmental Disorders*, 5, 43–57.

Muller, K., & Brady, N. (2016). Assessing early receptive language skills in children with ASD. *Perspectives of the ASHA Special Interest Groups*, 1(1), 12–19. https://doi.org/10.1044/persp1.sig1.12

Murray, S., & Noland, B. (2013). *Video modeling for young children with autism spectrum disorder: A practical guide for parents and professionals*. Jessica Kingsley Pub.

National Autism Center. (2015). *Autism interventions*. National Autism Center at May Institute. www.nationalautismcenter.org/autism/autism-interventions/

Nguyen, D.M., Lee, S.A., Hayakawa, T., Yamamoto, M., & Natsumef, N. (2021). Normative nasalance values in Vietnamese with southern dialect: Vowel and tone effects. *Journal of Speech, Language, and Hearing Research*, 64, 1515–1525.

Ohio Department of Education (2020). *Antecedent-based interventions*. Autism Internet Modules. https://autisminternetmodules.org/m/503

Partington, J.W. (2015). *The Assessment of Basic Language and Learning Skills – Revised (ABLLS-R)*. Educational & Psychological Assessments for Clinicians & Educators. www.partingtonbehavioranalysts.com/page/ablls-r-25.html

Partington, J.W., Bailey, A., & Partington, S.W. (2018). A pilot study on patterns of skill development of neurotypical children as measured by the ABLLS-R: Implications for educational programming for children with autism. *International Journal of Contemporary Education*, 1(2), 70–85. doi:10.11114/ijce.v1i2.3219

Prelock, P., Paul, R., & Allen, E.M. (2011). Evidence-Based Treatments in Communication for Children. In Reichow, B., Doehring, P., Cicchetti, D.V., & Volkmar, F.R. (Eds.), *Evidence-based practices and treatments for children with autism* (pp. 93–169). Springer Science+Business Media, LLC.

Pro-Ed. (2009). *SSI4 Stuttering Severity Instrument Fourth Edition*. Pro-Ed. www.proedinc.com/Products/13025/ssi4-stuttering-severity-instrument--fourth-edition.aspx.

Pro-Ed. (2009). *Test of childhood stuttering (TOCS)*. ATP: Test of Childhood Stuttering (TOCS). www.academictherapy.com/detailATP.tpl?eqskudatarq=DDD-2100.

Reichle, J., O'Neill, R.E., & Johnston, S.S. (2021). Advances in AAC intervention: some contributions related to applied behavior analysis. *Augmentative and Alternative Communication.* doi: 10.1080/07434618.2021.1962405

Reichle, J., & Wacker, D. (2017). *Functional communication training for problem behavior.* The Guilford Press.

Rickford, J.R., & King, S. (2016). Language and linguistics on trial: Hearing Rachel Jeantel (and other vernacular speakers) in the courtroom and beyond. *Language, 92*(4), 948–988. https:// doi.org/10.1353/lan.2016.0078

Robinson-Zañartu, C. (1996). Serving Native American children and families: Considering cultural variables. *Language. Speech, And Hearing Services In Schools, 27,* 373–384. https://pubs.asha.org/doi/pdf/10.1044/0161-1461.2704.373

Sam, A., & AFIRM Team. (2015a). *Prompting.* Chapel Hill, NC: National Professional Development Center on Autism Spectrum Disorder, FPG Child Development Center, University of North Carolina. http://afirm.fpg.unc.edu/prompting

Sam, A., & AFIRM Team. (2015b). *Task analysis.* Chapel Hill, NC: National Professional Development Center on Autism Spectrum Disorder, FPG Child Development Center, University of North Carolina. http://afirm.fpg.unc.edu/task-analysis

Scarpa, A., White, S.W., & Attwood, T. (2016). *CBT for children and adolescents with high-functioning autism spectrum disorders.* Guilford Press.

Schlosser, R.W. (2006). Evidence-based practice for AAC practitioners. *Perspectives on Augmentative and Alternative Communication, 15*(3), 8–9. doi:10.1044/aac17.3.113

Schlosser, R.W., & Wendt, O. (2008). Augmentative and alternative communication intervention for children with autism. In J.K. Luiselli, D.C. Russo, W.P. Christian, & S.M. Wilczynski (Eds.), *Effective practices for children with autism: Educational and behavioral support interventions that work* (pp. 325–389). Oxford University Press.

Shahidullah, J.D., McClain, M.B., Azad, G., Mezher, K.R., & McIntyre, L.L. (2020). Coordinating autism care across schools and medical settings: Considerations for school psychologists. *Intervention in School and Clinic, 56*(2), 107–114. doi:10.1177/1053451220914891

Shi, L.F., & Canizales, L.A. (2013). Dialectal effects on a clinical Spanish word recognition test. *American Journal of Audiology, 22*(1), 74–83. https://doi.org/10.1044/1059-0889(2012/12-0036)

Shire, S.Y., Goods, K., Shih, W., Distefano, C., Kaiser, A., Wright, C., Mathy, P., Landa, R., & Kasari, C. (2015). Parents' adoption of social communication intervention strategies: Families including children with autism spectrum disorder who are minimally verbal. *Journal of Autism and Developmental Disorders, 45*(6), 1712–1724. https://doi.org/10.1007/s10803-014-2329-x

Shumway, S., & Wetherby, A.M. (2009). Communicative acts of children with autism spectrum disorders in the second year of life. *Journal of Speech, Language, and Hearing Research, 52*(5), 1139–1156. https://doi.org/10.1044/1092-4388(2009/07-0280)

Sievers, S.B., Trembath, D., & Westerveld, M. (2018). A systematic review of predictors, moderators, and mediators of augmentative and alternative communication (AAC) outcomes for children with autism spectrum disorder. *Augmentative and Alternative Communication*, *34*(3), 219–229. https://doi.org/10.1080/07434618.2018.1462849

Sigafoos, J., Didden, R., & O'Reilly, M. (2003). Effects of speech output on maintenance of requesting and frequency of vocalizations in three children with developmental disabilities. *Augmentative and Alternative Communication*, *19*, 37–47.

Skinner, B.F. (1957). *Verbal behavior*. Copley Publishing Group.

Skinner, C., Pauly, R., Skinner, S.A., Schroer, R.J., Simensen, R.J., Taylor, H.A., Friez, M.J., DuPont, B.R., & Stevenson, R.E. (2021). Autistic disorder: A 20 year chronicle. *Journal of Autism and Developmental Disorders*, *51*, 677–684.

Spencer, T., Slim, L., Cardon, T., & Morgan, L. (2021). Interprofessional collaborative practice between behavior analysts and speech-language pathologists. *Association for Behavior Analysis International*. www.abainternational.org/constituents/practitioners/interprofessional-collaborative-practice.aspx

Steinbrenner, J.R., Hume, K., Odom, S.L., Morin, K.L., Nowell, S.W., Tomaszewski, B., Szendrey, S., McIntyre, N.S., Yücesoy-Özkan, S., & Savage, M.N. (2020). *Evidence-based practices for children, youth, and young adults with autism*. The University of North Carolina at Chapel Hill, Frank Porter Graham Child Development Institute, National Clearinghouse on Autism Evidence and Practice Review Team.

Stockman, I.J., Newkirk-Turner, B.L., Swartzlander, E., & Morris, L.R. (2016). Comparison of African American children's performances on a minimal competence core for morphosyntax and the index of productive syntax. *American Journal of Speech-Language Pathology*, *25*(1), 80–96. https://doi.org/10.1044/2015_ajslp-14-0207

Strasberger, S.K., & Ferreri, S.J. (2014). The effects of peer assisted communication application training on the communicative and social behaviors of children with ASD. *Journal of Developmental and Physical Disabilities*, *26*(5), 513–526.

Sundberg, M. (2014). The VB-MAPP: Conducting the assessment and identifying intervention priorities. Presentation retrieved from http://autism.outreach.psu.edu/sites/omcphplive.outreach.psu.edu.drpms.autismconference/files/18and30Presentation_0.pdf

Thompson, T. (2011). *Individualized autism interventions for young children: Blending discrete trial and naturalistic strategies*. Brookes Publishing.

Thunberg, G., Ahlsén, E., & Sandberg, A.D. (2007). Children with autistic spectrum disorders and speech-generating devices: Communication in different activities at home. *Clinical Linguistics & Phonetics*, *21*, 457–479.

Tincani, M., Crozier, S.E., & Alazetta, L. (2006). The picture exchange communication system: Effects on manding and speech development for school-aged children with autism. *Education and Training in Developmental Disabilities*, *41*(2), 177–184.

Trembath, D., Sutherland, R., Caithness, T., Dissanayake, C., Eapen, V., Fordyce, K., Frost, G., Iacono, T., Mahler, N., Masi, A., Paynter, J., Pye, K., Reilly, S., Rose, V., Sievers, S., Thirumanickam, A., Westerveld, M., & Tucker, M. (2021). Clinician proposed predictors of spoken language outcomes for minimally verbal children with autism spectrum disorder. *Journal of Autism and Developmental Disorders*, *51*, 564–575. doi:10.1007/s/10803-020-04550-z

Vietze, P., & Lax, L.E. (2020). Early intervention ABA for toddlers with ASD: Effect of age and amount. *Current Psychology*, *39*, 1234–1244. doi:10.1007/s12144-018-981-z

Wallace, G. (2015). *The English fluency formula*. Go Natural English.

Westby, C., Burda, A., & Mehta, Z. (2003, April 29). *Asking the right questions in the right ways: Strategies for ethnographic interviewing*. The ASHA Leader. www.asha.org/practice-portal/clinical-topics/late-language-emergence/assessm ent-tools-techniques-and-data-sources/

Wong, C., Odom, S.L., Hume, K., Cox, A.W., Fettig, A., Kucharczyk, S., Brock, M.E., Plavnick, J.B., Fleury, V.P., & Schultz, T.R. (2014). *Evidence-based practices for children, youth, and young adults with ASD Spectrum Disorder*. Chapel Hill: The University of North Carolina, Frank Porter Graham Child Development Institute, Autism Evidence-Based Practice Review Group.

WPS (2017). *Arizona™-4 Arizona Articulation and Phonology Scale™, Fourth Revision*. (Arizona™-4) Arizona Articulation Phonology Scale, Fourth Edition. WPS. www.wpspublish.com/arizona-4-arizona-articulation-and-phonology-scale-fourth-revision

WPS (2013). *CAAP-2 Clinical Assessment of Articulation and Phonology, Second Edition*. Educational & Psychological Assessments for Clinicians &Educators. WPS. www.wpspublish.com/caap-2-clinical-assessment-of-articulation-and-phonology-second-edition

Chapter 8

Building and Managing Appropriate Behaviors

E. Amanda DiGangi, Devon Ramey,[2] Sarah Robison,[1] and Samuel DiGangi[1]
[1]Mary Lou Fulton Teachers College, Arizona State University
[2]School of Social Sciences, Education and Social Work, Queen's University Belfast

Case Scenarios

Case 1, Jack:

Jack was diagnosed with ASD at age 3. He is currently 8 years old and attends a specialized program for children with ASD at his elementary school. Jack has minimal vocal communication and generally conveys his wants and needs through a series of gestures and vocal approximations. He has never had a formal augmentative or alternative communication system. Jack displays aggressive behaviors such as punching with his fist and open hand slapping. These behaviors are most often seen when Jack is trying to communicate something to someone who does not immediately comprehend what he wants. The behavior will continue and escalate until a picture-based choice board is offered and Jack can point to the item he wanted.

Case 2, Lana:

Lana is 4 years old and attends a special education preschool program for children with ASD. She was diagnosed at age 2.5 and has just begun to speak vocally. She has a vocabulary of approximately 15 words, mostly for things in her immediate environment (e.g., cracker, iPad, Mom, juice, etc.). Lana's challenging behavior is "throwing tantrums" – described as falling to the floor, kicking her feet on the floor or at anyone who comes near her, banging her head against the floor or nearby furniture, screaming, crying, and throwing materials. When anyone comes near her and tries to comfort her or offer help, she will often bang her head harder and try to kick or hit them. These behaviors typically occur when a task demand is placed on her. The behaviors continue until the teacher

DOI: 10.4324/9781003255147-10

moves on to another student or activity, leaving Lana to herself to calm down.

Case 3, Isaac:

Isaac is a 5th grade student attending mostly general education classes, with special education paraprofessional support for ASD. Isaac speaks clearly but is not on grade level academically and requires multiple accommodations and modifications to his assignments and instructions. Isaac engages in elopement behavior (i.e., leaving the area or room without permission) several times every day, often during work activities, but sometimes during free time as well. His paraprofessional follows him every time and they often end up walking and talking outside. The paraprofessional believes that Isaac needs these "breaks" from the classroom and enjoys going on walks with him.

Case 4, Bo:

Bo is a nonverbal 6-year-old boy attending a special education program for children with ASD. Bo was diagnosed at age 2. His home language is Mandarin, but there are no interpreters available in his school. Bo goes to inclusive Kindergarten classes each day for story time, lunch, and recess. Bo has no functional means of communication but he only engages in a few challenging behaviors. He is compliant with adult requests if they are accompanied by physical guidance, although it is assumed that he does not understand many of the commands being given. The only behavioral challenge that Bo has is disruptive behavior when he is in his general education classroom. This behavior includes making loud noises (e.g., "ooooo" and "eeeee"), accompanied by hand flapping and smacking his hands together in a loud and very distracting manner. Usually this behavior results in the reddening of his hands, and it makes the other children uncomfortable, according to his Kindergarten teacher. This behavior occurs throughout the day, regardless of the activity, who is present, or whether he is receiving attention or has been left alone. It is only an issue in Kindergarten because the staff feel it may be alienating for himself.

Building and Managing Appropriate Behaviors

Individuals diagnosed with autism spectrum disorder (ASD) can experience challenges in areas such as communication and social skills, which may inhibit their ability to be successful in a school, home, or community environment without appropriate supports to meet these needs (Horner et al., 2002). We refer to *challenging behaviors* as behaviors that challenge the person's ability to achieve success (Olive et al., 2017). More specifically, challenging behavior can be defined as:

> Culturally abnormal behavior(s) of such intensity, frequency or duration that the physical safety of the person or others is likely to be placed in serious jeopardy or behavior which is likely to seriously limit use of, or result in the person being denied access to, ordinary community facilities.
>
> (Emerson, 2001, p. 3)

Although it is not a core feature of the diagnosis, students with ASD can engage in challenging behaviors such as stereotypical/self-stimulatory behaviors, self-injurious behaviors, aggression, elopement, noncompliance, disruption, and tantrums (Hong et al., 2018). Key factors affecting challenging behaviors are the level of communication the individual has, the degree of structure within the environment, and the behavioral training of the adults working with the students.

The prevalence of challenging behaviors among children with ASD has been estimated to be anywhere between 22.5% and 94% (Hartley et al., 2008; Jang et al., 2011; Matson et al., 2009; McTiernan et al., 2011; Murphy et al., 2009). While the onset of challenging behavior is often seen during the toddler years, these behaviors can persist across the lifespan of individuals with ASD (Hong & Matson, 2021). Although males are four times more likely to be diagnosed with ASD than females (Maenner et al., 2020), gender does not affect rates of challenging behavior. Both females and males diagnosed with ASD will demonstrate challenging behaviors and there are no gender differences in their rates or presentation (Kozlowski et al., 2012).

Challenging behaviors can pose significant risks to individuals with ASD, their families, and educators. Such behaviors can cause physical harm to the individual and others, while hindering their learning and access to educational, vocational, and social settings (Emerson, 2001). Furthermore, these behaviors can result in the individual with ASD being placed in more restrictive settings and/or receiving more intrusive interventions such as chemical or mechanical restraint (Lydon et al., 2015). Parents of children with ASD who engage in challenging behaviors have reported high levels of family stress, financial strain, and feelings of isolation due to the social stigma surrounding the behaviors (Worcester et al., 2008). Challenging behaviors in the classroom can also interfere with instructional efforts and lead to more emotional exhaustion and burnout among educators (Kanne & Mazurek, 2011).

The purpose of this chapter is to discuss some of the major considerations when addressing challenging behaviors of students with ASD. We will first provide a rationale for identifying the *function* of challenging behaviors, as *function-based decision making* is critical to resolving these behaviors. Next, we will describe some *antecedent-based strategies* that can be used to create necessary structure and prevent challenging behaviors from occurring. We will also include a discussion of *consequence-based strategies*, paying particular attention to the difference between reinforcement- and punishment-based approaches and considerations for their use. We will conclude with *culturally and linguistically diverse considerations* when addressing challenging behaviors.

Function-Based Decision Making

Identifying the function of a challenging behavior is the necessary first step in the process of decreasing and/or stopping that behavior. Yet, despite procedural safeguards, schools continue to use punitive interventions (e.g., restraint, seclusion, corporal punishment) to eliminate challenging behaviors in the absence of appropriate assessment (Katsiyannis et al., 2017). Reading and math specialists would not attempt to address a reading or math difficulty without first completing an appropriate assessment to understand the issue; therefore, teachers addressing behavioral challenges must also conduct an assessment before beginning intervention. The process for identifying why a challenging behavior is occurring is known as the functional behavior assessment (FBA).

FBA Steps

A FBA is designed to provide as much information as possible about a specific behavior and the environment in which it occurs. The FBA makes it possible for professionals to form a hypothesis about the function the behavior serves an individual. According to Neitzel and Bogin (2008), there are six steps in the FBA process. First, a team of individuals who know the student well and are familiar with the challenging behavior should be assembled. An individual who has experience with FBAs should be designated as the FBA coordinator. Occasionally, outside experts or specialists may be called in to assist with the FBA, such as a Board Certified Behavior Analyst (BCBA).

In the second step, the team must identify the behavior that will be targeted for both assessment and intervention. If there are two or more behaviors, the team should select the one that is most interfering for the learner. Once this behavior is identified, it must be defined in observable and measurable terms. For example, instead of "Jason gets upset", the behavior might be defined as "Jason throws his lunch box across the room". In the third step, team members must collect data from multiple sources to identify a possible function. Some data collection methods commonly used in educational settings are described below.

The fourth step involves writing a hypothesis statement about the behavioral function using the data collected. In step five, the practitioner might test the hypothesis by modifying the environment to increase the likelihood that the behavior will occur. However, if this step could potentially cause injury or damage, the team should skip this and move to step six. The sixth step involves developing a comprehensive behavior intervention plan (BIP) that will be used to reduce the target behavior and increase the student's use of functional replacement behaviors. The BIP should include evidence-based strategies that match the hypothesized function. Finally, the team should collect progress monitoring data to determine the effectiveness of the BIP. If the BIP is effective, and the behavior is reduced or eliminated, the hypothesized function was likely correct.

Functions of Behavior

Identifying the hypothesized function of a challenging behavior is the goal of the FBA, but what do we mean by function? Another way to describe the process is to say that the FBA enables staff to determine why a behavior is occurring. According to behavioral theory, all behavior serves a purpose. The person engages in the behavior to either gain something of value or to avoid/escape something that is aversive or unpleasant (Peterson & Neef, 2020). We refer to this as positive reinforcement and negative reinforcement, respectively.

During the FBA, one of the critical areas of examination is the consequence that immediately follows the behavior. Does the behavior result in the student getting attention or a preferred item (i.e., tangible)? Does the behavior result in the student not having to do something (i.e., escape)? By examining the events that occur immediately before the behavior (i.e., antecedents) and the events that occur immediately after the behavior (i.e., consequences), the practitioner can identify the potential reinforcers maintaining the target behavior. It is also important to examine whether the behavior continues, escalates, or stops following the consequence. Generally, once someone has received what they wanted (e.g., attention, tangible, or escape), they no longer need it so their behavior will stop. If a behavior continues or escalates following the consequence, we can infer that it was not the reinforcing consequence sought by the learner.

The functions described above (e.g., attention, tangible, escape) are considered "socially mediated" because the consequences come from someone else in the environment other than the student themselves. However, a behavior with an automatic function does not require the action of another individual for reinforcement to occur. The behavior itself produces its own reinforcement. Automatically maintained behaviors can further be classified as either automatic positive or automatic negative. An example of a behavior with an *automatic positive* function would be a student practicing his violin because he enjoys it. An example of a behavior with an *automatic negative* function would be a student leaving a noisy classroom because it is too loud.

FBA Data Collection Procedures

Collecting and analyzing FBA data for the purpose of identifying a hypothesized function requires specialized training and experience and it is beyond the scope of this chapter. However, it is important that teachers are familiar with the various assessment methods so that they can assist when necessary. Once they have received the necessary training they can conduct such assessments on their own. There are three methods that can be used during an FBA: (1) indirect assessments, (2) descriptive assessments, and (3) functional (experimental) analyses. Here, we will focus on indirect and descriptive assessments, as functional analyses require a high level of specialized training. During these assessments, the behavior is intentionally evoked, so it is recommended that functional analyses are supervised by an experienced clinician, such as a BCBA (Tarbox et al., 2009). For more information on conducting functional analyses in schools, see Pennington et al. (2017).

Indirect Assessments

Indirect assessment methods include rating scales, interviews, or questionnaires to identify the environmental events that occur prior to and following the behavior. These assessments do not require direct observation of the target behavior; rather, they rely on the recollections of others to determine the possible function. They are quick and easy to administer, but some close-ended indirect assessments can be unreliable in determining the correct function of the behavior (Hanley, 2012). There are several rating scales available online, including the Functional Assessment Screening Tool (FAST; Iwata et al., 2013), the Questions About Behavioral Function (QABF; Paclawskyj et al., 2000), the Motivation Assessment Scale (MAS; Durand & Crimmins, 1992), and the Problem Behavior Questionnaire (PBQ; Lewis et al., 1994). Each consists of a series of questions to identify the potential reinforcing consequences maintaining a challenging behavior. Behavioral interviews can also provide insight into behavioral functions. Examples include the Functional Assessment Interview (FAI; O'Neill et al., 1997), the student version of the FAI (Kern et al., 1994), and the more recent open-ended semi-structured interview developed by Hanley et al. (2014). Each interview asks a series of questions that provide more detailed information about the behavior and its surrounding environmental events through structured and open-ended questions.

Descriptive Assessments

Descriptive assessments involve direct observations of the target behavior under naturally occurring conditions. The practitioner does not manipulate the environment in any way but records the proximal environmental events each time the target behavior occurs. While these assessments are more objective than indirect assessments, and less complicated than functional analyses, they can result in false positives for attention as the maintaining function as it is very difficult for educators to not react when the target behavior occurs (Peterson & Neef, 2020).

Antecedent-behavior-consequence (ABC) recording. One of the most common descriptive assessments is ABC recording. During this assessment, each time the behavior occurs, the practitioner documents what occurred immediately prior to the behavior (i.e., antecedents), the behavior itself, the events that occurred immediately after the behavior (i.e., consequences), and the response to the consequence (i.e., whether the behavior stopped, continued, or escalated). These data are then analyzed so that a functional hypothesis can be made. ABC recording can be done in a narrative or structured format. An example of a structured ABC data sheet is provided in Figure 8.1.

Case Reviews

Jack. Jack engaged in challenging behavior when he was trying to communicate and was not being understood by his communication partner. Once Jack had his needs met, his challenging behavior stopped. His ABC data might look like those in Table 8.1. Based on these data, and assuming this is a pattern that is commonly seen for Jack, we would hypothesize that the function of Jack's challenging behavior is access to tangibles.

Lana. Lana's challenging behavior was most often seen when task demands were placed, and it stopped only when the demand was removed. This suggests that the function of Lana's behavior is to escape task demands. Her ABC data might look like those in Table 8.2.

Isaac. Recall that Isaac engaged in elopement behavior during work or free time in the classroom, which was always followed by his paraprofessional going on a walk with him. While the topography, or form, of his behavior might make practitioners think the function is for escape, when

Student: _____ School: _____ Teacher: _____

Date	Time	Setting/staff	Antecedent	Behavior	Intensity	Consequence	Learner response
		☐1 ☐5 ☐2 ☐6 ☐3 ☐7 ☐4 ☐8 Staff:	☐1 ☐5 ☐2 ☐6 ☐3 ☐7 ☐4	☐1 ☐2 ☐3 ☐4 Duration:	Intensity ☐A ☐B ☐C	☐1 ☐5 ☐2 ☐6 ☐3 ☐7 ☐4 ☐8	☐1 ☐2 ☐3
		☐1 ☐5 ☐2 ☐6 ☐3 ☐7 ☐4 ☐8 Staff:	☐1 ☐5 ☐2 ☐6 ☐3 ☐7 ☐4	☐1 ☐2 ☐3 ☐4 Duration:	Intensity ☐A ☐B ☐C	☐1 ☐5 ☐2 ☐6 ☐3 ☐7 ☐4 ☐8	☐1 ☐2 ☐3
		☐1 ☐5 ☐2 ☐6 ☐3 ☐7 ☐4 ☐8 Staff:	☐1 ☐5 ☐2 ☐6 ☐3 ☐7 ☐4	☐1 ☐2 ☐3 ☐4 Duration:	Intensity ☐A ☐B ☐C	☐1 ☐5 ☐2 ☐6 ☐3 ☐7 ☐4 ☐8	☐1 ☐2 ☐3
		☐1 ☐5 ☐2 ☐6 ☐3 ☐7 ☐4 ☐8 Staff:	☐1 ☐5 ☐2 ☐6 ☐3 ☐7 ☐4	☐1 ☐2 ☐3 ☐4 Duration:	Intensity ☐A ☐B ☐C	☐1 ☐5 ☐2 ☐6 ☐3 ☐7 ☐4 ☐8	☐1 ☐2 ☐3
		☐1 ☐5 ☐2 ☐6 ☐3 ☐7 ☐4 ☐8 Staff:	☐1 ☐5 ☐2 ☐6 ☐3 ☐7 ☐4	☐1 ☐2 ☐3 ☐4 Duration:	Intensity ☐A ☐B ☐C	☐1 ☐5 ☐2 ☐6 ☐3 ☐7 ☐4 ☐8	☐1 ☐2 ☐3

Key:

Setting
1. Gen Ed
2. Special Ed
3. Specials/elective
4. Lunch
5. Recess/free time
6. Passing period
7. Playground/outside
8. Other: _____

Antecedent
1. Task demand
2. Redirection
3. Transition
4. Independent work
5. Group work
6. Break/free time
7. Other: _____

Behavior
1. _____
2. _____
3. _____
4. _____
Intensity:
A. Mild
B. Moderate
C. Severe

Consequence
1. Staff attention
2. Escape
3. Tangible item/activity
4. Offered choice
5. Peer attention
6. Planned ignore
7. Denied access/told no
8. Other: _____

Learner response
1. Behavior stops
2. Behavior continues
3. Behavior escalates

Figure 8.1 Structured ABC Data Sheet Example.

Table 8.1 Jack's ABC data

Date	Time	Activity	Antecedent	Behavior	Consequence	Response
11/22	12:30	Lunch	Lunch attendant said they did not know what Jack was trying to request	Open palm slapped the shoulder and upper arm of the lunch attendant 3 times	Lunch attendant tried to block the hitting and told Jack to "Use nice hands"	The behavior continued
11/22	12:30	Lunch	Lunch attendant tried to block Jack hitting her, and told him to "Use nice hands"	Jack open palm slapped the upper arm and head of the lunch attendant	Teacher came over and offered Jack a pictorial choice board with available items for lunch	Jack stopped hitting and pointed to pizza

Table 8.2 Lana's ABC data

Date	Time	Activity	Antecedent	Behavior	Consequence	Response
3/26	8:15	Writing Center	Paraprofessional began using hand-over-hand physical prompting to help Lana trace her name	Lana screamed, threw the marker and paper to the floor, fell to the floor, and began kicking her feet	Paraprofessional told Lana that she needed to get back in her seat and finish her tracing or she would not get to go to the next center (dress up)	The behavior continued
3/26	8:16	Writing Center	Paraprofessional repeated the request to get back in her seat and tried to physically help her up	Lana kicked the paraprofessional twice in the leg	Paraprofessional said, "Fine, we will do this later when you are more in the mood" and went to help another child	The behavior stopped

Table 8.3 Isaac's ABC data

Date	Time	Activity	Antecedent	Behavior	Consequence	Response
3/26	1:00	Independent math activity	Students working alone at their desks; teacher and paraprofessional helping a small group of students at the front of the room (Isaac at his desk)	Jumped up and ran from the classroom	Paraprofessional ran after him	Isaac stopped running as soon as he saw his paraprofessional exit the classroom
3/31	9:45	Students were having indoor recess because of inclement weather	Students were playing games in pairs and small groups; teacher and paraprofessional were putting up a bulletin board	Ran from the classroom	Paraprofessional ran after him	Isaac stopped running as soon as he saw his paraprofessional exit the classroom

one examines the ABC data in Table 8.3, it becomes clear that the function is more likely to access attention.

Bo. Bo's behavior of making loud sounds, flapping, and hitting his hands together was seen in all environments and in a variety of situations. The ABC data in Table 8.4 reveal that when Bo was receiving attention, had access to his preferred tangible (iPad), and no demands were placed, his behavior continued. Thus, it appears that Bo's behavior has an automatic function. We do not know whether this behavior has an automatic positive function (i.e., Bo is engaging in the behavior because it feels good) or an automatic negative function (i.e., Bo is engaging in this behavior because it provides him with relief) because we cannot see internal events and he cannot tell us.

Behavior Intervention Planning

The FBA is only the first part in addressing challenging behavior. Once the hypothesized function has been identified, function-based interventions must be developed to reduce or eliminate the behavior. Just as a reading or math specialist would base remedial instruction on assessment results, so should teachers who are working with students exhibiting challenging behaviors. The intervention selected is not based on the topography of the behavior, but by its function. Research over the last 50 years has demonstrated that function-based interventions have high efficacy (Iwata et al., 1994), support inclusion into general education (Reeves et al., 2013), and have greater preference among practitioners and learners alike (Hanley et al., 1997).

The FBA provides useful information for the BIP, such as the antecedents that may trigger the target behavior, reinforcement contingencies that can be altered, and replacement behaviors that can be taught (Peterson & Neef, 2020). Most importantly, the FBA identifies the reinforcer that should be used to teach a functionally equivalent replacement behavior. For example, if a student engages in challenging behavior to get attention from the teacher, the teacher might provide the student with attention only when he raises his hand.

What follows is a brief overview of the three types of interventions: antecedent-based interventions, reinforcement-based interventions, and punishment-based interventions. This is not meant to be an exhaustive list, nor does this chapter provide procedural details on how to implement each of these interventions. Teachers are encouraged to search the literature, but in particular, the evidence-based practices (EBP) reports from the National Professional Development Center on Autism Spectrum Disorders (Wong et al., 2014) and the National Clearinghouse on Autism Evidence and Practice (Steinbrenner et al.,

Table 8.4 Bo's ABC data

Date	Time	Activity	Antecedent	Behavior	Consequence	Response
5/22	10:10	Story time	Children seated on the floor after lunch; teacher reading a story	Rolled onto his back, made "oooooh" sound and hit his hands together (hard enough to leave a red mark and audible from several feet away)	Paraprofessional physically guided him back up and moved him to the "quiet corner" (an area of the room with a bean bag chair and books) and offered him his iPad	The behavior continued once he was in the quiet corner
5/26	11:50	Lunch	Children seated at a long table eating their lunch; students chatting around him	Bo made "oooooh" sound and hit his hands together (hard enough to leave a red mark and audible from several feet away)	Paraprofessional physically guided Bo into the hallway away from the other students	The behavior continued once he was in the hallway

2020). For a step-by-step guide on how to implement specific EBPs, please see the Autism Focused Intervention Resources & Modules (AFIRM, 2018).

Antecedent-Based Strategies

Antecedent-based strategies are designed to prevent the challenging behavior from occurring in the first place. They involve the "arrangement of events or circumstances that precede an activity or demand in order to increase the occurrence of a behavior or lead to the reduction of the challenging/interfering behaviors" (Steinbrenner et al., 2020, p. 28). Antecedent-based interventions are considered an evidence-based approach for individuals with ASD according to the most recent EBP report (Steinbrenner et al., 2020). The report refers to antecedent interventions more broadly, but it also includes specific antecedent-based strategies that can be useful for students with ASD, such as visual supports, social narratives, and modeling. Some examples of antecedent-based interventions for learners with ASD, based on function, are provided in Table 8.5. These supports can provide structure and predictability to students with ASD, the lack of which can be a trigger for challenging behaviors (Fuentes et al., 2021).

Case Reviews

Jack. Recall that the function of Jack's behavior was access to tangibles. The most obvious antecedent strategy for Jack, and certainly the most crucial for his overall well-being, is functional communication training (FCT). Jack urgently needs a communication system that is reliable enough to prevent his challenging behaviors. The staff should not wait until he is upset to offer him the choice board. A system such as the Picture Exchange Communication System (PECS; Frost & Bondy, 2002) is recommended to provide Jack with a more efficient way to communicate he needs.

Lana. The function of Lana's problem behavior was to escape demands. When addressing escape-maintained behaviors, the first and most important step is to identify *why* the learner wants or needs to escape. Looking at Lana's ABC data in Table 8.2, one can see that in addition to "work" being the most common activity, the immediate antecedent to the tantrum behavior is an adult physically prompting her to complete the task. This suggests that this type of prompt is aversive to her. Other possibilities include the difficulty of the task, the amount of work required/length of the task, lack of appropriate supports, lack of available reinforcement, or the aversiveness of the materials themselves (Geiger et al., 2010). Practitioners should attempt to identify why a learner

Table 8.5 Function-Based Antecedent Interventions

Attention Function	Tangible Function	Escape Function	Automatic Function
• Functional Communication Training (FCT) • Noncontingent attention • Check-in/Check-out • Social narratives • Assigning responsibilities • Increase proximity/change seating arrangements • Visual reminders	• FCT • Increased access to tangible • First-then • Visual schedules • Increased access to tangible • Social narratives • Use visual timers to show how much time they have with tangible • Visual reminders	• FCT • First-then • Noncontingent escape • Visual schedules • Activity choice • Curricular and instructional revision • Demand fading • Incorporate student interests • High-probability instructional sequences	• Visual behavioral reminders • Consistent routines • Visual schedules • Enriched environment • Incorporate sensory activities into instruction • Provide fidget toys/manipulatives • Sensory breaks

would want to escape in order to make changes that will prevent that need in the first place.

FCT is a highly effective approach when the function of behavior is escape. Instead of having to engage in a tantrum to escape demands, Lana could be taught to ask for a break. By decreasing the aversiveness of the task itself and teaching Lana a functional communicative response to escape tasks, a decrease in tantrums would be seen. Other antecedent interventions such as using a visual schedule, a "First-then" card, and/or providing choice could help Lana learn that there are times that work needs to be done, but she can choose the tasks she completes and she can engage in a preferred activity once it is completed.

Isaac. The function of Isaac's behavior was to gain attention. In examining the ABC data from Table 8.3, one can see that in each instance, Isaac was either working or playing alone. Eloping from the room provided him with 1:1 attention from his paraprofessional, which appears to be the reason for the elopement. Thus, an antecedent procedure that could be effective for Isaac is noncontingent attention. Noncontingent attention is a procedure where attention is provided freely and frequently throughout the day, but independent of any particular behavior, so that Isaac contacts the maintaining reinforcer (i.e., the paraprofessional's attention) on a regular basis. Another promising strategy for attention-maintained behaviors is "Check in-Check out" (CICO; Park & Blair, 2020). With this procedure, staff meet with the child regularly, at least twice a day, at the beginning and end of the day, to go over the rules and behavioral expectations. These expectations may be shown with visual supports (e.g., reminder cards, social narratives) or video models of the expected behaviors.

Bo. The function of Bo's behavior was automatic because he engages in the behavior in all circumstances throughout the day, although it is especially concerning to staff when he is in his general education classroom. An antecedent strategy that staff may attempt to use is a visual reminder to maintain "Quiet hands" (i.e., hands in his lap). Staff may also consider using video modeling to show Bo the expected behaviors during certain activities. Finally, staff could provide Bo with fidget items to manipulate with his hands throughout the school day to meet his sensory needs (e.g., stress ball, putty, keychains, etc.).

Consequence-Based Strategies

Reinforcement-Based Interventions

Reinforcement is the most important principle of behavior and the key element of most behavior change programs (Northup et al., 1993). From the child receiving praise for a job well done, to the teenager skipping class to avoid concepts he does not understand, reinforcement contingencies can be seen all around us in everyday situations. Reinforcement is considered a naturally occurring phenomenon, and a person does not need to be aware of the contingencies for reinforcement to work (Alberto & Troutman, 2012).

When most people think of reinforcement, they think of a person receiving something perceived as "good" (e.g., candy, high fives, praise). However, reinforcement is not about the perceived quality of the consequence provided; rather, it is concerned with how that consequence affects the future frequency of a behavior. For example, a consequence that one might find aversive (e.g., scolding, loud noises, painful stimulation) may be reinforcing for someone else depending on the situation. What makes a consequence a reinforcer is its ability to increase the future frequency of the behavior it follows (Alberto & Troutman, 2012).

There are two types of reinforcement: positive reinforcement and negative reinforcement. It is a common misconception for individuals unfamiliar with behavioral terminology to assume that "positive" means "good" and "negative" means "bad", but these terms are not synonymous. Reinforcement always means an *increase* in the future rate of a behavior, and the modifiers "positive" and "negative" only refer to the type of stimulus change (Cooper et al., 2020). Positive refers to the addition of something (e.g., attention or a tangible), while negative refers to the removal of something (e.g., escape or avoidance of something unpleasant). Each type of reinforcement increases the future likelihood of the behavior immediately preceding it.

Some examples of reinforcement-based interventions for learners with ASD, based on function, are provided in Table 8.6. The remainder of this section will provide more information on two commonly used reinforcement-based interventions: differential reinforcement and token economies.

Table 8.6 Function-Based Reinforcement-Based Interventions

Attention Function	Tangible Function	Escape Function	Automatic Function
• Differential reinforcement of alternative behavior (DRA) • Token economy • Differential reinforcement of other behavior (DRO) • Differential reinforcement of low rates (DRL)	• DRA • DRO • Token economy	• Differential negative reinforcement (DNRA) • DRO • Positive reinforcement for compliance • Token economy	• Differential reinforcement of incompatible behavior (DRI) • DRL • DRO • Token economy

Differential Reinforcement

Differential reinforcement involves reinforcing one behavior while withholding reinforcement for another behavior. Three types of differential reinforcement commonly used in applied settings are differential reinforcement of alternative behavior, differential reinforcement of incompatible behavior, and differential reinforcement of other behavior.

Differential reinforcement of alternative behavior (DRA). When using DRA, a practitioner reinforces a desirable alternative behavior while withholding or minimizing reinforcement for the problem behavior (Vollmer et al., 2020). The alternative behavior should be functionally equivalent to the problem behavior, meaning that it will result in the same reinforcer that was once provided for the problem behavior, but in a manner that is more socially acceptable. For example, the teacher might provide attention to a student raising his hand instead of shouting out.

Differential reinforcement of incompatible behavior (DRI). Procedurally, DRI is identical to DRA, except that the alternative behavior is incompatible with the problem behavior (Cooper et al., 2020). In other words, it is impossible for the alternative behavior to be performed at the same time as the problem behavior. An example of a DRI intervention would be to provide a break from academic work for appropriately engaging with the materials rather than throwing them.

Differential reinforcement of other behavior (DRO). During DRO, reinforcement is delivered contingent on the absence of the challenging behavior for a predetermined interval of time (Hedquist & Roscoe, 2020). If the challenging behavior occurs during the interval, reinforcement is withheld, and the interval is reset. DRO provides reinforcement for engaging in any other behavior *other* than the problem behavior. However, a specific alternative replacement behavior is not taught. In an example of a DRO procedure, a teacher sets her timer for 10 minutes. If the students do not get out of their seats for the entire 10 minutes, they are given extra recess time.

Token Economies

The token economy is a common evidence-based strategy for increasing appropriate behaviors (Bonfonte et al., 2020). Token economies have been used with a wide variety of individuals, from preschoolers through adulthood. In a token economy, a teacher first identifies the type of token that will be used. For example, a teacher may choose to award points on a point sheet or white board, use stickers, or use Velcro tokens on a token board. Some research suggests that special interest-based tokens can be highly effective for students with ASD (Carnett et al., 2014). Tokens, in whatever form, are given to the student or group of students contingent on specific appropriate behaviors (e.g., being on task, raising their hand, cooperating with peers).

For token economies to be effective, students must be able to "cash in" their earned tokens for a backup reinforcer (Cooper et al., 2020). Backup reinforcers are items or activities that the student finds valuable enough to work toward. Teachers using a token economy must decide what backup reinforcers they will use, often by asking the student what things they would like to work for, and then ensuring that those items or activities are available. Teachers must also decide how many tokens will be needed to purchase each backup reinforcer. Some teachers use a menu of backup reinforcers from which students can decide how much they want to spend.

Case Reviews

Jack. The function of Jack's behavior was access to a tangible, and FCT was identified as a necessary antecedent-based procedure. In Jack's case, FCT and DRA are both being used if staff reinforce the use of his communication system rather than aggression and they no longer provide access to tangibles when he does use aggression. Given the nature of the behavior, staff will need to ensure that Jack has ample opportunities throughout his day to access tangible items using his functional communication, so that he quickly learns that the PECS is a more efficient way to getting what he wants.

Lana. For Lana's escape-maintained tantrum behavior, staff may wish to increase the amount of positive reinforcement Lana receives for work that she does complete, which may include the use of a token board. Staff may combine the token board with a DRI procedure, whereby Lana can earn tokens for being in her seat and working, which is incompatible with throwing herself to the ground in a tantrum.

Isaac. Isaac's attention-maintained elopement behavior could be addressed through a token economy that with opportunities to go for walks with his paraprofessional contingent on certain behaviors, such as staying in the room. Staff could also reinforce him using the DRO procedure so that he earns tokens when he has not eloped for a certain amount of time.

Bo. A reinforcement-based intervention that could be effective for Bo is DRI. If Bo's hands were occupied with a fidget toy, it might reduce the number of hand smacks and flaps. Staff could provide reinforcement for Bo using the fidget toy. They could also use DRO for both his motor and vocal stereotyped behaviors. Both procedures could be combined with a token economy, whereby Bo can earn tokens for sensory activities.

Punishment-Based Interventions

Punishment is the opposite of reinforcement in that it *decreases* behavior rather than increasing it. Specifically, when a stimulus change immediately follows a response that then decreases the future frequency of that behavior, punishment has taken place (Cooper et al., 2020). However, we cannot define punishment based on the actions of the disciplinarian or the nature of the consequence itself. For example, just because a child is reprimanded for coloring on the walls, you cannot say punishment has occurred. This would only qualify as punishment if the child decreased the number of times he colored on the walls in the future or discontinued coloring on the walls altogether (Alberto & Troutman, 2012). As with reinforcement, there are two forms of punishment: positive and negative punishment. Just like with reinforcement, the terms "positive" and "negative" refer to the type of stimulus change taking place. Positive punishment involves the presentation or addition of an aversive stimulus, and negative punishment involves the removal of a preferred stimulus. The term punishment will always mean that there is a *decrease* in the future rate of the behavior.

When using behavioral interventions to decrease challenging behaviors, it is the ethical responsibility of the practitioner to implement the least-restrictive procedures. Reinforcement-based strategies – such as differential reinforcement – should always be implemented and found to be ineffective in reducing the problem behavior prior to the implementation of a punishment-based intervention. A punishment procedure may be considered once all the less restrictive options have been ruled out. Further, practitioners must consider the risks with using punishment, such as aggression, the escalation of the challenging behavior, and increases in the challenging behavior in environments where punishment is not being used (Cooper et al., 2020). Some examples of punishment-based interventions for learners with ASD, based on function, are provided in Table 8.7.

Table 8.7 Function-Based Punishment-Based Interventions

Attention Function	Tangible Function	Escape Function	Automatic Function
• Planned ignoring • Time-out • Overcorrection • Response cost	• Time-out • Overcorrection • Reprimands • Termination of activity/tangible access	• Overcorrection • Reprimands • Response cost	• Response blocking • Response interruption and redirection • Response cost • Overcorrection

There are several types of positive and negative punishment that are evidence-based and therefore, may be considered for certain behaviors or in certain circumstances. Response blocking is one such intervention that involves the practitioner physically intervening as soon as the individual begins an undesired behavior to prevent or block the completion of the response (Langone et al., 2013). A variation of response blocking is a procedure known as response interruption and redirection (RIRD). RIRD is considered an evidence-based strategy for reducing automatically maintained challenging behaviors, particularly those that involve motor and/or vocal stereotypy (Dowdy et al., 2020). During this procedure, the practitioner interrupts or blocks the stereotyped behavior and redirects the learner to a more functionally appropriate, high-probability behavior (Cooper et al., 2020).

Overcorrection is a form of punishment that requires the individual to engage in effortful behavior directly or logically related to the target behavior (Cooper et al., 2020). The two most common types of overcorrection are restitutional overcorrection and positive practice overcorrection. Restitutional overcorrection requires the individual to repair the damage caused by their misbehavior by returning the environment to its original state, and then engaging in additional behavior to bring the environment to a better condition than it was prior to the problem behavior (Miltenberger & Fuqua, 1981). An example would be a student throwing his box of crayons – he would then be required to pick up all the crayons and put them away, and then pick up all of the toys in the play area. With positive practice overcorrection, the individual is required to practice the appropriate behavior upon engagement in the inappropriate behavior. Positive practice overcorrection is useful in that it teaches the individual what is expected instead of the problem behavior. An example of positive practice overcorrection would be to have a student walk around the perimeter of the pool following an instance of running.

Time-out is a well-known form of negative punishment. Time-out is often the go-to disciplinary procedure, but unfortunately, it is often misused and misunderstood by practitioners and parents. Time-out is defined as the contingent withdrawal of the opportunity to earn positive reinforcement, or the loss of access to positive reinforcers following a problem behavior (Everett, 2010). This does not necessarily mean that the individual is being moved to an isolated setting – It only means that the individual is losing reinforcement for an amount of time following the problem behavior. The key to a successful time-out procedure is to ensure that the time-in setting is reinforcing for the student.

Finally, response cost is a procedure which involves the removal of generalized conditioned reinforcers (e.g., points, tokens), tangibles (e.g., stickers), or time from activities (e.g., minutes from a game) following a problem behavior. Response cost is a form of negative punishment in which the loss of a specific amount of reinforcers results in a decrease in the future frequency of the problem behavior (Silva & Wiskow, 2020).

Case Reviews

Jack, Lana, and Isaac. Punishment-based procedures would be contraindicated for these three students. As Jack's challenging behavior was aggression, a punishment-based intervention would not be appropriate as it could result in more aggression. Similarly, using punishment with either Lana or Isaac could lead to an escalation of their challenging behaviors. This could potentially result in injury to Lana or others, while an escalation of Isaac's elopement behavior could become a safety concern. For Lana, time-out would be highly inappropriate because time-out from the activity is exactly why she is engaging in the tantrums. Research has shown that the challenging behaviors demonstrated by these three students can be successfully eliminated through antecedent- and reinforcement-based interventions that are matched to the behavior's function.

Bo. Given the self-injurious nature of Bo's hand smacking behavior, he is the only student where punishment might be needed to reduce this behavior quickly, and in the most ethical way possible. Further, as this is an automatically maintained behavior, it is difficult to select a functional replacement behavior because we do not know if Bo's hand smacking has an automatic positive or automatic negative function. In such a situation, a case may be made that the RIRD intervention may be the most effective and efficient approach for decreasing this behavior, while also employing other antecedent-based and reinforcement-based interventions.

Culturally and Linguistically Diverse Considerations in FBA/BIP Processes

As inclusive practices for persons with ASD become commonplace in school settings throughout the world, there is also a need for practitioners to recognize the cultural and linguistic diversity (CLD) of their learners and apply this understanding into their behavioral assessments and intervention plans. According to a 2015 United States Census report, "60.4 million U.S. residents spoke a language other than English in the home, compared to 23.1 million in 1980, a 161.5% increase" (Neely et al., 2020, p.808). This diversity is recognized within the *Ethics Code for Behavior Analysts*. It states that "behavior analysts actively engage in professional development activities to acquire knowledge and skills related to cultural responsiveness and diversity" (BACB, 2020, p. 9).

The impact of culture on behavior is well-studied and supported in the literature. Sugai et al. (2012) suggested that students from CLD backgrounds were more likely to experience behavior-related negative outcomes at school, and this was likely attributable to the differences between home and school cultures. For many students with ASD, limited communication is a contributing factor to their challenging behaviors. However, for students who speak English as a second language, communication can be even more challenging. Neely et al. (2020) evaluated the effects of language on FCT for three children with ASD whose parents spoke Spanish at home. The results indicated that communication responses learned in English may lead to a resurgence of challenging behavior as the English responses did not contact reinforcement due to language differences between communication partners (Neely et al., 2020).

Moreno et al. (2017) found that teachers who lacked an understanding of the impact of CLD on their students' behaviors failed to identify these differences as potential factors during the FBA or the development of the BIP. Sugai and colleagues (2012) suggested that teachers who have limited experience with a student's culture should get to know the student and foster a positive relationship (Sugai et al., 2012). According to Moreno and colleagues, "the awareness of cultural existence does not automatically transfer into culturally attuned practices" (Moreno et al., 2017, p. 66). To achieve the best outcomes, educators "must align curriculum, methods, strategies, and supports with the culture, primary language, ethnicity, socioeconomic status, biological and physiological factors, and individual histories of their students" and then be aware of how "these factors are constantly influencing and being influenced by educational environments" (West et al., 2016, p. 152). To sustain behavior change across both the school setting and the natural environment, educators must be aware of the cultural and linguistic differences of their learners.

Recommendations for Educators and Practitioners

1. Conduct a FBA prior to designing or implementing any behavior change procedures.
2. Ensure that those who are conducting the FBA have the training and experience to do so.
3. Only use function-based interventions to address challenging behavior.
4. Collect data frequently to determine if the intervention was successful; if it is not, make the necessary changes to ensure progress is made.
5. Whenever possible, teach a functionally equivalent replacement behavior. For non-verbal learners or those with limited expressive communication, FCT should be a primary component of the BIP.

6. Consider cultural and linguistic differences when designing the BIP to ensure the FCT or other treatments are maintained, and challenging behavior is reduced in the learner's natural setting.
7. Use punishment only when antecedent- and reinforcement-based interventions have been used and found to be ineffective.
8. Choose the least restrictive and most effective intervention while ensuring that the procedure is safe and humane.
9. Ensure that only those who are trained in the procedures are responsible for implementing the intervention.

Conclusion

Students with ASD can exhibit behaviors that challenge their ability to be successful academically, socially, or functionally. In this chapter we discussed the FBA, which is the first and most important step in addressing challenging behaviors. The importance of the FBA is akin to the importance of an academic assessment when a student exhibits difficulties in math or reading. With behavior, however, the goal is to identify patterns of antecedents and consequences that point to a possible function for the behavior.

Teachers and other professionals are part of a multi-disciplinary team that will conduct the FBA, develop the BIP, and monitor the student's progress. When the student makes progress, the plan can be considered successful, and the hypothesized function was likely correct. If the student fails to make progress, however, there are numerous possible reasons. First, there is the possibility that the functional hypothesis was incorrect. In such cases, professionals are urged to complete the FBA again to determine if another function was present. Other possible reasons for failure to make progress include human error (e.g., someone on the team fails to implement the intervention correctly or consistently), poor or inconsistent progress monitoring data, inadequate consideration for cultural and linguistic differences in the natural environment, or a lack of buy-in from the professionals or family. Practitioners are encouraged to seek out specialists in their schools, districts, and communities to address severe problem behaviors that threaten the safety of the student, staff, or peers.

This chapter also outlined the importance of using only function-based interventions to address the challenging behavior of students, and to do so ethically and humanely in accordance with national and international standards and guidelines. We encourage educators to consult with other professionals and to seek the advanced knowledge and training necessary to conduct FBAs and implement function-based interventions that are evidence-based, culturally and linguistically responsive, and appropriate for their individual learners.

Discussion Questions

1. What are the major functions of behavior?
2. What are the six steps in the FBA process?
3. What are some antecedent, reinforcement-based, and punishment-based interventions for each of the major functions of behavior?
4. What are some ethical considerations in the use of punishment as an intervention for challenging behavior?
5. How can the consideration of cultural and linguistic diversity of a learner with ASD enhance the implementation of a behavior intervention plan?

References

Alberto, P. A., & Troutman, A. C. (2012). *Applied behavior analysis for teachers* (9th ed). Pearson.

Autism Focused Intervention Resources and Modules (AFIRM) Team. (2018). *Autism focused intervention resources and modules.* National Professional Development Center on Autism Spectrum Disorder, FPG Child Development Center, University of North Carolina. http://afirm.fpg.unc.edu

Behavior Analyst Certification Board. (2020). *Ethics code for behavior analysts.* Author. www.bacb.com/wp-content/uploads/2020/11/Ethics-Code-for-Behavior-Analysts-210902.pdf

Bonfonte, S.A., Bourret, J.C., & Lloveras, L.A. (2020). Comparing the reinforcing efficacy of tokens and primary reinforcers. *Journal of Applied Behavior Analysis, 53*(3), 1593–1605.

Carnett, A., Raulston, T., Lang, R., Tostanoski, A., Lee, A., Sigafoos, J., & Machalicek, W. (2014). Effects of a perseverative interest-based token economy on challenging and on-task behavior in a child with autism. *Journal of Behavioral Education, 23*(3), 368–377.

Cooper, J. O., Heron, T. E., & Heward, W. L. (2020). *Applied behavior analysis* (3rd ed.). Pearson.

Dowdy, A., Tincani, M., & Schneider, W. J. (2020). Evaluation of publication bias inresponse interruption and redirection: A meta-analysis. *Journal of Applied Behavior Analysis, 53* (4), 2151–2171.

Durand, V. M., & Crimmins, D. B. (1992). *The Motivation Assessment Scale (MAS) administration guide.* Monaco and Associates.

Emerson, E. (2001). *Challenging behavior: Analysis and intervention in people with severe intellectual disabilities* (2nd ed.). Cambridge University Press.

Everett, G. E. (2010). Time-out in special education settings: The parameters of previous implementation. *North American Journal of Psychology, 12*(1), 159–170.

Frost, L. A., & Bondy, A. S. (2002). *The picture exchange communication system training manual* (2nd ed.). Pyramid Educational Consultants.

Fuentes, J., Hervás, A., & Howlin, P. (2021). ESCAP practice guidance for autism: A summary of evidence-based recommendations for diagnosis and treatment. *European Child & Adolescent Psychiatry, 30*(6), 961–984.

Geiger, K. B., Carr, J. E., & LeBlanc, L. A. (2010). Function-based treatments for escape-maintained problem behavior: A treatment-selection model for practicing behavior analysts. *Behavior Analysis in Practice*, 3(1), 22–32.

Hanley, G. P. (2012). Functional assessment of problem behavior: Dispelling myths, overcoming implementation obstacles, and developing new lore. *Behavior Analysis in Practice*, 5(1), 54–72.

Hanley, G. P., Jin, C. S., Vanselow, N. R., & Hanratty, L. A. (2014). Producing meaningful improvements in problem behavior of children with autism via synthesized analyses and treatments. *Journal of Applied Behavior Analysis*, 47(1), 16–36.

Hanley, G. P., Piazza, C. C., Fisher, W. W., Construcci, S. A., & Maglieri, K. A. (1997). Evaluation of client preference for function-based treatment packages. *Journal of Applied Behavior Analysis*, 30(3), 459–473.

Hartley, S. L., Sikora, D. M., & McCoy, R. (2008). Prevalence and risk factors of maladaptive behaviour in young children with autistic disorder. *Journal of Intellectual Disability Research*, 52(10), 819–829.

Hedquist, C. B., & Roscoe, E. M. (2020). A comparison of differential reinforcement procedures for treating automatically reinforced behavior. *Journal of Applied Behavior Analysis*, 53(1), 284–295.

Hong, E., Dixon, D. R., Stevens, E., Burns, C. O., & Linstead, E. (2018). Topography and function of challenging behaviors in individuals with autism spectrum disorder. *Advances in Neurodevelopmental Disorders*, 2(2), 206–215.

Hong, E., & Matson, J. L. (2021). An evaluation of the functions of challenging behavior in toddlers with and without autism spectrum disorder. *Journal of Developmental and Physical Disabilities*, 33(1), 85–97.

Horner, R. H., Carr, E. G., Strain, P. S., Todd, A. W., & Reed, H. K. (2002). Problem behavior interventions for young children with autism: A research synthesis. *Journal of Autism and Developmental Disorders*, 32(5), 423–446.

Iwata, B. A., DeLeon, I. G., & Roscoe, E. M. (2013). Reliability and validity of the functional analysis screening tool. *Journal of Applied Behavior Analysis*, 46(1), 271–284.

Iwata, B. A., Pace, G. M., Cowery, G. E., & Miltenberger, R. G. (1994). What makes extinction work: An analysis of procedural form and function. *Journal of Applied Behavior Analysis*, 27(1), 131–144.

Jang, J., Dixon, D. R., Tarbox, J., & Granpeesheh, D. (2011). Symptom severity and challenging behavior in children with ASD. *Research in Autism Spectrum Disorders*, 5(3), 1028–1032.

Kanne, S. M., & Mazurek, M. O. (2011). Aggression in children and adolescents with ASD: Prevalence and risk factors. *Journal of Autism and Developmental Disorders*, 41(7), 926–937.

Katsiyannis, A., Losinski, M., Whitford, D. K., & Counts, J. (2017). The use of aversives in special education: Legal and practice considerations for school principals. *NASSP Bulletin*, 101(4), 315–330.

Kern, L., Dunlap, G., Clarke, S., & Childs, K. E. (1994). Student-assisted functional assessment interview. *Assessment for Effective Intervention*, 19(2–3), 29–39.

Kozlowski, A. M., Matson, J. L., & Rieske, R. D. (2012). Gender effects on challenging behaviors in children with autism spectrum disorders. *Research in Autism Spectrum Disorders*, 6(2), 958–964.

Langone, S. R., Luiselli, J. K., & Hamill, J. (2013). Effects of response blocking and programmed stimulus control on motor stereotypy: A pilot study. *Child & Family Behavior Therapy*, *35*(3), 249–255.

Lewis, T. J., Scott, T. M., & Sugai, G. (1994). The Problem Behavior Questionnaire: A teacher-based instrument to develop functional hypotheses of problem behavior in general education classrooms. *Assessment for Effective Intervention*, *19*(2–3), 103–115.

Lydon, S., Healy, O., Roche, M., Henry, R., Mulhern, T., & Hughes, B. M. (2015). Salivary cortisol levels and challenging behavior in children with autism spectrum disorder. *Research in Autism Spectrum Disorders*, *10*, 78–92.

Maenner, M. J., Shaw, K. A., Baio, J., Washington, A., Patrick, M., DiRienzo, M., Christensen, D. L., Wiggins, L. D., Pettygrove, S., Andrews, J. G., Lopez, M., Hudson, A., Baroud, T., Schwenk, Y., White, T., Robinson Rosenberg, C., Lee, L., Harrington, R. A., Huston, M., … Dietz, P. M. (2020). Prevalence of autism spectrum disorder among children aged 8 years — Autism and Developmental Disabilities Monitoring Network, 11 Sites, United States, 2016. *Centers for Disease Control and Prevention, Morbidity and Mortality Weekly Report*, *69*(4), 1–12.

Matson, J. L., Wilkins, J., & Macken, J. (2009). The relationship of challenging behaviors to severity and symptoms of autism spectrum disorders. *Journal of Mental Health Research in Intellectual Disabilities*, *2*(1), 29–44.

McTiernan, A., Leader, G., Healy, O., & Mannion, A. (2011). Analysis of risk factors and early predictors of challenging behavior for children with autism spectrum disorder. *Research in Autism Spectrum Disorders*, *5*(3), 1215–1222.

Miltenberger, R. G., & Fuqua, R. W. (1981). Overcorrection: A review and critical analysis. *The Behavior Analyst*, *4*(2), 123–141.

Moreno, G., Wong-Lo, M., & Bullock, L. M. (2017). Investigation on the practice of the functional behavioral assessment: Survey of educators and their experiences in the field. *The International Journal of Emotional Education*, *9*(1), 54–70.

Murphy, O., Healy, O., & Leader, G. (2009). Risk factors for challenging behaviors among 157 children with autism spectrum disorder in Ireland. *Research in Autism Spectrum Disorders*, *3*(2), 474–482.

Neely, L., Graber, J., Kunnavatana, S., & Cantrell, K. (2020). Impact of language on behavior treatment outcomes. *Journal of Applied Behavior Analysis*, *53*(2), 796–810.

Neitzel, J., & Bogin, J. (2008). *Steps for implementation: Functional behavior assessment*. The National Professional Development Center on Autism Spectrum Disorders, Frank Porter Graham Child Development Institute, The University of North Carolina. https://csesa.fpg.unc.edu/sites/csesa.fpg.unc.edu/files/ebpbriefs/FBA_Steps_0.pdf

Northup, J., Vollmer, T. R., & Serrett, K. (1993). Publication trends in 25 years of the *Journal of Applied Behavior Analysis*. *Journal of Applied Behavior Analysis*, *26*(4), 527–537.

Olive, M. L., Boutot, E. A., & Tarbox, J. (2017). Teaching students with autism using the principles of applied behavior analysis. In E. A. Boutot (Ed.), *Autism Education and Practice* (2nd ed.; pp. 79–95). Pearson.

O'Neill, R. E., Horner, R. H., Albin, R. W., Sprague, J. R., Storey, K., & Newton, J. S. (1997). *Functional assessment and program development for problem behavior: A practical handbook*. Brooks/Cole Publishing.

Paclawskyj, T. R., Matson, J. L., Rush, K. S., Smalls, Y., & Vollmer, T. R. (2000). Questions about behavioral function (QABF): A behavioral checklist for functional assessment of aberrant behavior. *Research in Developmental Disabilities*, 21(3), 223–229.

Park, E., & Blair, K. C. (2020). Check-in/check-out implementation in schools: Ameta-analysis of group design studies. *Education and Treatment of Children*, 43(4), 361–375.

Pennington, B., Pokorski, E. A., Kumm, S., & Sterrett, B. I. (2017). *Intensive intervention practice guide: School-based functional analysis*. US Department of Education, Office of Special Education Programs.

Peterson, S. M., & Neef, N. A. (2020). Functional behavior assessment. In J. O. Cooper, T. E. Heron, & W. L. Heward (Eds.), *Applied behavior analysis* (3rd ed.; pp. 678–706). Pearson.

Reeves, L. M., Umbreit, J., Ferro, J. B., & Liaupsin, C. J. (2013). Function-based intervention to support the inclusion of students with autism. *Education and Training in Autism and Developmental Disabilities*, 48(3), 379–391.

Silva, E., & Wiskow, K. M. (2020). Stimulus presentation versus stimulus removal in the Good Behavior Game. *Journal of Applied Behavior Analysis*, 53(4), 2186–2198.

Steinbrenner, J. R., Hume, K., Odom, S. L., Morin, K. L., Nowell, S. W., Tomaszewski, B., Szendrey, S., McIntyre, N. S., Yücesoy-Özkan, S., & Savage, M. N. (2020). *Evidence-based practices for children, youth, and young adults with autism*. The University of North Carolina at Chapel Hill, Frank Porter Graham Child Development Institute, National Clearinghouse on Autism Evidence and Practice Review Team.

Sugai, G., O'Keeffe, B. V., & Fallon, L. M. (2012). A contextual consideration of culture and school-wide positive behavior support. *Journal of Positive Behavior Interventions*, 14(4) 197–208.

Tarbox, J., Wilke, A. E., Najdowski, A. C., Findel-Pyles, R. S., Balasanyan, S., Caveney, A. C., Chilingaryan, V., King, D. M., Niehoff, S. M., Slease, K., & Tia, B. (2009). Comparing indirect, descriptive, and experimental functional assessments of challenging behavior in children with autism. *Journal of Developmental and Physical Disabilities*, 21(6), 493–514.

Vollmer, T. R., Peters, K. P., Kronfli, F. R., Lloveras, L. A., & Ibañez, V. F. (2020). On the definition of differential reinforcement of alternative behavior. *Journal of Applied Behavior Analysis*, 53 (3), 1299–1303.

West, E. A., Travers, J. C., Kemper, T. D., Liberty, L. M., Cote, D. L., McCollow, M. M., Stansberry Brusnahan, L. L. (2016). Racial and ethnic diversity of participants in research supporting evidence-based practices for learners with autism spectrum disorder. *The Journal of Special Education*, 50(3), 151–163.

Wong, C., Odom, S. L., Hume, K., Cox, A. W., Fettig, A., Kucharczyk, S., Brock, M. E., Plavnick, J. B., Fleury, V. P., & Schultz, T. R. (2014). *Evidence-based practices for children, youth, and young adults with autism spectrum disorder*. The University of North Carolina, Frank Porter Graham Child Development Institute, Autism Evidence-Based Practice Review Group.

Worcester, J. A., Nesman, T. M., Raffaele Mendez, L. M., & Keller, H. R. (2008). Giving voice to parents of young children with challenging behavior. *Exceptional Children*, 74(4), 509–525.

Chapter 9

Development of Academic Skills in Childhood

A. Leah Wood,[1] Jenny R. Root,[2] Julie L. Thompson,[3] and Deidre Gilley[2]

[1]School of Education, California Polytechnic University San Luis Obispo
[2]School of Teacher Education, Florida State University
[3]Department of Educational Psychology, Texas A&M University

Fatima is a seventh grade student at a local middle school. Her family moved to New York City from the Dominican Republic when Fatima was still a baby. Her parents and siblings are all bilingual, but they speak mostly Spanish at home. Fatima was diagnosed with autism when she was three years old and is currently receiving special education services. Fatima rarely uses spontaneous verbal language to communicate, though she can request basic needs and answer yes/no questions using a combination of verbal requesting, picture symbols, and approximated sign language. She is highly motivated to use her iPad, and she is beginning to use a new communication app (e.g., ProloQuo2GO) to augment her vocal speech. Fatima receives special education services in a separate setting for 20% of her school day for specially designed instruction in foundational and grade aligned academic skills in the areas of math and reading as well as communication skills.

Academic performance positively contributes to postschool outcomes, including employment and wages (Migliore et al., 2012). There are ever increasing opportunities for individuals with autism spectrum disorder (ASD) to access higher education through postsecondary education (PSE) programs, and students with disabilities who receive an education with a focus on academics are more than twice as likely to attend PSE after high school (Bouck & Joshi, 2015). For students with ASD specifically, academic achievement is significantly related to postsecondary education and overall success (Nasamran et al., 2017). Laying the foundation for preparing students with ASD for adult life is the responsibility of K-12 teachers. In-school predictors of post-school success for individuals with disabilities include (a) program of study, (b) inclusion in general

DOI: 10.4324/9781003255147-11

education, and (c) exit exam requirements and high school diploma (Mazotti et al., 2016).

There is heterogeneity across all aspects of individuals with ASD, including academic skill performance. Neither cognitive impairments nor academic difficulties are diagnostic characteristics of ASD, although intellectual disability was at one time thought to be a comorbidity (Evans, 2013). Current research indicates approximately 30% of individuals with ASD also have an intellectual disability as measured by an IQ below 70 and an additional 25% have an IQ in the borderline range of 71–85 (Christenson et al., 2016). While not all individuals with ASD have an intellectual disability, the severity of ASD characteristics in some individuals related to social interaction, social communication, and restricted, repetitive interests that may lead to problem behaviors such as aggression and/or withdrawal may cause practitioners to question the priority of academic instruction.

There is inherent value in providing academic instruction to all individuals with ASD, as well as dynamic instruction, and dynamic *explicit instruction* in academic skills can improve their quality of life. In addition to learning academic content, research shows that positive effects of academic instruction can include increased engagement, vocabulary, and communicative exchanges with others (Reutebuch et al., 2015). An undoubtable and unique challenge in writing about and implementing high-quality academic instruction is the broad range and abilities of students with ASD. Throughout this chapter on teaching academics, we will refer to students with ASD according to the type of academic content standards they access, and on which they are therefore assessed. The percentage of students who meet grade-level expectations is not readily available, though general estimates can be made based on graduation rates (Fleury et al., in press). Students with ASD who need less extensive academic support typically access their state's general state standards and assessments, while those who need extensive academic supports typically access alternate assessments based on alternate achievement standards (AA-AAS). In the 2017–2018 school year most students receiving special education services under the area of autism graduated with a regular diploma (72%), followed by 18% who graduated with an alternative certificate (likely indicating they took their state's AA-AAS). A remaining 10% either dropped out or aged out of the education system (National Center for Education Statistics, 2020). We will review and discuss research-based and evidence-based strategies for supporting the specific academic instructional needs of all students with ASD.

Academic Instructional Needs of Students with ASD

In planning academic instruction, it is important to consider how an individual's characteristics related to ASD may impact their learning.

A few well-researched areas to consider include executive functioning, joint attention, theory of mind, and central coherence. Executive functioning is an umbrella term for cognitive tasks that involve maintaining focus, switching between tasks, impulse control, and retention and application of information. Executive functioning is more strongly related to academic achievement than IQ. Learners with ASD who demonstrate markedly higher levels of distractibility, impulsivity, forgetfulness, and poor focus will likely need support strategies for academic tasks such as organizing outlines to develop expository texts, planning an inquiry-based process to answer a science question, or setting up an equation based on a word problem.

Joint attention (i.e., using eye gaze or gesture to attend along with another individual to an item or event of interest; Mundy et al., 1990) may interfere with a student's ability to detect when a teacher is emphasizing salient information. This could impact the information they receive and retain during instruction as well as the effectiveness of prompting. Learners with ASD characteristically also have limited perspective taking (i.e., Theory of Mind; Baron-Cohen et al., 1985). In academic tasks this may result in difficulty writing persuasive arguments, identifying an author or character's intent, and interpreting complex mathematical situations. Finally, weak central coherence results in strong bias towards details affecting focus on the whole task (Happe & Frith, 2006). This may be responsible for commonly noted strengths in processes requiring attention to detail such as mathematics procedures but can also result in challenges with reasoning abstractly and flexibly solving problems in unfamiliar contexts.

In addition to taking into consideration the cognitive profiles of individuals with ASD, it is also important to understand the academic achievement profiles of this population. The complexity of skills that contribute to decoding and linguistic comprehension are compounded by the heterogeneity of individuals with ASD in both their reading skills and general core characteristics. There is initial evidence of predictive patterns between autism symptomology in social communication and reading difficulties (e.g., Jones et al., 2009; McIntyre et al., 2017) and that reading abilities are impacted by cognition and communication modality (Davidson et al., 2021). There is not a single reading profile in ASD (Solari et al., 2019), and little is known about reading profiles for individuals with ASD with IQs below 70 (Charman et al., 2011). For the approximately 30% of learners with ASD who do not rely on speaking to communicate and/or use AAC (Tager-Flusberg & Kasari, 2011), reading serves an important dual communicative function. Thankfully, while there may be little research regarding the academic profile of this population, there is growing academic intervention research for individuals with ASD who do not rely on speaking to communicate. This is encouraging because reading comprehension is a pivotal skill that provides access to all other content areas as well as leisure, daily living, and employment activities (Spooner & Browder, 2015).

As with reading, it should be unsurprising that there is not a clear or agreed upon mathematics achievement profile of individuals with ASD. A conservative generalization is that the mathematical profile of students with ASD is uneven (Jones et al., 2009). Compared to peers without disabilities, students with ASD are up to five times more likely to exhibit mathematics difficulty (Oswald et al., 2016). There is a relationship between underachievement in mathematics and cognitive ability (Charman et al., 2011), though strengths in some areas (e.g., rote memory, procedural tasks) may mask some individuals' true understanding of operations during early elementary years. This suggests a complex and heterogeneous mathematics profile of students with ASD (Wei et al., 2014).

Using Education Science to Inform Academic Instruction

The focus of this chapter is on using evidence- and research-based practices to improve academic skills for learners with ASD. We define evidence-based practice (EBP) as an intervention that has been demonstrated successful through a number of rigorous research investigations, was carefully scrutinized through a systematic review using quality indicators, and was identified as meeting a high criterion of evidence and efficacy (Cook et al., 2015). Recently, Steinbrenner et al. (2020) conducted a comprehensive literature review of experimental studies conducted between 1990–2017 to identify approaches that support children and youth with ASD in achieving socially significant outcomes. This was an update to the review by Wong et al. (2014) of research conducted between 1990–2011 in response to the rapid growth of experimental research in this area. A total of 151 articles targeted academic or pre-academic skills, 96 of which were conducted since 2012. Whereas Wong et al. identified 13 EBPs to support academic outcomes for students with ASD, Steinbrenner et al. were able to identify 28 EBPs in all, with 24 having evidence to improve academic outcomes. This is evidence of expanding knowledge of how to teach academic skills to students with ASD.

The next section of the chapter includes descriptions of the big ideas of mathematics, reading, and science. The section also includes specific examples of instructional strategies derived from the research literature that can be applied to teach this content. Finally, the chapter concludes with a discussion of how asset-based instructional frameworks such as Universal Design for Learning and Culturally Sustaining Pedagogy can be used to draw on the strengths of students with ASD while acknowledging their intersectional identities.

Mathematics

Research conducted in the last 20 years has demonstrated that students with ASD can learn meaningful grade-aligned mathematics through high quality systematic instruction. We should reject the notion that students' education should be focused on a narrow view of what will be "functional" in their lives. Instead, a contextualized approach to mathematics should be used to make standards-based mathematics instruction meaningful and personally relevant (Root et al., 2018). The content of mathematics instruction for all students with ASD, including those who take their state's Alternate Assessment aligned with Alternate Achievement Standards (i.e., AA-AAS), should align with the general education mathematics standards of their grade. Learners with ASD will need specially designed instruction in mathematics due to characteristic challenges in executive functioning, metacognition, working memory, and language.

A critical factor in math performance is executive functioning (Bull & Scerif, 2001). It requires an individual to make a plan, organize information, attend a task for a prolonged amount of time, and self-monitor progress (Hart Barnett & Cleary, 2015). Additionally, executive functioning requires an individual to switch between cognitive sets using working memory, which is an executive challenge for many individuals with ASD that is required in mathematics tasks. Problem solving also requires metacognitive skills which include an individual's ability to plan, check, monitor, and evaluate their own performance (Montague, 1997). To be a proficient problem solver, students must be able to store and sequentially update important information (Fuchs et al., 2019). Language also plays a large role in mathematics (Hughes et al., 2016). Mathematical language is academic language that conveys mathematical ideas with more precise understanding than conversational or informal language used every day to communicate with others (Fuchs et al., 2021). In fact, word problem solving is its own form of text comprehension (Fuchs et al., 2015). Below we will outline specific considerations for providing high-quality instruction in mathematics to students with ASD related to their strengths and needs in the areas of number sense and problem solving.

Number Sense

Number sense, also called early numeracy, is to mathematics what phonics is to reading (Saunders, 2020). It includes the basic understanding of mathematical operations, which is necessary for students to understand and apply more complex mathematical concepts. Number sense is a key component to meaningful participation and access to mathematics for all students (NCTM, 2000). In fact, early mathematical understanding strongly influences later success in mathematics (Jordan et al., 2009), and students who struggle in mathematics often lack opportunities to learn critical early numeracy skills (Berch & Mazzocco, 2007). Given the broad definition of number sense, below we will give brief definitions and examples of number sense skills and how they can be developed for individuals with ASD.

Quantity. Children explore quantity before developing the ability to count. For example, young children evaluate quantity in objects outside of defining numbers (e.g., which piece of cake is larger; Van de Walle et al., 2016). Children later begin counting by sequentially listing numbers in order, referred to as rote counting (i.e., "one, two, three…") and then typically develop one-to-one correspondence, also called coordinated counting (Van de Walle et al.). One-to-one correspondence is the ability to apply one number quantity to a single object and give it only one count (Saunders, 2020). The recommended progression (Saunders et al., 2014) for teaching one-to-one correspondence includes first starting with a small number of objects (e.g., 1–5 of the same object) and slowly increasing the amount. Teachers can support students with ASD to visually organize the items they are counting by teaching them to count from left to right, as they would when reading, and to touch the items as they count. Teachers could also incorporate a line for students to organize the items as well as move them across the line as they count.

Next, students should practice counting nonmoveable objects in a line (i.e., stickers placed on a card) with the support of the line faded. After students have mastered this skill, teach them to count moveable, scattered objects (e.g., cube manipulatives on a table), which they can arrange into a line for themselves if needed. Lastly, if the students can count the scattered items without moving or touching them, provide practice opportunities for the student to count nonmoveable, scattered objects (i.e., stickers placed on a card). When the student can state the number of objects in a group without using one-to-one correspondence, they have developed the higher-level number sense skill of subitizing.

The development of subitizing, or the ability to look at an amount (e.g., five dots on a card) and identify the total (e.g., five) without counting, allows for more efficiency in working with quantities and sets. For students who are learning to subitize, begin with three objects organized in patterns that are symmetrical. Next, move on to larger numbers such as five with more challenging patterns (i.e., symmetrical and asymmetrical). An instructional strategy to teach subitizing is through systematic and errorless learning (i.e., response prompting; Jimenez & Saunders, 2019). Prompting (i.e., constant time delay, simultaneous prompting, system of least prompts) has also been identified as an evidence-based practice for teaching academic content to students with ASD (Wong et al., 2015) and specifically for mathematics for students with ASD who also have a moderate to severe intellectual disability (Spooner et al., 2019). Skip counting is also an efficient counting method (i.e., counting forward or backward from a number by a given quantity in a repeated fashion; e.g., 5, 10, 15). Instructional strategies that support skip counting include constant time delay, simultaneous prompting, and model-lead-test (Saunders, 2020).

Developing the understanding of cardinality is another critical aspect of number sense. Cardinality is the knowledge of how many items are in a set and the number name for that quantity. While cardinality is related to rote counting and one to one correspondence, it is developed separately. For example, a learner who can individually count six blocks in a set is demonstrating rote counting and one to one correspondence, but cardinality is not apparent until they can correctly answer "How many are there?" Thus, cardinality is a prerequisite skill for composing and decomposing sets using concrete (e.g., manipulatives) or representative (e.g., drawing) strategies. One way to help learners with ASD develop cardinality is to have them repeat the final number counted immediately after they finish counting. For example, when the learner finishes counting the teacher can immediately ask "how many?", have the learner repeat the last number stated (e.g., "6"), with the teacher following up with behavior-specific praise to reinforce the concept (e.g., "yes, you counted six blocks").

Related to cardinality is order and magnitude. This is the understanding of relationships between numerals and quantities (e.g., more than, less than, equal to). The recommended teaching sequence is *equal* (identifying and creating equal sets or numerals), *more* (identifying or creating a set that is greater than another), and *less* (identifying or creating a set that is less than another). Once the concept is understood at a concrete and representative level (e.g., manipulatives, items, drawings), it needs to be also assessed and, if needed, explicitly taught at the abstract level (e.g., numerals). Example/nonexample training is an efficient and effective strategy for teaching these concepts (Saunders et al., 2014).

Example/nonexample training is an explicit instructional strategy. In example/nonexample training, the instructor presents both examples and nonexamples (e.g., items that are same and items that are different). In the beginning, wide examples should be used with students (e.g., clearly equal and clearly unequal). Additionally with example/nonexample training, concepts should be grasped by the student before moving on to the next concept. At the start of instruction, the instructor models with rapid succession, pointing to an example and stating the concept (e.g., "These are the same") and then pointing to a non-example and stating that it is not the concept (e.g., "This is not same"). Massed trials are conducted with instructor models. After sufficient modeling, the instructor may test for either expressive or receptive understanding. To test expressive understanding, the instructor may say: "What is this?" and require the student to say "same" or "not same." To test receptive understanding, the instructor may say: "Touch same" or "Touch not same."

All of the previously discussed number sense skills did not require learners to be able to identify or write numerals. While these skills certainly should be priorities, they can be developed alongside other skills using the same instructional methods as identifying and writing letters. It is critical that delayed development of these skills does not prevent learners from making progress in other areas of mathematics. Additional skill areas that fall under the umbrella of number sense include patterning and units of measurement (Saunders, 2020). Patterning is a precursor to algebraic thinking and reasoning; it begins with visual patterns (e.g., colors, shapes, etc.) and then moves on to number patterns (e.g., 1, 3, 5 or 2, 4, 6, 2, 4, 6). Units of measurement include assessing the magnitude of an object such as length, weight, and height or comparing two or more objects. There are standard units of measurements (e.g., measuring someone's height in inches) and nonstandard units of measurements (e.g., measuring someone's height in soda cans).

Operational Understanding. The last skill area of number sense is operational understanding. It is the understanding of the basic operations, addition, subtraction, multiplication, and division. This allows students to see mathematical situations in their everyday lives and apply their understanding of appropriate operations in real-world settings. There is a difference in operational understanding related to conceptual understanding and procedural understanding. Procedural understanding is where an individual knows which procedures to apply to a specific problem type and in turn arrive at the right answer; comparatively, conceptual understanding is the student understanding what they just did, why they did it, and why it makes sense within the context of the situation (Van de Walle et al., 2016).

The use of manipulative-based instructional sequences, an evidence-based practice for students with ASD (Spooner et al., 2019), is one way to develop students' operational understanding. This can be done through concrete (i.e., physical) or virtual (i.e., digital) manipulatives (Bouck & Long, 2020). Manipulative-based instructional sequences provide instruction to students by slowly shifting from learning from a manipulative (i.e., concrete or virtual), to representations (i.e., drawings), and then with abstract strategies (i.e., numerals; Agrawal & Morin, 2016). Manipulative based instruction can be delivered in a range of similarly structured formats (e.g., VR, VRA, CR, CRA; Bouck & Long, 2020). The concrete sequence can include manipulatives such as base ten blocks, money (i.e., coins, dollar bills), or tiles, while virtual manipulatives are technology based (i.e., computer, website, app). The representational sequence can include the student drawing or using pictures to represent the problem. Lastly, the abstract sequence can include numerical strategies and procedures to help solve the problem (i.e., counting up from $1.97 to $2.00 in order to know how much change is needed or showing your work" by solving 2 + x = 10). The manipulative-based instructional sequence is reliant on the incorporation of explicit instruction (Agrawal & Morin, 2016). Students must first be shown how to use the manipulatives (i.e., model), then guided with the manipulatives (i.e., lead), and then given the opportunity to practice with the manipulatives independently (i.e., test).

Problem Solving

Both number sense and problem solving need to be built up together. Students with ASD need the opportunity to practice the development of both mathematical skills collectively; however, limits on number sense will also constrain the development of problem solving. According to NCTM (2000), problem solving is the cornerstone of mathematical learning. Browder et al. (2018) maintain problem solving instruction for learners with ASD, and other developmental disabilities, must explicitly give students the tools they need to go beyond the "how" (i.e., procedures) but also the *when* and *why* to apply them (i.e., conceptual understanding). Not all problem solving needs to be taught through word problems, but this is how problem solving is most often taught and assessed in schools.

According to Mayer (1985), there are four phases to solving a mathematical word problem: (a) problem translation, (b) problem integration, (c) solution planning, (d) and solution execution. Root et al. (2016) outlined barriers students with ASD and other developmental disabilities may face at each phase of problem solving that need to be considered during instruction. For example, each phase requires cognitive skills for successful completion (Krawec et al., 2013). At the problem translation phase, students need literacy and semantic language skills to be able to construct meaning from the problem. The problem integration phase requires the student to be able to select important parts from the problem and translate them to the mathematical structure. The solution planning and execution phases both require the student to select the operationally correct procedure and successfully execute it to arrive at the correct answer. Each phase is dependent on the previous for the student to arrive at the correct solution. If the student makes an error at any point of the process, it may prevent them from demonstrating conceptual understanding and/or procedural knowledge. To support development of problem solving skills, teachers need to provide students with the appropriate strategies for attacking word problems.

While there is a range of strategies students can use to solve problems with corresponding instructional strategies for teachers, we believe instructional time is a precious commodity (Heward, 2003) and therefore only the most effective and efficient should be deployed. In contrast, the keyword strategy is neither effective nor efficient (Spooner et al., 2017). The faulty keyword strategy teaches students to rely on "signal" words (e.g., more indicates addition, difference indicates subtraction) when word problem solving. The keyword strategy only works for a little more than half of one-step problems that include one keyword, a third of one-step problems that includes more than one keyword, and less than 10% of multi-step word problems (Powell et al., 2022). This strategy does not provide students with the conceptual understanding needed for problem solving skills to generalize to real-world scenarios (Jitendra & Star, 2011).

Evidence-based Problem Solving Strategies. Root et al. (2021) recently conducted a systematic review to synthesize the evidence on teaching mathematical word problem solving skills to students with ASD. Root and colleagues identified 18 studies that met the Council for Exceptional Children's threshold as "high quality." They identified the following strategies as evidence-based practices: task analysis, system of least prompts, graphic organizers, explicit instruction, schema-based instruction, and technology-assisted instruction. While these six practices met the CEC standards to be evidenced-based practices, they were consistently used together in treatment packages. All included studies that used at least two of the evidence-based strategies together with several studies incorporating all six strategies together in an intervention package called modified schema-based instruction (MSBI) to teach mathematical word problem solving.

MSBI supplements the essential features of schema-based instruction (SBI), an EBP for students with learning disabilities (Jitendra et al., 2016), with the addition of (a) a task analysis and chant with hand motions to serve as a heuristic, (b) enhanced visual supports on graphic organizers, and (c) incorporation of systematic instruction along with explicit instruction (Root et al., 2020). In SBI (Jitendra et al., 2016), students are taught to follow a heuristic to visually diagram the problem on a schematic diagram (i.e., graphic organizer) and solve the problem using explicit instruction. Schema-based instructional techniques are consistent with schema theory in supporting students to recognize the semantic structure of a mathematical problem; this is a critical step in problem comprehension (Jitendra et al., 2016). Schemas are broken up into additive and multiplicative problem types. There are three general schemas for additive (group or combine, change, compare) and four for multiplicative (equal groups, multiplicative comparison, ratio, and proportion).

The MSBI package is like all other schema-based instructional techniques by teaching students to recognize the mathematic problem structure (i.e., schema) and use that knowledge to devise a plan to find the answer. The MSBI intervention package makes problem solving more accessible by supporting students to (a) access the problem, (b) conceptualize the problem and mathematical content, (c) solve the problem procedurally, and (d) generalize multiple ways (Spooner et al., 2017). Discrimination training should be taught to students with ASD in order for them not to overgeneralize. It is a form of explicit instruction, and it involves teaching students when to and when not to apply problem solving strategies (Browder et al., 2018; Saunders, 2014). It involves teaching students to identify key features of each problem type to determine their next steps of problem solving. However, while a few past MSBI research studies demonstrate that some individuals with ASD have needed explicit discrimination training (e.g., Browder et al., 2018; Root et al., 2020), not all individuals with ASD may need this.

In math, Fatima can rote count to 50, demonstrates an understanding of cardinality for sets up to 10, tells time using a digital clock, adds and subtracts given manipulatives and numbers to 10, and identifies coins and bills. To address Fatima's needs in math, her teacher plans to design intensive instruction in foundational skills, co-plan and co-teach accessible grade-aligned lessons related to 7th grade math standards, and continue teaching mathematical practices, like making sense of problems and modeling with mathematics, both in her small group intensive intervention classes and within her inclusive math class.

To continue building Fatima's foundational math, or early numeracy skills, her teacher designs intensive instruction routines to ensure Fatima receives daily practice to build both conceptual understanding and fluency of basic computations. These lessons are short but frequent, occur in small group settings, and are carefully monitored with curriculum-based measures her teacher administers once a week. Her special education teacher and general education math teacher co-plan a unit for the 7th grade inclusive math class that will allow Fatima to access content related to ratios and proportions. Her teachers start with the Achieve the Core website and identify "Analyze proportional relationships and use them to solve real-world and mathematical problems" as a prioritized 7th grade math standard. They then use the learning progressions table from the website to work backwards across previous grade levels and identify any prerequisite skills students will need in order to fully understand the target grade level standards. Related prerequisite standards included "Understanding ratio concepts and use ratio reasoning to solve problems" (6th grade), "Understanding fraction equivalence" (5th grade), "Building fractions from unit fractions" (5th grade), and "Developing an understanding of fractions as numbers" (4th grade). Based on this information, Fatima's special education teacher knows that she needs to pre-teach the concept of fractions, ratios, and proportions, the concept of equivalency, the ability to build fractions and ratios, and finally, the ability to solve problems about proportional relationships. She will start with brief, intensive and explicit lessons in which she teaches the concept of fractions, ratios and proportions.

Fatima's teacher considers how to design lessons using concrete representations of the core concept to support conceptual development She chooses a variety of concrete manipulatives to teach the concept of fractions. She selects multiple exemplars, varying in size, shape, and color. She includes 3-D objects using both real world objects, like pizza slices, and generic objects, like cuisenaire rods. She decides to promote generalization across formats and includes virtual fraction tiles from the free website Toy Theater. Through carefully designed instruction that begins with explicit vocabulary instruction and review, her teacher builds understanding of fractions, ratios, proportions, and equivalency. Fatima is not the only student in her class who benefits from explicit instruction in foundational concepts, and she receives this instruction in a small group of three students during regular math center rotations.

To give Fatima the opportunity to apply what she's learning in a meaningful way, her teachers write personally relevant word problems that use Fatima's name and the names of her family and friends. They include scenarios that have to do with activities or events Fatima enjoys. For example, during their current unit focusing on ratios, some of Fatima's problems are relevant to cooking because it is an activity she enjoys with her Abuela and others are related to art because it is her favorite elective. As a result of ongoing modified schema-based instruction (MSBI), Fatima understands equal group and multiplicative comparison types, setting her up for the next unit on ratios. Fatima's math word problems are displayed on the GoWorksheet app, which allows her to access read alouds for all word problems and to type her answers, using the keyboard like a number line (Table 9.1).

Table 9.1 Summary of Recommended Practices for Teaching Mathematics to Students with ASD

Practices for Teaching	Description and Examples
Follow scaffolded teaching sequence to support visual organization needed for counting with 1:1 correspondence	First start by teaching students to count movable objects in a line. Next, progress to counting non-movable representations/drawings in a line, scattered moveable objects, and then non-movable scattered representations/drawings while increasing quantities as the student demonstrates mastery.
Use example/ nonexample training to teach order and magnitude	Use the recommended teaching sequence of more, less, and equal (same) by providing clear examples and non-examples of quantities. Initial quantities should have wide examples (e.g., 1 and 10) and then become more narrow to make discrimination more difficult as students develop fluency.
Use manipulative based instructional sequences to support operational understanding	Support the development of operational, procedural, and conceptual understanding through manipulative-based teaching sequences. First begin with virtual (i.e., counters on iPad application) or concrete (i.e., unifix cubes) manipulates and then progress to representational (i.e., drawings, tallies). Once the student is ready, incorporate abstract strategies (i.e., numerals).
Use explicit instruction (i.e., model, guided practice, independent practice) to support operational understanding	All variations of manipulative based instructional sequences (i.e., VR, VRA, CR, CRA) should be taught explicitly. First show students how to use the manipulatives (i.e., model) and then guide them while they use them (i.e., lead). Lastly, provide students with the opportunity to use the manipulatives independently with feedback.
Use modified schema-based instruction (MSBI) to support mathematical problem solving	First make sure word problems are meaningful and accessible (i.e., appropriate reading level, predictable format) with visual supports if needed. Next, explicitly teach students a problem solving routine or attack strategy that is displayed to student as a task analysis (with visual supports as needed) that they can use to self-monitor as they complete steps. The task analysis can further support student independence by providing them with a "by myself" and "with help" column to self-monitor independence rather than simply completion. Teach students to follow the problem solving routine (e.g., steps of task analysis) to represent the quantities from the word problem onto the schematic diagram through modeling and think alouds as well as opportunities to practice and receive feedback. Some students may need the support of a system of least prompts during guided and/or independent practice.

Reading

There has been a substantial increase in research on reading instruction for individuals with ASD over the past decade. The broad application of extensive reading research has led to an emphasis on the empirical "science of reading" defined as "accumulated knowledge about reading, reading development, and best practices for reading instruction obtained by the use of the scientific method" (Petscher, p. 268, 2020). The Simple View of Reading is a theoretical framework for understanding how the skill of reading is acquired (Gough & Tunmer, 1986). Reading is defined as the construction of meaning from text (Hoover & Gough, 1990). Through the lens of the Simple View of Reading this meaning is constructed by the additive combination of linguistic comprehension and decoding skills. As linguistic comprehension and decoding skills are improved, so is the construction of meaning from text (hereafter referred to as reading or reading skills). Unsurprisingly, reading is impacted by difficulties in language and communication often seen in individuals with ASD.

Given the heterogeneity of autism characteristics in individuals with ASD, it is not surprising reading characteristics of individuals with ASD are also heterogeneous (Solari et al., 2019). Bullen et al. (2022) examined reading achievement of elementary aged students with ASD without co-occurring intellectual disability and described two subgroups in reading performance: low achievement and high achievement readers. Low achievement readers comprised approximately 70% of the sample and were described as having average intelligence but performing at least one standard deviation below the mean performance of all readers in comprehension skills. Additional characteristics of the low achievement group included (a) a negative predictive correlation of working memory on reading fluency and (b) a negative predictive correlation between working memory and inferential thinking on reading comprehension. High achievement readers comprised approximately 30% of the sample, had above average intelligence, and average performance in reading fluency and comprehension.

In summary, assessment of reading skills of individuals with ASD has demonstrated the reading profiles of this population are heterogeneous. However, some consistent findings have included weaknesses in decoding skills for individuals with ASD and co-occurring intellectual disability and weakness in comprehension skills for approximately 70% of all individuals with ASD with or without intellectual disability. These weaknesses may be impacted by difficulties in working memory and inferential thinking as a result of the core characteristics of ASD. Interventions which address these difficulties are necessary to ameliorate reading skills for individuals with ASD.

An evidenced-based practice for teaching skills across a variety of skill domains to individuals with ASD, including reading skills, is systematic instruction (Browder, Wood, Thompson, Ribuffo, 2014). Systematic instruction is "teaching focused on specific, measurable responses that may either be discrete (singular) or a response chain (e.g., task analysis), and that are established through the use of defined methods of prompting and feedback based on the principles and research of applied behavior analysis" (Browder, 2001, p. 95). Many of the evidence-based practices identified in Steinbrenner (2020) for individuals with autism are specific components of systematic instruction (e.g., time delay, task-analysis, modeling, prompting, time-delay, and reinforcement). A recent meta-analysis of reading interventions for students with autism (Thompson et al., 2022) found that all of the studies identified as meeting WWC quality indicators and demonstrating moderate or strong evidence of positive outcomes on reading for students with ASD used systematic instruction alone or in combination with other strategies including naturalistic instruction, graphic organizers, and technology-based instruction (Thompson et al., 2022). Below we will provide definitions and examples of research or evidence-based strategies for effective instruction in decoding and comprehension.

Decoding

Decoding is word recognition and involves the combination of phonological awareness, alphabetic knowledge, and letter-sound correspondence. While individuals with ASD and without co-occurring intellectual disability often perform similarly to the norm in decoding, those with ASD that do not will need explicit instruction in decoding strategies to support their acquisition of these critical skills. In this section we will describe the application of the evidence-based strategy naturalistic instruction which has been used to successfully teach decoding skills. In addition, we will review two readily available published curricula with research demonstrating their effectiveness in teaching decoding skills students with ASD.

Naturalistic instruction paired with systematic instruction has been successfully used with preschool and elementary school children with ASD to learn phonemic awareness, letter sound correspondence, and sight word vocabulary. Naturalistic instruction is an evidence-based practice defined as "a collection of techniques and strategies that are embedded in typical activities and/or routines in which the learner participates to naturally promote, support, and encourage target skills/behaviors" (Steinbrenner et al., 2020, p. 28). Hanson et al. (2014) used naturalistic instruction to teach phonemic awareness (individual sounds in words) during 15-minute play sessions with elementary students with ASD and the ability to imitate words. When a student with ASD would approach or interact with a toy the instructor would gain the child's attention, label the object the child was playing with, and prompt the child to engage in three activities: clapping the syllables, say the first sound of the object, and sound out the full word. Benedek-Wood et al. (2016) used naturalistic instruction to teach letter-sound correspondence (understanding the relationship of graphemes and phonemes) to preschool students with ASD and limited verbal ability. First the instructor used model-lead-test procedures to teach one target letter-sound correspondence at a time by placing the target letter and a distractor on the floor and saying "I am going to say a sound …and point to the letter that makes the sound" (model), then asked the child to point to the corresponding letter along with the instructor (lead), and finally asked the student to independently point to the sound (test). If the child made an error the instructor would repeat the model-lead-test until the student was able to independently point to the correct letter. Following the brief instructional session, the child was given time to engage in a preferred activity that included opportunities for the instructor to emphasize and prompt the student to indicate the letter-sound correspondence in their natural environment. McGee et al. (1986) T taught sight word identification in the context of a play activity by making available two toys to the student, one of which was the target vocabulary word. Whenever the child reached for or requested the target toy, the instructor would place five index cards with words, one of which was the name of the toy. Then the instructor would say "Give me the word [name of toy]" and use a system-of-least prompts (independent → model → partial physical) to teach the target vocabulary word.

Curricula have also been shown to be effective in teaching early reading and decoding skills. Reading Mastery is a Direct Instruction program. Steinbrenner et al. (2020) identified Direct Instruction as an evidence-based practice and defined it as "a systematic approach to teaching using a sequenced instructional package with scripted protocols or lessons. It emphasizes teacher and student dialogue through choral and independent student responses and employs systematic and explicit error corrections to promote mastery and generalization" (p. 28). In Kamps et al. (2017) study, elementary-aged students with ASD and vocal imitation skills who received Reading Mastery small group instruction demonstrated significant improvements on word identification and letter-sound correspondence when compared to those who did not receive the intervention.

Other curricula, Early Literacy Skill Builder (ELSB; Browder, Gibbs, Alhgrim-Delzell, Courtade, & Lee, 2007), include a researched-based curriculum for teaching phonological awareness to students with ASD and ID. The ELSB has evidenced-based practices as instructional strategies within the scripted curricula including time-delay, prompting, and task analysis. Hunt et al. conducted a conceptual replication study examining the effects of ELSB on reading skills of students with severe disabilities. All participants were identified as having a moderate to severe intellectual disability and were in kindergarten to fourth grade. While the primary focus was not specifically ASD, the authors disaggregated performance by disability type enabling examination of the efficacy of the curricula on learning of students identified with ASD. Students with ASD who received the ELSB instruction performed significantly better than the students with ASD who received business as usual instruction. In addition, data were disaggregated for students who were verbal and those who were non-verbal and both made significant gains compared to those with similar characteristics in the control group. Significant differences were found in reading conventions, listening comprehension, phonics, phonological awareness, and letter sound correspondence. There was not a significant difference between the experimental and control groups in vocabulary performance.

Students who complete the ELSB are ready for instruction in decoding. Many students can begin a program like Reading Mastery, but for students with complex communication needs, curricula that require expressive response modes ("What sound does 'm' make?") is not accessible. The Early Reading Skills Builder (ERSB; Ahlgrim-Delzell, Wood, & Browder, 2015) was designed to address the need of articulatory feedback, or the process of hearing oneself blend and segment speech sounds out loud. The vocalization of blending and segmenting allows people with vocal speech to evaluate and self-correct as they learn to sound out words. The ERSB is an app-based curriculum that provides students with complex communication needs, including some students with ASD, the ability to produce speech sounds to blend and segment using technology. Students who complete the ERSB can decode at a second grade reading level.

Comprehension

Not surprisingly, given the characteristics of autism impacting communication and social language as well as reading assessment research indicating difficulties with reading comprehension, the bulk of reading research for individuals with ASD has focused on comprehension instruction. In this section we will describe research and evidence-based practices for teaching comprehension to students with ASD.

Story-based instruction for reading comprehension and language skills. Boyle et al. (2019) conducted a systematic review and meta-analysis to examine the effects of shared reading on early reading and language skills of individuals with ASD. Using the National Autism Center evidence of classification system (NAC, 2015) they indicated that story-based instruction is an emerging treatment for individuals with ASD, meaning that there is evidence that story-based instruction provides positive outcomes for individuals with ASD, but additional research is needed to determine whether it can be considered an established evidence-based practice. Below we will describe two representative examples of the research on story-based instruction to teach reading comprehension and language skills to students with ASD.

Fleury and Schwartz (2017) examined the effects of a modified version of dialog shared-story reading on vocal initiation and responding, and text specific vocabulary with preschool-aged children with ASD. Dialogic reading is an evidenced-based strategy identified by the What Works Clearinghouse (WWC, 2007) as effective for improving oral language for at-risk preschoolers. Dialogic reading instruction involves the adult's use of two acronyms to guide their reading instruction with the students as they read the story. The first acronym is CROWD which stands for: (1) C – "completion", the adult reads a sentence and pauses before saying a key word in the sentence to prompt the child to say the word; (2) R – "recall", after reading one or more pages the adult pauses and asks the child a question about what has been read; (3) O – "open-ended", the adult asks the child to describe the pictures in the text; (4) W – "wh-questions", the adult asks the child wh questions about the story; and (5) D – "distancing", the adult describes how the events in the story relate to the child's own experiences. The second acronym is PEER which is used at each stage of the CROWD acronym, meaning that as the adult addresses the "C" they use PEER to support the child in "completing" the sentence. PEER stands for: (1) P – "prompt", the adult prompts the child to respond; (2) E – "evaluate," the adult evaluates the child's response; (3) E – "expand," the adult repeats the child's response and expands on the response with, for example, additional details; and (4) R – "repeats," the adult provides the child an additional opportunity to demonstrate the targeted skill. Fluery et al. modified the traditional dialogic reading intervention by replacing the PEER component with a system of least prompts, which included (a) providing a follow up question when the child was incorrect or unresponsive to the initial CROWD prompt; if still not correct, (b) providing a choice of two options; if still not correct, (c) changing the question to a yes/no option; if still not correct, (d) asking the child to repeat the target word; if still not correct, (d) requesting child to point to the image in the book that represented the target term; and finally, if still not correct, (e) prompting the child with physical assistance to point to the correct response. Students in the study demonstrated an immediate increase in their frequency of responding to adult questions but demonstrated only minimal increases in verbal initiations. Students also increased their acquisition of story-book specific vocabulary words which was measured by showing illustrations of the key vocabulary words and asking the students to label the pictures.

Mims et al. (2012) examined the effects of task-analyzed read-alouds with systematic prompting on text specific listening comprehension of middle school students with autism and moderate to severe intellectual disability. Three of the students used pictures and objects to communicate and one student used vocal language. Some were able to read a few sight words but none were fluent readers. Teachers were previously trained to follow a story-based instruction task analysis (Browder et al., 2007; see table below for example) and for this study a modified system-of-least prompts to support the students with autism in answering comprehension questions about the text was added to the task analysis as the primary intervention. Researchers adapted grade-aligned biographies into summaries so that the biography could be read aloud by the instructor in a single session. The adapted text included Writing With Symbols 2000 pictures symbols paired with key vocabulary in the text. Each student was given their own biography summary to refer to in the lesson. For each biography summary, 11 questions were developed consisting of eight wh-questions and three sequencing questions. Two graphic organizers were used: one was used as a template for sequencing three events and was labeled with "first, next, last"; the other was a t-chart with rules for determining how to answer wh-questions (e.g., when you year "what," listen for a thing). All students demonstrated an increase in the number of unprompted correct listening comprehension responses following the intervention.

Following a series of conceptual and systematic replications (e.g., Browder et al., 2013; Hudson et al, 2014), the modified system of least prompts for passage comprehension was refined into what is consistently used today. For literal questions (where answers can be found directly in the text) the instructor asks the literal comprehension question and waits for the student to answer. If the student does not answer or answers incorrectly the instructor begins the modified system of least prompts for passage comprehension beginning with (a) rereading the paragraph with the answer (or approximately three sentences; whichever is briefest) and repeating the question, then (b) rereading the sentence with the answer and repeating the question, then (c) rereading the key word or phrase with the answer and repeating the question, and then (d) providing a controlling prompt so that the student points to the correct answer (on a response board if using one or in the passage). The instructor provides a brief wait time (usually 5 s) between prompts to allow for students to provide the answer without receiving additional prompting. For inferential questions the steps are the same except the instructor models thinking aloud prior to rereading text selections with pertinent information.

Graphic organizers with systematic instruction. Graphic organizers are "visual templates that assist a student in grouping and categorizing information. The visual representations aid comprehension by providing a concrete picture of the organization of ... information" (Browder et al., 2011, p. 158). Given students with autism have difficulties with working memory, graphic organizers can be particularly helpful with the organization of story grammar in narrative texts and organizing text structure and key points in expository texts.

Bethune and Wood (2013) examined the effects of using system least-to-most prompts, in this case independent, verbal, gesture, and physical, to complete a graphic organizer on answering comprehension questions with elementary-aged students with autism who were early readers. Students read brief passages from their current reading level and then were taught to use a graphic organizer to sort the information from the text. The graphic organizer was a table with four columns labeled "who? (person), where? (place), what? (thing), and what doing? (event)" (p. 239). The students were given a list of typed words or phrases related to the text and asked to sort them by writing them under the corresponding column. The instructor provided prompting as needed to support them to complete the task. Following the graphic organizer activity, the students read the passage that corresponded with the graphic organizer. Then, the students were asked eight literal recall questions, two of each "wh" question type. They were allowed to refer to the graphic organizer when answering questions. All the students demonstrated an immediate increase in accurately answering comprehension questions and maintained the skill at a high level in subsequent weekly maintenance probes following the system-of-least prompts with graphic organizer intervention.

Williamson et al. (2015) used a graphic organizer and think-alouds during group instruction to improve reading comprehension of high school students with ASD who read at approximately a 5th grade level. Students would follow along in their novel as the novel was read aloud via audio recording. Then the teacher would present the character event map, identify an event from the passage that was read, and then use a think-aloud strategy to model her thoughts as she completed the first row of the graphic organizer. The graphic organizer contained three columns with the following headings: "who is involved", "what happened", "what it means." In the initial lesson she also explained the purpose and utility of the graphic organizer. During the think alouds, she would model referencing the text to identify who was involved in the event and describe how she made meaning of the event in its relation to the broader context of the story. Then she would identify another event from the passage and guide the students in the group to complete the graphic organizer for that event. Following the completion of the graphic organizer students were given 10 comprehension questions (9 inferential and one literal) related to the passage. The teacher read aloud the questions and the students could either write or speak their answers. They were allowed to refer back to the text or the graphic organizer as needed.

Technology-based systematic instruction. Technology is "an electronic item/equipment, application, or virtual network" (Odom et al., 2015,

p. 3806). The predictability and consistent presentation of information provided by technology can be especially useful for students with ASD (Root et al., 2017). Also, many evidence-based practices can be embedded into technology to provide clear and consistent instruction and error correction such as time-delay, system of least prompts, graphic organizers, and reinforcement. In this section we will review one representative study of how technology-based systematic instruction is used to teach comprehension to students with ASD.

Browder et al. (2015) examined the effects of a technology-based story-mapping procedure on the comprehension of narrative texts. All of the texts were derived from elementary-level texts typically taught to all students, adapted to a reading level of 2nd–3rd grade, and written in length of 100 to 120 words. In addition, the texts selected included the five story elements targeted for instruction which included character, setting, problem, solution, and outcome. Students were taught the definitions of the story elements using constant time delay. The elements and definitions were presented on the iPad with the element centered on the screen and the definition and distractors displayed in the four corners for the students to select. In the study the instructor implemented the time delay procedure with the iPad essentially providing access to the answer choices, however, in future studies the research team embedded the time-delay into the iPad application using GoTalkNow, a communication application which allows for a variety of programming options which can be used to develop time-delay instruction. After the students practiced learning the definitions, the instructor then read aloud the passage while the students followed along with their own copy of the passage. Then students were taught to use the story-map on the iPad which was created using the SMART notebook© application. The story map was similar to a paper graphic organizer with the labels of each element (e.g., character) and a box for the students to fill in the element related to the current text. However, there were several additional features unavailable to a simple paper/pencil graphic organizer including a small microphone icon just below each story map element which when pressed indicated the story element and provided its definition. In addition, students were able to choose between three response modes: writing their answer, typing their answer, or recording their answer to each element. Students were taught to complete the story map using a system of least prompts where the instructor directed the student to complete a story element component, waited 10s and then if the student did not respond or responded incorrectly the instructor "(a) prompted the student to activate the read-aloud of the story element definition on the story map and reviewed completed story map, (b) reread portion of the text (two to three sentences) that contained the answer, (c) reread the sentence or phrase from the story that contained the answer, and (d) read the answer and had the participant fill it in on his or her story map" (pp. 248–249). After the students completed the story map the instructor asked the students comprehension questions related to the text. If the students did not answer or answered incorrectly the instructor followed the system-of-least prompts described above with one exception, the first prompt involved prompting the student to refer to the story map for the answer. The remaining steps were the same. All of the students in this study demonstrated an immediate and large increase in the total number of correct answers to the comprehension questions. Additional studies have extended the work of Browder 2015 and have included embedding the story in the iPad, as well as programming the iPad to provide the system of least prompts for passage comprehension instead of the instructor (e.g., Allison et al., 2017). When a student does not respond or responds incorrectly, the application is programmed to systematically move through the system-of-least prompts and following the student answering correctly provides praise and/or reinforcement.

Fatima can decode at a first grade level, but she struggles to comprehend what she reads. Fatima can write lists of words but does not yet write complete sentences, though she is beginning to write words in context given a sentence template and a word bank. Each day Fatima participates in group instruction where the group collectively reads a passage of a narrative or expository text, and when it is Fatima's turn to read aloud she enjoys using the text-to-speech feature on her iPad to read her assigned section of the passage. After the passage is read all the students are given skill-appropriate independent work to summarize and answer comprehension questions from the passage. First, Fatima is given a graphic organizer relevant to the current selected passage (e.g. problem solution, comparison, story elements) and a list of details relevant to the passage and is asked to write the details onto the graphic organizer. Previously Fatima's teacher worked with her individually to teach her how to complete the graphic organizer using a system of least prompts. Now, because her teacher consistently uses the same text-structure graphic organizers, Fatima is familiar with how to complete them and is able to complete this activity independently with a few reminders to stay on task and reinforcement via the "caught you being good" tickets provided to all students as a part of the school wide positive behavior support system.

Once Fatima finishes her graphic organizer she shows it to her teacher who then hands her the iPad which has a completed

graphic organizer. Fatima compares her answers to the an-
swers on the iPad and makes corrections. Then Fatima follows
the programmed story-based lesson. Her teacher developed
a story-based lesson template which is easy to fill in for each
new passage and also includes comprehension questions. Savvy
teacher that she is, her teacher also realized it could be a good
passage summary activity for other students, so students who
read the same passage at grade level can choose as their final
project for each text to create an adapted text activity by filling
in the pre-developed template. It is great for the students to
learn how to tell the story in their own words, and it saves the
teacher time. Fatima benefits from this because she gets to listen
to her same-age peer voices as she listens to the text and follows
along with the text highlighted on the screen as the words are
read. Then she answers the comprehension questions provided
to her via technology with a system-of-least prompts and is
happy because she always eventually gets every question cor-
rect (Table 9.2).

Science

To address the need for improved outcomes for all students, the Committee on a Conceptual Framework for New K-12 Science Education Standards formulated a guide for teaching science to school-aged students. This framework includes the skills and processes students need to develop an appreciation for science, gain employment skills based on scientific principles, acquire knowledge of scientific content, and hone the life-long skill of thinking critically about scientific information (NGSS Lead States, 2013). Collectively, the practices, concepts, and core ideas of this framework form the basis for the Next Generation Science Standards (NGSS), a set of performance standards intended to promote deep understanding and application of science.

Overall, only a small amount of research has been done on teaching science to students with developmental disabilities. Within this body of research, an even smaller amount has focused on outcomes for students with ASD. Even so, the findings and implications within this emerging body of research suggest students with ASD can learn core vocabulary and concepts, comprehension, science practices (e.g., asking questions, interpreting data), and an inquiry-based process for scientific understanding. The overall implication is the potential to pique interest in scientific content, increase the capacity of students to communicate about scientific phenomena, and teach students problem solving skills that could possibly promote independence and quality of life outcomes. The

Table 9.2 Summary of Recommended Practices for Teaching Reading to Students with ASD

Practices for Teaching	Description and Examples
Embed instruction in phonological awareness, including phonemic awareness, by teaching students to identify initial sounds, clapping syllables, and sounding out words during daily activities	When a student is engaged in a preferred activity or with a preferred object, label the preferred object and indicate the initial sound, prompt the student to say the sound, do the same with clapping out the syllables, and sounding out the words. For example if a student is putting together a puzzle. Initial sounds practice: [Teacher gains students' attention and says] "I see you are playing with the puzzle. Puzzle starts with the "p" sound. Say it with me [Teacher pauses and signals for the student to respond with them] "p" . If the student is unable to vocalize, the teacher may use a preprogrammed button (e.g. BIGmack or SoundingBoard iPad app [free]) and prompt the student to say the sound by pressing the button.
Use time-delay to teach sight word vocabulary and/or vocabulary definitions	Systematically teach sight words at the students reading level. Work through established lists like Dolch words or Fry words, teaching words in groups of 3-5 at a time. Once students have mastered words, plan to promote skill mastery over time by reviewing learned words periodically. Before students learn to decode, all words are sight words. Once students learn to decode, they should only be memorizing irregular words that cannot be sounded out phonetically. Pick words that allow you to write connected text composed of the letter sounds and sight words students have learned. For instance, if you teach the sounds /s/ /a/ and /m/ and teach the sight words "is," "a," and "boy," students can learn to independently read the sentence "Sam is a boy." For academic language, teach the words and definitions for key grade appropriate vocabulary that will support comprehension of books students read or listen to read aloud.
Use naturalist instruction to teach phonemic awareness and letter-sound correspondence and sight word instruction	Plan times to purposely embed naturalistic instruction in reading, and elicit others to do this as well (e.g., paraprofessionals, peers, families). In addition to increasing the amount of opportunities to practice, which leads to fluency of skills, students are learning to generalize reading skills across environments, people, and materials.
Select reading programs that use explicit instruction in reading, and ensure it matches the student's response mode	If your student does not use vocal speech to respond expressively, ensure students can fully participate in the reading curriculum you select. All students need to be able to blend and segment letter sounds and hear the output as they practice mastering these skills. Technology can support students with complex communication needs by voicing letter sounds for them.

Table 9.2 Cont.

Practices for Teaching	Description and Examples
Provide explicit story-based instruction	Story-based reading can include dialogic reading and task analyzed read alouds with systematic prompting. Read alouds can be done with original grade level texts or adapted grade-level texts, and the format can be paper-based or on an iPad.
Support comprehension by using a system of least prompts to answer WH questions either in the book or in their head	Consider preaching the meaning of WH words (e.g., "who tells about people"). Remember to develop an instructional task analysis that differentiates between the type of question (literal or inferential) and either includes prompts and a model for finding the answer in the book (for literal questions) or uses think aloud modeling to show students how to construct the answer in their head. Consider also teaching students to ask their own questions, which is another strategy for promoting comprehension.
Use graphic organizers to help students organize and understand story grammar	Use systematic prompting like a system of least prompts to teach students to complete a graphic organizer; be sure to teach students how to use the information in their graphic organizers, either as reference for a writing project or to help answer comprehension questions about the text.
Consider using tech-based tools to teach literacy	Use apps like GoTalk NOW to embed instructional formats, like time delay procedures to teach vocabulary or a system of least prompts to support comprehension. Graphic organizers built in apps like SMART Notebook allow students to listen to audio definitions of key words and use voice dictation features to complete the graphic organizer.

body of research on science for students with ASD is embedded primarily in research for students with severe disabilities, or students with moderate to severe ID. For this reason, the majority of research reviewed in this section includes science practices that were developed for students who access AA-AAS.

Research on science content practices for students with ASD continues to evolve. Spooner et al. (2011) conducted a review of literature in which science skills were taught to students with severe disabilities (including students with ASD). The findings from this review indicated this population of students was most typically taught science content or skills related to recall of science vocabulary terms, cooking, or health and safety. Since the Spooner et al. review, research on science education for students with ASD has expanded to include more academic and grade-aligned content (e.g., understanding chemical reactions) *and* scientific practices (e.g., asking questions). Knight et al. (2020) reviewed recent research (2009–2018) on teaching science and identified 15 studies that were deemed methodologically sound. Knight et al. examined both the content and intervention practices and identified an encouraging shift in the focus of student outcomes. Instead of teaching skills that were primarily focused on daily living, recent research includes teaching not only grade-level science standards but scientific practices as well. Specifically, scientific practices included asking questions; developing or using models; planning and carrying out investigations; reporting, analyzing, or interpreting data; and using mathematical computational thinking.

Knight et al. identified several instructional practices (i.e., techniques used to teach content) for teaching both science content and science practices to students with ASD. They identified *multiple exemplar training, task analytic instruction*, and *time delay* as evidence-based practices for teaching both scientific content and practices. Potentially evidence-based practices (i.e., practices supported by two to four studies with positive effects and no studies with neutral, mixed, or negative effects) included *example/nonexample training, model-lead-test procedures*, and the use of *graphic organizers*.

Common elements across the research on teaching science to students with ASD includes an emphasis on scientific literacy (building knowledge of science terms and comprehension of science text) and guided inquiry (systematic and explicit instruction in how to apply science knowledge to answer questions or explore phenomena about the natural world). First, there are several examples from recent research for teaching science vocabulary and core concepts to students with ASD. Teaching science vocabulary, including scientific academic language (e.g., cause, effect), scientific descriptors (e.g., cold, hot), and scientific concepts (e.g., force, velocity) can be used to support comprehension of scientific content, including that presented through texts, video examples, and dialogue during in-class experiments and demonstrations. Equipping students with ASD with the vocabulary necessary to receptively understand the content and expressively communicate ideas related to the content is an important prerequisite to engaging in scientific activities and experiences. The following section includes specific descriptions and examples of research-based instruction for teaching both science content and practices to students with ASD.

Multiple Exemplar Training

Scientific content consists of many scientific concepts, which are often complex, with varying critical features or characteristics. Using multiple exemplars or pictorial representations of concepts during instruction allows teachers to emphasize and promote the generalization of the critical features of the core concepts (Cooper et al., 2007). For example, the concept of "habitat" involves several critical features that must be present but can also vary in many ways. When teaching an understanding of the vocabulary word "habitat" or when reading a science text about habitats with embedded picture symbols of core vocabulary, teachers should vary the visual stimuli used to represent the concepts. For "habitat," teachers might have multiple pictorial examples to show that all habitats have a climate, certain geographical features, and specific plant and animal species present, but the range of these features is broad. Teaching habitat using images of different species in different geographic regions helps students generalize the concepts and understand the critical features of the definition. Using multiple exemplars in teaching science is particularly effective for students with ASD who may be likely to memorize photos of images instead of comprehending the characteristics that are necessary for the depiction of a particular concept (Knight et al., 2013). By teaching concepts in this way, teachers promote the likelihood that students will generalize knowledge concepts in order to identify novel examples across contexts (e.g., see an untrained picture of an arctic habitat and label it as a "habitat").

Task Analytic Instruction

In addition to conceptual knowledge of science, students need to learn procedural knowledge related to scientific practices and processes. For example, asking a question is a multistep process that may include several discrete steps, like 1. Think about the material you see, 2. Decide if there is something you don't understand or would like to know more about, 3. Choose a question word to ask about your topic (see Wood et al., 2015). In other cases, carrying out an experiment can include following a series of steps (e.g., building a balloon rocket and measuring the time the balloon travels across the string). Whether students are learning how to do a scientific practice or combine practices to engage in a process (e.g., an experiment or demonstration), receiving discrete instruction in a chained series of steps is an evidence-based practice for promoting learning. Students benefit when task analyses are provided in student-friendly language (e.g., matching their reading level and or containing picture symbols for core words or to illustrate each step). Students can use task analyses as a checklist to perform practices or processes as independently as possible, especially after the steps have been explicitly modeled to the student in a step-by-step format. Teachers can use explicit instruction (like model-lead-test procedures) to initially teach a chained task and then embed response-promoting strategies, like time delay, as needed. Finally, teachers can use task analytic instruction to teach guided inquiry to students with ASD. Recommendations from Courtade, et al.

(2010) include using task analytic instruction across four phases of the guided inquiry process: (a) promote engagement, (b) investigate and describe relationships, (c) construct explanation, and (d) report.

Time Delay

Response prompting strategies like time delay are versatile in that this type of instruction can be used to teach both conceptual and procedural knowledge. Time delay is a technique in which a discrete skill or step is first modeled to the student several times. Students repeat the model during this teaching round so that they can practice performing the target behavior correctly. Next, students are given opportunities to perform the behavior independently. If students cannot perform the behavior independently and correctly within a short amount of time (usually 4 to 5 s), the instructor provides a prompt that will ensure the student can perform the behavior (e.g, a model prompt). Time delay is an efficient way to teach initial vocabulary identification. For example, before a student is ready to learn the conceptual understanding of a word, students need to be able to identify the target word. Teachers can use time delay procedures to teach recognition of words (e.g., show me the word "habitat") or to memorize the definitions of words (e.g., Show me the word that means "the natural home of an animal or plant"). Time delay procedures are also useful when teaching the discrete steps of a chained behavior. For example, when learning how to collect data, teachers can use time delay procedures to teach and then test knowledge of each step of a task analysis for how to collect data.

Potentially Evidence-based Practices

Additional research-based strategies include example/non-example instruction, model-lead-test procedures, and the use of graphic organizers. Similar to multiple exemplar training, example/non-example instruction is a specific training procedure that combines multiple representations of a target concept with non-examples of the same concept to further illustrate the boundaries of a concept. For example, to demonstrate the concept of the "core" of something, like the core of the Earth, teachers can present examples of the center or central part of different objects (core of the Earth, core of an apple, core of the human body). To illustrate that the critical feature is not the type of object but rather the central location, non-examples could include the crust of the Earth and human extremities. Teachers can use explicit instruction, like model-lead-test procedures, to teach students to label visual stimuli as either examples or non-examples (see Knight et al., 2012). Model-lead-test procedures can also be used to teach procedural knowledge, like carrying out the steps to an experiment or investigation, or scientific practices, like how to build a model or interpret data. Finally, graphic organizers can be used to support conceptual or procedural knowledge. Teachers can display multiple exemplars using a concept map. Or teachers can use model-lead-test procedures to guide students to complete a KWHL chart. This type of graphic organizer helps students both organize information and follow specific steps to an investigation by prompting them to consider what they already (K) *know* about a topic, (W) consider what they *want* to know, (H) determining *how* they will figure it out, and finally (L) reviewing what they *learned* (e.g., Jimenez et al., 2014).

Fatima's special education teacher collaborates with the general education teacher to adapt and modify 7th grade science content for Fatima. Fatima shows a high level of engagement in the class when she can touch or manipulate materials (e.g., construct a model roller coaster to demonstrate potential and kinetic energy). She has received very little science education in the past and has limited background knowledge related to science content. Her teachers review grade-aligned state science standards, which in the state of New York are based on the Next Generation Science Standards.

When preparing for an upcoming unit on energy, her teachers notice that the vocabulary words "heat," "thermal energy," "temperature," and "transfer" are central concepts across the related grade level standards. The teachers will build literacy-based supports to ensure this content is accessible to Fatima, but they first think ahead and develop an idea for a hands-on investigation that will allow all students to engage in science practices and cross-cutting concepts. In their review of the New York State Science Middle School Learning Standards, the teachers see that "planning and carrying out investigations" is a science practice associated with the disciplinary core ideas related to energy. They also notice that "compare and contrast" is a relevant cross cutting concept. Together, the teachers plan an accessible activity that will integrate content knowledge (core ideas about energy), opportunities to plan and carry out an investigation, and continued practice with comparing and contrasting. This activity will include task analytic instruction in how to plan and carry out an investigation about thermal energy. Teachers will model using the task analysis to ask a question and find the answer. The teachers will include the concept of cause and effect relationships by modeling how to ask and answer cause and effect questions about thermal energy, temperature, and altering variables, such as different surface materials. Over iterations of the investigation, teachers will gradually release responsibility to their students, who will make their own decisions about how to manipulate variables, collect data, and identify answers to their questions. Fatima may require additional explicit prompting, but the student-friendly task analysis with picture supports will allow her to participate with a high level of independence.

To ensure Fatima learns the vocabulary and concepts needed to engage in the investigation, Fatima's special education teacher develops companion materials to augment the general education science textbook, such as multiple versions of vocabulary cards with pictures and student-friendly definitions to support generalization. Finally, her teacher programs the words into her communication app in both English and Spanish. Her teacher will use English and Spanish when using time delay, and if Fatima responds with vocal speech, she can answer in whichever language she prefers. Finally, her teacher reviews the content from the 7th grade textbook and writes a chapter summary using supportive text (e.g., 1st to 2nd grade readability level, embedded picture symbols). She writes 4-5 comprehension questions with response options to check for understanding.

As they are team-teaching, the teachers show images and video clips to the whole group to pique students' interest and introduce the topic of thermal energy. Next, students work in small groups to preview the text and teach each other core vocabulary words. Fatima's teacher works with her group and embeds 1:1 constant time delay instruction and example/ nonexample training for Fatima while the other students are completing related vocabulary building activities. Students read the science text on their own and turn and talk to peers about what they've learned. During this time, Fatima's teacher works 1:1 with her to read the adapted companion text and check for understanding with comprehension questions. As a whole group, the class is led through another brainstorming session to produce inquiry-worthy questions. Fatima works with a small group of peers to investigate thermal energy and ask questions of her own. Fatima's special education teacher checks for understanding by asking Fatima to identify what she learned from an array of four response options. Her findings are programmed into her communication app and she is able to share what she learned with the whole group (Table 9.3).

Table 9.3 Summary of Recommended Practices for Teaching Science to Students with ASD

Practices for Teaching	Description and Examples
Develop literacy-based science materials and instruction	Scan grade level standards for key words and concepts from grade level standards (e.g., precipitation, convection) and write student friendly definitions for these words. Preteach vocabulary identification and student-friendly definitions. Next, select one or two core concepts to teach explicitly. Select multiple images to represent each key word or concept as well as nonexamples. Create an adapted text or create a grade level text companion that deepens understanding by embedding science vocabulary words and concepts in the text. Check for understanding by asking comprehension questions about the target concepts.
Apply conceptual understanding by asking questions or solving problems about the natural world using task analytic instruction	Develop instructional formats and materials for explicitly teaching students how to engage in science and engineering practices. For example, develop a list of procedures for each practice, like how to ask a question. Include internal thoughts, such as "Pick something you are *most* interested in." Write these procedural lists using student friendly language (at about a 1st to 2nd grade readability level) and consider adding picture support to illustrate each step or picture symbols over key words. Use chaining procedures to model each step of the task analysis and have students repeat the model.
Use constant time delay procedures to teach vocabulary identification and definitions	Develop materials, like vocabulary word cards with words and images and student friendly definitions. First, teach students to identify words (e.g., "Show me the word ___." or when shown a word card, "What word?"). Next, teach students to define words or match words to the definition. For each skill, start with a 0-s delay teaching round in which the teacher models the response immediately. After several trials, switch to a 4-s delay testing round in which students have a brief opportunity to respond independently. Provide a controlling prompt (e.g., model prompt) if the student cannot respond correctly within 4 s.
Use multiple exemplar training to teach understanding of core concepts	Use multiple representations of all vocabulary words by varying the pictures that are used across materials. For example, when teaching vocabulary identification and definitions using time delay, use several versions of each vocabulary card. When teaching a deeper conceptual understanding of core concepts, select multiple representations of the word and carefully explain why all of the pictures represent the same concept, even though some characteristics vary. If needed, create non-examples to help build understanding of what characteristics are critical and what are extraneous.

(continued)

Table 9.3 Cont.

Practices for Teaching	Description and Examples
Use explicit model-lead-test procedures and graphic organizers to promote both conceptual and procedural understanding	Use graphic organizers like KWHL charts and use think-aloud modeling to show how you complete each step. For example, teacher's could say, "What do I already <u>know</u> about this topic? Hmm. I remember learning about something similar last year. And I remember reading about this with my family a while ago too. I'll write down what I can remember about it..."

Putting It All Together

Academic instruction for students with ASD needs to prepare them for positive adult outcomes. Our society continues to progress and provide meaningful and inclusive opportunities for employment, leisure, and living. Since the publication of the prior edition of this text there is increased awareness of systemic ableism and the impact of intersectional identities on the lived experiences of individuals with ASD. The neurodiversity movement that recognizes neurologically based conditions such as ASD as a variation of the human condition (instead of something to be cured) solidifies the importance of using identity-affirming and strengths-based approaches to instruction that have been in line with our values for decades.

Asset-based pedagogies such as Universal Design for Learning (UDL) and Culturally Sustaining Pedagogy (CSP) align with the values we hold in special education as they draw on the strengths of individuals rather than focusing on skill deficits as the fault of an individual. UDL aims to reduce barriers to learning by proactively centering learner variability in the design of curriculum, assessment, and learning environments (Rose & Meyer, 2002). A distinction is made between the desired learning outcome and the means by which learners can achieve those outcomes so that there are flexible options for access that meet the needs and preferences of all learners (Smith, 2012). Out of a desire to provide practitioners with a way to meaningfully value and maintain the current practices of students while extending their repertoires, Paris (2012) defined CSP as instruction that "seeks to perpetuate and foster linguistic, literate, and cultural pluralism as part of the democratic project of schooling" (p. 95). Waitoller and King Thorius (2016) argued that UDL and CSP benefit from "cross-pollination" to support intersectional identities of students with disabilities. That is, educators should recognize the multiple intersectional identities that influence the lived experience of students with ASD – for example how their gender, race, religion, geographic location, family structure, native language, and communication modality can be an asset to draw on but also not a barrier within the classroom.

These instructional frameworks do not replace the use of evidence-based practices or specific interventions for learners with ASD, but rather are intended to increase inclusion and sense of belonging, which may in turn increase effectiveness of instruction and interventions (Shmulsky et al., 2021). Educators can use a critical disability viewpoint to combine understanding of ASD from a medical perspective (i.e., communication, social, behavioral, and sensory aspects of disorder) and social perspective (e.g., degree to which environment is universally designed, impact of systemic ableism). This nuanced viewpoint can positively impact the academic instruction provided to students with ASD. Culturally-focused educators can adopt a social-justice lens in each aspect of instruction by recognizing biases that create disadvantages and making these connections explicit for learners with ASD (Harkins Monaco et al., 2022). Paired with this social-justice focus, should be a focus on self-determination and self-advocacy in order to provide students with ASD the social skills needed to continue recognizing and advocating for change in future environments.

References

Agrawal, J., & Morin, L. L. (2016). Evidence-based practices: Applications of concrete representational abstract framework across math concepts for students with mathematics disabilities. *Learning Disabilities Research & Practice*, 31 (1), 34–44.

Ahlgrim-Delzell, L., Wood, L., & Browder, D. M. (2015). *Early Reading Skills Builder*. Verona, WI: Attainment Company.

Alison, C., Root, J. R., Browder, D. M., & Wood, L. (2017). Technology-based shared story reading for students with autism who are English-language learners. *Journal of Special Education Technology*, 32 (2), 91–101. http://dx.doi.org/10.1177/0162643417690606

Bailey, B., & Arciuli, J. (2019). Reading instruction for children with autism spectrum disorders: A systematic review and quality analysis. *Review Journal of Autism and Developmental Disorders*. Advance online publication. https://doi.org/fp49

Baron-Cohen, S., Leslie, A. M., & Frith, U. (1985). Does the autistic child have a "theory of mind"? *Cognition*, 21, 37–46.

Benedek-Wood, E., McNaughton, D., & Light, J. (2016). Instruction in letter-sound correspondences for children with autism and limited speech. *Topics in Early Childhood Special Education*, 36 (1), 43–54. http://dx.doi.org/10.1177/0271121415593497

Berch, D. B., & Mazzocco, M. M. (2007). *Why is math so hard for some children? The nature and origins of mathematical learning difficulties and disabilities*. Paul H. Brookes Publishing Co.

Bethune, K. S., & Wood, C. L. (2013). Effects of wh-question graphic organizers on reading comprehension skills of students with autism spectrum disorders. *Education and Training in Autism and Developmental Disabilities*, 48 (2), 236–244. http://dx.doi.org/doi:10.1177/0271121415593497

Blair, C., & Razza, R. P. (2007). Relating effortful control, executive function, and false belief understanding to emerging math and literacy ability in kindergarten. *Child Development*, 78(2), 647–663. https://doi.org/10.1111/j.1467-8624.2007.01019.x

Bouck, E. C., & Joshi, G. S. (2015). Does curriculum matter for secondary students with autism spectrum disorders: Analyzing the NLTS2. *Journal of Autism and Developmental Disorders*, 45, 1204–1212.

Bouck, E. C., & Long, H. (2020). Manipulatives and manipulative based instructional sequences, In Bouck, E., Root., J., & Jimenez (Ed.), *Mathematics education and students with autism, intellectual disability, and other developmental disabilities* (pp. 138–171). Published (DADD)

Boyle, S. A., McNaughton, D., & Chapin, S. E. (2019). Effects of shared reading on the early language and literacy skills of children with autism spectrum disorders: A systematic review. Focus on Autism and Other Developmental Disabilities, 34 (4), 205–214. https://doi.org/fp5b

Browder, D. (2001). Curriculum and assessment for students with moderate and severe disabilities. New York: Guilford Press.

Browder, D. M., Gibbs, S., Ahlgrim-Delzell, L., Courtade, G., & Lee, A. (2007). Early Literacy Skills Builder (ELSB). Verona, WI: Attainment Company.

Browder, D.M., Spooner, F., & Meyer, C. (2011) Comprehension across the curriculum. In Browder, D. M. & Spooner, F. *Teaching students with moderate and severe disabilities* (pp. 141–167). Guilford Publications.

Browder, D. M., Hudson, M. E., & Wood, A. L. (2013). Teaching students with moderate intellectual disability who are emergent readers to comprehend passages of text. *Exceptionality*, 21(4), 191–206.

Browder, D. M., Wood, L., Thompson, J., & Ribuffo, C. (2014). Evidence-based practices for students with severe disabilities. *Ceedar Document NO. IC-3. Ceedar Center*.

Browder, D. M., Root, J. R., Wood, L., & Allison, C. (2015). Effects of a story-mapping procedure using the ipad on the comprehension of narrative texts by students with autism spectrum disorder. Focus on Autism and Other Developmental Disabilities, 1–13. http://dx.doi.org/doi:10.1177/1088357615611387

Browder, D. M., Spooner, F., Lo, Y. Y., Saunders, A. F., Root, J. R., Ley Davis, L., & Brosh, C. R. (2018). Teaching students with moderate intellectual disability to solve word problems. *The Journal of Special Education*, 51(4), 222–235.

Bull, R., & Scerif, G. (2001). Executive functioning as a predictor of children's mathematics ability: Inhibition, switching, and working memory. *Developmental Neuropsychology*, 19 (3), 273–293.

Bullen, J. C., Zajic, M. C., McIntyre, N., & Solari, E. (2022). Patterns of math and reading achievement in children and adolescents with autism spectrum disorder. *Research in Autism Spectrum Disorders*, 92(2022). Advanced online publication. https://doi.org/10.1016/j.rasd.2022.101933

Charman, T., Jones, C. R., Pickles, A., Simonoff, E., Baird, G., & Happé, F. (2011). Defining the cognitive phenotype of autism. *Brain Research*, 1380, 10–21. doi:10.1016/j. brainres.2010.10.075

Charman, T., Pickles, A., Simonoff, E., Chandler, S., Loucas, T., & Baird, G. (2011). IQ in children with autism spectrum disorders: Data from the Special

Needs and Autism Project (SNAP). *Psychological Medicine*, 41, 619–627. http://dx.doi.org/10.1017/S0033291710000991

Christenson, D. L., Braun, K. V. N., Baio, J., Bilder, D., Charles, J., Constantino, J. N., Daniels, J., Durkin, M. S., Fitzgerald, R. T., Kurzius-Spencer, M., Lee, L., Pettygrove, S., Robinson, C., Schulz, E., Wells, C., Wingate, M. S., Zahorodny, W., & Yeargin-Allsopp, M. (2018). Prevalence and characteristics of autism spectrum disorder among children aged 8 years. *Morbidity and Mortality Weekly Report: Surveillance Summaries*, 65(3), 1–23. https://doi.org/10.15585/mmwr.ss6503a1

Cook, B. G., Buysse, V., Klingner, J., Landrum, T. J., McWilliam, R. A., Tankersley, M., & Test, D. W. (2015). CEC's standards for classifying the evidence base of practices in special education. *Remedial and Special Education*, 36, 220–234. http://doi.org/10.1177/0741932514557271

Cooper, J. O., Heron, T. E., & Heward, W. L. (2007). Applied behavior analysis. Pearson.

Courtade, G., Browder, D. M., Spooner, F., & DiBiase, W. (2010). Training teachers to use an inquiry-based task analysis to teach science to students with moderate and severe disabilities. *Education and Training in Developmental Disabilities*, 45, 378–399.

Davidson, M. M. (2021). Reading comprehension in school-age children with autism spectrum disorder: Examining the many components that may contribute. *Language, Speech, and Hearing Services in Schools*, 52(1), 181–196.

Evans, B. (2013). How autism became autism: The radical transformation of a central concept of child development in Britain. *History of the Human Sciences*, 26 (3), 3–31. https://doi.org/10.1177/0952695113484320

Fleury, V. P., & Schwartz, I. S. (2017). A modified dialogic reading intervention for preschool children with autism spectrum disorder. *Topics in Early Childhood Special Education*, 37(1), 16–28.

Fleury, V. P., Root, J. R., Whalon, K., Stover, E., & Williams, A. (In press). Evidence based practices to teach academic skills. In L. C. Chezan, K. Wolfe, & E. Drasgow's (Eds.) *Guide to Evidence-Based Practices for Practitioners Working with Individuals with Autism Spectrum Disorder*. Rowman & Littlefield.

Fuchs, L. S., Fuchs, D., Compton, D. L., Hamlett, C. L., & Wang, A. Y. (2015). Is word-problem solving a form of text comprehension?. *Scientific Studies of Reading*, 19(3), 204–223.

Fuchs, L. S., Seethaler, P. M., Sterba, S. K., Craddock, C., Fuchs, D., Compton, D. L., ... Changas, P. (2019). Word-problem intervention with and without embedded language comprehension instruction: Causal evidence on language comprehension's contribution to word-problem solving. Manuscript submitted for publication.

Fuchs, L. S., N. Bucka, B. Clarke, B. Dougherty, N. C. Jordan, K. S. Karp, J. Woodward et al. (2021) "Assisting Students Struggling with Mathematics: Intervention in the Elementary Grades. Educator's Practice Guide. WWC 2021006." *What Works Clearinghouse.*

Gough, P. B., & Tunmer, W. E. (1986). Decoding, reading, and reading disability. *Remedial and special education*, 7(1), 6–10.

Hansen, B. D., Wadsworth, J. P., Roberts, M. R., & Poole T. N. (2014). Effects of naturalistic instruction on phonological awareness skills of children with intellectual and developmental disabilities. *Research in Developmental Disabilities*, 35, 2790–2801. http://dx.doi.org/10.1016/j.ridd.2014.07.011

Happe, F., & Frith, U. (2006). The weak coherence account: detail-focused cognitive style in autism spectrum disorders. *Journal of Autism and Developmental Disorders*, 36, 5–25. doi: 10.1007/s20803-005-0039-0

Harkins Monaco, E. A., Brusnahan, L. S., & Fuller, M. (2022). Guidance for the Antiracist Educator: Culturally Sustaining Pedagogies for Disability and Diversity. *TEACHING Exceptional Children*, Advance online publication. https://doi.org/ 00400599211046281

Hart Barnett, J. E., & Cleary, S. (2015). Review of evidence-based mathematics interventions for students with autism spectrum disorders. *Education and Training in Autism and Developmental Disabilities*, 50, 172–185.

Heward, W. L. (2003). Ten faulty notions about teaching and learning that hinder the effectiveness of special education. *The Journal of Special Education*, 36(4), 186–205.

Hojnoski, R. L., Caskie, G. I., & Miller Young, R. (2018). Early numeracy trajectories: Baseline performance levels and growth rates in young children by disability status. *Topics in Early Childhood Special Education*, 37(4), 206–218.

Hoover, W. A., & Gough, P. B. (1990). The simple view of reading. *Reading and Writing*, 2, 127–160.

Hudson, M. E., Browder, D. M., & Jimenez, B. A. (2014). Effects of a peer-delivered system of least prompts intervention and adapted science read-alouds on listening comprehension for participants with moderate intellectual disability. *Education and Training in Autism and Developmental Disabilities*, 60–77.

Hughes, E. M., Powell, S. R., & Stevens, E. A. (2016). Supporting clear and concise mathematics language: Instead of that, say this. *Teaching Exceptional Children*, 49(1), 7–17.

Jimenez, B. A., Lo, Y., & Saunders, A. F. (2014). The additive effects of scripted lessons plus guided notes on science quiz scores of students with intellectual disability and autism. *The Journal of Special Education*, 47, 231–244.

Jimenez, B., & Saunders, A. (2019). Increasing efficiency in mathematics: teaching subitizing to students with moderate intellectual disability. *Journal of Developmental and Physical Disabilities*, 31(1), 23–37.

Jitendra, A. K., & Star, J. R. (2011). Meeting the needs of students with learning disabilities in inclusive mathematics classrooms: The role of schema-based instruction on mathematical problem-solving. *Theory into Practice*, 50 (1), 12–19.

Jitendra, A. K., Nelson, G., Pulles, S. M., Kiss, A. J., & Houseworth, J. (2016). Is mathematical representation of problems an evidence-based strategy for students with mathematics difficulties? *Exceptional Children*, 83, 412–438. https://doi.org/10.1177/002246699703000404

Jones, C. R., Happé, F., Golden, H., Marsden, A. J., Tregay, J., Simonoff, E., ... & Charman, T. (2009). Reading and arithmetic in adolescents with autism spectrum disorders: Peaks and dips in attainment. *Neuropsychology*, 23(6), 718.

Jordan, N. C., Kaplan, D., Olah, L. N., & Locuniak, M. N. (2006). Number sense growth in kindergarten: A longitudinal investigation of children at risk for mathematics difficulties. *Child Development, 77,* 153–175.

Jordan, N. C., Kaplan, D., Ramineni, C., & Locuniak, M. N. (2009). Early math matters: kindergarten number competence and later mathematics outcomes. *Developmental Psychology, 45*(3), 850.

Kamps, D. M., Mason, R., & Heitzman-Powell, L. (2017). Peer mediation interventions to improve social and communication skills for children and youth with autism spectrum disorders. In *Handbook of social skills and autism spectrum disorder* (pp. 257–283). Springer, Cham.

Knight, V. F., Smith, B. R., Spooner, F., & Browder, D. M. (2012). Using explicit instruction to teach science descriptors to students with autism spectrum disorders. *Journal of Autism and Developmental Disorders, 42,* 378–389.

Knight, V., Spooner, F., Browder, D. M., Smith, B. R., & Wood, C. L. (2013). Using systematic instruction and graphic organizers to teach science to students with autism spectrum disorders and intellectual disability. *Focus on Autism and Other Developmental Disabilities, 28,* 115–126.

Knight, V. F., Wood, L., McKissick, B. R., & Kuntz, E. M. (2020). Teaching Science Content and Practices to Students with Intellectual Disability and Autism. *Remedial and Special Education, 41*(6), 327–340.

Krawec, J., Huang, J., Montague, M., Kressler, B., & Melia de Alba, A. (2013). The effects of cognitive strategy instruction on knowledge of math problem-solving processes of middle school students with learning disabilities. *Learning Disability Quarterly, 36*(2), 80–92.

Mayer, R. E. (1985). Implications of cognitive psychology for instruction in mathematical problem solving. *Teaching and learning mathematical problem solving: Multiple research perspectives,* 123–138.

Mazzotti, V. L., Rowe, D. A., Sinclair, J., Poppen, M., Woods, W. E., & Shearer, M. L. (2016). Predictors of post-school success: A systematic review of NLTS2 secondary analyses. *Career Development and Transition for Exceptional Individuals, 39,* 195–215.

McGee, R., Williams, S., Share, D. L., Anderson, J., & Silva, P. A. (1986). The relationship between specific reading retardation, general reading backwardness and behavioural problems in a large sample of Dunedin boys: A longitudinal study from five to eleven years. *Journal of Child Psychology and Psychiatry, 27*(5), 597–610.

McIntyre, N. S., Solari, E. J., Grimm, R. P., Lerro, L. E., Gonzales, J. E., & Mundy, P. C. (2017). A comprehensive examination of reading heterogeneity in students with high functioning autism: Distinct reading profiles and their relation to autism symptom severity. *Journal of Autism and Developmental Disorders, 47,* 1086–1101. https://doi.org/10.1007/s10803-017-3029-0

Migliore, A., Timmons, J., Butterworth, J., & Lugas, J. (2012). Predictors of employment and postsecondary education of youth with autism. *Rehabilitation Counseling Bulletin, 55,* 176–184.

Mims, P. J., Hudson, M. E., & Brower, D. M. (2012). Using read-alouds of grade-level biographies and systematic prompting to promote comprehension for students with moderate and severe developmental disabilities. Focus on

Autism and Other Developmental Disabilities, 27(2), 67–80. http://dx.doi.org/10.1177/1088357612446859

Montague, M. (1997). Cognitive strategy instruction in mathematics for students with learning disabilities. *Journal of Learning Disabilities*, 30, 164–177.

Mundy, P., Sigman, M., & Kasari, C. (1990). A longitudinal study of joint attention and language development in autistic children. *Journal of Autism and Developmental Disorders*, 20, 115–128.

Nasamran, A., Witmer, S. E., & Los, J. E. (2017). Exploring predictors of postsecondary outcomes for students with autism spectrum disorder. *Education and Training in Autism and Developmental Disabilities*, 52(4), 343–356.

National Center for Education Statistics (2020). https://nces.ed.gov

National Council of Teachers of Mathematics. (2000). Principles and standards for school mathematics. Reston, VA: NCTM.

NGSS Lead States. (2013). *Next Generation Science Standards: For states, by states*. Washington, DC: The National Academies Press.

Odom, S., Thompson, J. L., Boyd, B., Dykstra, J., Duda, M., Hedges, S., Szidon, K., Smith, L., Bord, A. (2015). Technology-aided interventions and instruction for adolescents with autism spectrum disorder. *Journal of Autism and Developmental Disorders*, 45, 3805–3819. https://doi.org/f72h2x

Oswald, T. M., Beck, J. S., Iosif, A. M., McCauley, J. B., Gilhooly, L. J., Matter, J. C., & Solomon, M. (2016). Clinical and cognitive characteristics associated with mathematics problem solving in adolescents with autism spectrum disorder. *Autism Research*, 9(4), 480–490

Paris, D. (2012). Culturally sustaining pedagogy: A needed change in stance, terminology, and practice. *Educational Researcher*, 41(3), 93–97.

Petscher, Y., Cabell, S. Q., Catts, H. W., Compton, D. L., Foorman, B. R., Hart, S. A., Lonigan, C. J., Philips, B. M., Schatschenider, C., Stacey L. M., Terry, N. P., & Wagner, R. K. (2020) How the science of reading informs 21st-century education. *Reading Research Quarterly*, 55(1), 267–282. https://doi.org/10.1002/rrq.352 [doi.org]

Powell, S. R., Namkung, J. M., & Lin, X. (in press). An investigation of using keywords to solve word problems. *The Elementary School Journal*.

Reutebuch, C. K., El Zein, F., Kim, M. K., Weinberg, A. N., & Vaughn, S. (2015). Investigating a reading comprehension intervention for high school students with autism spectrum disorder: A pilot study. *Research in Autism Spectrum Disorders*, 9, 96–111.

Root, J. R., Cox, S. K., Hammons, N., Saunders, A. F., & Gilley, D. (2018). Contextualizing mathematics: Teaching problem solving to secondary students with intellectual and developmental disabilities. *Intellectual and Developmental Disabilities*, 56(6), 442–457.

Root, J. R., Cox, S. K., Saunders, A., & Gilley, D. (2020). Applying the universal design for learning framework to mathematics instruction for learners with extensive support needs. *Remedial and Special Education*, 41(4), 194–206.

Root, J. R., Henning, B., & Boccumini, E. (2018). Teaching students with autism and intellectual disability to solve algebraic word problems. *Education and Training in Autism and Developmental Disabilities*, 53(3), 325–338.

Root, J. R., Ingelin, B., & Cox, S. K. (2021). Teaching mathematical word problem solving to students with autism spectrum disorder: A best-evidence synthesis. *Education and Training in Autism and Developmental Disabilities*, 56(4), 420–436.

Root, J., Browder, D. M., & Jimenez, B. (2016). Access to algebra for students with moderate and severe developmental disabilities. *Bridging the gap between arithmetic and algebra*, 171–193.

Root, J., Clausen, A., & Spooner (2020). Teaching Problem Solving Using Modified Schema-Based Instruction, In Bouck, E., Root, J., & Jimenez (Ed.), *Mathematics education and students with autism, intellectual disability, and other developmental disabilities* (pp. 138–171). Published (DADD).

Root, J. R., Stevenson, B. S., Davis, L. L., Geddes-Hall, J., Test, D. W. (2017). Establishing computer assisted instruction to teach academics to students with autism and an evidence-based practice. *Journal of Autism and Developmental Disorders*, 47, 275–284. https://doi.org/f9tq7d

Rose, D. H., & Meyer, A. (2002). *Teaching every student in the digital age: Universal design for learning*. Association for supervision and Curriculum Development.

Saunders, A. (2020). Building early numeracy and problem solving. In Browder, D., Spooner, F., & Courtade, G. (Ed.), *Teaching students with moderate and severe disabilities* (pp. 209–232). New York, NY: Psychology Press.

Saunders, A., Lo, Y., & Polly, D. (2014). Beginning numeracy skills. In B Browder, D. M., & Spooner, F. (Eds.). (2014). *More language arts, math, and science for students with severe disabilities*. Paul H. Brookes Publishing Company.

Schreibman, L., Dawson, G., Stahmer, A. C., Landa, R., Rogers, S. J., McGee, G. G., . . . Halladay, A. (2015). Naturalistic developmental behavioral interventions: Empirically validated treatments for autism spectrum disorder. Journal of Autism and Developmental Disorders, 45, 2411–2428. https://doi.org/gf5mg5

Shmulsky, S., Gobbo, K., & Vitt, S. (2021). Culturally Relevant Pedagogy for Neurodiversity. *Community College Journal of Research and Practice*, 1–5. https://doi.org/10.1080/10668926.2021.1972362

Smith, F. G. (2012). Analyzing a college course that adheres to the Universal Design for Learning (UDL) framework. *Journal of the Scholarship of Teaching and Learning*, 12 (3), 31–61.

Solari, E. J., Grimm, R. P., McIntyre, N. S., Zajic, M., & Mundy, P. C. (2019). Longitudinal stability of reading profiles in individuals with higher functioning autism. *Autism*, 23(8), 1911–1926.

Spooner, F., & Browder, D. M. (2015). Raising the bar significant advances and future needs for promoting learning for students with severe disabilities. *Remedial and Special Education*, 36, 28–32. http://doi.org/10741932514555022

Spooner, F., Root, J. R., Saunders, A. F., & Browder, D. M. (2019). An updated evidence-based practice review on teaching mathematics to students with moderate and severe developmental disabilities. *Remedial and Special Education*, 40(3), 150–165.

Spooner, F., Saunders, A., Root, J., & Brosh, C. (2017). Promoting access to common core mathematics for students with severe disabilities through mathematical problem solving. *Research and Practice for Persons with Severe Disabilities*, 42(3), 171–186.

Spooner, F., Knight, V., Browder, D. M., Jimenez, B., & DiBiase, W. (2011). Evaluating evidence-based practice in teaching science content to students with severe developmental disabilities. *Research and Practice in Severe Disabilities*, 36, 62–75.

Steinbrenner, J. R., Hume, K., Odom, S. L., Morin, K. L., Nowell, S. W., Tomaszewski, B., ... & Savage, M. N. (2020). Evidence-Based Practices for Children, Youth, and Young Adults with Autism. *FPG Child Development Institute*.

Tager-Flusberg, H., & Kasari, C. (2013). Minimally verbal school-aged children with autism spectrum disorder: The neglected end of the spectrum. *Autism Research*, 6, 468–478. http://dx.doi.org/10.1002/aur.1329

Thompson, J., Root, J. R., Ko, E. H., Tarlow, K., Foster, M., Kang, A., & Harrod, H. (2022). *A meta-analysis and evidence-based review of reading interventions for students with autism spectrum disorder*.

Titeca, D., Roeyers, H., Josephy, H., Ceulemans, A., & Desoete, A. (2014). Preschool predictors of mathematics in first grade children with autism spectrum disorder. *Research in Developmental Disabilities*, 35(11), 2714–2727.

Van de Walle, J. A., Karp, K. S., & Bay-Williams, J. M. (2016). *Elementary and middle school mathematics*. Pearson Education UK.

Waitoller, F. R., & King Thorius, K. A. (2016). Cross-pollinating culturally sustaining pedagogy and universal design for learning: Toward an inclusive pedagogy that accounts for dis/ability. *Harvard Educational Review*, 86 (3), 366–389.

Wei, X., Christiano, E. R., Yu, W. J., Wagner, M., & Spiker, D. (2014). Reading and math achievement profiles and longitudinal growth trajectories of children with an autism spectrum disorder. *Autism*, 1–11. doi: 10.1177/1362361313516549

Williamson, P., Carnahan, C. R., Birri, N., & Swoboda, C. (2015). Improving comprehension of narrative using character event maps for high school students with autism spectrum disorder. *The Journal of Special Education*, 49(1), 28–38. http://dx.doi.org/10.1177/0022466914521301

Wong, C., Odom, S. L., Hume, K. A., Cox, A. W., Fettig, A., Kucharczyk, S., ... & Schultz, T. R. (2015). Evidence-based practices for children, youth, and young adults with autism spectrum disorder: A comprehensive review. *Journal of autism and developmental disorders*, 45(7), 1951–1966.

Wong, C., Odom, S. L., Hume, K., Cox, A. W., Fettig, A., Kucharczyk, S...Schultz, T. R. (2014). *Evidence-based practices for children, youth, and young adults with autism spectrum disorder*. Chapel Hill: The University of North Carolina, Frank Potter Graham Child Development Institute, Autism Evidence-Based Practice Review Group.

Wood, L. Browder, D. M., & Spooner, F. (2015). Teaching students with moderate intellectual disability to use a self-questioning strategy and iPad to comprehend science e-text. *Manuscript in preparation*.

Chapter 10

Developing Social Interaction Competence

Cate C. Smith, David F. Cihak, and Michael C. Morrow
Department of Theory and Practice in Teacher Education,
The University of Tennessee, Knoxville

DSM-V: Social Communication

The DSM-5 represents ASD symptoms across two domains (a) social communication differences and (b) restricted, repetitive behaviors. The text of DSM-5 offers more detail on the topography of core characteristics of ASD at different ages including toddlers, school-aged children, and adults. Social communication criteria provide examples of how differences may appear in individuals with limited language or cognitive disability. Examples relevant for different ages are also provided. For example, a possible indicator within the social relationships criterion is an apparent lack of interest in peers. This would be an irrelevant characteristic in toddlers for whom establishing and maintaining friendships are not yet developmentally expected.

While DSM-IV social interaction and communication domains were collapsed and reorganized in DSM-5, individual characteristics are largely retained. Constantino et al.'s (2004) landmark factor analytic study revealed that symptoms representing the DSM-IV clusters, Social Interaction and Communication, were best represented by a single "social communication" factor. Furthermore, stereotyped speech related more to the repetitive behaviors factor rather than social communication. The DSM-5 identifies a smaller number of more general principles in social communication that are expected to be present in all individuals with ASD regardless of age or developmental level, but that can be manifested in many different ways (Mahjouri & Lord, 2012). Additionally, social communication symptoms have been reconfigured as a dimensional continuum of behaviors representing social-emotional reciprocity, coordination of verbal and nonverbal communication, and establishing, maintaining, and understanding social relationships.

The DSM-5 includes modifications to the descriptions of social interaction contained in the DSM-IV. The DSM-5 requires that all social communication criteria have been met, either currently or by history, for a diagnosis of ASD. These changes were made to improve diagnostic specificity.

DOI: 10.4324/9781003255147-12

Levels of support are rated separately for social communication in the DSM-5. Because a diagnosis requires that symptoms impact functioning, even the lowest level of support indicates the presence of noticeable impairments or interference with independent functioning. Three levels of support are available: Level 1, Requiring support; Level 2, Requiring substantial support; and Level 3, Requiring very substantial support. Each level provides descriptions of the extent to which social communication and adaptive behavior differences affect an individual's functioning. The DSM-5 support ratings are designed to provide information on the extent to which ASD impacts daily functioning. The DSM-5 attempts to provide objective information for clinicians to use in choosing a rating. For example, a Level 2 repetitive behavior should appear frequently enough to be noticed by the "casual observer" (APA, 2013, p. 52). Although support ratings are based on current behavior, the DSM-5 recognizes that a child's level of needed support and independence may be fluid over time or vary by context.

Support ratings in the DSM-5 may provide a useful structure for summarizing information from observation and interview measures in evaluation reports, to lead to service and support decisions. For example, social communication support ratings describe a child's ability to interact with peers and teachers in general education settings. A child with low impacts in the area of social communication may do well with coaching and instruction given within inclusive settings, while a child with significant social communication needs may need a service plan that includes assistive/augmentative communication supports.

Social Differences

Both Leo Kanner (1943) and Hans Asperger (1944) described children and youth with ASD as having a marked difference in their abilities to interact socially. For many individuals with ASD, strong preferences for objects and non-social stimuli are in sharp contrast with opportunities to interact with people around them (Gale et al., 2019). By three to five years of age, children with ASD may show preferences for their caregivers over strangers (Sigman et al., 2004), but the way they show these preferences may be unusual and can place added stress on parents and guardians (Keenan et al., 2016). From early childhood, many individuals with ASD are less engaged with others (verbally and nonverbally), make fewer self-initiated requests, focus on preferred topics, and usually remain removed from direct play and social interactions, which ultimately limits opportunities for meaningful social interactions with same-aged peers (Wolfberg et al., 2014). However, each individual with ASD demonstrates unique social needs and skills which make generalizations difficult.

For individuals with ASD, the acquisition of social skills can be quite challenging due to difficulties with interpersonal communication. Ultimately, this can lead to difficulties in interaction skills necessary for success later in life (Whalen et al., 2010). In addition, struggles with flexibility, attention, organization, turn-taking, and generalizing or transferring social skills to novel circumstances, further complicate social and adaptive skill challenges (Lydon et al., 2011; Rieth et al., 2014). Social competency of some individuals with ASD may be further impacted by difficulty expressing and perceiving their own emotions and those of others (Myles & Adreon, 2001). They may in-turn engage in challenging or maladaptive behaviors, as well as restricted and repetitive stereotypical behaviors (Ledford et al., 2021; Losinski et al., 2017). As breakdowns occur in communication that compound internalized struggles with self-regulation, individuals with ASD have fewer opportunities to develop and maintain friendships and they may experience social isolation (Dovgan & Mazurek, 2019). As individuals with ASD engage less with peers, fewer attempts are made by peers to initiate with them, which then provides fewer opportunities for individuals with ASD to interact socially, resulting in more time away from their peers.

Some individuals with ASD do not understand social conventions and expectations of people without ASD. Most people without ASD learn behavioral expectations to demonstrate or to avoid in order to stay out of trouble or "blend in" with the crowd. The "hidden curriculum," or the skills that are generally learned covertly as they are unwritten and unofficially present in the social learning environment, are often lost on individuals with ASD (Sulaimani & Gut, 2019). Most individuals with ASD do not have the ability to access the hidden social curriculum due to their neurological differences. Therefore, individuals with ASD may not have any concept of how people are expected to behave in different contexts and at times may appear to have no behavioral inhibitions. However, many people with ASD may decide not to follow the hidden curriculum "rules" and may choose to embrace their unique qualities and skills. People without ASD should consider that social skill differences may not always be deficits and in fact, people without ASD may need to change their understanding and expectations of what is "acceptable" to include the unique skills found in people with ASD.

Individuals with ASD who have average or above-average IQ may be successful in applying the correct communicative skills in very specific social situations, but those same soft skills are often lost when the context of the situation changes, even if similar responses would be appropriate (Sung et al., 2019). Unfortunately, since many with ASD can repeat social rules, teachers and employers assume they should be able to apply those same skills at any time. Difficulties recognizing emotional states, initiating, maintaining, or even joining existing conversations limit social experiences and may cause misconceptions about others, and in turn, ostracize those with ASD (Huang et al., 2017). It may also be difficult to recognize that telling others how to follow the rules may be perceived as rude or bossy, resulting in unnecessary disciplinary actions and additional peer and adult rejection. Sulaimani & Gut (2019) point to a lack of social interactional opportunities in and out of school, which further exacerbates matters associated with the "hidden curriculum."

Social and communication skill differences, engaging in repetitive or other behaviors considered inappropriate, and difficulties with emotional recognition often lead to increased bullying and a loss of socially meaningful skill building opportunities for children with ASD (Forrest et al., 2020). The perception of or actual experience of being bullied as a result of social differences associated with ASD can lead to individuals developing mental health concerns such as anxiety and depression (Rodriguez et al., 2021). Students who demonstrate social differences may experience fewer opportunities for lasting friendships, limited access to social activities, and less options for employment and recreational activities (Babb et al., 2021). All of this can lead to poor school performance and lower self-esteem in adulthood without additional support (Cooper et al., 2017).

Nonverbal Communication

Developing and understanding nonverbal communication is a common barrier for people with ASD. Nonverbal communication includes a variety of gestures, facial expressions, and body postures that can be difficult to comprehend. Additionally, the difficulty with determining how these unspoken forms of communication work together to convey an implicit meaning may contribute to feelings of frustration.

A lack of understanding facial expressions also leads to poor social communication for those with ASD. Varying intensity levels in the facial expressions conveyed can lead to misunderstandings of the emotions recognized by individuals with ASD. While neutral, low, and medium intensity facial expressions are difficult to interpret, high intensity expressions are easier to recognize (Wingenbach et al., 2017). This lack of understanding also leads to misused or unused facial expressions on the part of the child. Children with ASD may appear to have a flat affect or to be detached from the conversation. If the child is unable to gain information from the faces of those around him, he is unlikely to use his own face to convey information to others. Or, the child may engage in inappropriate facial expressions as he is unsure which expression matches the current situation.

Limited understanding of nonverbal communication can lead to difficulty structuring and maintaining conversations with others. Children with ASD often engage in atypical eye contact (e.g., holding the gaze of others for too long, or not long enough) (Paul et al., 2009). This increased eye contact or lack thereof can be uncomfortable for a communicative partner. This can also be remarkably difficult for the individual with ASD to understand (Trevisan et al., 2017). Children with ASD may also infringe upon the personal space of others without understanding the social ramifications.

Verbal and nonverbal communication skill differences in children with ASD contribute to misunderstandings or missed opportunities to engage with others socially. Rather than avoiding interactions with others on purpose, a child with ASD may be unaware of the attempt to socialize and inadvertently ignore the other child. Additionally, many children with ASD do not understand the use of gestures to indicate meaning and will ignore these attempts to communicate (e.g., pointing, waving). They may also ignore facial expressions such as smiling and miss opportunities to develop relationships with others.

Many children with ASD have a variety of social and language limitations. These include difficulty making inferences and understanding implicit information (Reichow & Volkmar, 2010). Additionally, nonliteral and ambiguous meanings of language can be difficult. These difficulties are referred to as deficits in pragmatic language, which includes linguistic (referential utterances, tone) and non-linguistic components (eye contact, body language, facial expressions), along with cognitive-linguistic components (auditory and visual perception) (Levinson et al., 2020). Understanding abstract concepts that are not presented visually is difficult for those with autism (Reichow & Volkmar, 2010). When teaching and interacting with children who have autism, it is best to limit the use of nonliteral or ambiguous language.

Understanding Relationships

Social impairments also lead to problems engaging in and understanding relationships with others. Developing meaningful relationships is imperative to creating social connectedness and gaining emotional support (Daughrity, 2019). Many people with ASD long to have friendships and share connections with others. However, difficulty processing social information leads to problems in making, keeping, and understanding relationships with others. Relating to others and engaging in relationships requires emotional reciprocity, which is difficult for students with ASD.

Many children with ASD have difficulty engaging in symbolic or "pretend" play. Pretend play involves exploratory uses of toys that involve imaginary characteristics and functions (Campbell et al., 2016). Children engaged in pretend play may gather rocks to make "dinner" or use a banana as a phone. In contrast, a child with ASD may stack building blocks in size order or categorize them by shape and color (i.e., using the toys for their literal purpose). Children with ASD may play with toys in very different ways from their peers without disabilities (e.g., flipping cars over to spin the wheels repeatedly, or lining up toys around the perimeter of the room) (Jung & Sainato, 2013). These differences in play may lead to fewer opportunities to engage with peers without disabilities and to develop friendships.

The unspoken "rules" of communicating with others include: matching the context and needs of the listener, using appropriate tone and language (both verbal and nonverbal), and avoiding the use of overly formal language (Paul et al., 2009). Conversation rules also include the need to adjust behavior to meet social contexts. For example, when speaking in a library, it is appropriate to whisper or speak softly; however, a conversation at a party would be loud and energetic. Understanding embedded environment cues (e.g., a "no talking" sign in the library) helps one to use the appropriate volume, gestures, and body language. These embedded cues may be difficult for people with ASD to understand.

Other limited social skills contribute to problems relating to others. Many people with ASD lack the ability to be flexible and may become rigid in the need for order and structure, which can lead to distress over changes in routine and potential struggles relating to others (Adams et al., 2020). Children with ASD may also have difficulty expressing and regulating their emotions and often express frustration using less constructive strategies (e.g., venting or avoidance-related strategies) (Zantinge et al., 2017). Behaviors caused by difficulty regulating emotions such as physical actions toward others may lead to isolation in both school and home settings. Other behaviors such as unusual language (e.g., overly formal), fixations with favorite objects, and a lack of understanding social norms can lead to a higher incidence of bullying. Research indicates that children with ASD are more likely to be bullied than their peers without disabilities (Humphrey & Symes, 2010; Maïano et al., 2016). In turn, bullying can lead to low self-esteem and higher rates of depression and anxiety (Forrest et al., 2020; Rodriguez et al., 2020; Zablotsky et. al., 2013).

As children with ASD become adolescents, they may choose to engage in friendships and dating relationships. However, social and communication differences often lead to trouble connecting appropriately with others. Adolescents and young adults with ASD may have difficulty understanding the unspoken rules of dating (Volkmar et al., 2014). For example, calling or texting someone repeatedly is considered rude or even "stalking" behavior. However, to a teen with ASD, this may be a demonstration of sincere interest in the other person. Limited awareness of nonverbal cues such as body language may also lead to unwanted physical advances such as hugging without permission. Social media is another outlet in which unspoken rules of common courtesy apply.

Technology and social media are embedded in every facet of our lives. Misunderstanding the needs, desires, and intentions of others often leads to behaviors such as contact that is too frequent or unwanted (Volkmar et al., 2014).

Social Communicative Assessments

Often children and youth with ASD exhibit limitations in communication skills, reduced social interactions, and may engage in behaviors toward others. The first step in teaching any new skill, including social skills, is to measure present skill levels of functioning and subsequently plan for appropriate interventions. Researchers refer to behaviors that serve as a threshold to other, more advanced behaviors as "behavioral cusps" (Rosales-Ruiz & Baer, 1997). An example of a behavioral cusp is teaching a child to push a button on a switch. By learning to press the button, the child has unlocked the potential to indicate choices, identify objects, and communicate via the device (or similar devices) in the future. Similarly, social skills and behaviors should be assessed to identify the target behavioral cusps that will lead to long-term positive outcomes. For example, will the skill lead to increased friendships and reduced isolation for the individual? Or, does the target skill have the potential to be generalizable (used in more than one setting with a variety of people)? These criteria allow for the focus to be on potential goals and interventions for behavior change that might have lasting impacts on the individual with ASD (Robertson, 2015).

There are both formal and informal assessments available for social skills. Both formal and informal assessments involve gathering information about the present level of skills, interpreting this data, and taking action based on the results of the assessment. Formal assessments are standardized measures designed to assess student knowledge, whereas informal assessments generate evidence of skills learned over time through informal day-to-day interactions and observations (Ruiz-Primo, 2011). Formal assessments include standardized and norm-referenced measures such as an intelligence or IQ test where students are compared to other students of the same age. Informal assessments include direct observations, interviews, and portfolio assessments.

There are many commercially available formal assessments for the purpose of assessing social skills. For children between the ages of 3–18, the Assessment of Social and Communication Skills for Individuals with Autism Spectrum Disorder, Revised (ASCS-2; Quill & Brusnahan, 2017) allows parents and teachers to assess social and communication skills. For older children and adolescents, ages 8 to 18, the Social Skills Improvement System Rating Scales (SSIS; Gresham & Elliot, 2008) measures social skills, problem behaviors, and academic competency.

Using parent, teacher, and student questionnaires, the SSRS assesses skills including cooperation, empathy and self-control. Similarly, the Social Responsiveness Scale- Second Edition (SRS-2; Constantino & Gruber, 2012) uses feedback from parents and teachers to assess social skills. Used in screening and diagnosis of ASD, the SRS-2 measures skills including social awareness, social cognition, social communication, social motivation, and restricted interests and behaviors. To assess initial needs and progress post-intervention, the Autism Social Skills Profile 2 (ASSP; Bellini, 2016) uses a Likert scale to measure social reciprocity, social participation/avoidance, and detrimental social behaviors. The ASSP also provides a total score of social functioning. These assessment tools must be given by qualified personnel, usually a school or clinical psychologist.

Informal assessments also yield valuable information about the present levels of children with ASD. Information is gained by observing the student in various academic or social experiences. The experiences may occur naturally or be created by the observer. Often, informal assessments are teacher-created checklists making them inexpensive and easy to obtain. A variety of individuals may gather data for informal assessments. Teachers, parents, or other professionals who work with the child may conduct informal assessments. See Table 10.1 for examples of informal assessments.

Early social competence and meaningful friendships have long been associated with positive outcomes in adaptive functioning in childhood (Blandon et al., 2010). Social competence is the ability to understand others' perspectives regarding various situations and to learn from our own experiences in navigating the evolving social landscapes

Table 10.1 Examples of Informal Assessments for Social Skills

Assessment Strategy	Description
Observation	Observing child engaging with others in natural settings
Interview	Engaging child in discussion through questions
Anecdotal record	Record notes of observed behaviors during interactions with peers
Event sampling	Record data of target behavior occurrence during a specific period (e.g., hitting others at lunchtime or talking out during reading group)
Time sampling	Record target behavior occurrence or nonoccurrence at the end of specific time intervals (e.g., five minutes, ten minutes)
Checklist	A list of target or ideal behaviors which allows teachers to check off behaviors that are present or absent
Work Sample	May be a drawing or writing sample chosen by the child
Portfolio	A collection of the child's work samples and other products such as videos and test scores

(Semrud-Clikeman, 2007). Furthermore, people are considered socially competent if others view their behavior as appropriate. In their landmark research, Crick and Dodge (1994) identified three predictors for social competence in students: (1) the extent to which students are accepted by their peers, (2) the degree to which students demonstrate physical behaviors towards their peers, and (3) the degree to which students withdraw from peer interactions. Crick and Dodge (1994) also determined that the inability to understand others' emotions and solve problems, academic failure, social rejection, and the inability to get along in a group to form friendships are major risk factors that interfere with the performance of social skills.

Teaching Social Skills: Practical Application

Once social skills are assessed, the results should be discussed with the child and family in order to develop goals and identify specific areas of need to reach these goals. Social skills should be targeted for instruction based on priority of importance for long-term success of the child (Bosch & Fuqua, 2001; Radley et al., 2014). There are specific social skills that can be taught to increase the chances of acceptance by others. These skills may be categorized as: (1) nonverbal behaviors, (2) social interactions, and (3) relationship skills.

The first category of skills to teach is nonverbal behaviors. These include eye contact, gestures, joint attention, proximity, and understanding the body language of others. Eye contact can be difficult for those with autism for a myriad of reasons and is often over-emphasized as an area of concern (Cook et al., 2017). In fact, emphasis on eye contact may be unnecessary and in many instances may detract from learning more valuable academic and adaptive skills. Educators and families should model appropriate eye contact without overreacting to differences seen in people with ASD.

Another area of nonvervbal behaviors to teach is gestures. Understanding that gestures indicate meaning or add to the content of the discussion is also necessary to develop nonverbal behavior skills. Another important nonverbal behavior is joint attention. Joint attention is the parallel participation in dialogue of two or more individuals that is key in the development of social awareness between social partners and topics of conversation (Murza et al., 2016). Taking the time to share attention on an object or conversation topic is helpful in teaching this skill. Proximity and personal space are other nonverbal behaviors to teach children with ASD. Understanding the concept of "my space" and "your space" is crucial to establishing conversations and ultimately relationships with others. Finally, awareness of the meanings of body language and facial expressions in others is a critical skill.

The second category of skills to teach is social interaction skills. Social interaction skills include recognizing social cues, conversational and emotional reciprocity, empathy, and perspective taking (Stichter et al., 2010). Teaching children with ASD to recognize and respond to cues such as facial expressions, tone, and body language enables them to establish conversations with others. Social and emotional reciprocity instruction should also be incorporated. Social reciprocity involves maintaining the conversation by taking turns and continuing the back and forth pattern of conversing. Emotional reciprocity entails recognizing emotions and demonstrating empathy and understanding toward others. Finally, perspective taking requires the use of environmental cues, emotional cues from others, and the understanding that the beliefs and perspectives of others may differ from our own (Stichter et al., 2010). When combined, social interaction skills allow individuals to participate in meaningful conversations and relationships with others.

Finally, the third category of social skills for target instruction is relationship skills. Relationship skills include intrapersonal skills (e.g., self-esteem, self-regulation) and interpersonal skills (e.g., friendships, group interactions, dating, and digital social skills). It is important to establish positive self-esteem for children with ASD. Self-regulation involves awareness of one's own emotions and using coping strategies to deal with difficult situations. Establishing these two intrapersonal skills enables a child with ASD to develop interpersonal skills with others. Friendship skills include developing relationships and interacting with friends. In a related skill set, group skills include sharing, turn taking, listening, and following directions. Teaching group skills enables children with ASD to benefit from positive social interactions with their peers.

Building Relationships

For teens and young adults with ASD, navigating relationships with others can be especially difficult. Understanding appropriate social contact is one of the first dating skills to develop (Sala et al., 2019). This begins with an awareness of one's own body and the difference in appropriate and inappropriate touching. Communicating with a partner is another crucial dating skill. Knowing the acceptable forms of communication (e.g., texting once per day or sending one message via a social networking platform) versus unacceptable communication (e.g., calling or messaging repeatedly) are important differentiations. Digital social skills and networking skills must also be established. From creating an email account to using "netiquette" online, digital platforms are readily available and helpful in establishing and maintaining connections with others. Table 10.2 lists social skills categories to develop for children and youth.

Table 10.2 Social Skills to Teach Children with Autism Spectrum Disorders

Category	Social skills
Nonverbal behaviors	Eye contact
	Gestures
	Joint Attention
	Proximity
	Body language
Social interaction skills	Social cues
	Conversational reciprocity
	Emotional reciprocity
	Empathy
	Perspective taking
Intrapersonal relationship skills	Self-regulation
	Self-esteem
Interpersonal relationship skills	Friendships
	Group interactions
	Dating
	Digital social skills

Case Study: Meet Amir

Amir is eight years old and in the second grade. He was diagnosed with an autism spectrum disorder at 18 months of age. Amir's parents noticed he had difficulty connecting with them and rarely smiled as a baby. He had no spoken words at the age of twelve months and was not able to communicate his needs other than by crying. Due to his limited communication, his parents wondered if he had a hearing impairment before he was diagnosed with autism. Now they understand that his autism impacted his ability to connect and communicate.

Every day Amir is fully included in the general education setting with support. He is slightly behind his peers academically but has age-appropriate communication and vocabulary skills. Amir's greatest needs are behavioral and social. He struggles to complete non-preferred tasks and often "shuts down" or cries when presented with challenging requests. During classroom instruction, Amir often blurts out the answer and becomes upset if other children answer a question.

Amir has one acquaintance in his class whom he sits with in the classroom and at lunch. When other children approach Amir he turns and walks away without speaking or pushes them. On the playground, Amir walks around by himself or demands access to the playground equipment other children are using. Recently, when asked about friendships, Amir responded he has no friends. His parents and IEP team are concerned about his lack of friendships and social skills.

Teaching Social Skills

Teaching social skills to individuals with ASD can be one of the most challenging and rewarding areas of instruction. Often communication skills carry little influence if social skills are not developed for effective communication to take place. Social difficulties for people with autism are diverse. Some are mild and some involve severe behavior towards self or others. All involve problems with social understanding and may be affected by difficulties with attention, communication, problem solving, cognition, sensory processing, and motor problems. According to the National Professional Development Center on Autism Spectrum Disorder, evidence-based practices (EBPs) are techniques and interventions shown to be effective for teaching skills to children with ASD (Steinbrenner et al., 2020). In this section of the chapter we will describe the following evidence-based practices to teach social skills: positive reinforcement, differential reinforcement, priming, prompts, antecedent-based interventions, parent-implemented practices, visual supports, video modeling, social narratives, peer-mediated interventions, and cognitive behavioral interventions.

Positive Reinforcement

Reinforcement is an evidence-based practice used to increase appropriate behavior and teach new skills (e.g., replacement behavior in place of an interfering behavior). Positive Reinforcement describes a relation between learner behavior and a consequence that follows the behavior. For example, children learn to ask for something politely if they want to receive it in return. The ultimate goal of reinforcement is to help learners with ASD learn new skills and maintain them over time in a variety of settings with many different individuals.

Differential Reinforcement

Differential reinforcement is another evidence-based practice used to shape behavior by reinforcing only the desired replacement behavior (Savage et al., 2017). When using differential reinforcement, the undesired (target) behavior is identified first. After identifying the target behavior to change, a replacement behavior is selected. Following the identification of the target (undesired) and replacement (desired) behavior, reinforcement is provided only for the desired behavior and withheld for the undesired behavior. For example, if Amir's target behavior is blurting out answers during instruction and the replacement behavior is for Amir to raise his hand before speaking, Amir's behavior of hand raising would be reinforced and no reinforcement would be provided for blurting out answers.

Priming

Priming is another strategy used to provide a person with information and answers before they are presented with an activity or before they enter a social situation. The positive effects of priming to facilitate social behavior are supported by researchers, who used priming to increase the social initiations of children with ASD (Gengoux, 2015; Sancho et al., 2010) and to decrease problem behaviors (Hume et al., 2014). Social behaviors (e.g., greeting others) can be primed by presenting behavioral expectations just prior to performance of the skill in the natural environment.

Prompts

Prompts are highly effective in facilitating child-adult and child-child interactions in children with ASD (Sam et al., 2015a). Prompts are supports that provide assistance to the child to successfully perform behaviors and skills. Prompts may be used to teach new social skills and to enhance performance of previously acquired skills. A limitation of prompting strategies is that the child with ASD may only engage in social interactions in which prompting is provided. As such, a prompt-fading plan needs to be implemented to systematically fade prompts from most-to-least assistance. Types of prompts (from least-to-most supportive):

- Natural: saying or doing what would typically happen before a behavior
- Gestural: pointing to, looking at, moving, or touching an item or area to indicate a correct response
- Verbal: providing a verbal instruction, cue, or model
- Modeling: the acting out of a target behavior with the hope the child will imitate
- Physical: moving the child through the behavior; can be full, which is doing the whole behavior, or partial, such as just touching the hand.

Antecedent-Based Interventions

Antecedent-Based Interventions (ABI) are evidence-based practices used to address both interfering and on-task behaviors (Sam, 2016). These practices are most often used after a functional behavior assessment (FBA) has been conducted to identify the function of the interfering behavior. Many interfering behaviors continue to occur because the environmental conditions in a particular setting have become linked to the behavior over time. The kinds of behavioral interventions that are widely used when antecedent factors are identified as the precipitating factors in challenging behavior, are often described as prevention-focused interventions.

Reszka et al. (2012) indicated increased social engagement of preschool children with ASD with their peers when they were in a classroom book area. Books may provide a more concrete basis for initiating and sustaining interactions (e.g., showing pictures or discussing topics from a book) than materials requiring more imaginative play. In addition, children may select books that relate to their interest areas. Often the interest areas of children with ASD are related to joint attention and engagement with others (Adamson et al., 2010). Furthermore, research has indicated that large motor activities can assist in increasing appropriate play behaviors in children with ASD and often are preferred activities for them (Case-Smith & Kuhaneck, 2008). In the case of Amir, increasing his physical activity each day while incorporating peers may provide increased social opportunities.

Parent-Implemented Practices

Parent-implemented practices or parent-implemented interventions (PII), provide options for parents in supporting their children's direct acquisition of social skills or to build towards behavior change (Bearss et al., 2015). PII focuses on the improvement of children's skill sets, including social skills, behavior, and personal competencies, using evidence-based practices during daily routines and activities (Amsbary et al., 2017). Following a coaching model developed by Rush and Shelden (2020), parents and practitioners collaborate through joint planning, then practitioners observe, engage in action steps to encourage and reinforce parent practices, allow time for reflection, and then feedback is provided to further progress towards child-centered goals. A major advantage of parent-mediated interventions is the opportunity for improved generalization of skills in a wide variety of natural environments (Pacia et al., 2021).

Visual Supports

Visual supports are tools presented visually that provide information to enhance an individual's access to a variety of environments and/or communicate information (Rutherford et al., 2020; Sam et al., 2015b). Visual supports might include, but are not limited to, pictures, written words, objects within the environment, arrangement of the environment or visual boundaries, schedules, maps, labels, organization systems, timelines, and scripts. They are useful across settings (e.g., school, home, community) in encouraging social interaction (Rutherford et al., 2020). Many students with ASD have difficulty thinking about abstract concepts, and respond better to visual information (Kellems et al., 2016b; Postorino et al.,

2016). Visual supports have been proven to be effective in increasing play skills, social interaction skills, and social initiation (Steinbrenner et al., 2020). Visual supports meet the evidence-based practice criteria within the early childhood, elementary, and middle school age groups.

Video Modeling

Video modeling is an evidence-based practice that uses video recording and display equipment to provide a visual model of the targeted behavior or skill (Cihak et al., 2010; Cihak et al., 2012). There are a variety of ways to present a video model: basic video modeling, or other as a model (e.g., a peer, an adult or teacher); video self-modeling (the individuals themselves acts as the model for the video); and point-of-view video modeling, where a specific first-person view, often of the hands, acts as the model (Park et al., 2019). Video prompting is a video modeling strategy that involves breaking the behavior skill into steps and recording each step with incorporated pauses during which the learner may attempt the step before viewing subsequent steps (Kellems et al., 2016a). Video prompting may be done with either the learner or another person acting as a model. Going back to our case study, Amir may benefit from the use of a video model on how to engage in a conversation with friends or how to share equipment on the playground.

Social Narratives

Social narratives are interventions that describe social situations in detail by highlighting relevant cues and offering examples of appropriate responding. In general, social narratives are read to the child before they enter the difficult situation being described in the story. Their purpose is to support learners in adjusting to changes in routine and adapting their behaviors based on the social and physical cues of a situation, or in teaching specific social skills or behaviors. Social narratives are individualized according to learner needs and typically are quite short, and often incorporate illustrations, pictures or other visual aids, and songs. Social narratives encompass a variety of interventions that function to introduce and teach appropriate behavior through written story form, such as Social Stories, Power Cards, and other written story-based prompts.

The most common of these are Social Stories, developed by Carol Gray (Gray, 1995, 2004, 2005, 2010; Gray & Garand, 1993). A Social Story describes a situation, skill, or concept in terms of relevant social cues, perspectives, and common responses. Specific sentence types that are often used when constructing Social Stories include: descriptive, directive, perspective, affirmative, control, and cooperative. Evidence-based research suggests that social narratives can be used effectively with learners with ASD, especially when positive reinforcement is applied (Steinbrenner et al., 2020). Another type of social narrative is Power Cards. The primary difference between Social Stories and Power Cards is that Power Cards incorporate the child's special interest area (Daubert et al., 2014; Gagnon, 2001). Power Cards have demonstrated effectiveness in developing social behaviors, such as increasing the percentage of time that adolescents engage in conversation outside of their preferred topic (Davis et al., 2010).

In a meta-analysis on the effectiveness of Social Stories, researchers discovered low to questionable effects on improving participant behavior and skill levels (Kokina & Kern, 2010). This low to questionable effect is surprising given the popularity of Social Stories. However, the authors concluded that most of the studies reviewed either resulted in a high degree of effectiveness or were not effective at all, suggesting that not all youth may benefit equally from this intervention. Social Story effects were greater when the child was their own agent of the intervention, as opposed to having the story read by a parent, teacher, or researcher, and when it was read just before the situation described. In addition, simple stories presented within a brief time frame resulted in better outcomes for the child.

Peer-mediated Interventions (PMI)

PMI has been identified as a versatile and potentially effective intervention approach to teach a variety of skills to individuals with ASD (Chang & Locke, 2016; Odom & Strain, 1984; Odom et al., 2003; Reichow & Volkmar, 2010; Zagona & Mastergeorge, 2018). PMI components include training peers to implement pivotal response training techniques (Harper et al., 2008), training participants to use scripted phrases related to different play themes (Ganz & Flores, 2008), and implementing high probability request sequences with embedded peer-modeling during play sessions (Jung et al., 2008). Developing peer modeling of social skills has been successfully applied in inclusive environments and can be used to promote social interaction between students with ASD and their peers (Chan et al., 2009; Koegel et al., 2012). PMI offers unique advantages that are particularly beneficial in inclusive settings. Peers acting as intervention agents may increase access to the intervention for the individual with ASD while also potentially placing fewer demands on teachers to serve as the sole intervention provider (Chan et al., 2009). Furthermore, PMI potentially creates opportunities for students with ASD to interact and practice social skills with a variety of communication partners, thus possibly increasing the likelihood that these acquired skills will generalize across settings and individuals. Finally, PMI can be incorporated into the natural context of daily activities, making it particularly well suited to inclusive settings. PMI would be appropriate to use for our case study student, Amir. By providing opportunities for peers to model appropriate play and social interactions, Amir could practice needed skills throughout the day.

Cognitive Behavioral Therapy

Cognitive Behavioral Therapy (CBI) is a method that focuses on targeting positive and negative thought processes to change behavior. Some researchers have posited that social skill limitations occur as a function of avoidance due to increased social anxiety (Mussey et al., 2017). CBI is used primarily with those who experience anxiety or difficulty controlling expressions of anger and behavior toward others. White et al. (2010) suggest that CBI alleviates anxiety experienced by youth with ASD and increases social competence. It is effective with youth from elementary school age to high school (Brock, 2013). Individuals using CBI are taught to identify their feelings and the thoughts associated with those feelings and then use strategies to express their behavior in a more prosocial manner. CBI requires students to self-evaluate the social situation and determine an appropriate plan of action. Therefore, the student learns to function in a more positive manner by addressing the thoughts and feelings associated with social anxiety. Additionally, other studies reported that the use of CBI was effective in increasing executive functioning skills, facial recognition, problem-solving, Theory of Mind, reading nonverbal cues, and accurately describing how to respond in a social situation (Koning et al., 2011; Stitcher et al., 2010).

Case Study: Meet Mateo

Mateo is an 11-, almost 12-year-old, transitioning from elementary school into middle school next school year. He is slightly older than his peers in 5th grade as his family and IEP team decided to delay his start in Kindergarten to continue work on his communication and social skills as a preschool student. Mateo was diagnosed with ASD when he was 3 years old. As a young child, Mateo would often react to frustrations by lashing out physically or with high emotions when he was unable to make his needs known or express his feelings.

Mateo has been attending a rural elementary school that does not have many options for extracurricular activities outside of sports, of which Mateo has no interest. His family applied for, and was granted a transfer to a local STEM Academy within the public school system, and he is excited for this change due to a large number of clubs that fit his direct interests. Mateo is also nervous about moving to a new school.

Mateo is often considered an average student in core subjects such as math and English, but excels in elective courses such as art and music classes that were available in his elementary school. He prefers hands-on learning, and tends to be better in individual work situations as opposed to group projects. Mateo also finds teacher-led presentations hard to follow without visual representations of the content.

Mateo is profoundly rigid to routines, and struggles to engage with peers of a similar age as a result of not having many opportunities to make meaningful connections with those in his direct community. Mateo experienced bullying at a young age due to his social skill differences, and approaches peer relationships with caution. He gets along well with adults in school and in the community, but discloses to his parents and mentors that he would like to have friendships with other kids his age.

Becoming Socially Competent

Social competence can be defined as independently and successfully engaging with others, understanding social situations, and establishing and maintaining relationships (Stichter et al., 2010). Social competence also involves taking the perspective of others, learning from social interactions, and applying this knowledge to future interactions. Socially competent individuals enjoy relationships with others, have increased levels of self-esteem and self-confidence, and are adaptable to a variety of environments. At each stage of development, the goals for social competence will vary.

For young children, social competency focuses on getting along with others. Goals at this stage of development include increasing communicative attempts, learning to respect the boundaries of others, and interacting with peers in play and group settings. Many early skills are learned through play, specifically pretend play. Pretend play contributes to cognitive as well as social development. Play also encourages perspective-taking and empathy. Families play a critical role in encouraging the development of these skills (Carter et al., 2014). Research indicates that peers without disabilities can be useful in supporting social skill development in children with ASD through the use of prompting and visual supports (Rutherford et al., 2019). As children mature and develop these skills, they can expand upon the basics by adding conversation skills, practicing empathy for others, and developing friendships with peers. Children in elementary and middle school should begin to develop self-regulation skills including identifying their own emotions and using self-control.

Adolescents with ASD face increased expectations to act in socially competent ways, along with a desire to develop relationships with others. Social demands become more complex, requiring an expanding skill set and increasing awareness for social success. Middle and high school students often engage in social banter including joking, teasing, and conversing about popular music or events. For adolescents with ASD, it is crucial to understand the context to engage in these socially fluid interactions. The adolescent period is full of both physical and emotional changes for all teenagers. From evolving relationships with parents and peers, to shifting school and leisure environments, youth with ASD are forced to confront change. Adding to the complexities of adolescence, many teens with ASD report feeling lonely, isolated, or bullied by peers (Humphrey & Symes, 2010).

As adolescents become young adults, the focus on achieving social competence shifts to a need for developing relationships with others, pursuing employment or higher education, and engaging in community recreation and leisure activities. Teaching students to become socially competent is especially critical during the transition from school to adulthood (Carter & Draper, 2010). In addition to giving students the skills to be successful during high school and in higher education settings, educators must give students with ASD the tools to be socially successful in everyday life (Carter et al., 2014).

Overall, the desired outcome for students with ASD is to achieve high levels of social functioning, engage in fulfilling relationships with others, and develop self-esteem. "Social functioning" is a global term encompassing employment, friendships, and independence (Gillespie-Lynch et al., 2011). Social functioning skills including communication, self-regulation, and understanding the social expectations of new settings are critical skills to obtain and maintain employment and pursue an independent adult life.

Case Study: Mateo at the New School

It has been six months since Mateo moved to the STEM Academy and began 6th grade. At the beginning of the year, Mateo struggled to find his place and often felt lonely and lost at the new school. The lunchroom and hallways were crowded and noisy. Transitions between classes were difficult and unplanned events caused a great deal of anxiety for Mateo. Seeing Mateo struggle, his IEP team convened to plan for ways to help Mateo acclimate and thrive at his new school. The IEP team asked Mateo and his family for their input too.

The IEP team recommended some simple accommodations for Mateo to use throughout the school day. First, the team recommended the use of a visual schedule on a tablet to help Mateo deal with unexpected events. Each morning, Mateo's teacher would update the schedule to indicate any changes to the usual routine such as class parties or field trips. The team also recommended the use of noise-canceling headphones for Mateo to access as needed.

After finding out from his parents that Mateo preferred hands-on learning, the team recommended an industrial arts (woodworking) class. This led to the most successful intervention which was incorporating the use of peers in peer-mediated intervention. Mateo's classmates in the woodworking class were excited to help him learn new skills. His woodworking teacher, Mr. Hernandez, provided time at the end of each class period for the students to talk. This time provided much-needed opportunities for Mateo to make friends and build social connections.

Conclusion

Differences in communication and social skills can contribute to problems relating to others. Gaining social competence through the teaching of social skills and the application of interventions gives individuals with autism spectrum disorders a better chance at getting along with others, making friends, and being able to obtain and sustain a job. Learning how to initiate, reciprocate, and think about social interactions is key to decreasing the challenges persons with ASD experience. People on the spectrum need to be assessed and have an individualized program developed for them to move toward a higher level of social competence. There are many interventions described in this chapter to assist with teaching social interaction competence. Adults supporting the social skill development of children and youth with ASD should remember to fade the use of strategies over time and teach skill generalization and maintenance to increase independence and long-term success.

Additional Resources

- Autism Internet Modules (AIM) https://autisminternetmodules.org/
- Autism Focused Intervention Resources & Modules (AFIRM) is an extension of the National Professional Development Center (NPDC) https://afirm.fpg.unc.edu/
- Endow, J. (2019). *Autistically Thriving: Reading Comprehension, Conversational Engagement, and Living a Self-Determined Life Based on Autistic Neurology*. Lancaster, PA: Judy Endow.
- Endow, J. (2012). *Learning the Hidden Curriculum: The Odyssey of One Autistic Adult*. Shawnee Mission, KS: AAPC Publishing.
- Fleming, J. (2021). *How to Be Human: An Autistic Man's Guide to Life*. Simon & Schuster. SBN-13:9781501180507
- IRIS Center https://iris.peabody.vanderbilt.edu/
- NeuroClastic https://neuroclastic.com/

References

Adams, R. E., Taylor, J. L., & Bishop, S. L. (2020). Brief report: ASD-related behavior problems and negative peer experiences among adolescents with ASD in general education settings. *Journal of Autism and Developmental Disorders*, *50*(12), 4548–4552. https://doi.org/10.1007/s10803-020-04508-1

Adamson, L. B., Deckner, D. F., & Bakeman, R. (2010). Early interests and joint engagement in typical development, autism, and Down syndrome. *Journal of Autism and Developmental Disorders, 40*, 665–676.

American Psychiatric Association (2013). *Diagnostic and statistical manual of mental disorders, fifth edition (DSM-5)*. Arlington, VA: American Psychiatric Publishing.

Amsbary, J., & AFIRM Team. (2017). *Parent implemented interventions*. Chapel Hill, NC: National Professional Development Center on Autism Spectrum Disorder, FPG Child Development Center, University of North Carolina. Retrieved from http://afirm.fpg.unc.edu/parent-implemented-interventions.

Asperger, H. (1944). Die Autistischen Psychopathen im Kindesalter. *European Archives of Psychiatry and Clinical Neuroscience, 117*(1), 76–136.

Babb, S., Raulston, T., McNaughton, D., Lee, J., & Weintraub, R. (2021). Social interaction interventions for adolescents with autism: A meta-analysis. *Remedial and Special Education, 42*(5), 343–357. https://doi.org/10.1177/0741932520956362

Bearss, K., Burrell, T. L., Stewart, L., & Scahill, L. (2015). Parent training in autism spectrum disorder: What's in a name? *Clinical Child and Family Psychology Review, 18*(2), 170–182. https://doi.org/10.1007/s10567-015-0179-5

Bellini, S. (2016). *Building social relationships 2: A systematic approach to teaching social interaction skills to children and adolescents on the autism spectrum*. Lenexa, KS: AAPC Publishing.

Blandon, A. Y., Calkins, S. D., Grimm, K. J., Keane, S. P., & O'Brien, M. (2010). Testing a developmental cascade model of emotional and social competence and early peer acceptance. *Development and Psychopathology, 22*(4), 737–748. https://doi.org/10.1017/S0954579410000428

Bosch, S., & Fuqua, R. W. (2001). Behavioral cusps: A model for selecting target behaviors. *Journal of Applied Behavioral Analysis, 34*(1), 123–125.

Brock, M. E. (2013). *Cognitive behavioral intervention (CBI) fact sheet*. Chapel Hill (NC): The University of North Carolina; Frank Porter Graham Child Development Institute; The National Professional Development Center on Autism Spectrum.

Campbell, S. B., Leezenbaum, N. B., Mahoney, A. S., Moore, E. L., & Brownell, C. A. (2016). Pretend Play and Social Engagement in Toddlers at High and Low Genetic Risk for Autism Spectrum Disorder. *Journal of Autism and Developmental Disorders, 46*(7), 2305–2316. https://doi.org/10.1007/s10803-016-2764-y

Carter, E. W., Common, E. A., Sreckovic, M. A., Heartley, B. H., Bottema-Beutel, K., Gustafson, J. R., Dykstra, J., & Hume, K. (2014). Promoting social competence and peer relationships for adolescents with autism spectrum disorders. *Remedial and Special Education, 35*(2), 91–101.

Carter, E. W., & Draper, J. (2010). Making school matter: Supporting meaningful secondary experiences for adolescents who use AAC. In McNaughton & D. R. Buekelman (Eds.), *Transition strategies for adolescents and young adults who use augmentative and alternative communication* (pp. 69–90). Baltimore, MD: Brookes.

Case-Smith, J., & Kuhaneck, H. M. (2008). Play preferences of typically developing children and children with developmental delays between ages 3 and 7 years. *OTJR: Occupation, Participation and Health, 28,* 19–29.

Chan, J. M., Lang, R., Rispoli, M., O'Reilly, M., Sigafoos, J., & Cole, H. (2009). Use of peer-mediated interventions in the treatment of autism spectrum disorders: A systematic review. *Research in Autism Spectrum Disorders, 3*(4), 876–889.

Chang, Y. C., & Locke, J. (2016). A systematic review of peer-mediated interventions for children with autism spectrum disorder. *Research in Autism Spectrum Disorders, 27,* 1–10. https://doi.org/10.1016/j.rasd.2016.03.010

Cihak, D. F., Fahrenkrog, C.D., Ayres, K. M., & Smith, C. (2010). The use of video modeling via a video iPod® and a system of least prompts to improve transitional behaviors for students with autism spectrum disorders in the general education classroom. *Journal of Positive Behavior Interventions, 12,* 103–115.

Cihak, D. F, Kildare, L., Smith, C., McMahon, D. D., & Quinn-Brown, L. (2012). *Using video* Social Stories™ to *increase task engagement for middle school students with autism spectrum disorders. Behavior Modification, 36,* 399–425.

Cohen, M. J., & Sloan, D. L. (2007). *Visual supports for people with autism: A guide for parents and professionals.* Bethesda, MD: Woodbine House.

Constantino, J. N., & Gruber, C. P. (2012). *Social Responsiveness Scale, Second Edition.* Los Angeles: Western Psychological Services.

Constantino, J. N., Gruber, C. P., Davis, S., Hayes, S., Passanante, N., & Przybeck, T. (2004). The factor structure of autistic traits. *Journal of Child Psychology and Psychiatry and Allied Disciplines, 45*(4), 718–726.

Cook, J. L., Rapp, J. T., Mann, K. R., McHugh, C., Burji, C., & Nuta, R. (2017). A practitioner model for increasing eye contact in children with autism. *Behavior Modification, 41*(3), 382–404. https://doi.org/10.1177/014544551 6689323

Cooper, K., Smith, L. G. E., & Russell, A. (2017). Social identity, self-esteem, and mental health in autism. *European Journal of Social Psychology, 47*(7), 844–854. https://doi.org/10.1002/ejsp.2297

Crick, N. R., & Dodge, K. A. (1994). A review and reformulation of social-information-processing mechanisms in children's social adjustment. *Psychological Bulletin, 115,* 74–101.

Daubert, A., Hornstein, S., Tincani, M. (2014). Effects of a modified power card strategy on turn taking and social commenting of children with autism spectrum disorder playing board games. *Journal of Developmental and Physical Disabilities, 27*(1): 93–110. https://doi.org/10.1007/s10882-014-9403-3

Daughrity, B. L. (2019). Parent perceptions of barriers to friendship development for children with Autism spectrum disorders. *Communication Disorders Quarterly, 40*(3), 142–151. https://doi.org/10.1177/1525740118788039

Davis, K. T., Boon, R. T., Fore, C., & Cihak, D. F. (2010). Improving the conversational skills among adolescents with Asperger's syndrome via the use of power cards. *Focus on Autism and Other Developmental Disabilities, 25*, 12–22.

Dovgan, K. N., & Mazurek, M. O. (2019). Relations among activity participation, friendship, and internalizing problems in children with autism spectrum disorder. *Autism, 23*(3), 750–758. https://doi.org/10.1177/136236131 8775541

Forrest, D. L., Kroeger, R. A., & Stroope, S. (2019). Autism spectrum disorder symptoms and bullying victimization among children with Autism in the United States. *Journal of Autism and Developmental Disorders, 50*(2), 560–571. https://doi.org/10.1007/s10803-019-04282-9

Gagnon, E. (2001). *Power cards: using special interests to motivate children and youth with Asperger syndrome and autism.* Shawnee Mission (KS): Autism Asperger Publishing.

Gale, C., Eikeseth, S., & Klintwall, L. (2019). Children with Autism show atypical preference for non-social stimuli. *Scientific Reports, 9*(1), 1–10. https://doi.org/10.1038/s41598-019-46705-8

Ganz, J. B., & Flores, M. M. (2008). Effects of the use of visual strategies in play groups for children with autism spectrum disorders and their peers. *Journal of Autism and Developmental Disorders, 38*(5), 926–940.

Gengoux, G. W. (2015). Priming for social activities: Effects on interactions between children with autism and typically developing peers. *Journal of Positive Behavior Interventions, 17*(3), 181–192.

Gillespie-Lynch, K., Sepeta, L., Wang, Y., Marshall, S., Gomez, L., Sigman, M., & Hutman, T. (2011). Early childhood predictors of the social competence of adults with autism. *Journal of Autism and Developmental Disorders, 42*, 161–174.

Gray, C. (1995). Teaching children with autism to "read" social situations. In K. Quill (Ed.), *Teaching Children with Autism: Strategies to Enhance Communication and Socialization* (pp. 219–241). Albany, NY: Delmar.

Gray, C. (2004) Social Stories 10.0. *Jenison Autism Journal, 15*(4), 2–21.

Gray, C. (2005) Social Stories. www.thegraycenter.org/

Gray, C. (2010). *The new social story book.* Future Horizons.

Gray, C. A., & Garand, J. D. (1993). Social stories: Improving responses of students with autism with accurate social information. *Focus on Autistic Behavior, 8*, 1–10.

Gresham, F. M., & Elliott, S. N. (2008). *Social Skills Improvement Rating Scales.* Minneapolis, MN: Pearson.

Harper, C. B., Symon, J. B. G., & Frea, W. D. (2008). Recess is time-in: Using peers toimprove social skills of children with autism. *Journal of Autism and Developmental Disorders, 38*, 815–826.

Huang, A.X., Hughes, T. L., Sutton, L. R., Lawrence, M., Chen, X., Ji, Z., & Zeleke, W. (2017). Understanding the self in individuals with Autism spectrum disorders (ASD): A review of literature. *Frontiers in Psychology*, 8, 1422–1422. https://doi.org/10.3389/fpsyg.2017.01422

Hume, K., Sreckovic, M., Snyder, K., & Carnahan, C. (2014). Smooth transitions: Helping students with autism spectrum disorder navigate the school day. TEACHING Exceptional Children, 47(1), 35–45. https://doi.org/10.1177/0040059914542794

Humphrey, N., & Symes, W. (2010). Perceptions of social support and experience of bullying among pupils with autism spectrum disorders in mainstream secondary schools. *European Journal of Special Needs Education*, 25, 77–91.

Jung, S. & Sainato, D. M. (2013). Teaching play skills to young children with autism. *Journal of Intellectual & Developmental Disability*, 38(1), 74–90. https://doi.org/10.3109/13668250.2012.732220

Jung, S., Sainato, D. M., & Davis, C. A. (2008). Using high-probability request sequences to increase social interactions in young children with autism. *Journal of Early Intervention*, 30(3), 163–187.

Kanner, L. (1943). Autistic disturbances of affective contact. *Nervous Child*, 2, 217–250.

Keenan, B. M., Newman, L. K., Gray, K. M., & Rinehart, N. J. (2016). Parents of children with ASD experience more psychological distress, parenting stress, and attachment-related anxiety. *Journal of Autism and Developmental Disorders*, 46(9), 2979–2991. https://doi.org/10.1007/s10803-016-2836-z

Kellems, R. O., Frandsen, K., Hansen, B., Gabrielsen, T., Clarke, B., Simons, K., & Clements, K. (2016a). Teaching multi-step math skills to adults with disabilities via video prompting. *Research in Developmental Disabilities*, 58, 31–44. https://doi.org/10.1016/j.ridd.2016.08.013

Kellems, R. O., Gabrielsen, T. P., & Williams, C. (2016b). Using visual organizers and technology: supporting executive function, abstract language comprehension, and social learning. In T. A. Cardon (Ed.), *Technology and the Treatment of Children with Autism Spectrum Disorder* (pp. 75–86). Springer International Publishing. https://doi.org/10.1007/978-3-319-20872-5_7

Koegel, L., Matos-Freden, R., Lang, R., & Koegel, R. (2012). Interventions for children with autism spectrum disorders in inclusive school settings. *Cognitive and Behavioral Practice*, 19, 401–412.

Kokina, A., & Kern L. (2010). Social story interventions for students with autism spectrum disorders: a meta-analysis. *Journal of Autism and Developmental Disorders*, 40, 812–826.

Koning, C., Magill-Evans, J., Volden, J., & Dick, B. (2011). Efficacy of cognitive behavior therapy-based social skills intervention for school-aged boys with autism spectrum disorders. *Research in Autism Spectrum Disorders*, 7, 1280–1290.

Ledford, J. R., Lambert, J. M., Barton, E. E., & Ayres, K. M. (2021). The evidence base for interventions for individuals with ASD: A call to improve practice conceptualization and synthesis. *Focus on Autism and Other Developmental Disabilities*, 36(3), 135–147. https://doi.org/10.1177/10883576211023349

Levinson, S., Eisenhower, A., Bush, H. H., Carter, A. S., & Blacher, J. (2020). Brief report: Predicting social skills from semantic, syntactic, and pragmatic language among young children with Autism spectrum disorder. *Journal of*

Autism and Developmental Disorders, 50(11), 4165–4175. https://doi.org/10.1007/s10803-020-04445-z

Losinski, M., Cook, K., Hirsch, S., & Sanders, S. (2017). The effects of deep pressure therapies and antecedent exercise on stereotypical behaviors of students with Autism spectrum disorders. *Behavioral Disorders*, 42(4), 196–208. https://doi.org/10.1177/0198742917715873

Lydon, H., Healy, O., & Leader, G. (2011). A comparison of video modeling and pivotal response training to teach pretend play skills to children with Autism spectrum disorder. *Research in Autism Spectrum Disorders*, 5(2), 872–884. https://doi.org/10.1016/j.rasd.2010.10.002

Mahjouri, S., & Lord, C. E. (2012). What the DSM-5 portends for research, diagnosis, and treatment of autism spectrum disorders. *Current Psychiatry Reports*, 14(6), 739–747.

Maïano, C., Normand, C. L., Salvas, M.-C., Moullec, G., & Aimé, A. (2016). Prevalence of School Bullying Among Youth with Autism Spectrum Disorders: A Systematic Review and Meta-Analysis. *Autism Research*, 9(6), 601–615. https://doi.org/10.1002/aur.1568

Murza, K. A., Schwartz, J. B., Hahs-Vaughn, D. L., & Nye, C. (2016). Joint attention interventions for children with autism spectrum disorder: A systematic review and meta-analysis. *International Journal of Language & Communication Disorders*, 51(3), 236–251. https://doi.org/10.1111/1460-6984.12212

Mussey, J., Dawkins, T., & AFIRM Team. (2017). Cognitive behavioral intervention. Chapel Hill, NC: National Professional Development Center on Autism Spectrum Disorder, FPG Child Development Center, University of North Carolina. Retrieved from http://afirm.fpg.unc.edu/cognitive-behavioral-intervention

Myles, B. S., & Adreon, D. (2001). *Asperger syndrome and adolescence: Practical solutions for school success*. AAPC Publishing.

Odom, S. L., Brown, W. H., Frey, T., Karasu, N., Smith-Canter, L. L., & Strain, P. S. (2003). Evidence-based practices for young children with autism contributions for single-subject design research. *Focus on Autism and Other Developmental Disabilities*, 18(3), 166–175.

Odom, S. L., & Strain, P. S. (1984). Peer mediated approaches to promoting children's social interaction: A review. *American Journal of Orthopsychiatry*, 54, 544–557.

Pacia, C., Holloway, J., Gunning, C., & Lee, H. (2021). A systematic review of family-mediated social communication interventions for young children with Autism. *Review Journal of Autism and Developmental Disorders*.

Park, J., Bouck, E., & Duenas, A. (2019). The effect of video modeling and video prompting interventions on individuals with intellectual disability: A systematic literature review. *Journal of Special Education Technology*, 34(1), 3–16. https://doi.org/10.1177/0162643418780464

Paul, R., Orlovski, S. M., Marcinko, H. C., & Volkmar, F. (2009). Conversational behaviors in youth with high-functioning ASD and Asperger syndrome. *Journal of Autism and Developmental Disorders*, 39(1), 115–125.

Postorino, V., Fatta, L. M., Sanges, V., Giovagnoli, G., De Peppo, L., Vicari, S., & Mazzone, L. (2016). Intellectual disability in Autism Spectrum Disorder: Investigation of prevalence in an Italian sample of children and adolescents. *Research in Developmental Disabilities, 48*, 193–201. https://doi.org/10.1016/j.ridd.2015.10.020

Quill, K. & Brusnahan, L. (2017). *DO-WATCH-LISTEN-SAY: Social and communication intervention for autism spectrum disorder* (2nd ed.). Baltimore: New York: Brookes Publishing.

Radley, K. C., Jenson, W. R., Clark, E., Hood, J. A., & Nicholas, P. (2014). Using a multimedia social skills intervention to increase social engagement of young children with autism spectrum disorder, *Intervention in School and Clinic, 50*, 22–28.

Reichow, B. & Vokmar, F. R. (2010). Social skills interventions for individuals with autism: Evaluation for evidence-based practices within a best evidence synthesis framework, *Journal of Autism and Developmental Disorders, 40*, 149–166.

Reszka, S. S., Odom, S. L., & Hume, K. A. (2012). Ecological features of preschools and the social engagement of children with autism. *Journal of Early Intervention, 34*, 40–56.

Rieth, S. R., Stahmer, A. C., Suhrheinrich, J., Schreibman, L., Kennedy, J., & Ross, B. (2014). Identifying critical elements of treatment: examining the use of turn taking in Autism intervention. *Focus on Autism and Other Developmental Disabilities, 29*(3), 168–179. https://doi.org/10.1177/1088357613513792

Robertson, R. E. (2015). The acquisition of problem behavior in individuals with developmental disabilities as a behavioral cusp. *Behavior Modification, 39*(4), 475–495. https://doi.org/10.1177/0145445515572185

Rodriguez, G., Drastal, K., & Hartley, S. L. (2021). Cross-lagged model of bullying victimization and mental health problems in children with autism in middle to older childhood. *Autism, 25*(1), 90–101. https://doi.org/10.1177/1362361320947513

Rosales-Ruiz, J., & Baer, D. M. (1997). Behavioral cusps: A developmental and pragmatic concept for behavior analysis. *Journal of Applied Behavioral Analysis, 30*(3), 533–544.

Ruiz-Primo, M. A. (2011). Informal formative assessment: The role of instructional dialogues in assessing students' learning. *Studies in Educational Evaluation, 37*(1), 15–24. https://doi.org/10.1016/j.stueduc.2011.04.003

Rush, D. D., & Shelden, M. L. L. (2020). *The early childhood coaching handbook*. Paul H. Brookes Publishing Co.

Rutherford, M., Baxter, J., Grayson, Z., Johnston, L., & O'Hare, A. (2020). Visual supports at home and in the community for individuals with autism spectrum disorders: A scoping review. *Autism, 24*(2), 447–469. https://doi.org/10.1177/1362361319871756

Sala, G., Hooley, M., Attwood, T., Mesibov, G., & Stokes, M. (2019). Autism and intellectual disability: A systematic review of sexuality and relationship education. *Sexuality and Disability, 37*, 353–382.

Sam, A. (2016). Antecedent-Based Intervention (ABI). EBP Brief Packet. *National Professional Development Center on Autism Spectrum Disorders.*

Sam, A., & AFIRM Team. (2015a). *Prompting.* Chapel Hill, NC: National Professional Development Center on Autism Spectrum Disorder, FPG Child Development Center, University of North Carolina. Retrieved from http://afirm.fpg.unc.edu/prompting

Sam, A., & AFIRM Team. (2015b). *Visual supports.* Chapel Hill, NC: National Professional Development Center on Autism Spectrum Disorder, FPG Child Development Center, University of North Carolina. Retrieved from http:// afirm.fpg.unc.edu/visual-supports

Savage, M. N., & AFIRM Team. (2017). *Differential reinforcement.* Chapel Hill, NC: National Professional Development Center on Autism Spectrum Disorder, FPG Child Development Center, University of North Carolina. Retrieved from http://afirm.fpg.unc.edu/differential-reinforcement

Sancho, K., Sidener, T. M., Reeve, S. A., & Sidener, D. W. (2010). Two variations of video modeling interventions for teaching play skills to children with autism. *Education and Treatment of Children, 33,* 421–442.

Semrud-Clikeman, M. (2007). *Social competence in children.* Springer Science + Business Media.

Sigman, M., Dijamco, A., Gratier, M., & Rozga, A. (2004). Early detection of core deficits in autism. *Mental retardation and developmental disabilities research reviews, 10*(4), 221–233.

Steinbrenner, J. R., Hume, K., Odom, S. L., Morin, K. L., Nowell, S. W., Tomaszewski, B., Szendrey, S., McIntyre, N. S., Yücesoy-Özkan, S., & Savage, M. N. (2020). *Evidence-based practices for children, youth, and young adults with Autism.* The University of North Carolina at Chapel Hill, Frank Porter Graham Child Development Institute, National Clearinghouse on Autism Evidence and Practice Review Team.

Stichter, J. P., Herzog, M. J., Visovsky, K., Schmidt, C., Randolph, J., Schultz, T., & Gage, N. (2010). Social competence intervention for youth with Asperger syndrome and high-functioning autism: An initial investigation. *Journal of Autism and Developmental Disorders, 40,* 1067–1079.

Sulaimani, & Gut, D. M. (2019). Hidden curriculum in a special education context: T case of individuals with Autism. *Journal of Educational Research and Practice, 9*(1), 30–39. https://doi.org/10.5590/JERAP.2019.09.1.03

Sung, C., Connor, A., Chen, J., Lin, C.-C., Kuo, H.-J., & Chun, J. (2019). Development, feasibility, and preliminary efficacy of an employment-related social skills intervention for young adults with high-functioning autism. *Autism, 23*(6), 1542–1553. https://doi.org/10.1177/1362361318801345

Trevisan, D., Roberts, N., Lin, C., & Birmingham, E. (2017). How do adults and teens with self-declared Autism spectrum disorder experience eye contact? A qualitative analysis of first-hand accounts. *PloS One,* 12(11), e0188446–e0188446. https://doi.org/10.1371/journal.pone.0188446

Whalen, C., Moss, D., Ilan, A. B., Vaupel, M., Fielding, P., Macdonald, K., ... & Symon, J. (2010). Efficacy of TeachTown: Basics computer-assisted intervention for the intensive comprehensive autism program in Los Angeles unified school district. *Autism, 14*(3), 179–197.

White, S. W., Albano, A., Johnson, C., Kasari, C., Ollendick, T., Klin, A., Oswald, D., & Scahill, L. (2010). Development of a cognitive-behavioral intervention program to treat anxiety and social deficits in teens with high-functioning autism. *Clinical Child and Family Psychology Review, 13*(1), 77–90.

Wingenbach, T. S. H., Ashwin, C., & Brosnan, M. (2017). Diminished sensitivity and specificity at recognising facial emotional expressions of varying intensity underlie emotion-specific recognition deficits in autism spectrum disorders.

Research in Autism Spectrum Disorders, *34*, 52–61. https://doi.org/10.1016/j.rasd.2016.11.003

Wolfberg, P., DeWitt, M., Young, G. S., & Nguyen, T. (2014). Integrated play groups: Promoting symbolic play and social engagement with typical peers in children with ASD across settings. *Journal of Autism and Developmental Disorders*, *45*(3), 830–845. https://doi.org/10.1007/s10803-014-2245-0

Volkmar, F. R., Rogers, S., Paul, R., & Pelphrey, K.A. (2014). *Handbook of Autism and Pervasive Developmental Disorders. 4th ed.* Hoboken, NJ: John Wiley & Sons, Inc.

Zablotsky, B., Bradshaw, C. P., Anderson, C., & Law, P. A. (2013). The association between bullying and the psychological functioning of children with autism spectrum disorders. *Journal of Developmental and Behavioral Pediatrics*, *34*(1), 1–8.

Zagona, A. L., & Mastergeorge, A. M. (2018). An empirical review of peer-mediated interventions: Implications for young children with autism spectrum disorders. *Focus on Autism and Other Developmental Disabilities*, *33*(3), 131–141. https://doi.org/10.1177/1088357616671295

Zantinge, G., van Rijn, S., Stockmann, L., & Swaab, H. (2017). Physiological arousal and emotion regulation strategies in young children with Autism spectrum disorders. *Journal of Autism and Developmental Disorders*, *47*(9), 2648–2657. https://doi.org/10.1007/s10803-017-3181-6

Section III

Adolescent and Young Adult Years

Chapter 11

Self-Determination in School and Community

Karrie A. Shogren,[1] Sheida K. Raley,[1] Ben Edwards,[1] and Michael L. Wehmeyer[1]
[1]University of Kansas

Self-Determination in School and Community

Self-determination has received significant attention in the disability field since the early 1990s, particularly in the context of school-based transition services to prepare young people with disabilities for the transition from school to the community and ongoing education and employment (Ward, 1996). The impetus for the attention directed to self-determination in the transition from school to adult life was national data suggesting highly disparate post-school outcomes for young people with disabilities in employment, postsecondary education, and community participation after they exited school, compared to their peers without disabilities (Blackorby & Wagner, 1996). The simple proposal forwarded at that time was that one of the reasons that students with disabilities were not succeeding after high school was that they were not aware of or engaged in their transition planning. The 1992 amendments to the Individuals with Disabilities Education Act (IDEA) required, for the first, time that transition goals be discussed and that students with disabilities become involved in their transition planning (Wehmeyer & Ward, 1995). The emphasis on transition services and supports has remained in subsequent reauthorizations of IDEA.

Promoting and enhancing self-determination was recognized as a means of enabling students to become more engaged in their transition planning. Since the early 1990s an array of research-based practices to support student self-determination in transition planning as well as in other aspects of their education have emerged (Algozzine et al., 2001; Burke et al., 2020). Self-determination has been identified as a predictor of postschool outcomes for students with a wide range of disabilities, including autism (Mazzotti et al., 2021). Despite compelling data suggesting that promoting self-determination is an essential component of secondary special education and transition planning for students with disabilities, access to effective self-determination instruction and supports remains limited in today's schools. This is particularly true for young

DOI: 10.4324/9781003255147-14

people with autism; school-based transition and self-determination instruction has been limited (Odom et al., 2010), although there has been increased attention to the critical need to focus on the transition to adulthood for youth with autism in recent years, by multiple groups (Interagency Autism Coordinating Committee (IACC, 2017).

Young people with autism continue to have some of the most negative post-school outcomes, which have prompted a more substantial focus on promoting self-determination in transition in this population. For example, young adults with autism face particular challenges with accessing community participation supports, employment opportunities, and social networks (Hume et al., 2018; Kim, 2019). Longitudinal studies have suggested that about one third of young adults with autism are unemployed, and those that are employed often fail to maintain employment or struggle with employment over time (Taylor et al., 2015). The data highlights the need for evidence-based interventions that support young people with autism as they transition that can be delivered in schools and communities. Promoting and enhancing self-determination is key to these efforts (Shogren, Mosconi, et al., in press).

What is Self-Determination?

> *Tom is 19 years old and identifies as male and autistic. He is currently engaging in career design activities in a school-based program that supports students aged 18-22 years old. Tom's deepest desire is to become a private investigator (PI), which he always had an interest in during high school and expressed during transition planning and IEP meetings; however, he didn't know how to start working toward his goal and did not always think he had the support from his IEP team. Currently, Tom is unsure what the professional or educational requirements are to achieve his career goal of being a PI. Tom decides to talk to his family about wanting to be a PI and his family suggests that he talk to his college and career counselors from the 18-22 program to see how to go about exploring this career option. Tom sets up a time to talk to a college and career counselor and the counselor shares that there is a registry of all the PIs in Tom's town that can be found online. The college and career counselor suggests that Tom talk to one of the PIs to find out what it takes to become a PI. She also suggests that Tom learn about the different types of PIs there are and that he see if one of the local PIs would be willing to have Tom shadow him.*

The term self-determination is widely used in the disability field, and advocates with disabilities have recognized the importance of self-determination not only during the transition to adulthood, but throughout the life course to actualize the values of the disability rights and self-advocacy movements, namely the inherent right of people with disabilities to direct their own lives with the supports needed to do so (Shogren, Wehmeyer, et al., 2015; Ward, 1996). The concept of self-determination has consistently been used by advocates across disability populations to articulate their vision for their lives. Self-determination is recognized as a critical value and outcome in the autistic community. The Autistic Self-Advocacy Network (ASAN) states, "disability is a natural part of human diversity. Autism is something we are born with, and that shouldn't be changed. Autistic children should get the support they need to grow up into happy, self-determined autistic adults" (Autistic Self-Advocacy Network, n.d.).

Causal Agency Theory

Causal Agency Theory (Shogren, Wehmeyer, et al., 2015) was introduced to advance existing self-determination theories that emerged in the disability field in the late 1990s and early 2000s, namely the functional model of self-determination (Wehmeyer, 1999, 2003). To establish a clear operational definition of self-determination and a theoretical framework to inform assessment and intervention, Casual Agency Theory integrated research across education and psychology, and was guided by the perspectives of people with disabilities on the meaning of self-determination in their lives (Shogren, Abery, et al., 2015; Shogren & Broussard, 2011; Shogren & Ward, 2018). A specific focus was to determine the abilities that could support the actualization of calls from the disability community on how supports are delivered, namely shifting the focus from other-directed to self-directed actions. This shift enables people with disabilities, including youth and young adults with autism, to receive supports that empower them to use self-determination abilities and skills (e.g., decision making, problem solving, self-advocacy) and to navigate environments that are supportive (or not supportive) of self-determination.

Causal Agency Theory defines self-determination as a psychological construct within the organizing structure of theories of human agentic behavior (Shogren et al., 2017; Shogren, Wehmeyer, et al., 2015). Agentic theories recognize that humans are active contributors to, or agents of, their behavior. An agentic person engages in self-regulated and goal-directed action that leads to a sense of causal agency (Little et al., 2002). Causal Agency Theory holds that people – including people with autism and other disabilities – shape their lives and behaviors, and that this is more effective when environments are supportive and do not create barriers through ableist policies and practices.

Causal Agency Theory defines self-determination as a "dispositional characteristic manifested as acting as the causal agent in one's life" (Shogren, Wehmeyer, et al., 2015, p. 258). A *dispositional characteristic* is an enduring tendency that is expressed differently across people and time. Causal Agency Theory asserts that self-determination can be expressed in different ways and at various times across the life course and that it can be measured with variability seen across individuals and within individuals over time. The purpose of assessing self-determination should be to inform supports in the environment and identify ways to build personal capacities and skills to further enhance self-determination. Additionally, Causal Agency Theory assumes that cultural values and beliefs influence the expression of self-determination, particularly how goals are defined and actions are taken to move toward goals. Causal Agency Theory rejects the notion that there is a "right" way to engage in self-determined action, and instead presumes that with supportive environments that *all people* can determine the most effective, interdependent ways to engage in self-determined actions that embrace their values, beliefs, visions, and self and communal goals. It is critical to recognize that self-determined people identify their vision for their future and engage in self-determined actions to move toward that vision, but self-determination does not imply control over events or outcomes. In fact, actions can be self-determined even when they do not lead to the intended outcome so long as the person learns more about themselves and their goals and visions for the future. Self-determination, therefore, is not an end, but a continuously evolving process.

Engaging in self-determined *action* is central to becoming self-determined, and Causal Agency Defines three key self-determined actions – *volitional action, agentic action,* and *action-control beliefs.* The three self-determined actions refer not to specific actions, but to the *function* the action serves for the person; that is, whether the action enabled the person to act as a causal agent. Volitional actions are defined by self-initiation and autonomy; this involves making intentional, conscious choices based on one's preferences. Agentic actions are defined by self-regulation, self-direction, and pathways thinking; when acting agentically a person is working towards their goals, self-directing their actions, and identifying and navigating pathways to make progress. Action-control beliefs reflect each person's beliefs about the relationship between their actions and the outcomes they experience, or their control expectancies; when a person has adaptive action-control beliefs they can act with self-awareness and self-knowledge in an empowered, and goal-directed way.

The three self-determined actions emerge across the life course as children and adolescents learn abilities, skills, and attitudes that enable them

Table 11.1 Self-Determined Action as Defined by Causal Agency Theory

Self-determined actions	Abilities and Attitudes	Skills
Volitional action (Decide)	Autonomy Self-initiation Inhibitory control	Choice making Decision making Goal setting
Agentic action (Act)	Self-regulation Self-direction Pathways thinking Cognitive flexibility	Self-management (e.g., self-monitoring, self-evaluation) Planning Goal attainment Problem solving Self-advocacy
Action-control beliefs (Believe)	Psychological empowerment Self-realization Control expectancy	Self-awareness Self-knowledge

Note: Copyright 2021 Kansas University Center on Developmental Disabilities.

to be causal agents in their lives. Table 11.1 highlights key abilities and skills that are associated with self-determined actions. Young people grow in their self-determination as they have opportunities to develop the abilities and skills shown in Table 11.1. Transition planning provides a context for learning self-determination abilities, skills, and attitudes, accessing opportunities for self-determined actions and building the supports that will enable progress toward self-directed goals.

Importance of Promoting Self-Determination

Tom sets out to learn what it takes to become a private investigator (PI) and works with his college and career counselor to learn more about what a career as PI would look like. His college and career counselor recently learned about an evidence-based intervention designed to promote self-determination, the Self-Determined Learning Model of Instruction (SDLMI) and thinks Tom would benefit from using the SDLMI to set and work toward a goal to become a PI. The SDLMI provides a framework for Tom to grow in his self-determination abilities while determining if a career as a PI is the goal he wants to pursue, or if he wants to adjust his goal as he learns more. In SDLMI Phase 1: Set a Goal, Tom decides to set a goal to learn three new things about the requirements for becoming a PI and find out about the different types of PI so he can decide what type he wants to be. In SDLMI Phase 2: Take Action, Tom

*creates his action plan to set aside time to research PI profes-
sional requirements and the different types of PI focus areas.
As he creates his action plan, Tom identifies some potential
barriers like finding it difficult to not get anxious as he is researching with all of the information he might find. To identify
a solution to remove this barrier, Tom talks to his family and
his 18-22 year program college and career counselor, and they
come up with a plan where Tom makes a deadline for himself
to research online in 15 minute increments over an hour for a
couple of days, and if he has done so, he will reward himself
with a Frappuccino from his favorite local coffee shop.*

*After implementing his action plan and self-evaluating what
he has learned in SDLMI Phase 3: Adjust Goal or Plan, Tom
now knows that there are over 35 types of PIs, including arson,
computer forensics, legal, corporate, financial, and insurance.
Tom decides he wants to become a criminal private investigator, whose job is similar to a detective, investigating criminal
acts in order to bring evidence forward at a trial. Tom also finds
out that one of the hard and fast requirements for becoming
a PI is a high school degree. He also learns that being a PI
requires having a license in every state except Alaska, Idaho,
Mississippi, South Dakota, and Wyoming, and that he must be
at least 21 years of age (in some states 25) and possess U.S. citizenship or residency. For his next SDLMI goal, Tom decides
he wants to find a PI in his area who is a criminal PI so he can
learn how they started their career and perhaps see if he can get
an internship or job.*

Promoting the self-determination of youth and young adults with disabilities is important for several reasons. First, there is ample research
to show that if provided adequate instruction, youth with disabilities can become more self-determined. A recent meta-analysis of self-
determination interventions identified a range of strategies that can be
used to teach key self-determination skills and abilities (e.g., problem-
solving skills, decision-making skills, goal-setting and attainment skills,
self-advocacy skills, self-management skills) (Burke et al., 2020). And,
specific instructional approaches that target multiple self-determination
skills like the *Self-Determined Learning Model of Instruction* (SDLMI;
Shogren, Raley, et al., 2018) have their basis in strong research in transition planning (Hagiwara et al., 2017). Researchers have found that
the SDLMI leads to positive student outcomes, including enhanced self-
determination (Raley, Shogren, et al., 2021; Shogren, Burke, et al., 2019),

access to the general education curriculum for students with disabilities (Agran et al., 2001; Shogren et al., 2012), and academic- and transition-related goal attainment (Shogren, Burke, et al., in press; Shogren, Hicks, Raley, et al., in press; Shogren et al., 2012).

Importance of Promoting Student Involvement

> *With support from his family and the rest of his IEP team, Tom takes several steps to be more active in his next IEP by presenting his strengths and advocating for his support needs. He decides he wants to create a presentation that highlights what he has learned during his first year in the 18-22 program and his progress on his first SDLMI goal focused on having the career he wants as a PI. During his presentation, Tom feels comfortable sharing with his IEP team that he deals with social anxiety and needs support approaching new social situations. He describes how practicing role-playing in the various types of social situations he might encounter, talking on the telephone, and introducing himself to people helps a lot. By working with his college and career counselor, Tom learns various "tools" and options he has when in social interactions that can support him as he pursues a career as a PI.*

IDEA requires that students ages 16 must receive transition services, including supports to develop and take steps toward goals to promote the movement from school to college, vocational training, employment, and community living. IDEA also requires that if transition services are discussed at the IEP meeting, the student receiving special education services must be invited to the meeting. Since the IEP of every student ages 16 and over must include transition services, then technically, every student aged 16 and over must be invited to the IEP meeting. Further, the transition services definition in IDEA highlights that transition services should be based on student needs, taking into account student interests and preferences. These amendments, referred to as the student-involvement requirements in IDEA, established the importance of student involvement in transition planning. This creates a natural context to promote self-determination and enable students to self-direct their IEP meeting and their transition goals, with supports from their IEP and transition planning team.

Researchers have documented a number of benefits of active student involvement in transition planning, including enhanced self-determination and student participation (Martin et al., 2006; Shogren, Hicks, Burke, et al., in press). However, there is often a disconnect between professionals approaches to promoting self-determination in the context of student involvement in transition planning (Dean, Kirby, et al., 2021). Scott and colleagues (2021) interviewed Black youth with intellectual and developmental disabilities and their families about opportunities for self-determination during transition planning. Both youth and families expressed that schools were not always respectful of students' and families' values and needs. Youth especially emphasized the importance of having teachers who understood and empowered them to use their voices to self-advocate (Scott et al., 2021).

Self-Determination and Students with Autism

Early research on self-determination tended to focus broadly on students who received special education services or targeted youth with intellectual disability or learning disabilities (Burke et al., 2020; Hagiwara et al., 2017). However, there is a growing body of work focused on self-determination and young people with autism, given data suggesting that adolescents with autism not only experience disparities in postschool outcomes, but also disparities in self-determination outcomes (Shogren, Shaw, et al., 2018). Such work has emphasized the power of self-determination interventions for supporting self-determination and goal directed actions in young people with autism (Dean et al., in press; Dean, Hagiwara, et al., 2021) as well as the growing research-base on effective self-determination supports for young people with autism (Morán et al., in press; Shogren & Wehmeyer, 2018).

The SDLMI, for example, has been identified as a potential way to deliver and personalize self-determination intervention for students with varying disabilities and support needs (Hagiwara et al., 2017), including young people with autism (Shogren, Mosconi, et al., in press). Research studies are currently underway that address the needs of young people with autism during self-determination intervention in school and community-based settings, as well as ways to combine interventions like the SDLMI with other evidence-based practices and supports in autism, like peer supports. A strong focus has been on ensuring that evidence-based practices in autism (Hume et al., 2021) are infused through the SDLMI intervention delivery. A guide for SDLMI implementers, created in partnership with autistic advocates and professionals in the autism field, highlights ways that specific evidence-based supports (i.e., modeling, prompting, self-management, visual supports) and best practices (i.e., commitment to neurodiversity, focus on high expectations) in autism can be used to enhance engagement in the SDLMI in school and community settings for young people with autism (Raley, Wallisch, et al., 2021). This guide of strategies for SDLMI implementers also highlights that although evidence-based supports and best practices are particularly useful when implementing the SDLMI with students with autism, decisions about strategies and supports should be based on each individual student's needs, preferences, and priorities.

Promoting the Self-Determination of Youth and Young Adults with Autism: Practical Strategies

In the following sections, we highlight research-based self-determination assessment and intervention approaches that can be used to support young people with autism as they transition from school to the community.

Assessing Self-Determination

> When Tom's college and career counselor was trained to use the SDLMI, he also learned about the Self-Determination Inventory: Student Report [SDI:SR]) that is designed to inform SDLMI implementation. Tom's college and career counselor shared that Tom can take the SDI:SR and use the SDI:SR results to direct his goal development, including his IEP and transition planning goals. The counselor highlighted how they could use information from the SDI:SR to inform his identification of goals and the steps he wants to take as he explores careers during his transition to adulthood. Tom takes the SDI:SR and learns that he has strengths in the areas of Decide and Believe, and Act is an area for growth. After talking over his SDI Report with his college and career counselor, Tom reflects that Decide and Believe are probably strengths because he is excited about setting goals for his future and likes to do that with support from his family. He also thinks that using deadlines to motivate himself might support him in implementing his action plan, and that, in doing so, he can give himself an extra incentive (treat himself from a coffee shop, reward himself with an hour or so of TV, or make his own "trophies" or plaques to celebrate his achievement).

The Self-Determination Inventory System (SDIS; Shogren & Wehmeyer, 2017) was developed to assess the self-determination people with and without disabilities across the life course. The SDIS is aligned with Causal Agency Theory and leverages technology to enhance delivery and accessibility options. It also provides more immediate feedback to students, families, teachers, and researchers. The SDIS includes a suite of measures designed to collect data from youth and adults, including youth and young adults with autism and their teachers and family members (SDI: Student Report [SDI:SR]), parents and teachers (SDI: Parent/Teacher Report [SDI:PTR]), and adults (SDI: Adult Report [SDI:AR]). The SDIS was developed for people with and without disabilities, which allows for self-determination assessment in inclusive settings as well as the identification of disparities across different groups. For example, researchers have found that young people with autism tend to score lower on the SDI:SR than students without disability labels and with other disabilities labels, like learning disabilities (Shogren, Shaw, et al., 2018). This highlights the importance of creating opportunities for self-determination during the transition to adulthood for adolescents with autism.

The SDI includes 21 items that are rated in a customized, online platform using a slider scale that the computer scores between 0 (Disagree) and 99 (Agree). The custom online system includes embedded accessibility features (e.g., in-text definitions, audio playback). An overall self-determination score, as well as scores for the self-determined actions defined by Causal Agency Theory (i.e., volitional action, agentic action, action-control beliefs), are automatically calculated and provided to users via a user-friendly report and saved in a secure data management system for tracking and analysis. After completing a measure within the SDIS, adolescents, parents/teachers, or adults receive an automatic report that describes strengths and areas for growth. The report uses user-friendly language aligned with each of three self-determined actions: Decide (volitional action), Act (agentic action), and Believe (action-control beliefs). The SDI Report Guide provides specific recommendations on how people can strengthen self-determined actions across school, home, and community environments.

The SDI can be accessed at www.self-determination.org and is currently available in English, Spanish, and American Sign Language. Table 11.2 provides a sample of items from the SDI:SR and Figure 11.1 shows a sample SDI Report.

Table 11.2 Alignment of Causal Agency Theory and SDI:SR Items

Self-Determined Action	Sample SDI:SR items
Volitional Action (Decide)	I choose activities I want to do. I look for new experiences I think I will like.
Agentic Action (Act)	I think of more than one way to solve a problem. I think about each of my goals. I have what it takes to reach my goals.
Action-Control Beliefs (Believe)	I keep trying even after I get something wrong. I know my strengths.

Note. SDI:SR = *Self-Determination Inventory: Student* Report. Copyright 2021 Kansas University Center on Developmental Disabilities.

MY SELF-DETERMINATION INVENTORY

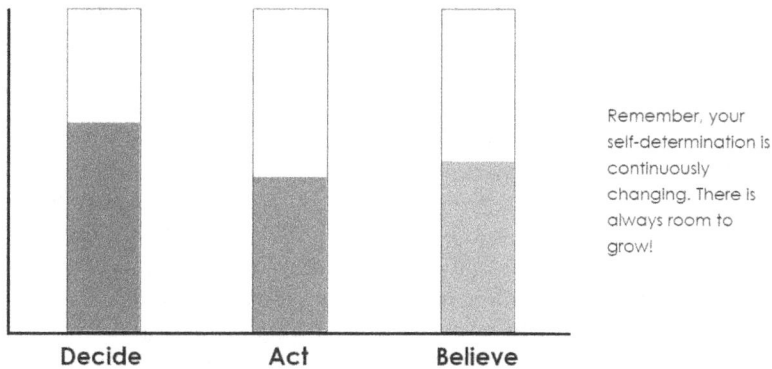

Remember, your self-determination is continuously changing. There is always room to grow!

Decide   Act   Believe

Figure 11.1 SDI:SR Report Results.

Resources have also been created, like the SDI:SR 3-2-1 Snapshot (see Figure 11.2) that students, teachers, and families can complete together to guide self-determination instruction. This can be a time for students, teachers, and families to discuss their ratings on the SDI, as researchers have found low correlations between student and teacher ratings, with greater discrepancies for students with disabilities and from other marginalized identities (Shogren, Shaw, et al., 2018). These conversations can be critical to developing shared understandings of self-determination, particularly as interventions are personalized and implemented based on student needs.

Promoting Self-Determination: The Self-Determined Learning Model of Instruction

After achieving this first SDLMI goal focused on learning three new things about the requirements for becoming a PI and finding out about the different types of PI as well as sharing his progress with his IEP team, Tom uses the SDLMI for a second cycle and in Phase 1: Set a Goal, he decides he wants to set a new goal focused on looking up online PI training courses, one of the requirements to get a PI license which he learned in his first SDLMI cycle. In Phase 2: Take Action, Tom decides that he will use the strategies he learned in his first cycle of the SDLMI (e.g., researching online in 15 minute increments, rewarding himself after completing action steps) to remove barriers, demonstrating his self-awareness and self-knowledge growth as he uses the SDLMI iteratively. Also, because sharing his progress with IEP team members went so well during the first cycle of the SDLMI, Tom decides that part of his action plan will be sharing his progress more regularly with his family members and college and career counselor as we he works toward this new goal so they can support him in taking steps toward his long-term of becoming a PI. When Tom self-evaluates his progress in Phase 3: Adjust Goal or Plan, he reflects that he made some progress toward his goal focused on looking up online PI training courses; however, he felt quite anxious when learning how many hours he would have to be online (e.g., 20+ hours) and, after discussing what he learned with his college and career counselor and family, he also now thinks that an in-person training course would be more engaging for him than an online course. Overall, Tom feels good about what he has learned about himself through using the SDLMI, is excited about taking the SDI:SR again to see if he has grown in Decide, Act, and Believe based on his SDI Report, and feels like he is on his way of becoming a criminal PI.

The SDLMI is a model of instruction designed to enable trained facilitators (e.g., general or special educators, related service providers, family members, self-advocates) to teach self-regulated problem-solving skills. The SDLMI has been used during transition planning (Burke et al., in press), as is the focus of this chapter, as well as in inclusive academic classes to support students with and without disabilities in setting academic goals (Raley et al., 2018; Raley et al., 2020) and in the community to guide career design and development of youth with autism (Dean, Hagiwara, et al., 2021). The goal of the SDLMI is to engage people in directing their goal setting and attainment by learning the steps necessary to identify goals, develop action plans, and evaluate attainment, solving problems and navigating barriers encountered along the way. This approach differs from how instruction and supports are typically provided in the secondary transition field, where there has been a strong and historic focus on other-directedness in goal setting and action planning. The SDLMI focuses on shifting this model, providing the person with autism supports rooted in high expectations to direct the learning process toward goals that are important in their life. The SDLMI is also designed to be used repeatedly, supporting young people with autism to explore

SDLMI

Self-Determined Learning
Model of Instruction

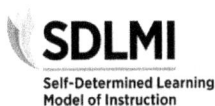

My SDI:SR on _____(*date*): A self-determination **3-2-1** snapshot

3 What are **3 actions** I can take by _____(*day/date*) **to improve my self-determination?**

DECIDE **What it means to me:**	One **action** I can take to grow:
ACT **What it means to me:**	One **action** I can take to grow:
BELIEVE **What it means to me:**	One **action** I can take to grow:

2 What are **2 self-determination skills** (like decision making, goal setting) **I want to make stronger?**

Skill: _____ **What this skill looks like for me:**	One way I will **grow** in this skill:
Skill: _____ **What this skill looks like for me:**	One way I will **grow** in this skill:

1 What is **one reflection** about discovering and developing your self-determination?

("Ah-ha!" statement, question, celebration, comment, or drawing?)

Figure 11.2 SDI:SR 3-2-1 Snapshot.

goals, learn about the steps they can take to act as causal agents, and use their past learning to revise future goals and plans for the future.

There are three distinct phases of the SDLMI (see Figure 11.3): Set a Goal (Phase 1), Take Action (Phase 2), and Adjust Goal or Plan (Phase 3). These phases directly align with Causal Agency Theory and the domains assessed on the SDI: volitional action (Decide), agentic action (Act), and

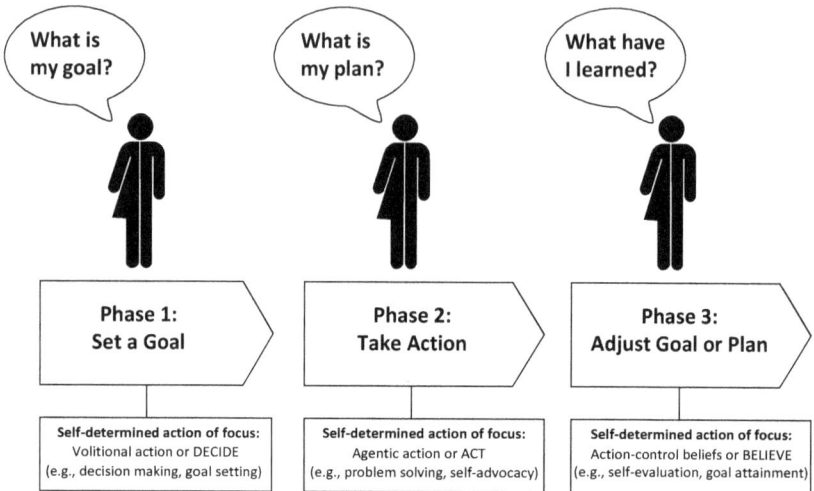

Figure 11.3 Self-Determined Learning Model of Instruction Alignment with Self-Determined Actions.

action-control beliefs (Believe). Therefore, information from the SDI can be used to identify critical SDLMI Educational Supports based on each student's past learning and experiences. In each SDLMI phase, students are supported to solve an overall problem (Phase 1: What is my goal?; Phase 2: What is my plan?; Phase 3: What have I learned?). There are three core components of the SDLMI and its implementation: Student Questions, Teacher Objectives, and Educational Supports. Students solve the overall question in each phase by answering a series of four Student Questions in each phase (for a total of 12 Student Questions) that support them in moving from where they are (i.e., not have a goal and a plan for achieving it) to where they want to be (i.e., achieving their goal or learning more about the goal or action plan they need to act as a causal agent). Each Student Question is associated with Teacher Objectives that provide SDLMI facilitators with a road map of what they must do to support students in answering the targeted Student Question. To meet Teacher Objectives, SDLMI facilitators utilize Educational Supports (e.g., goal-setting, decision-making, or self-scheduling instruction) to enable students to learn the abilities and skills needed to answer the Student Questions and self-direct learning (see Figure 11.4 for an overview of SDLMI and its core components).

In school settings, students typically work through the 12 SDLMI Student Questions once during an academic semester; in subsequent semesters and years students are supported to continue to build on

Self-Determined Learning Model of Instruction
Phase 1: Set a Goal
Student Problem to Solve: What is my goal?

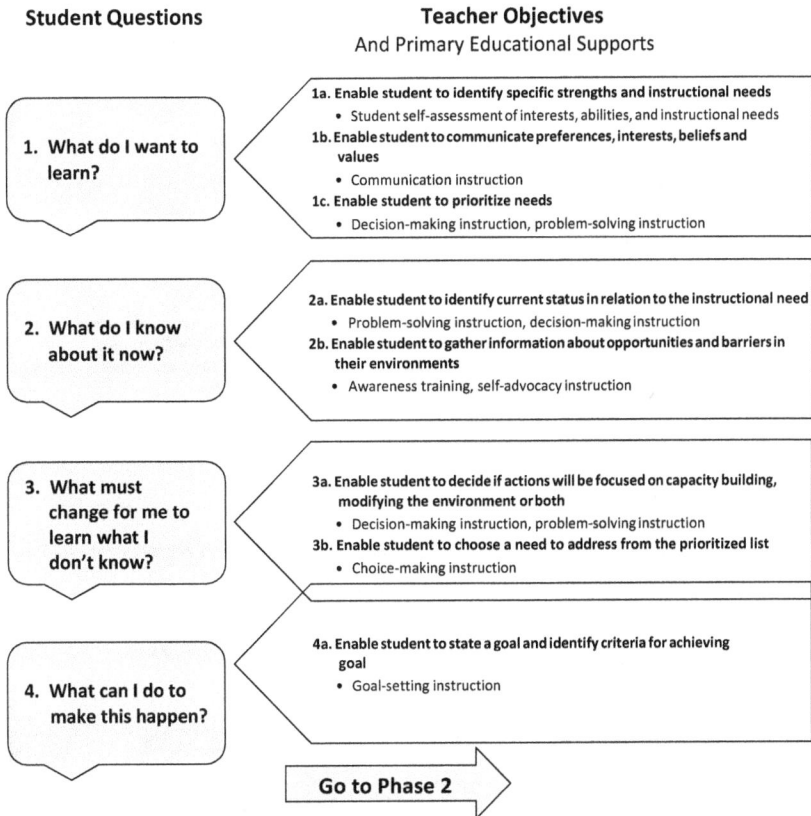

Student Questions	Teacher Objectives
	And Primary Educational Supports

1. What do I want to learn?

1a. Enable student to identify specific strengths and instructional needs
- Student self-assessment of interests, abilities, and instructional needs

1b. Enable student to communicate preferences, interests, beliefs and values
- Communication instruction

1c. Enable student to prioritize needs
- Decision-making instruction, problem-solving instruction

2. What do I know about it now?

2a. Enable student to identify current status in relation to the instructional need
- Problem-solving instruction, decision-making instruction

2b. Enable student to gather information about opportunities and barriers in their environments
- Awareness training, self-advocacy instruction

3. What must change for me to learn what I don't know?

3a. Enable student to decide if actions will be focused on capacity building, modifying the environment or both
- Decision-making instruction, problem-solving instruction

3b. Enable student to choose a need to address from the prioritized list
- Choice-making instruction

4. What can I do to make this happen?

4a. Enable student to state a goal and identify criteria for achieving goal
- Goal-setting instruction

Go to Phase 2

Figure 11.4 Self-Determined Learning Model of Instruction: Student Questions, Teacher Objectives and Educational Supports.

Note. Reprinted with permission from Shogren et al. (2018).

their learning by working through the Student Questions again to identify new or different goals and action plans. The SDLMI is considered a multicomponent intervention as it targeted multiple self-determination abilities, skills, and attitudes (see Table 11.1) simultaneously, enabling young people to grow in their causal agency and self-determination as they begin to make connections between their learning and the attainment of valued outcomes.

Self-Determined Learning Model of Instruction
Phase 2: Take Action
Student Problem to Solve: What is my plan?

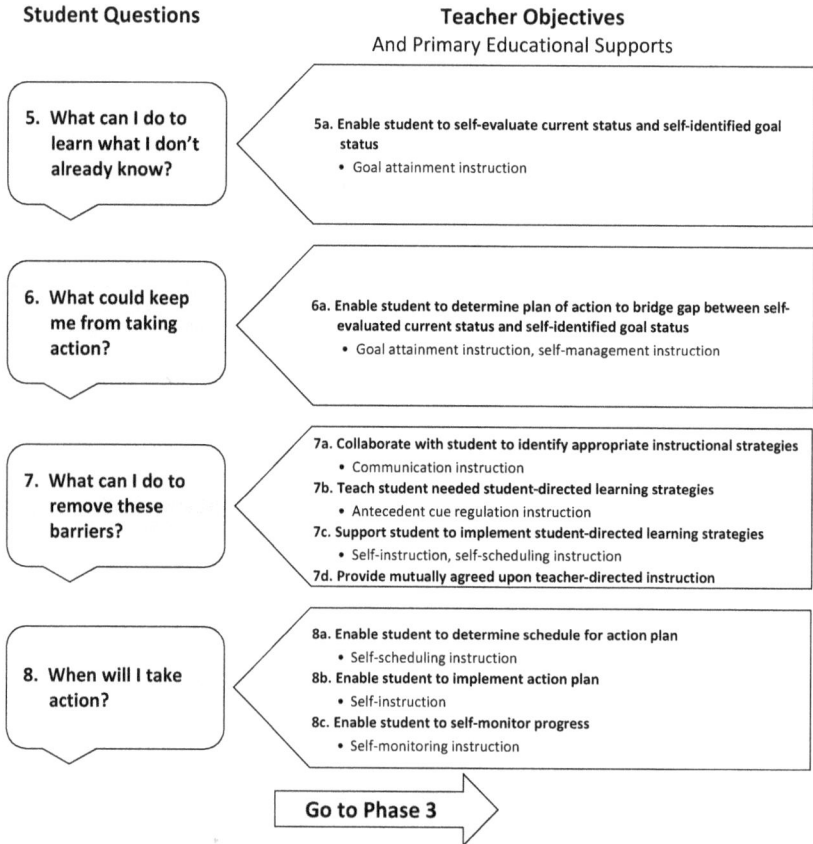

Student Questions	Teacher Objectives And Primary Educational Supports
5. What can I do to learn what I don't already know?	5a. Enable student to self-evaluate current status and self-identified goal status • Goal attainment instruction
6. What could keep me from taking action?	6a. Enable student to determine plan of action to bridge gap between self-evaluated current status and self-identified goal status • Goal attainment instruction, self-management instruction
7. What can I do to remove these barriers?	7a. Collaborate with student to identify appropriate instructional strategies • Communication instruction 7b. Teach student needed student-directed learning strategies • Antecedent cue regulation instruction 7c. Support student to implement student-directed learning strategies • Self-instruction, self-scheduling instruction 7d. Provide mutually agreed upon teacher-directed instruction
8. When will I take action?	8a. Enable student to determine schedule for action plan • Self-scheduling instruction 8b. Enable student to implement action plan • Self-instruction 8c. Enable student to self-monitor progress • Self-monitoring instruction

Go to Phase 3

Figure 11.4 (Continued)

A variety of resources are available to support trained SDLMI facilitators to deliver the SDLMI with fidelity in the classroom and community (Shogren, Raley, et al., in press). Researchers have found that with training and ongoing coaching teachers perceive themselves as able to implement the SDLMI, and that their self-perceptions of their fidelity are directly linked to self-determination outcomes (Shogren et al., 2020). SDLMI facilitators receive standardized training (visit

Self-Determined Learning Model of Instruction
Phase 3: Adjust Goal or Plan
Student Problem to Solve: What have I learned?

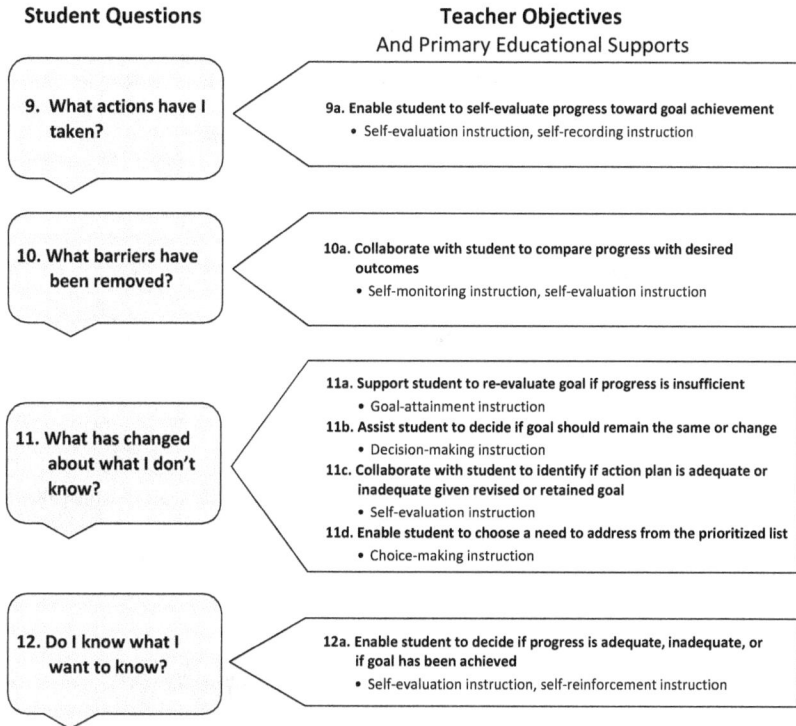

Student Questions	Teacher Objectives And Primary Educational Supports
9. What actions have I taken?	**9a. Enable student to self-evaluate progress toward goal achievement** • Self-evaluation instruction, self-recording instruction
10. What barriers have been removed?	**10a. Collaborate with student to compare progress with desired outcomes** • Self-monitoring instruction, self-evaluation instruction
11. What has changed about what I don't know?	**11a. Support student to re-evaluate goal if progress is insufficient** • Goal-attainment instruction **11b. Assist student to decide if goal should remain the same or change** • Decision-making instruction **11c. Collaborate with student to identify if action plan is adequate or inadequate given revised or retained goal** • Self-evaluation instruction **11d. Enable student to choose a need to address from the prioritized list** • Choice-making instruction
12. Do I know what I want to know?	**12a. Enable student to decide if progress is adequate, inadequate, or if goal has been achieved** • Self-evaluation instruction, self-reinforcement instruction

Did I finish my goal? *Please mark in the bubble*   ◯ Yes ◯ No

If YES
How did I feel about the results? _____
Now I will go back to Phase 1 and set a new goal.
If NO
I will look back at Phase 1 again. If the goal is still a good one for me, I will move on to Phase 2 to revise my plan **OR** I can rewrite my same goal or change it to a new goal.

Note. Reprinted with permission from Shogren et al. (2018).

Figure 11.4 (Continued)

www.self-determination.org for online resources and more information) and there is an array of implementation supports, including the SDLMI Teacher's Guide (Shogren, Raley, et al., 2018) which provides key guidelines for infusing the model into instruction. Further, a variety of additional resources are available including resources specific to students with autism (Raley, Wallisch, et al., 2021), strategies to make the Student Questions accessible for students with complex communication needs (Shogren & Burke, 2019) as well as strategies to use the SDLMI to engage students in transition planning (Burke et al., 2019) and in inclusive general education classrooms (Raley et al., 2018; Shogren, Raley, et al., 2019). Overall, the SDLMI has wide applicability for adolescents with autism, and provides an evidence-based practice to support students with autism and other disabilities to grow in their self-determination and their goal attainment across multiple life domains relevant to the transition from school to the community.

Conclusion

An ever-expanding body of research documents that promoting and enhancing self-determination during the transition from school to the community leads to enhanced outcomes. However, self-determination assessment and intervention must be integrated into broader efforts to create systems of supports for young people with autism that address the continued, highly disparate post-school outcomes. Ongoing work is needed to integrate evidence-based supports for young people with autism into self-determination instruction and to ensure effective systems of supports that respect and value the cultural identities of young people with autism, enabling them to go after their goals, dreams, and visions for their future across the life course.

References

Agran, M., Blanchard, C., Wehmeyer, M. L., & Hughes, C. (2001). Teaching students to self-regulate their behavior: The differential effects of student- vs. teacher-delivered reinforcement. *Research in Developmental Disabilities*, 22(4), 319–332. www.elsevier.com/inca/publications/store/8/2/6/

Algozzine, B., Browder, D., Karvonen, M., Test, D. W., & Wood, W. M. (2001). Effects of interventions to promote self-determination for individuals with disabilities. *Review of Educational Research, 71*, 219–277. https://doi.org/ 10.3102/00346543071002219

Autistic Self-Advocacy Network. (n.d.). Changing how people think about autism. https://autisticadvocacy.org/about-asan/position-statements/

Blackorby, J., & Wagner, M. (1996). Longitudinal postschool outcomes of youth with disabilities: Findings from the National Longitudinal Transition Study. *Exceptional Children, 62*, 399–413.

Burke, K. M., Raley, S. K., Shogren, K. A., Hagiwara, M., Mumbardó-Adam, C., Uyanik, H., & Behrens, S. (2020). A meta-analysis of interventions to promote self-determination for students with disabilities. *Remedial and Special Education, 41*(3), 176–188. https://doi.org/10.1177/074193251 8802274

Burke, K. M., Shogren, K. A., Antosh, A. A., LaPlante, T., & Masterson, L. H. (2019). Implementing the SDLMI with students with significant support needs during transition planning. *Career Development and Transition for Exceptional Individuals, 43*(2), 115–121. https://doi.org/10.1177/216514341 9887858

Burke, K. M., Shogren, K. A., Raley, S. K., Wehmeyer, M. L., Antosh, A. A., & LaPlante, T. (in press). Implementing evidence-based practices to promote self-determination: Lessons learned from a state-wide implementation of the Self-Determined Learning Model of Instruction. *Education and Training in Autism and Developmental Disabilities.*

Dean, E. E., Burke, K. M., & Shogren, K. A. (in press). Understanding career design goals set by youth with autism spectrum disorder. *American Journal of Occupational Therapy.*

Dean, E. E., Hagiwara, M., Shogren, K. A., Wehmeyer, M. L., & Shrum, J. (2021). Promoting Career Design in Youth and Young Adults with ASD: A Feasibility Study. *Journal of Autism and Developmental Disorders.* https://doi.org/10.1007/s10803-021-05146-x

Dean, E. E., Kirby, A. V., Hagiwara, M., Shogren, K. A., Ersan, D. T., & Brown, S. (2021). Family role in the development of self-determination for youth with intellectual and developmental disabilities: A scoping review. *Intellectual and Developmental Disabilities, 59*(4), 315–334. https://doi.org/10.1352/1934-9556-59.4.315

Hagiwara, M., Shogren, K., & Leko, M. (2017). Reviewing research on the Self-Determined Learning Model of Instruction: Mapping the terrain and charting a course to promote adoption and use. *Advances in Neurodevelopmental Disorders, 1*, 3–13. https://doi.org/10.1007/s41252-017-0007-7

Hume, K., Dykstra Steinbrenner, J., Sideris, J., Smith, L., Kucharczyk, S., & Szidon, K. (2018). Multi-informant assessment of transition-related skills and skill importance in adolescents with autism spectrum disorder. *Autism, 22*, 40–50.

Hume, K., Steinbrenner, J. R., Odom, S. L., Morin, K. L., Nowell, S. W., Tomaszewski, B., Szendrey, S., McIntyre, N. S., Yücesoy-Özkan, S., & Savage, M. N. (2021). Evidence-Based Practices for Children, Youth, and Young Adults with Autism: Third Generation Review. *Journal of Autism and Developmental Disorders.* https://doi.org/10.1007/s10803-020-04844-2

Interagency Autism Coordinating Committee (IACC). (2017). *2016-2017 IACC Strategic Plan for Autism Spectrum Disorder.* U.S. Department of Health and Human Services.

Kim, S. Y. (2019). The experiences of adults with autism spectrum disorder: Self-determination and quality of life. *Research in Autism Spectrum Disorders, 60*, 1–15. https://doi.org/https://doi.org/10.1016/j.rasd.2018.12.002

Little, T. D., Hawley, P. H., Henrich, C. C., & Marsland, K. W. (2002). Three views of the agentic self: A developmental synthesis. In E. L. Deci & R. M. Ryan (Eds.), *Handbook of self-determination research* (pp. 389–404). University of Rochester Press.

Martin, J. E., van Dycke, J. L., Christensen, W. R., Greene, B. A., Gardner, J. E., & Lovett, D. L. (2006). Increasing student participation in IEP meetings: Establishing the self-directed IEP as an evidenced-based practice. *Exceptional Children*, 72, 299–316.

Mazzotti, V. L., Rowe, D. A., Kwiatek, S., Voggt, A., Chang, W.-H., Fowler, C. H., Poppen, M., Sinclair, J., & Test, D. W. (2021). Secondary Transition Predictors of Postschool Success: An Update to the Research Base. *Career Development and Transition for Exceptional Individuals*, 44(1), 47–64. https://doi.org/10.1177/2165143420959793

Morán, M. L., Hagiwara, M., Raley, S. K., Alsaaed, A. H., Shogren, K. A., Qian, X., Gómez, L. E., & Alcedo, M. A. (in press). Self-determination of students with autism spectrum disorder: a systematic review. *Journal of Developmental and Physical Disabilities*.

Odom, S. L., Boyd, B., Hall, L. J., & Hume, K. (2010). Evaluation of comprehensive treatment models for individuals with autism spectrum disorders. *Journal of Autism and Developmental Disorders*, 40(425–436). https://doi.org/0.1007/s10803-009-0825-1

Raley, S. K., Shogren, K. A., & McDonald, A. (2018). How to implement the Self-Determined Learning Model of Instruction in inclusive general education classrooms. *Teaching Exceptional Children*, 51(1), 62–71. https://doi.org/10.1177/0040059918790236

Raley, S. K., Shogren, K. A., Rifenbark, G. G., Lane, K. L., & Pace, J. R. (2021). The Impact of the Self-Determined Learning Model of Instruction on Student Self-Determination in Inclusive, Secondary Classrooms. *Remedial and Special Education*, 42(6), 363–373. https://doi.org/10.1177/0741932520984842

Raley, S. K., Shogren, K. A., Rifenbark, G. G., Thomas, K., McDonald, A. F., & Burke, K. M. (2020). Enhancing secondary students' goal attainment and self-determination in general education mathematics classes using the Self-Determined Learning Model of Instruction. *Advances in Neurodevelopmental Disorders*, 4(2), 155–167. https://doi.org/10.1007/s41252-020-00152-z

Raley, S. K., Wallisch, A., Shogren, K. A., & Boyd, B. (2021). *SDLMI Teacher's Guide Supplement: Supporting Students with Autism and Related Developmental Disabilities to Engage with the SDLMI*. Kansas University Center on Developmental Disabilities.

Scott, L. A., Thoma, C. A., Gokita, T., Bruno, L., Ruiz, A. B., Brendli, K., ... & Vitullo, V. (2021). I'm Trying to Make Myself Happy: Black Students With Intellectual and Developmental Disabilities and Families on Promoting Self-Determination During Transition. *Inclusion*, 9(3), 170–188.

Shogren, K. A., Abery, B., Antosh, A., Broussard, R., Coppens, B., Finn, C., Goodman, A., Harris, C., Knapp, J., Martinis, J., Neeman, A., Nelis, T., & Wehmeyer, M. L. (2015). Recommendations of the self-determination and self-advocacy strand from the National Goals 2015 conference. *Inclusion*, 3(4), 205–210. https://doi.org/10.1352/2326-6988-3.4.205

Shogren, K. A., & Broussard, R. (2011, Apr). Exploring the perceptions of self-determination of individuals with intellectual disability. *Intellectual and Developmental Disabilities*, 49(2), 86–102. https://doi.org/10.1352/1934-9556-49.2.86

Shogren, K. A., & Burke, K. M. (2019). *Teacher's Guide Supplement: Supporting Students with Complex Communication Needs to Engage with the SDLMI*. Kansas University Center on Developmental Disabilities.

Shogren, K. A., Burke, K. M., Anderson, M. A., Antosh, A. A., LaPlante, T., & Hicks, T. A. (2020). Examining the relationship between teacher perceptions of implementation of the SDLMI and student self-determination outcomes. *Career Development and Transition for Exceptional Individuals, 43*(1), 53–63. https://doi.org/10.1177/2165143419887855

Shogren, K. A., Burke, K. M., Antosh, A. A., Wehmeyer, M. L., LaPlante, T., Shaw, L. A., & Raley, S. K. (2019). Impact of the Self-Determined Learning Model of Instruction on self-determination and goal attainment in adolescents with intellectual disability. *Journal of Disability Policy Studies, 30*, 22–34. https://doi.org/10.1177/1044207318792178

Shogren, K. A., Burke, K. M., Antosh, A. A., Wehmeyer, M. L., LaPlante, T., Shaw, L. A., & Raley, S. K. (in press). Impact of the Self-Determined Learning Model of Instruction on self-determination and goal attainment in adolescents with intellectual disability. *Journal of Disability Policy Studies.* https://doi.org/10.1177/1044207318792178

Shogren, K. A., Hicks, T. A., Burke, K. M., Antosh, A. A., LaPlante, T., & Anderson, M. H. (in press). Examining the impact of the SDLMI and Whose Future Is It? over a two-year period with students with intellectual disability. *American Journal on Intellectual and Developmental Disabilities.*

Shogren, K. A., Hicks, T. A., Raley, S. K., Pace, J. R., Rifenbark, G. G., & Lane, K. L. (in press). Student and Teacher Perceptions of Goal Attainment During Intervention With the Self-Determined Learning Model of Instruction. *The Journal of Special Education.* https://doi.org/10.1177/0022466920950264

Shogren, K. A., Mosconi, M. W., Raley, S. K., Dean, E. E., Edwards, B., Wallisch, A., Boyd, B., & Kiblen, J. C. (in press). Approaches for advancing the personalization of assessment and intervention in young adults with autism by targeting self-determination and executive processes. *Autism in Adulthood.*

Shogren, K. A., Palmer, S. B., Wehmeyer, M. L., Williams-Diehm, K., & Little, T. D. (2012). Effect of intervention with the Self-Determined Learning Model of Instruction on access and goal attainment. *Remedial and Special Education, 33*, 320–330. https://doi.org/10.1177/0741932511410072

Shogren, K. A., Raley, S. K., & Burke, K. M. (2019). *SDLMI Teacher's Guide Supplement: Implementing the SDLMI with the Whole Class.* Kansas University Center on Developmental Disabilities

Shogren, K. A., Raley, S. K., Burke, K. M., & Wehmeyer, M. L. (2018). *The Self-Determined Learning Model of Instruction: Teacher's Guide.* Kansas University Center on Developmental Disabilities.

Shogren, K. A., Raley, S. K., Rifenbark, G. G., Lane, K. L., Bojanek, E. K., Karpur, A., & Quirk, C. (in press). *The Self-Determined Learning Model of Instruction: Promoting implementation fidelity. Inclusion.*

Shogren, K. A., Shaw, L. A., Raley, S. K., & Wehmeyer, M. L. (2018). Exploring the effect of disability, race/ethnicity, and socioeconomic status on scores on the Self-Determination Inventory: Student Report. *Exceptional Children, 85*, 10–27. https://doi.org/10.1177/0014402918782150

Shogren, K. A., & Ward, M. J. (2018). Promoting and enhancing self-determination to improve the post-school outcomes of people with disabilities. *Journal of Vocational Rehabilitation, 48*(2), 187–196. https://doi.org/https://doi.org/10.3233/jvr-180935

Shogren, K. A., & Wehmeyer, M. L. (2017). *Self-Determination Inventory: Student-Report.* Kansas University Center on Developmental Disabilities.

Shogren, K. A., & Wehmeyer, M. L. (2018). *How to facilitate and support self-determination.* Pro-ED.

Shogren, K. A., Wehmeyer, M. L., & Palmer, S. B. (2017). Causal agency theory. In M. L. Wehmeyer, K. A. Shogren, T. D. Little, & S. J. Lopez (Eds.), *Handbook on the development of self-determination* (pp. 55–70). Springer.

Shogren, K. A., Wehmeyer, M. L., Palmer, S. B., Forber-Pratt, A. J., Little, T. J., & Lopez, S. (2015). Causal agency theory: Reconceptualizing a functional model of self-determination. *Education and Training in Autism and Developmental Disabilities, 50*(3), 251. https://doi.org/10.1007/978-94-024-1042-6_5

Taylor, J. L., Henninger, N. A., & Mailick, M. R. (2015). Longitudinal patterns of employment and postsecondary education for adults with autism and average-range IQ. *Autism: the international journal of research and practice, 19*(7), 785–793. https://doi.org/10.1177/1362361315585643

Ward, M. J. (1996). Coming of age in the age of self-determination: A historical and personal perspective. In D. J. Sands & M. L. Wehmeyer (Eds.), *Self-determination across the life span: Independence and choice for people with disabilities.* Paul H. Brookes.

Wehmeyer, M. L. (1999). A functional model of self-determination: Describing development and implementing instruction. *Focus on Autism and Other Developmental Disabilities, 14,* 53–61.

Wehmeyer, M. L. (2003). A functional theory of self-determination: Model overview. In M. L. Wehmeyer, B. Abery, D. E. Mithaug, & R. Stancliffe (Eds.), *Theory in self-determination: Foundations for educational practice* (pp. 182–201). Charles C. Thomas Publishing Company.

Wehmeyer, M. L., & Ward, M. J. (1995). The spirit of the IDEA mandate: Student involvement in transition planning. *The Journal for Vocational Special Needs Education, 17,* 108–111.

Chapter 12

Universal Design for Transition for Students on the Spectrum

Linking Academic and Transition Education to Improve Postschool Outcomes

Colleen A. Thoma,[1] Irina Cain,[1] Andrew Wojcik[2], Monica Grillo,[3] LaRon A. Scott,[3] and Kathryn Best[4]

[1]Virginia Commonwealth University
[2]Kings College
[3]Virginia Commonwealth University
[4]Collegiate School, Richmond, VA

Introduction

The teacher began the interview. "Yvonne, after high school, where do you want to work?" Yvonne waited before shrugging her shoulders and saying, "I don't know." The teacher persisted. "Your father works as a gardener. I hear you like growing items in the garden. Perhaps you would like to get a job at the local nursery?" Yvonne nodded her head reluctantly, and the teacher went about planning and building activities for Yvonne's to practice watering plants, measuring, writing labels, planting seeds, and transplanting plants. Yvonne didn't say anything, but deep inside she wished she didn't have to get dirty. When presented with gardening tasks, Yvonne would push the dirt with her pinky finger before running to the bathroom to wash her hands.

After observing Yvonne's reluctance, the teacher gave Yvonne a camera and asked her family to remind Yvonne to take pictures of activities and places that she found interesting. Yvonne took her camera to recreational events with the family. She amassed pictures of friends, and from stores where they shopped. The family noted that Yvonne "seemed excited" when visiting an electronics store with her brother. Her picture book contained dozens of close-up photos of computer parts from an electronic supply store. The teacher didn't recognize the images, but a representative from the computer store told

DOI: 10.4324/9781003255147-15

him they were computer parts, "These are the types of computer parts enthusiasts use to build computers. I see graphics cards, sound cards, network cards, memory chips, CPUs and coolers. Hey, we hire people that have this sort of hobby to work with our Prodigy Posse. The job pays $18.00 per hour."

When they talked to Yvonne, she nodded her head, smiled, and said, "Yes, yes, computer to game." The teacher, unfamiliar with computer assembly/repair, worked with the supply store to make a list of common jobs (e.g. upgrading memory, reimaging a disk drive, replacing a screen). The teacher built activities to engage and help Yvonne with these skills while completing her academics. For example, reading activities included "how to" guides and computer magazines. Science lessons about electricity included how to read a multimeter, and math activities included solving problems using computer programming. In Yvonne's 2nd year of high school she began apprenticing with the school technology office, and in her 3rd year of high school she started an internship with the computer parts store.

Yvonne's story illustrates how using multiple means of assessment can help a teacher to develop a program to leverage a student's interests into a post-secondary skill (in this case employment and recreation). Yvonne's teacher integrated both academic (reading, math and science) and non-academic (job skills) components to develop a comprehensive transition plan. Seamless integration of academic and transition goals can be difficult; Best et al. (2015) noted that teachers have reported struggling to include students with disabilities in the general education curriculum while preparing them for their transition to adult life (i.e. employment, independent living, vocational and training). It is for this reason that a new framework for educational planning, instructional design, and assessment was developed: Universal Design for Transition (Thoma et al., 2009).

Universal Design for Transition (UDT) is a framework for instructional design that promotes successful transitional outcomes for students with disabilities by combining academic and transition education for all students. The framework maximizes accessibility to transition services for the greatest number of individuals with needs (Scott, & Bruno, 2018). The UDT model also adopts strategies from the Universal Design from Learning framework, which promotes student achievement with educational activities that employ: (a) multiple means of engagement, (b) multiple means of representation, and (c) multiple means of action and expression (Meyer et al., 2013). Most importantly, UDT focuses on blending transition and academic education to maximize the individual's future opportunities, in accordance with their cultural identity and values. UDT helps develop a more adaptable, flexible individual who can find and utilize multiple natural supports. For example, instead of the complexity of developing individual transition supports for employment or postsecondary programs for a number of individual students, the UDT method focuses on building the student's adaptability to a variety of different environments. While these individualized experiences may ultimately be needed, they do not need to be done at the expense of teaching academic skills that can also promote and support the transition to adult life for students with disabilities.

For Yvonne, the assessment activity helped the team focus on academic and nonacademic skills development to develop Yvonne's ability to generalize problem-solving skills used to "troubleshoot" computer issues. Although her program was inspired by a computer parts store, her lessons will allow her to explore vocational training related to computer and network repair, website, application development, or something not invented as yet. To maximize the adaptability of the individual, UDT focuses on developing barrier-free transition experiences in the areas of postschool life, self-advocacy, and academic skills. Specifically, UDT helps improve the design, delivery, and assessment related to transition (Thoma et al., 2009).

Traditionally, transition services for individuals with autism spectrum disorder (ASD) have been set by a team of individuals (parents, teachers, the student, and school-based staff). The student's interests and goals were matched to "*realistic*" outcomes, and individuals were "trained" to acquire, generalize, and maintain a limited number of discrete or sequential skills customized to individual students (e.g. see Collins, 2012). For example, a student may learn to restock or organize products in a grocery store, and academic activities were limited to the skills identified as necessary for the particular job (See Thoma et al., 2009). This approach is limiting the student in both breadth of experiences and also type of skills acquired, which are based on the planners' narrow vision of what future employment might look like. Teachers, parents, and students may focus on outcomes they believe are *realistic* and attainable for the student (Ayres et al., 2011; 2012), but too often these outcomes prove to be unnecessarily limiting. In the short run, s/he might have access to community education services (e.g. gardening), but in the long-run, they might miss new opportunities (e.g. the computer class). The focus on *realistic* outcomes may prevent students with disabilities from participation in academics. UDT assumes that the *realistic* outcomes for students expand when both academic and post-secondary skills instruction takes place, and the UDT approach encourages the individual to develop a broad range of academic skills that can be applied flexibly to future situations.

UDT encourages the participation of all students in academic curriculums; the philosophy also includes and encourages instruction in functional and vocational skills. In general, UDT encourages flexibility by embracing multiple teaching methodologies and practices to promote long-term outcomes. This chapter will review the principles of Universal Design for Transition, and provide examples and details of each component.

How Does UDT Apply to Students with ASD?

Research across multiple domains reveals persons with autism spectrum disorder (ASD) experience poorer outcomes in the transition to adulthood compared with their peers without disabilities and even peers with other developmental disabilities (Friedman et al., 2013). Specific to the three domains targeted by transition services stipulated in IDEA, when compared to adults with other developmental disabilities those with ASD have the lowest rates of independent living (Braddock et al., 2017), postsecondary education participation (Newman et al., 2011), and employment. In addition, Black youth with disabilities, including ASD experience lower rates of employment, higher rates of poverty, and a greater degree of isolation than their peers (Flexer et al., 2011). In academic post-secondary settings, individuals with ASD participate at lower rates than students with other disabilities (Newman et al., 2011). Similarly, individuals with ASD and intellectual disability are more likely to be isolated from the general education environment and curriculum (Kleinert et al., 2015). In the isolated environment, the three pedagogical approaches used (a) community based instruction, (b) basic academic skills instruction, and (c) functional skills instruction have proven to be equally ineffective (Bouck, 2012).

Clearly, a different, more robust approach to transition is required (Friedman et al., 2013). The UDT framework used research to identify the conditions that create barriers or restrict flexibility for students. Also, UDT borrows the best evidence-based practices related to pedagogy, technology, and self determination to help build new higher standards for students with ASD. As an open philosophy, UDT seeks out information from a diverse group of formal and informal transition team members (like having Yvonne's family help with gathering information about her interests and goals for the future), encouraging a fuller integration of the complexities of students' identities.

UDT aims to eliminate the obstacles preventing access for students with disabilities, especially those with intersectional identities. Just as implementing a UDL framework provides an opportunity for teachers to design curriculum that is accessible to all and eliminates the need to retro-fit a number of individual accommodations, the UDT framework infuses broad transition educational goals and assessments into academic lessons.

Outcomes and High Expectations

Although our field consistently urges special educators to hold high expectations for students with disabilities, perceptions have remained that students with ASD are unable to participate in academic situations. Low expectations create a barrier to success for students with significant disabilities, including ASD, especially for culturally and linguistically diverse individuals (Kieran & Anderson, 2019). The research clearly documents low expectations as an obstacle to success for students with significant disabilities like autism and an association between outcomes and expectations has been established (see Mazzotti et al., 2021). Mazzotti and colleagues built upon prior research, continuing to document a link between parent expectations and student outcomes, and similar research has been conducted by other researchers (see Rojewski et al., 2014; Wehman et al., 2015). UDT builds on the research that encourages all students to meet high standards because they are provided with instruction designed to develop academic skills (Darling-Hammond, 2010) as well as meet their individual transition goals for the future (Best et al., 2015). UDT embraces the best practices across all environments for a variety of students, leaving space for culturally and linguistically diverse students to flourish.

Evidence Based Practices

One of the greatest obstacles to successful postsecondary academic transition continues to be the lack of consistent evidence-based practices for students with ASD across a variety of environments, particularly those born out of studies with a diverse sample of participants. Because researchers supporting students with ASD come from a variety of different disciplines (e.g. medicine, alternative communication science, psychology, rehabilitation science, and education), cross-field communication can sometimes be awkward if not confusing. Each field has different terms, different standards for evaluating evidence, and different goals. Because small samples of students are frequently studied, researchers will often cluster many studies together to get a bigger picture of the effectiveness of a strategy. In addition, it has only been recently that researchers have conducted studies designed to determine the effectiveness of educational practices for specific under-represented minority populations of students with disabilities. For example, de Bruin and colleagues (2013) found at least three approaches to be effective when they grouped single subject studies into one of three categories: (a) Consequence Based Instruction (e.g. time delay, task analytic feedback, TEACCH, Lovaas, and errorless learning),

(b) Self-management strategies (self-determination, self-monitoring, and self-reinforcement), and (c) video based strategies (e.g. video modeling). Data from this meta-analysis was not disaggregated by race/ethnicity. Although clustering can help to determine the relative effectiveness of a strategy, in the real world practitioners often need to blend, mix, and match strategies together. It is also worth noting that youth with autism experience disparities in participating in their transition planning based on their race/ethnicity status (Eilenberg et al., 2019), thus introducing more confusion in gauging the effectiveness of different approaches.

As a result of this confusion, an effective practitioner might use a combination of strategies and approaches simultaneously. For example, Agran et al. (2010) encouraged the field of special education to recognize that approaches like Self-Determination and UDL overlap, blend, and blur together. Kuhn and colleagues (2020) adapted an existing transition program using the ecological validity framework (Bernal et al., 1995) to better fit the needs of Latinx individuals with ASD, as no programs exist which are designed with culturally and linguistically diverse youth in mind. The UDT model encourages the use of a variety of strategies and views this blending as an opportunity to link academic and transition skill development by building on the UDL framework. Table 12.1 highlights the various components of the UDT model: multiple means of representation; multiple means of expression; multiple means of engagement; multiple transition domains; multiple transition assessments; self-determination; and multiple sources of information (Thoma et al., 2009), and provides guidance for how a culturally responsive approach can be infused throughout.

Component 1: Multiple Means of Representation (UDL)

The most recognizable component of both UDL and UDT frameworks is multiple means of representation, which refers to presenting instruction in multiple ways so that students with a variety of learning support needs can participate (Thoma et al., 2013).

The CAST group has identified three different types of options to consider under multiple means of representation. They include: options for perception; language/mathematical expression and symbols; and comprehension. The use of instructional technology can assist with the implementation of multiple means of representation as it provides individuals with ASD a variety of ways that material can be adapted. For example, electronic versions of text can be modified so that a student could "hear" the information, or pictures could be added to assist with comprehension, or definitions and/or symbols for keywords could be embedded in the text. In addition, links could be added to web-based content that can provide a more concrete example of the concepts

Table 12.1 Culturally Responsive Universal Design for Transition

Universal Design for Transition Domain	Transition Focus	Culturally Responsive Approach
Multiple life domains	Focus is on the transition to a complete, integrated plan for life rather than on multiple, divided life segments.	A student's culture is viewed as a strength and therefore the multiple life domains are planned for in the rich context of the student's intersectional identity. The transition team interrogates oppressive systems within the plan and equips the student with navigational tools.
Multiple means of assessment	Focus is on collecting an array of information about the student that provides holistic data upon which decisions are made.	A student's ability, gender, cultural, linguistic, and racial diversity is affirmed through consistent, high expectations during the assessment process. The team encourages student choice and assesses the whole person while increasing access to those assessments with examples from the student's lived experience.
Individual self-determination	Student is the focus of the process, with his or her preferences and interests serving as the basis for transition services. Student is the causal agent.	A student's background is authentically integrated into e aspect of transition services. The student's cultural values and traditions are prioritized. The transition team critically reflects on their understanding of culture and intentionally acts to minimize their individual biases.
Multiple means of representation	Transition planning and services are developed so that they include materials, services, and instruction that include a range of methods.	A student's ability, gender, cultural, linguistic, and racial diversity is viewed as a strength and therefore represented positively in all aspects of the transition process. Transition team members plan services that align with the student's diverse strengths, challenging the dominant perspective.
Multiple means of engagement	Transition planning and services are developed to assure that there are multiple ways that students can be involved in the process.	The community's cultural capital is aligned to the student's background and identity so the student engages with transition planning and services in a way that they can live out their values. The transition team environment is nonthreatening to the student and they prioritize mutual respect.

(continued)

Table 12.1 Cont.

Universal Design for Transition Domain	Transition Focus	Culturally Responsive Approach
Multiple means of expression	Transition planning and services are developed to assure that students can communicate their preferences and interests, and demonstrate progress in multiple ways.	A student's traditions and experiential knowledge are viewed as integral to the planning process. Students are explicitly taught code-switching skills in alignment with their goals for transition. The transition team welcomes the student and their input in the form most convenient for the student.
Multiple resources/ perspectives	Transition planning and services are developed collaboratively, pooling resources (financial, human, and/or material), using natural supports and/or generic community services, as well as disability specific ones.	The resources and support from a student's home culture and community are prioritized during the planning process. The transition team interrogates inequity within the community systems and resources, providing the student with tools to disrupt oppression.

Source: *Adapted from Thoma et al., 2009.*

included in the text. These types of options can assist students with a range of learning challenges, including students with autism. In addition, for students who need few distractions while learning, these options can be "turned off." For many students with ASD hyper focus is one of the characteristics that make transition between activities problematic. Technology can alleviate some of these issues by embedding prompts for transition within the content, or providing a tool for self-pacing. Another useful tool for students with ASD, many of whom experience anxiety in new situations, is to prepare by using simulated environments or augmented reality. In fact, augmented reality and modified-schema based instruction were successful means for training students with ASD in a variety of skills, including mathematical problem-solving skills (Root et al., 2021).

The CAST group lists the following guidelines for providing instructional materials that use multiple means of representation that address the three different types of options: perception; language, mathematical expressions, and symbols; and comprehension (CAST, 2011). The first option for perception is that teachers consider ways of customizing the display of information. Culturally responsive representation calls for the intentional communication of diversity and non-dominant culture as a strength (Kieran & Anderson, 2019). As previously stated, CAST recommends that multiple options be available and be flexible enough for students to choose which options best meet their needs for learning a particular academic lesson. This is important because learning needs can change based on the type of information being shared and the goals for a specific lesson. Yvonne, the student described earlier, had no problem learning by reading text-based information for most academic content, particularly in math or science. However, when learning how to participate in a debate in her history class, Yvonne needed concrete examples of how to debate, and web-based links to video-taped debates provided an option to represent that information. Those links, however, were not required for all students in the class; they could be used if needed, or ignored if not. Many teachers report that higher academic expectations can result in fewer opportunities for community-based activities and an elimination of field trips. There are a number of virtual field trips that can be used to bring art, history, and science lessons to life for students. They also bring benefits to the education of students with autism who may find actual field trips too overwhelming; students can participate in these virtual field trips over multiple and shorter timeframes. These types of experiences can also be used to prepare students for community-based engagement, including opportunities for learning employment or independent living skills.

The final area teachers need to address under multiple means of representation is comprehension (CAST, 2011). Options to support students' comprehension can include providing background knowledge; highlighting patterns, relationships, critical features, and big ideas; guiding information processing, visualization, and manipulation; and maximizing transfer and generalization. These learning goals can be particularly important for a student like Yvonne who may learn a vast array of factual information but struggles with generalizing that information in new situations. Yvonne was able to learn to calculate the area of a rectangle, but could not use that to determine the size of a room to be painted, and the amount of paint she needs to purchase to complete that task. So, Yvonne's teacher used multiple practical examples of tasks that required her to determine the area of a rectangle in order to complete a project (e.g., painting, purchasing a rug for a room, determining whether furniture will fit in a room). Yvonne's teacher also used online resources to provide an opportunity for her to manipulate items to see if her calculations were correct, and to find resources to learn about other projects that require learning to calculate area (including jobs that use this skill regularly).

Component 2: Multiple Means of Expression (UDL)

The second component of UDT, based on UDL characteristics, is the provision of multiple means of action and expression (CAST, 2011). This refers to providing multiple ways for students to communicate what they know or have learned. Students with ASD can face challenges in communication, so this component of a UDL approach provides a way to determine more accurately what they learned and how effectively a lesson reached a specific benchmark or learning goal. Done well, the use of multiple means of expression ensures that the strategic networks of the brain are activated, addressing the "how" of learning. In general terms, the strategic networks of the brain focus on how one organizes and expresses ideas, plans, and performs tasks. Examples of multiple means of action can include engaging in problem-solving activities, writing an essay, working collaboratively on a project, and/or building a model. This is particularly relevant for students with autism, who often experience executive dysfunction (Demetriou et al., 2018) and might struggle with performing complex tasks without support.

Guidelines for teachers from CAST (2011) recommend the following considerations that are part of providing multiple means of action and expression: provide options for physical action; provide options for expression and communication; and provide options for executive functions. Providing options for physical action includes not only opportunities to demonstrate through performance, but also varying the technology tools (including assistive technology) that can be used to access the lesson and demonstrate understanding. Technology also helps provide options for communication, from using an alternative communication system to using tools such as word prediction software to support efforts to communicate in writing. Lastly, there are a number of tools that can be used to support executive functions such as planning, goal-settings, and monitoring of progress. Teachers use many of these tools as ways to provide multiple means of representation during lessons, but they also can be used to support the assessment process, and these processes can be implemented in both classroom tasks and in the community. For example, a flow chart used to help students take notes of the key concepts from a history lesson can also be used to help students organize their answers on a test of the material, and organizing notes during a field trip to a museum.

Students with ASD often struggle with communication and collaborative work. While that does not mean that they shouldn't have opportunities to engage in these activities, their performance in such activities should not be the only way that teachers assess progress in learning academic content or meeting individualized learning goals. Pairing these experiences with an opportunity to work independently in completing a more concrete assessment of their learning (a written test, writing an essay, or completing an online assessment) would be an effective way to provide multiple means of representation.

Component 3: Multiple Means of Engagement (UDL)

The third characteristic of UDL is that it provides multiple means of engagement (CAST, 2011), which centers on the affective networks of the brain and focuses on the "why of learning" (CAST, 2011). This emphasis helps students become purposeful, motivated learners. Teachers focus on increasing student interest in the learning activity; providing options for sustaining effort and persistence; and allowing students to self-regulate their learning. Through a culturally responsive lens, this includes intentionally minimizing threats and distractions for students traditionally marginalized and oppressed by the systems and structures within education (Kieran & Anderson, 2019).

Typically, students with ASD have strengths when it comes to persistence in learning when the activity or content is highly motivating. In fact, "talking about preferred topics" and "seeking out objects or activities that offer desired stimulation to the exclusion of other activities" are listed as challenges students on the autism spectrum face (Schall et al., 2013, p. 452). Those same challenges can be also regarded as strengths. For example, in a study by Reis and collaborators (2021) students with ASD attribute their successful post-secondary matriculation to the autonomy they were afforded to pursue content and activities of interest to them that were closely aligned to their strengths in academic content and social skills experiences. Teachers can increase engagement for all students when they take a strengths-based approach to their students' diversity, intentionally incorporating their cultural capital seamlessly into the curriculum and classroom environment (Kieran & Anderson, 2019). Similarly, the neurodiversity characteristics at the core of autism can be used as a way to find new meaning in content, including in areas that do not fall match their preferred domains of engagement.

A UDL approach provides a framework for scaffolding new content or new learning experiences by linking to those that are highly engaging. Strategies that overlap with components of self-determination are particularly relevant options for increasing student motivation to learn academic content. Students are less likely to be engaged in learning academic content that is difficult, particularly when they do not see how it is something they will need to use in the future. Finding ways for students to have a choice in how they engage with academic content, to solve problems, to assess and reward their progress, all can increase student motivation in learning.

Yvonne's history teacher could have increased student engagement in learning about the Civil War by having students explore what it was like to live in that era: what jobs were available, how people traveled to work or town, and how daily chores were done without many of our modern technologies. Students would still learn about the war itself, the timelines, and the key battles, but they could do so by also learning about the realities of life at the time, and comparing those to options available now (jobs, transportation, chores, technologies). This provides an opportunity to not only learn about the civil war era, but also reflect on their own lives and their hopes for what their adult world could be.

Component 4: Multiple Transition Domains

Students with ASD, regardless of their level of support needs, have considerably more postsecondary options today than a few decades ago. Support and programs specifically designed for people with disabilities have taken root in most major universities (Grigal et al., 2013), while competitive integrated employment has become the standard in legislation (WIOA, 2014). However, when we design transition services for students with ASD, who can experience difficulty with communication, social skills, and the ability to generalize across settings, keeping in mind the variety of transition domains becomes essential.

"Multiple transition domains" refer to preparing students with disabilities for an adult life that reflects their goals, preferences, and interests. These include options such as employment or postsecondary education, and the functional facets of life composed of community living, recreation, self-care, communication, self-determination, and transportation. A student's cultural identity and traditions should be celebrated through these domains, intentionally preparing students with the tools needed to navigate inequitable systems. These domains have been identified from the Transition Planning Inventory (TPI) and are generally accepted as covering both academic and functional skills (Carter et al., 2009).

UDT advocates for targeting an array of skills that enable youth to access all areas of life, not just academic skills. Reis and colleagues (2021) found that 90% of students with ASD who matriculated to competitive colleges had participated in extracurricular activities while in high school and 50% had participated in residential camps or other immersive experiences. These students gravitated strongly toward individual-oriented sports (e.g., swimming and track) and STEM content (e.g., robotics clubs). A high school student with ASD with minimal educational support needs might be proficient in core academic skills, and therefore may not be seen as needing educational services for transition. However, the same student might need extensive support to access transportation, live in the community, communicate effectively, and engage in meaningful relationships with peers. Community participation drops sharply after high school for individuals because the support from school systems is no longer in place (Myers et al., 2015). It is very likely for someone who does not have access to transportation to engage in solitary and sedentary leisure activities, such as watching TV, which would directly impact his ability to interact with same-aged youth or maintain a healthy weight (Wagner, 2005).

The example in Figure 12.1 below is a one-page summary developed as part of the *I'm Determined* curriculum available through the Virginia Department of Education (www.imdetermined.org). This one-page summary provides a snapshot that a student can use to communicate his or her goals for an adult life with transition team members, as well as adult support providers. It demonstrates clearly that most individuals picture an adult life that includes more than just a job or going to college after high school.

Component 5: Multiple Means of Transition Assessment

Multiple means of assessment of needs during the transition period means that the planning team for a student uses a variety of formal, informal, and alternative/performance-based transitional assessments to gather information about the student's interests, needs, and strengths as

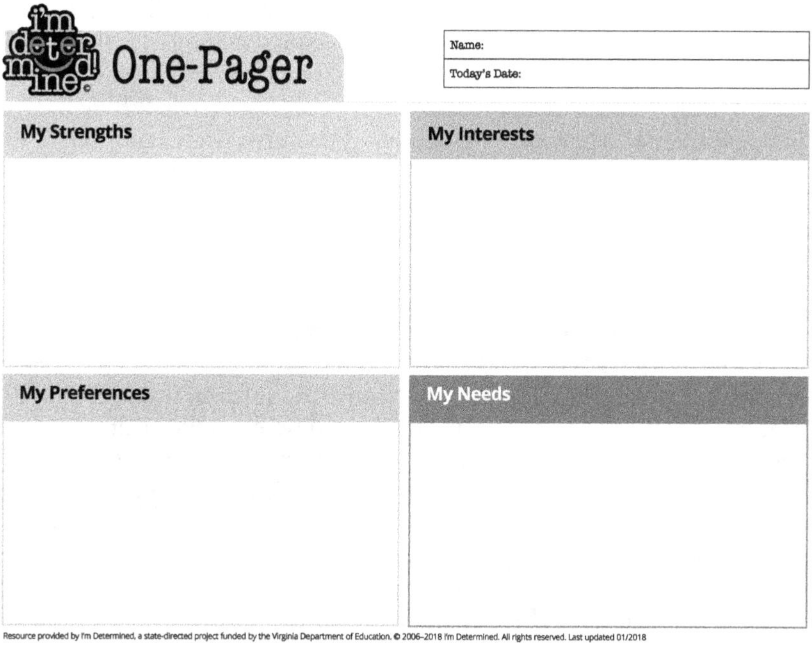
One-Pager

Name:

Today's Date:

My Strengths

My Interests

My Preferences

My Needs

Resource provided by I'm Determined, a state-directed project funded by the Virginia Department of Education. © 2006–2018 I'm Determined. All rights reserved. Last updated 01/2018

Figure 12.1 Sample Self Determination One-Pager Worksheet.

they apply to their future. Formal assessments are often commercially produced or normed by researchers; they are typically administered to all of the students within a school. The assessments might include career interest inventories (e.g. Career Opportunities Assessment (COPS), vocational placement tests (e.g. Armed Services Vocational Battery – ASVAB), the Brigance Transitional Skills Activities, or educational placement tests (e.g. Scholastic Aptitude Test – SAT). Formal transition assessments might also be part of eligibility screening for government services like community living services Social Security Disability Insurance (SSDI), or state or regional employment commissions. Formal assessments may have a cultural bias and care must be taken to affirm a student's identity during the process. Informal assessments might include interviews with parents and students, observations of the student in the community, or teacher-made surveys. One way to support students from racial/ethnic and socioeconomically diverse backgrounds is to encourage student input in selecting or creating assessments and ensure availability of brokering or transition services during the assessment process.

There are some examples of accessible transition assessments. One option for students with communication or reading difficulties is the *Choose and Take Action* software package (Martin & Marshall, 1995). This assessment shows the student short clips of individuals working in the community; two videos are shown consecutively and the student is asked to choose the job they like best. Over a short period of time, the student will have narrowed his or her job choices. Similarly, the COPS picture inventory assesses a student's interest in a career after viewing images of individuals in different careers. Another example is *Whose Future Is It Anyway?* (Wehmeyer et al., 2004). This curriculum and assessment product includes a student reader, workbook, software package, and instructor guide, providing information in multiple formats for use in the classroom.

While these assessments can provide valuable information about student transition needs and goals, they can be difficult to infuse into the classroom where academic instruction is occurring. The UDT model encourages special educators to identify opportunities in those academic classes to gather relevant transition information that can be used to inform student transition plans. For example, using a class presentation in a history class to identify whether Yvonne will need support to be effective in her interactions with customers who need help with their computers along with her performance in the computer class to determine if she can identify next steps in updating a memory card, or if she needs to have instructions nearby to guide her through the process. These kinds of informal assessment procedures can be invaluable to helping Yvonne make a smooth transition to her future employment.

Informal Parent Inventory for Post-Secondary Education Options

Directions

There are many college/university programs available for students with autism. Please take a moment to answer the following questions. The questions will be used to direct you to future transitional support services.

Which educational options would you be interested in exploring?

❑ Adult continuing education programs
❑ Parks and recreation educational options
❑ Vocational opportunities
❑ 2 year college programs
❑ 4 year college programs
❑ I am not sure.
❑ Other: [   ]

Have you ever taken a "tour" of a post educational organization with your child?

❑ Yes
❑ No
❑ I am not sure.
❑ Other: [   ]

Which of the following post-secondary funding options would you like to explore?

❑ Federal Financial Aid
❑ Social Security (SSI/SSDI)
❑ Achieving a Better Life Experience (ABLE) account
❑ Apprentice programs
❑ Scholarship options
❑ Other: [   ]

Figure 12.2 Informal Parental Inventory (Part 1).

There are a number of examples of informal transition assessments that can be useful in following a UDT framework. Figure 12.2 presents a teacher-made informal survey to assess parental interest in postsecondary educational options. The assessment asks parents to choose options for postsecondary goals that the teacher uses to start conversations with the family. The first question invites the parents to explore a variety of post-secondary educational options, ranging from recreational educational programs to college programs designed for students with ASD. The second and third questions encourage the parents to explore different educational options with their child. The second part of the assessment, Figure 12.3, contains questions related to the admissions requirements for some of the local programs (e.g. transportation and a history of employment is sometimes stipulated by the college admissions teams). Involving parents in the process whenever possible can

Check the statements which describe your child's transportation experiences.

❑ My child has a driver's license.
❑ My child has qualified for para-transportation services?
❑ My child can use mass transit.
❑ My child can use/access a van pooling or carpooling service.
❑ My child can navigate independently on a campus.
❑ I am not sure.
❑ Other: [＿＿＿＿＿＿＿＿＿]

Check the statements which would describe your child's employment experiences.

❑ No experience.
❑ Some volunteer experience < 100 hours.
❑ Extensive volunteer experience > 100 hours.
❑ Part-time summer employment
❑ Full-time summer employment
❑ Supported employment (part or full time)
❑ Experience within a family business
❑ Other: [＿＿＿＿＿＿＿＿＿]

From Project BASE (Building Autism Supports with Evidence)

Created by A. Wojcik

Figure 12.3 Informal Parental Inventory (Part 2).

be extremely valuable for all students with disabilities, but particularly for students with ASD who are racially, culturally, and/or linguistically diverse. It can be translated to reach families who are learning English and can allow for an open dialogue between school personnel, students and their families.

Regardless of the accessibility, formal off-the-shelf assessments have significant weaknesses. First, commercial publications are based on the job market at the time of publication and they may not reflect recent changes in cultural and linguistic diversity, the economy, technological advances, and job market. Additionally, commercial publications are not familiar with the local jobs market, and jobs unique to localities will often be overlooked. For instance, oyster farmers might be needed in the maritime regions of Virginia, while gas attendants might be more readily employed in New Jersey. Another disadvantage to some of the off-the-shelf transitional assessments is that they might not focus on post-secondary educational options. A fourth disadvantage is that such formal assessments are typically inventory-like assessments that assume individuals have had sufficient experiences to identify their preferences; they are often only as accurate as the degree to which an individual has had these experiences and can identify preferences. Care should be taken to see that under-represented minority students are not disadvantaged by the inventory-like options available in the assessment. For many students with disabilities, including students with ASD, opportunities to gain experiences are very limited, and the level of self-awareness necessary to make such inventories valid is often a challenge. Lastly, preferences for certain activities are often contextual. That is, what may be an undesirable activity could be acceptable if required as part of a larger picture that is highly preferred. For example, Yvonne answered that she preferred jobs that were done with minimal interaction. However, when working in the computer store, she was able to interact with others by talking about computer parts, video games, and software developers.

Similar local issues can surface related to the postsecondary educational options located within each community. Each locality is likely to have unique educational and vocational options. For example, a large urban area might have multiple postsecondary education programs and adult support agencies that provide vocational and educational services for young adults with ASD; this may be very different from rural and suburban areas that might have more limited agency support but whose communities might be more inclusive and supportive. Transition assessments must include a survey of the communities in which students plan to live, to identify the opportunities, supports, services, and barriers to their goals for adult life. A strategy known as community resource mapping (Crane & Mooney, 2005) provides a structure for investigating what is available in a specific community in terms of multiple transition domains. See the resource list at the end of this chapter for a link to this information and a way to collect this important information.

Documenting student abilities should include assessments that observe their skills, strengths, and needs in real-world settings. For students with intersectional identities often marginalized by the dominant culture, this calls for the transition team to be critically conscious, critically reflective, and intentionally inclusive, both in developing and administering assessments. More importantly, the student should be an integral part of the discussion and decision-making. These informal assessments can help to expand the long-term goals considered for students, while providing information that is more useful in planning supports and services needed to be successful in the new settings. Assessments should be used to start the conversation about transition, and the assessments should be used to help the team explore all available options, especially those central to the student's culture and values. Teams should avoid using the results of transitional assessments to limit the post-secondary opportunities for students.

Component 6: Multiple Means to Support Student Self-determination

Student self-determination, a concept reflecting the belief that all individuals have the right to direct their own lives (Bremer et al., 2003), lies at the heart of quality transition planning. In fact, student self-determination has emerged as a best practice in transition (Test et al., 2009) since it has been linked to a variety of desired postschool outcomes (Shogren et al., 2012; Wehmeyer & Palmer, 2003).

Using a UDT framework for instructional planning, students play a more active role in creating their own learning experiences than they would in a more traditional program. Students are encouraged to make and express choices based on their goals, learning preferences, strengths and weaknesses, and preferences, fostering growth in understanding themselves and their own needs and goals for the future. This approach not only supports improved academic achievement, it also prepares them to make decisions about their adult life (Wehmeyer et al., 2013).

According to the principles of UDT, transition planning and services are designed to give students multiple ways to be engaged in the process, beginning with setting goals and working in a "backward-planning process" (Bowen, 2017) to identify the skills, resources, needs, or modifications necessary for students to achieve those goals. There are many ways students can participate in this process, whether using a student-led or person-centered approach, depending on the student's level of comfort and the availability of supports (Thoma et al., 2002). Involving parents, facilitating hands-on, authentic community experiences, and accommodating autistic young adults' anxiety related to transition planning meetings can foster increased motivation and participation for the student (Lee & Kim, 2021).

Self-determination involves the student's involvement in both the setting of goals and in the steps taken to achieve them (Landmark et al., 2010). Improving the self-determination of culturally and linguistically diverse individuals calls for a culturally responsive transition planning approach wherein each team member and the student are critically conscious and reflective, interrogating existing systems which pose barriers for successful planning and outcomes (Brown Ruiz & Scott, 2021).

An example of a tool to include self-determination in any curriculum is the Self-Determined Learning Model of Instruction (SDLMI; Wehmeyer et al., 2002) provides a framework to foster self-determination through a problem-solving approach. The SDLMI involves three phases of questions to help students set a learning goal, construct a learning plan, and adjust behaviors (Wehmeyer et al., 2002). The SDLMI is an effective organizational tool that facilitates students' roles as "the causal agent in their transition planning" (Shogren et al., 2012). While it teaches students to use a problem-solving strategy that increases their self-determination, it can be used to address multiple goals or problems, including academic learning, choosing transition goals, and/or identifying options for approaching problem-solving. Students with autism need both a structured approach and explicit instruction to support learning. The SDLMI can offer the needed structure to teach the concept of self-determination, and to practice this skill in a variety of contexts, which is essential for generalization.

See the example below of Phases 1 and 2 of the SDLMI for Yvonne's request for accommodations in her Math Class (Figure 12.4).

Component 7: Multiple Sources of Information

Transition planning requires teamwork, more so than any other type of educational planning process (Thoma, 1999). It is for this reason that stakeholders outside the school system are required to be invited to the transition IEP meeting, including a representative from any agency that will (or might) provide services to the student after graduation (Individuals with Disabilities Education Improvement Act (IDEA), 2004). One person alone cannot know the student's preferences, the postsecondary options available, and the means to make the connection between the two. Students and their families know how they envision their futures, teachers know the legal mandates and the steps to planning for transition, while other agency representatives are familiar with the types of postsecondary services available. For this very reason, interdisciplinary planning has been determined to be a critically important part of the transition planning process for youth with disabilities, including those on the autism spectrum (Noonan et al., 2012).

The UDT framework encourages transition teams to expand the network of individuals they consider including in the planning process and involving in instructional lessons. This includes an intentional consideration and integration of the student's cultural and linguistic diversity. As Yvonne considered life after high school, she expressed an interest in working with technology. While his teachers had some knowledge of the different types of positions working in the field of technology, like software engineer or computer programmer, they did not know all the types of jobs that are available. The teacher correctly realized that only using the teacher's and student's prior knowledge and experience can limit opportunity. Job markets change. New technologies are developed, and new skills generalize to new opportunities.

Yvonne's teacher invited a software engineer from a local firm to meet with the team to discuss a range of different positions in the field, as well as the educational requirements for each. This information provided guidance for high school course planning, as well as part-time jobs to gain valuable experience, and helped guide decisions about post school options. Not only did this collaboration provide a way to improve the individual transition planning process, it also provides opportunities to improve educational lessons. This software engineer worked with teachers to identify computer skills that all students would need to enter the job market, and incorporated opportunities for students to work on those skills in academic courses. Using spreadsheets to present and analyze data, social media to communicate with the world, and the internet to research relevant information to guide decisions are all twenty-first

Phase 1: What is my goal? *Identify technology supports that work for me.*
  1. What do I want to learn?
  How does my disability impact my ability to learn? What supports work to help overcome/minimize the impact of my disability in school? At home?
  How can I advocate for the supports I need?
  2. What do I know about it now?
  I know that I struggle with remembering dates.
  I know that I struggle with learning math.
  I know that I am good at English and writing.
  I know that I am easily distracted.
  I know that I get extra time on tests and assignments.
  3. What must change for me to learn what I don't know?
  I need to find out more about my disability and my strengths and weaknesses/needs.
  I need to determine my ability to do my homework.
  I need to learn more about my own strengths and preferences.
  I need help with matching my strengths/preferences and needs with available supports that can help me learn.
  4. What can I do to make this happen?
  I can work with my teacher to identify steps to determine the impact of my disability on learning and transition goals.
  I can research possible supports the searching the Internet, teachers, and other resources that my school identifies.

Phase 2: What is my plan? *Identify ways to reach my goal and barriers I may need to overcome them.*
  1. What five things can I do this week to work toward my goal?
  a. I will meet with my teacher to develop a plan of action.
  b. I will meet with the school psychologist to identify an assessment of the impact of my disability after receiving approval from my family.
  c. I will list the things that I struggle with in school, at home, and in the community.
  d. I will list anything that has worked for me in the past.
  e. I will meet with an assistive technology specialist to determine if there are supports/technologies that I should try to better meet my needs.
  2. What could keep me from taking action?
  I might get distracted searching the web.
  I might not find websites that have enough information to help me make a decision.
  People might not have time to meet with me.
  The school psychologist might not be able to administer additional assessments.
  My family might not want me to have additional testing.
  3. What can I do to remove these barriers?
  I can work really hard on accomplishing these goals/steps.
  I can schedule meetings with key people, as far in advance as possible.
  I can learn my rights and how to advocate for what I need.
  I can explain the purpose for additional testing to my family.
  4. When will I take action?
  I will use my study hall time this week to organize my meetings.
  I will take the online assessment on Friday during my technology lab.
  I will schedule meetings with the school psychologist, the assistive technology specialist, and my teacher within the next week.
  I will talk with my family about this plan today.

Figure 12.4 Yvonne's SDLMI for Math Class (Phases 1 & 2).

century skills that students need to be competitive for employment. Teachers should be able to call on experts to help with lesson planning that incorporates useful strategies, and when possible, to teach these hands-on practical aspects of the lesson. Skills like these would have prepared Yvonne for a specific job after graduation, but also would have helped her have other options for the future if he changed his mind, or if he wanted or needed to move onto other options later.

One of the barriers to inviting community resources into the transition planning process is the formality of the IEP process. It is also important to mitigate the barriers to participation for individuals who have been historically marginalized by our education systems. For example, people of color in the United States have a unique history of oppression within public education systems. People experiencing poverty have roadblocks often invisible to people who have never experienced poverty. Nevertheless, there are alternative meeting approaches that are designed to be more conducive to participation for a range of individuals, including the school personnel who are required to be there. To encourage the participation of students, parents, school and adult agency personnel, as well as community resources, one might consider using person-centered planning approaches (Mount, 1992). These strategies have been used widely in community service agencies for many years, but have not been incorporated into many of the school-based IEP meeting procedures. Special educators can explore these options as a way to make the IEP meeting process more welcoming to families and other community agency support staff. Person-centered planning approaches to consider include McGill Action Planning Systems (MAPS; Forest & Lusthaus, 1989); Planning Alternative Tomorrows with Hope (PATH; Pearpoint et al., 1993); or Group Action Planning (GAP; Turnbull & Turnbull, 1996). There are also a range of student-led planning processes (i.e. Thoma & Wehman, 2010) that can more easily support student involvement in those meetings. Research on the impact of these types of training processes found that not only did students and their parents interact more during IEP meetings that used these approaches, but teachers and school administrators also increased their communication during those meetings (Martin et al., 2006).

Incorporating a student-directed IEP approach can be viewed as a continuum of student involvement in the meeting (Thoma et al., 2010), from student presence at the meeting through having the student lead all or part of the meeting. Facilitating student involvement for those with diverse experiences requires that a student's language and communication style is valued by the team. This is especially relevant for students with ASD, whose main challenge often revolves around effective communication. Learning how to communicate with the transition team and become part of the planning process is in itself a challenge and opportunity for growth for this population. It is worthwhile to consider the use of technology to support student involvement in the transition planning process and in academic assignments that facilitate goal setting, understanding the impact of a disability on strengths and needs, and developing self-advocacy skills. See Figure 12.5 below for a planning tool that can be used with students and their parents to improve the participation of student direction of the planning process.

International Applications for UDT & Autism

Although the principles of UDT should work in any area, there are some factors to consider when implementing UDT internationally, as UDT

UDT Template

Breakdown of the learner, setting, and framework for lesson
1. Who are the students for whom you are responsible?
2. What are their learning needs?
3. What are their transition needs/priorities?

Goals and Standards
1. What are the academic standards you are responsible to teach?
2. What are the transition goals you are trying to meet?
3. What are the UDL components for teaching and assessing these goals?

Transition Domains
1. What transition links do you see?
2. Are there transition links beyond work?
3. What skills can you link to instruction that can serve multiple purposes?

Assessment Methods (one or multiple options)
1. What are we currently doing?
2. What other strategies could you use?
3. What assessments provide information useful for transition planning?

Resources (one or multiple) – (technology, adaptive, etc.)
1. Who do you involve now?
2. Who else could be involved
3. What are the resources that could be used to provide greater access for a range of students?

Self-determination
1. What do you already do to facilitate self-determination (instruction)?
2. What do you already do to facilitate self-determination (beyond lessons)?
3. What else could you do?
4. What is your overall approach to supporting student self-determination?

Figure 12.5 Universal Design for Transition Template.
Source: Thoma, Bartholomew, Tamura, Scott & Terpstra (2009).

strategies for individuals with autism may require adjustments for different international locations. Considerations may require adjustments related to the geographic infrastructure, government policies, and the availability of resources.

Teachers and caregivers may need to consider the geographic infrastructure when implementing UDT for individuals with autism. In particular, the issue may arise in the areas of transportation where navigation can hinder an individual's ability to get to and from work (Lubin & Feeley, 2016). For example, cities with older transit systems may lack the communication structures to make cities accessible via taxis, trains, and streetscapes (see Wong et al., 2020). Teachers and caregivers may need to consider multiple means of transportation that includes walking, carpooling, mass transit, or ridesharing, or multiple employment options may need to be considered to avoid transportation issues. For instance, Hsieh and colleagues (2019) described the use of in-home self-employment as a tool that addresses transportation concerns. The real advantage to the UDT framework is its ability to flex to different individuals in different environments.

Similarly, teachers and caregivers may need to flexibly adapt to international laws, and policies. Internationally, the range of laws and policies covering employment for individuals with disabilities is pretty vast. For instance, some countries, provide constitutional protections against employment discrimination (e.g. Kenya and Uganda), whereas, other countries like Uganda provide incentives to companies that employ individuals with disabilities, and still other countries offer little to no governmental guidance for the employment of individuals with disabilities (Griffiths et al., 2020; Wickenden et al., 2020). Even countries that have similar historic or cultural backgrounds can display variations in laws and policies. Geiger et al. (2018) noted that some countries provide individuals with qualifying disabilities regular financial payments in lieu of work and others provide discrete vocational training to qualified individuals. Additionally, the written policies and laws may differ from the practices or customs. Kang (2013) noted that employers regularly disregarded South Korean policies related to employment of individuals with disabilities out of liability concerns or local customs or cultural perceptions. Regardless of the variation of legislation or policy, within a particular country, UDT can be practiced, and multiple means of support may require assistance from non-governmental agencies. Families, peers, or nongovernmental agencies can strengthen plans. Wickenden et al. (2020) noted that multiple non-governmental organizations are available in most countries, and access to employment for individuals with disabilities may require accessing support from the different organizations.

Admittedly, there isn't much research directly examining the UDT approach for individuals with ASD, and given the patchwork of laws,

Table 12.2 Resources

SCIENCE & SOCIAL SCIENCE

1. The CAST Science Writer guides students through the steps of creating a science report. The following is the website: http://sciencewriter.cast.org/
2. Building prior knowledge can be important, and virtual field trips can help students explore historic or scientific places of merit. The following is the website: www.middleweb.com/22188/virtual-field-trips-spice-up-learning/

MATH

CAST has created a number of resources to help students learn Algebra. This resource has developed a number of computer aided instructional tools for teaching Algebra skills to students. Website: http://iSolveIt.cast.org

READING/LANGUAGE ARTS

CAST has created a public library of UDL books. The books contain hyperlinks, read aloud, and prompting cues. The demonstration texts are available at website and links to a library of electronic books are available at websites: http://udleditions.cast.org, and http://bookbuilder.cast.org .

TEACHER PLANNING TOOLS

Graphic organizers can help students structure information. There are a couple of free options available at the following websites:www.dailyteachingtools.com/free-graphic-organizers and www.dailyteachingtools.com/free-graphic-organizers-readerizer2

Jigsaw reading assignments can help to strengthen comprehension skills. teachers can use screenshots of text to create digital jigsaws using the following website: www.jigsawplanet.com.

TECHNOLOGY

Universal Design features are available on most computers. However, there are a number of free publicly available resources.

(1) The Massachusetts Institute of Technology has created a Freedom Stick to help teachers and students to activate different features like text-to-speech, speech-to-text, and visual contrast options. The software can be stored on a USB drive or downloaded to a hard drive on the a computer. The information is available at the following website: http://mits.cenmi.org/Resources/MITSFreedomStick.aspx

(2) The CAST website has developed a tool to help teachers and students to build UDL books. In addition, a library of free texts is available at the following website: http://bookbuilder.cast.org

(3) Natural Voice Reader is another option. The software recognizes text with optical character recognition and the software can read text aloud. The software is available at website: www.naturalreaders.com/.

(4) Similar software is available for the Mac computers at the following website: www.pure-mac.com/access .

(5) A group of educators have created an interactive wiki to share UDL resources. The group collectively edits the resources using the following website: http://udltechtoolkit.wikispaces.com

SELF-DETERMINATION RESOURCES

1. The I'm Determined project promotes student self-advocacy. The program encourages students to advocate for services, promote policy reform, and participation in the individual's IEP. The following website provides more information: www.imdetermined.org/

Table 12.2 Cont.

2. The National Gateway to Self-Determination provides information about self-determination. The organization provides general information and resources for teachers and parents. The website is as follows: www.ngsd.org.
3. The Beach Center provides many resources for working with students with disabilities. The library provides a teacher's guide to self-determination. The resources are available at the following website: www.beachcenter.org
4. The National Resource Center for Supported Decision-Making provides state specific information related to issues for individuals with disabilities. The information is available at the following: http://supporteddecisonmaking.org .

TRANSITION ASSESSMENT
1. The National Secondary Transition Technical Assistance Center (NSTTAC) provides information related to the evidence based practices in the world of transition and the organization has provided a toolkit for age appropriate transition assessment. The website is as follows: http://nsttac.org/.
2. The Zarrow Center for Learning Enrichment has multiple transitional assessment resources including a preference assessment, a self-determination assessment, a curriculum, and a transitional goals generator. The information can be found at http://tagg.ou.edu/tagg

INFORMATION FOR PARENTS
Parents are important team members, and they often need support in the form of information. The PACER Center regularly publishes information for parents. Past publications have examined self-determination, issues associated with the age of majority, and other transition issues. The resources can be found at the following website: www.pacer.org/publications .

policies, and support, Wickenden and colleagues' (2020) suggestion to connect with international non-government organizations would provide individuals, teachers, and caregivers with the networking links necessary to establish UDT programs or interventions for individuals with ASD. The advocacy organization, Autism Speaks, provides a list of non-governmental organizations that support the cause of inclusion for individuals with autism. Resources can be accessed at www.autismspeaks.org/international-autism-organizations.

Pulling It All Together

There are a number of resources available for teachers to help them incorporate a UDL framework in their lesson planning process, but how does a special educator expand that to include these critically important aspects of transition education and planning? Thoma et al. (2002) have developed a lesson planning template that teachers can use to link transition and academic education for youth with disabilities (see Figure 12.5 below). It provides a way to consider all of the possible links that can and do exist between academic and transition education. It should be noted, of course, that not all lessons will incorporate all of the seven components of UDT. Instead, each of these should be considered for the most relevant links, with the ultimate goal of addressing each over time.

Of course, since goals for adult life are individual, there will come a time when the focus will be more individualized and less universal; however, the more that middle and early high school academic instruction infuses knowledge and skills that students will need to prepare for their future, the better the foundational preparation for life will be for all students. And that's ultimately the goal of education for all, isn't it? The following list of resources (see Table 12.2) will help to identify the ways that academic and transition education can be linked for secondary school students.

REFERENCES

Agran, M., Wehmeyer, M., Cavin, M., & Palmer, S. (2010). Promoting active engagement in the general education classroom and access to the general education curriculum for students with cognitive disabilities. *Education and Training in Autism and Developmental Disabilities*, 163–174.

Ayres, K. M., Lowrey, K. A., Douglas, K. H., & Sievers, C. (2011). I can identify Saturn but I can't brush my teeth: What happens when the curricular focus for students with severe disabilities shifts. *Education and Training in Autism and Developmental Disabilities*, 46, 11–21.

Ayres, K. M., Lowrey, K. A., Douglas, K. H., & Sievers, C. (2012). The question still remains: What happens when the curricular focus for students with severe disabilities shifts? A reply to Courtade, Spooner, Browder, and Jimenez (2012). *Education and Training in Autism and Developmental Disabilities*, 47, 14–22.

Bernal, J., & Hollins, S. (1995). Psychiatric illness and learning disability: a dual diagnosis. *Advances in Psychiatric Treatment*, 1(5), 138–145.

Best, K., Scott, L., & Thoma, C.A. (2015). Starting with the end in mind: Inclusive education designed to prepare students for adult life. In E. Brown, R.G. Craven, & G. McLean (Eds.). *International Advances in Education: Global Initiatives for Equity and Social Justice: Vol. 9, Inclusive education for students with intellectual disabilities* (pp. 45–72). Charlotte, NC: Information Age Press.

Bouck, E. C. (2012). Secondary students with moderate/severe intellectual disability: considerations of curriculum and post-school outcomes from the National Longitudinal Transition Study-2. *Journal of Intellectual Disability Research*, 56(12), 1175–1186.

Bowen, R. S. (2017). *Understanding by Design.* Vanderbilt University Center for Teaching. Retrieved from https://cft.vanderbilt.edu/understanding-by-design.

Braddock, D. L., Hemp, R. E., Tanis, E. S., Wu, J., & Haffer, L. (2017). State of the states in intellectual and developmental disabilities. American Association on Intellectual and Developmental Disabilities.

Bremer, C., Kachgal, M., & Schoeller, K. (2003). Self-Determination: Supporting successful transition (National Center on Secondary Education and Transition

Research to Practice Brief). *Improving Secondary Education and Transition Services through Research*, 2(1), 1–6.

Carter, E. W., Trainor, A. A., Sun, Y., & Owens, L. (2009). Assessing the transition-related strengths and needs of adolescents with high-incidence disabilities. *Exceptional Children*, 76(1), 74–94.

CAST. (2011). *Universal Design for Learning Guidelines version 2.0.* Wakefield, MA.

Collins, B. C. (2012). *Systematic Instruction for Students with Moderate and Severe Disabilities*. Paul H. Brooks Publishing.

Crane, K. & Mooney, M. (2005). *Essential tools: Community resource mapping*. Retrieved from: www.ncset.org/publications/essentialtools/mapping/defa ult.asp.

Darling-Hammond, L. (2010). *The flat world and education: How America's commitment to equity will determine our future*. New York, NY: Teachers College Press.

De Bruin, C. L., Deppeler, J. M., Moore, D. W., & Diamond, N. T. (2013). Public school–based interventions for adolescents and young adults with an Autism Spectrum Disorder: A meta-analysis. *Review of Educational Research*, 0034654313498621.

Demetriou, E. A., Lampit, A., Quintana, D. S., Naismith, S. L., Song, Y. J. C., Pye, J. E., ... & Guastella, A. J. (2018). Autism spectrum disorders: A meta-analysis of executive function. *Molecular Psychiatry*, 23(5), 1198–1204.

Eilenberg, J. S., Paff, M., Harrison, A. J., & Long, K. A. (2019). Disparities based on race, ethnicity, and socioeconomic status over the transition to adulthood among adolescents and young adults on the autism spectrum: A systematic review. *Current Psychiatry Reports*, 21(5), 1–16.

Flexer, R. W., Daviso, A. W., Baer, R. M., Queen, R. M., & Meindl, R. S. (2011). An epidemiological model of transition and postschool outcomes. *Career Development for Exceptional Individuals*, 34(2), 83–94.

Forest, M., & Lusthaus, E. (1989). Promoting educational equality for all students: Circles and MAPS. in S. Stainback, W. Stainback, & M. Forest (Eds.), *Educational all students in the mainstream of regular education* (pp. 43–57). Baltimore: Paul H. Brookes Publishing Co.

Friedman, N. D., Warfield, M. E., & Parish, S. L. (2013). Transition to adulthood for individuals with autism spectrum disorder: Current issues and future perspectives. *Neuropsychiatry*, 3(2), 181–192.

Geiger, B. B., Garthwaite, K., Warren, J., & Bambra, C. (2018). Accessing work disability for social security benefits: International Models for direct assessment of work capacity. *Disability and Rehabilitation*, 40(24), 2962–2970. https://doi.org/10.1080/09638288.2017.1366556

Griffiths, A., Bechange, S., Loryman, H., Iga, C., & Schmidt, E. (2020). How do legal and policy frameworks support employment of people with disabilities in Uganda? Findings from a qualitative policy analysis study. *Journal of International Development*, 32(8), 1360–1378. https://doi.org/10.1002/jid.3508

Grigal, M., Hart, D., & Weir, C. (2013). Postsecondary education for people with intellectual disability: Current issues and critical challenges. *Inclusion*, 1(1), 50–63.

Higher Education Opportunity Act of 2008, Pub. L. No. 110–315, 20 U.S.C. § 1003 (2008).

Hsieh, Y., Molina, V. M. J., Weng, J. (2019). The road to entrepreneurship with impairments: A challenges-adaptive mechanisms-results model for disabled entrepreneurs. *International Business Journal: Researching Entrepreneurship*, *37*(8), 761–779. https://doi.org/10.1177/0266242619867654

Individuals with Disabilities Education Improvement Act of 2004, Pub. L. No. 108-446, 20 U.S.C. § 1400.

Kang, S. (2013). Coverage of autism spectrum disorder in the US television news: An analysis of framing. *Disability & Society*, *28*(2), 245–259.

Kieran, L., & Anderson, C. (2019). Connecting universal design for learning with culturally responsive teaching. *Education and Urban Society*, *51*(9), 1202–1216. https://doi.org/10.1177/0013124518785012

Kleinert, H., Towles-Reeves, E., Quenemoen, R., Thurlow, M., Fluegge, L., Weseman, L., & Kerbel, A. (2015). Where students with the most significant cognitive disabilities are taught: Implications for general curriculum access. *Exceptional Children*, doi: 0014402914563697.

Kuhn, J. L., Vanegas, S. B., Salgado, R., Borjas, S. K., Magaña, S., & Smith DaWalt, L. (2020). The cultural adaptation of a transition program for Latino families of youth with Autism Spectrum Disorder. *Family Process*, *59*(2), 477–491. https://doi.org/10.1111/famp.12439

Landmark, L. J., Ju, S., & Zhang, D. (2010). Substantiated best practices in transition: Fifteen plus years later. *Career Development for Exceptional Individuals.*

Lee, C. E., & Kim, J. G. (2021). Person-centered transition planning for youth on the Autism Spectrum: What are we still missing? *Exceptionality*, 1–14. https://doi.org/10.1080/09362835.2021.1938065

Lubin, A. & Feeley, C. (2016). Transportation issue of adults on the Autism Spectrum: Findings from focus group discussions. *Journal of the Transportation Research Board*, *2542(1)*, 1–8. https://doi.org/10.3141/2542-01.

Martin, J. E., & Marshall, L. H. (1995). ChoiceMaker: A comprehensive self-determination transition program. *Intervention in School and Clinic*, 30, 147–156.

Martin, J. E., Van Dycke, J. L., Christensen, W. R., Greene, B. A., Gardner, J. E., & Lovett, D. L. (2006). Increasing student participation in their transition IEP meetings: Establishing the *Self-Directed IEP* as an evidenced-based practice. *Exceptional Children*, *72*(3), 299–316.

Mazzotti, V. L., Rowe, D. A., Kwiatek, S., Voggt, A., Chang, W.-H., Fowler, C. H., Poppen, M., Sinclair, J., & Test, D. W. (2021). Secondary transition predictors of postschool success: An update to the research base. *Career Development and Transition for Exceptional Individuals*, *44*(1), 47–64. https://doi.org/10.1177/2165143420959793

Meyer, A., Rose, D. H., Gordon, D. (2013). *Universal Design for Learning: Theory and Practice*. Wakefield, MA: Cast Professional Publishing.

Mount, B. (1992). *Person-centered planning: A sourcebook of values, ideas, and methods to encourage person-centered development*. New York: Graphic Futures.

Myers, E., Davis, B. E., Stobbe, G., & Bjornson, K. (2015). Community and social participation among individuals with Autism Spectrum Disorder transitioning to adulthood. *Journal of Autism and Developmental Disorders*, *45*(8), 2373–2381. https://doi.org/10.1007/s10803-015-2403-z

Newman, L., Wagner, M., Knokey, A. M., Marder, C., Nagle, K., Shaver, D., & Wei, X. (2011). *The Post-High School Outcomes of Young Adults with Disabilities up to 8 Years after High School: A Report from the National Longitudinal Transition Study-2 (NLTS2)*.

Noonan, P. M., Erickson, A. G., & Morningstar, M. E. (2012). Effects of community transition teams on interagency collaboration for school and adult agency staff. *Career development and transition for exceptional individuals*, 2165143412451119

Pearpoint, J., O'Brien, J., & Forest, M. (1993). *PATH (Planning Alternative Tomorrows with Hope): A workbook for planning positive futures.* Toronto: Inclusion Press.

Reis, S. M., Gelbar, N. W., & Madaus, J. W. (2021). Understanding the academic success of academically talented college students with Autism Spectrum Disorders. *Journal of Autism and Developmental Disorders*. https://doi.org/10.1007/s10803-021-05290-4

Rojewski, J. W., Lee, I. H., & Gregg, N. (2014). Intermediate work outcomes for adolescents with high-incidence disabilities. *Career Development and Transition for Exceptional Individuals*, *37*(2), 106–118.

Root, J. R., Cox, S. K., Davis, K., & Gonzales, S. (2021). Using augmented reality and modified schema-based instruction to teach problem solving to students with autism. *Remedial and Special Education*, 07419325211054209

Ruiz, A.B., & Scott, L. A. (2021). Guiding questions for a culturally responsive framework during preemployment transition services. *TEACHING Exceptional Children*, *53*(5), 369–375. https://doi.org/10.1177/0040059920982312

Schall, C., Targett, P., & Wehman, P. (2013). Applications for youth with autism spectrum disorders. In P. Wehman, *Life beyond the classroom: Transition strategies for young people with disabilities* (pp. 447–471). Baltimore: Paul Brookes Publishing.

Scott, L. A., & Bruno, L. (2018). Universal design for transition: A conceptual framework for blending academics and transition instruction. *The Journal of Special Education Apprenticeship*, *7*(3), 1–15.

Test, D. W., Fowler, C. H., Richter, S. M., White, J., Mazzotti, V., Walker, A. R., Kohler, P., & Kortering, L. (2009). Evidence-based practices in secondary transition. *Career Development for Exceptional Individuals*, *32*, 115–128.

Thoma, C. A., Baker, S. R., & Saddler, S. J. (2002). Self-determination in teacher education: A model to facilitate transition planning for students with disabilities. *Remedial and Special Education*, *23*(2), 82–89.

Thoma, C. A., Bartholomew, C. C., & Scott, L. A. (2009). *Universal design for transition: A roadmap for planning and instruction.* Paul H. Brookes Publishing.

Thoma, C.A., Boyd, K., & Austin, K. (2013). Teaching for Transition. In P. Wehman. *Life beyond the classroom: Transition strategies for young people with disabilities* (5th ed.) (pp. 201–236). Baltimore: Paul H. Brookes.

Thoma, C. A., & Wehman, P. (2010). *Getting the Most out of IEPs: An Educator's Guide to the Student-Directed Approach.* Brookes Publishing Company. Baltimore, MD.

Turnbull, A. & Turnbull, H.R. (1996). Group Action Planning as a strategy for providing comprehensive family support. In L.K. Koegel, R.L. Koegel, & G. Dunlap (Eds.), *Positive behavioral support: Including people with difficult behavior in the community* (pp. 99–114). Baltimore: Paul H. Brookes Publishing Co.

Wagner, M., Newman, L., Cameto, R., Garza, N., & Levine, P. (2005). After high school: A first look at the postschool experiences of youth with disabilities. A report from the National Longitudinal Transition Study-2 (NLTS2). *Online submission.*

Wehman, P., Sima, A. P., Ketchum, J., West, M. D., Chan, F., & Luecking, R. (2015). Predictors of successful transition from school to employment for youth with disabilities. *Journal of Occupational Rehabilitation, 25*(2), 323–334.

Wehmeyer, M. L., Lance, G. D., & Bashinski, S. (2002). Promoting access to the general education curriculum for students with mental retardation: A multilevel model. *Education and Training in Mental Retardation and Developmental Disabilities, 37*(3), 223–234.

Wehmeyer, M. L., Lawrence, M., Kelchner, K., Palmer, S. B., Garner, N., & Soukup, J. H. (2004). Whose future is it anyway? A student-directed transition planning process. Lawrence, KS: Kansas University Center on Developmental Disabilities.

Wehmeyer, M. L., & Palmer, S. B. (2003). Adult outcomes for students with cognitive disabilities three-years after high school: The impact of self-determination. *Education and Training in Developmental Disabilities,* 131–144.

Wehmeyer, M. L., Palmer, S. B., Shogren, K. A., Williams-Diehm, K., & Soukup, J. H. (2013). Establishing a causal relationship between interventions to promote self-determination and enhanced student self-determination. *Journal of Special Education, 46,* 195–210. Doi: 10.1177/0022466910392377

Wickenden, M., Thompson, S., Mader, P., Brown, S., & Rohwerder, B. (2020). Accelerating disability inclusive formal employment in Bangladesh, Kenya, Nigeria, and Uganda: What are the vital ingredients? Brighton: Institute of Development Studies. https://opendocs.ids.ac.uk/opendocs/handle/20.500.12413/15198

Wong, S., McLafferty, S. L., Planey, A. M., & Preston V. A. (2020). Disability, wages, and commuting in New York. *Journal of Transportation Geography, 87,* https://doi.org/10.1016/j.jtrangeo.2020.102818

Workforce Innovation and Improvement Act of 2014 Pub. L. *113-128* 128 USC § 1425 (2014).

Chapter 13

Positive Behavior Supports in Middle and Secondary School

Shannon L. Sparks[1]* and Debra L. Cote[2]

[1]Department of Special Education, Rehabilitation & Counseling, California State University, San Bernardino
[2]Department of Special Education, California State University, Fullerton
*Correspondence Author: Email: shannon.sparks@csusb.edu

Positive Behavior Supports in Middle and Secondary School

Mathias is a middle school student who was diagnosed with autism spectrum disorder (ASD) at the age of three. While Mathias is fully included in general education classrooms, he struggles academically, behaviorally, and socially. Mathias has severe delays in both syntax and academic language and deficits in behavior. During conversations, he does not use more than three or four words in a sentence. He can become agitated or disturbed when teachers or peers do not understand him. Reading aloud or negative social interactions may elicit inappropriate behaviors of throwing objects, hitting, yelling, refusals to the demand/request, or elopement. A calm redirecting voice does not appear to affect the behavior, nor does Mathias accept consequences in a socially acceptable manner. Mathias's explosive behaviors are highly disruptive to the general education environment.

Due to increased numbers of children with autism participating in inclusionary settings, changes have occurred in school-wide expectations for these students and in corresponding supports needed. Middle and secondary-age students with autism often struggle with maladaptive behaviors (e.g., communication, social interactions, stereotypic repetitive behaviors) and in managing their feelings and/or emotions (Viezel et al., 2020). Some students with ASD may exhibit high levels of aggression, escape behaviors, and difficulties with transitions (Kern et al., 2006). Individuals with ASD often engage in aggressive behaviors due to anxiousness or changes in one's routine (Gonzalez et al., 2017). Inappropriate and challenging behaviors often prevent these students from making adequate academic progress, developing friendships, and learning basic skills (Bryant et al., 2020).

DOI: 10.4324/9781003255147-16

Hence, students with ASD require educational supports that are scientifically sound, grounded in evidence-based practice (EBP), and based on research (Steinbrenner et al., 2020; Test et al., 2020). As a response to these special needs, teachers and parents should adopt comprehensive and established teaching practices with histories that suggest they hold promise for preventing and managing the problematic behaviors.

A comprehensive practice, positive behavior support (PBS), has strong evidence to support its use with students exhibiting challenging behaviors (Sugai et al., 2000). PBS is a behaviorally based systems approach that enhances the environment using research practices that improve student teaching and learning (Sugai et al., 2000). A PBS approach developed within the context of the student and his or her family directly impacts one's quality of life (Becker-Cottrill et al., 2003). It is important to present a valid picture of a student's behaviors and what PBS approaches are utilized in various settings.

While Mr. Dominguez utilized PBS within the classroom, he was also aware of his limited knowledge of Mathias's behaviors across settings/environments. Hence, he spoke with those who were familiar with Mathias and the overt behaviors in order to design an effective behavior support plan. During a parent interview, Mathias's father shared that it was easier to 'give in' than to deal with the anger or yelling. During afternoon PE, often Mathias did not participate and told the teacher he was tired; his father confirmed a similar pattern repeated from last year. Mr. Dominguez interviewed three previous teachers to ascertain how long the behaviors had been occurring, when and where they occurred, and what positive behavior supports were used.

Basic Concepts of Positive Behavior Supports

Positive behavior support strategies foster school and classroom environments that value and reinforce appropriate behaviors. An overall positive learning environment stimulates academic and behavioral achievement. PBS is an EBP that includes primary, secondary and tertiary level supports (Center on Positive Behavioral Interventions & Supports, 2021). The core values of PBS are founded on prevention, application of EBP and creating supportive contexts that are person-centered (Alberto et al., 2022). A PBS approach is a practice that decreases problem behaviors, since it reduces the negative impact often associated with consequences (Alberto et al., 2022). The preventative approach involves providing supports that increase student success and engagement. PBS extends the elements of applied behavioral analysis utilizing several key principles: (1) behaviors that are learned can be changed, (2) intervention follows a functional behavior assessment, (3) intervention targets prevention and teaching a communicative replacement behavior, (4) interventions are of social significance to the individual, and (5) multicomponent supports are involved (Bambara et al., 2015). Two additional goals of PBS are: to improve one's quality of life and to make the challenging behavior ineffective by replacing it with a socially acceptable behavior (Alberto et al., 2022; Carr et al., 2014).

While a PBS approach (i.e., assessment, intervention strategies) is best practice for supporting individual students and their behaviors, it can also be used within districts, schools and groups of students with ASD. The framework of PBS stresses prevention, a supportive environment with predictable routines, the teaching and reinforcing of positive behaviors and reliance on EBP (Scheuermann et al., 2022).

Philosophical Foundations and Research

The underlying philosophical foundation for PBS is applied behavior analysis (ABA), taken from Skinner's operant conditioning model. The model helps explain, predict and change human behavior (Alberto et al., 2022). Some assumptions of ABA are that behavior is learned, behavior can be improved by altering antecedents and consequences, and systems of support can be put into place to increase/support appropriate behaviors and decrease undesirable behaviors (Olive et al., 2017). Thus, children with challenging behaviors may benefit from educational systems of support that utilize positive behavioral teaching principles (e.g., ABA, PBS, discrete trial training) in design and delivery of instruction (de Boer, 2018). The use of positive behavioral practices/principles can facilitate student quality of life (Carr & Horner, 2007).

Ethical Issues and Laws That Address Behavior

Student behavior is addressed under federal law in the Individuals with Disabilities Education Act (IDEA, 1997). The act mandates that an IEP team identify strategies, supports, and positive behavior interventions when a child's challenging behavior impedes learning (IDEA, 1997). Additionally, practitioners must address ethical issues when making decisions as to which method or intervention to use with a student. Ethical issues that can/may influence practitioner's behavior includes: one's personal history, cultural biases/and or religious rearing and the context in which the behavior occurs (Council for Exceptional Children, 2015). Practitioners need to approach a student and the challenging behavior from an ethical perspective when deciding which practice or treatment to implement. This approach further connects the value and worth of the intervention to the student (Cooper et al., 2007).

Operant Principles

Principles of operant conditioning suggest that behavior is voluntary, measurable, discrete, verifiable, and functional relationships are formed between the behavior and consequence (Alberto et al., 2022). Practitioners should clearly define observable behaviors that give evidence of a functional relationship between treatment and the results (Alberto et al., 2022).

Positive reinforcement. A positive reinforcement system focuses on catching students when they display desired behaviors and reinforcing them, thereby increasing or maintaining the behaviors (Scheuermann et al., 2022). Teachers should set up positive class-wide reinforcing systems that teach and reinforce appropriate behaviors (Sayeski & Brown, 2014). Positive reinforcement allows for the chosen item, preferred activity, or social consequence being offered subsequent to the behavior and the behavior increasing in future settings (Tincani et al., 2018). All students should experience positive and supportive teacher-student relationships. It is even more imperative for a student who struggles academically and behaviorally (Jones & Jones, 2021).

Negative reinforcement. Negative reinforcement is the contingent removal of an aversive or negative stimulus following a response that leads to an increase in the future occurrence of the behavior (Alberto et al., 2022; Scheuermann et al., 2022; Tincani et al., 2018). For example, Mr. Dominguez tells Mathias he will not need to journal if he finishes the reading assignment by the end of the period (Shea & Bauer, 2012). Mathias may be negatively reinforced by the removal of journal writing which he perceives as an aversive stimulus (Tincani et al., 2018). Although negative reinforcement may be effective in the short term, teachers should utilize positive reinforcement procedures to increase and teach appropriate behaviors (Zirpoli, 2016).

Punishment. Punishment is mistakenly confused with negative reinforcement. When educators utilize punitive methods, the behavior decreases, reducing future occurrences of the challenging behavior (Alberto et al., 2022). Challenging behaviors often are maintained by positive and negative reinforcement. It is vital to understand the 'why' and the consequences (Tincani et al., 2018). It is a short-term solution that does not get at the function of a behavior (Bambara et al, 2015). Without addressing the function, students are left without a communicative replacement behavior (Alberto et al., 2022). In an attempt to avoid punishment, a student may stop performing the challenging target behavior and choose a replacement, one that is just as challenging as the original behavior (Chandler & Dahlquist, 2015). Sometimes teachers unknowingly punish students for appropriate behaviors as well as behaviors that may be seen as inappropriate (Zirpoli, 2016). For example, a student may raise their hand and want to be called on for every question. While raising one's hand to answer is an appropriate behavior it can be viewed as inappropriate when in excess.

Mr. Dominguez wanted to better support Mathias, thus he conducted observations during different times of the day and within various environments (e.g., lunchtime, PE, assigned classrooms). Mathias struggled with expressing his ideas or protests on several occasions. He then became exasperated, angry, and eloped.

Operational Definition of Behavior

When observing a student with ASD who displays challenging behaviors, it is crucial to provide a clear operational definition of the behavior prior to collecting data. Observations need to remain objective and include examples of what is being observed (Alberto et al., 2022). For instance, when defining talk outs, a concise description would be "When one student or a group of students makes an outward comment or begins talking to others about on-task or off-task topic. This would be considered as one talking out occurrence" (Gongola & Daddario, 2010, p.17). The success of data collection includes a well-defined description of the behavior so as to assist everyone (e.g., educator, paraeducator, parent, student) involved. Significant consideration should be given to clearly describing the operational definition of the behavior as this enables data collection.

Methods for Observing and Recording Behavior

Practitioners must consider the data collection method they will use. They are encouraged to match the recording method to the type/characteristics of the desired or maladaptive behavior, while cognizant of time and staffing constraints. If the appropriate method is chosen, it will increase the likelihood that data collection is effective and remains consistent. Trustworthy recording methods include: event, interval, latency, and duration (LeBlanc et al., 2016). When using an event recording method, practitioners can measure behaviors that have a clear beginning and end (Cooper et al., 2007). Interval recording (e.g., whole, partial) is best used during brief amounts of time (e.g.,15 seconds) to record whether or not a student exhibited a specific behavior. Latency recording assist teachers in noting how much time elapses from the presentation of the antecedent stimulus to the student initiating the corresponding behavior (LeBlanc et al., 2016). Educators may find duration recording practical in identifying how long a student exhibits a behavior. For example, duration recording can reveal how long a student with ASD engages in a particular stereotypic behavior, remains in seat, or engages in independent reading.

Mathias gets overwhelmed with loud noises, close proximity to other students, reading in small groups and/or negative social interactions with other students. Mr. Dominguez conducted a functional assessment to determine the function of Mathias's maladaptive behaviors. From the assessment, it was evident that Mathias engaged in several overt behaviors in a predictable chain on more than one occasion. More than 45% of the time, Mathias's yelling resulted in additional behaviors of hitting, name calling, and elopement from class. Data revealed the discriminative stimuli of a transition, demand/request, social interactions and/or reading aloud as antecedents to the maladaptive behaviors. Based on the assessment findings, Mr. Dominguez hypothesized that the aggressive behavior served to meet the function of escape or avoidance when feeling misunderstood or following a negative social interaction.

Data Collection and Analysis

Routinely, teachers of students with ASD conduct formative assessments and collect and analyze data to assess the effectiveness of an instructional practice. Data collection is required by law to determine whether a student has made successful gains as a result of the academic or behavioral intervention (IDEA, 1997). As a result of regular analysis, teachers' responses to the data can be purposeful, in whether the intervention should be continued or stopped. Data analysis may reveal the following about an EBP: (a) treatment fidelity (i.e., instruction was not implemented as described by the researcher) was lacking, (b) adaptations should have been made based on the teacher's teaching style and/or student needs, and (c) the EBP did not match the context in which it was taught (Cook et al., 2008).

Functional Assessment and Analysis

Educators may conduct functional assessments to gain insight as to the setting events, antecedents, activities, and consequences that directly impact behavior (Bryant et al., 2020). Communication, learning styles, teacher/ peer relationships, classroom environment, time of the day, delivery of instruction, and presence of certain individuals can set the stage for challenging behaviors to occur. Indirect and direct observations help educators determine the function(s) of a student's behavior (e.g., sensory, tangible, escape, attention) and form a hypothesis (Travers & Nunez, 2017).

Mathias rips up a reading passage during a group activity. A hypothesis is that he destroys the worksheet to avoid/escape reading words that are unfamiliar to him. To test the hypothesis, Mr. Dominguez could pre-read the passage with Mathias, to familiarize him with new vocabulary prior to the next day's group activity.

Functional analysis manipulations should not be carried out unless appropriate safeguards are available (O'Neill et al., 2015). It involves manipulating the conditions and observing the effects on the behavior before developing an intervention (Scheuermann et al., 2022). Given the serious challenging behaviors (e.g., aggression, head banging, biting, property destruction) that students with ASD may exhibit, expert teachers know that qualified staff must be present when conducting a functional behavior analysis (O'Neill et al., 2015). A qualified team who embraces a PBS approach is beneficial when creating a positive behavior support plan for those students who require the most intensive individualized (i.e., tertiary) supports.

Behavior Support Plans

As previously stated, goals and objectives are developed into a well-written behavior support plan (BSP) based on the results of a functional behavioral assessment and functional behavior analysis. Once developed, teachers continue to collect data, evaluate the results and make changes to the BSP (Bryant et al., 2020). The BSP is fluid in that resources, student development, peers, staffing, and contexts are ever-changing (Travers & Nunez, 2017; Wheeler & Richey, 2019). Within the BSP, is a cohesive program that supports a student's quality of life. The program is based on information gathered by a functional assessment and details the intervention strategies to be used in addressing individual need (Travers & Nunez, 2017; Wheeler & Richey, 2019).

Positive Behavior Support in Middle School

A PBS environment is especially important in middle school due to the size and sophistication of the students, as well as the social demands. The behaviors may occur in areas of the school where teachers have less influence and control (e.g., hallways, restrooms, cafeteria, during passing periods, gym, bus, lunchroom) (Rusby et al., 2011). Positive behavior management practices need to occur at the middle school level, so that all students experience positive social interactions and feel supported and safe at school. Data suggests schools that implement PBS at the middle school level decrease the following: office discipline referrals, time spent sitting at the office, and school suspensions (Scheuermann et al., 2022). Students with ASD can and do benefit from school wide PBS environments when IEP teams carefully design plans based on the components of a functional behavioral assessment and identify goals and objectives that focus on the problem behaviors (e.g., talk outs, disregard for personal space, out of seat) (Turnbull et al., 2002). In order for PBS to be effective, educators must create a positive learning environment for all students with ASD to thrive in, incorporate EBP into teaching, and utilize behavior reduction techniques. Indeed, PBS takes into account what challenges diverse students/families face, the stressors, and the overall impact of ASD (Boutot & Walberg, 2017; Papoudi et al., 2021).

Mr. Dominguez learned from Mathias's father that any changes in his routine at home results in aggressive behavior (e.g., yelling, throwing objects). Mathias is keenly aware of the class schedule and knows what class he will be going to depending on the day. He watches the clock and does not respond well to any changes regardless of the surroundings. The problem behaviors are more likely to occur when Mathias is interrupted from a desired event or a modification in the daily schedule/routine. In order to best support Mathias, Mr. Dominguez provides enough warning regarding any changes to the normal schedule.

Creating a Positive Learning Environment

Students thrive in positive learning environments, when they are reinforced to develop and apply needed skills. Therefore, practitioners should reflect on how they can utilize direct instruction, modeling, role play, positive classroom management, high expectations, teacher with-it-ness, positive reinforcement contingent on student performance, guided practice, explicit teaching practices, structured transitions, corrective feedback, formative and summative assessments that guide instruction, appropriate wait time/pacing, pre-corrects, task analysis, established routines and procedures to engage students (Alberto et al., 2022; Sayeski & Brown, 2014; Scheuermann et al., 2022; Smith & Yell, 2013). Middle school students make better academic and behavioral gains when teachers engage in the following: address learning preferences/modality strengths, arrange the environment to decrease sensory stimulation (e.g., provide a quiet area, soften the lighting), provide alternatives/choice (i.e., time of the day), assess students' physical needs, and encourage movement when working (Jones & Jones, 2021; White et al., 2022). Students who struggle with change often exhibit challenging behaviors associated with transitions. Teachers should prepare students with ASD for changes in advance, signal upcoming events, and incorporate the use of timers (Chandler & Dahlquist, 2015). The following subsections list those elements that go into creating a positive learning environment.

Differential Reinforcement

Differential reinforcement is an EBP that adheres to the principles of the Office of Special Education Programs (OSEP) and IDEA (1997) and is used to decrease challenging target behaviors (Steinbrenner et al., 2020), while simultaneously building adaptive desirable behaviors and skills. Teachers can use differential reinforcement to reinforce appropriate behaviors that are already in students' repertoires, but are displayed inconsistently (Savage & AFIRM Team, 2017). For example, using differential reinforcement of other behavior (DRO), Mathias learns to engage in behaviors other than the undesired behavior. He is reinforced for the absence of screaming, exiting quietly, remaining quiet, and putting away books when the bell rings. Mr. Dominguez rewards Mathias for independent reading, turning in the assignment, and asking to break four times (i.e., differential reinforcement of lower rate, DRL), as an alternative of asking to break eight times (i.e., excess rate) throughout the day (The IRIS Center, 2005). When substituting an undesired behavior with a topographically incompatible behavior, teachers can use differential reinforcement of incompatible behavior (DRI) (Zirpoli, 2016). Reinforcement is provided when Mathias walks quietly to a designated area of the classroom to journal vs yelling and walking out of the classroom (The IRIS Center, 2005). Mr. Dominguez employs differential reinforcement of an alternative (DRA) behavior when teaching Mathias to point to the break card and take a 2-minute sensory break. Pointing to the break card is a socially appropriate behavior and meets the same function as escape, as he is immediately reinforced (Robinson et al., 2019). Regardless of the differential reinforcement used, teachers must refrain from reinforcing a student's challenging behavior (i.e., extinction) (Chandler & Dahlquist, 2015).

Extinction

Extinction is an EBP shown to be successful in removing or reducing challenging behavior in order to reduce the future occurrence of that behavior in students with ASD (Steinbrenner et al., 2020). Sullivan and Bogin (2010a) defined extinction as the act of withdrawing a positive reinforcement, one that is maintaining the behavior. Extinction helps eliminate an undesired behavior and is often used in conjunction with differential reinforcement to encourage appropriate behaviors in individuals with ASD from early childhood to middle school (Steinbrenner et al., 2020; Wong et al., 2013). In order to effectively extinguish challenging behaviors, educators must: (a) identify the behavior (i.e., outbursts, attention seeking, task avoidance, (b) identify data collection procedures to be used, and the method for obtaining baseline data, (c) identify the function of the behavior and what it looks like, (d) create an intervention plan or plan of action, (e) implement the intervention or plan of action, (f) compile the results of data, and (g) review the results of the intervention plan to see if it needs revision or modification (Sullivan & Bogin, 2010b).

A behavior that is put on extinction requires that the educator ignore the behavior that was previously reinforced (Zirpoli, 2016). Extinction can be effectively used with students with ASD when the behavior is extrinsically reinforced (e.g., teacher attention for escaping). However, teachers of students with ASD will find that extinction is not effective for behaviors that are intrinsically reinforcing to the student (e.g., rocking, humming, hand flapping). Severely aggressive behaviors should never be ignored (i.e., extinction) when they are harmful to the student or others (O'Neil et al., 2015; Robinson et al., 2019; Zirpoli, 2016). Extinction practices should be used only when the teacher or clinician will be able to tolerate escalation of the targeted undesirable behavior before it is reduced.

Functional Communication Training

Functional communication training (FCT) involves conducting a functional behavior assessment to identify the stimuli that reinforce the challenging/maladaptive behavior and teaching an appropriate communicative replacement behavior that meets the function (Andzik et al., 2016; Steinbrenner et al., 2020; Wheeler & Richey, 2019). The appropriate communicative replacement behavior may be an action, response, or a communication (e.g., place a picture in someone's hand, vocalize break please, gesture). For example, a high school student is reinforced with teacher attention when he or she raises a hand to answer/ask a question and ignored when talking out without permission (Wheeler & Richey, 2019; Zirpoli, 2016). Teachers may begin FCT once data are collected (i.e., following a functional behavior assessment) and the function has been determined. During FCT teachers can use differential reinforcement with the new functionally equivalent behavior and extinction with the challenging behavior (Robinson et al., 2019; Scheuermann et al., 2022).

Video Modeling

Video modeling has been found to be effective with students with ASD who struggle with generalizing skills across different settings (Franzone & Collet-Klingenberg, 2008; Monaco & Wolfe, 2018). Video modeling allows students with ASD to view a task in its entirety, and then perform the skill set they previously viewed (Bellini & Merrill, 2017) There are a variety of video modeling methods: (a) basic modeling involves recording a video of someone modeling or performing a task or skill set, after which the learner watches the video at a later date, (b) video self-modeling involves the learner being recorded performing the desired task or skill, after which the video is viewed, (c) point-of-view modeling involves the task or skill set being recorded through the eyes of the learner, and (d) video

Table 13.1 Video Modeling

Example: Video Modeling
Mathias is a 13-year-old middle school student with ASD who attends a public school. Data revealed Mathias has difficulty responding to peers during typical conversations in the general education classroom. He struggles with conducting a conversation, understanding wait time or choosing appropriate topics to discuss. Mr. Dominguez decides to implement video modeling by creating a short video with the help of two same age peer mentors. Next, Mr. Dominguez introduces conversational steps to Mathias and a classroom peer mentor. After viewing the video Mathias and the peer practice/review the steps for conducting a conversation.

Source: Adapted from Ogilvie, 2011.

prompting involves a skill or desired task being broken down into smaller chunks that allows the learner to view the video through a visual task analysis (Bellini & Merrill, 2017; Franzone & Collet-Klingenberg, 2008; Monaco & Wolfe, 2018). Video modeling has been successfully noted in the literature to teach students with ASD how to perform daily/functional life skills (Bellini & Merrill, 2017; Huaqing et al., 2018; Kim et al., 2022; Ogilvie, 2011; Steinbrenner et al., 2020). See Table 13.1 for an example of how video modeling was used with Mathias.

Positive Behavior Support in High School

Mr. Dominguez meets with the high school special education program specialist to review the names of incoming freshmen. He presents Mathias's goals and objectives and shares the strategies (e.g., access to sensory reinforcers; video prompting) that best meet his needs. Together they plan and strategize how Mathias's goals and objectives can be maintained in the high school environment.

The dynamics of high school become more complex as students with ASD transition from middle to high school (Kirby et al., 2020). During the high school years, students must interact with multiple staff and administrators, and a larger population of students. In addition, rules and behavioral expectations may vary from classroom to classroom (Flannery et al., 2009). PBS focuses on prevention, provides consistency for high school students with ASD, thus reducing problematic behaviors and prevents future reoccurrences (Carr et al., 2014).

High school students with ASD face many challenges when it comes to daily routines, environmental changes, mental health (i.e., anxiety), and the transition into adulthood (Kirby et al., 2020). Since PBS enhances the capacity of a student, family and community, practitioners should look beyond the constraints of the classroom as the principles help meet the present and future needs of students and better prepare them for adult living and employment (Sugai et al., 2000; Test et al., 2014). In order to meet the needs, educators can help to: (a) build social and communication skills with peers and community members, (b) prepare others to work collaboratively in social settings with youth with ASD, and (c) foster supportive environments (Carter et al., 2013). Research provides evidence that youth with ASD must play an active role in their individualized transition plan, have opportunities to explore postsecondary options, and receive ongoing instruction in the areas of self-management, decision making, problem solving, independent living, and functional skills (Carter et al., 2013). By preparing transition-age youth with ASD in high school for the real world educators can help improve their overall quality of life (Lee & Carter, 2012; Test et al., 2020). What follows are aspects and or examples of PBS in high school.

Structured Learning Environments and Visual Supports

High school youth with ASD are best supported in structured learning environments with supports that include visual schedules, prompts and picture cues (Martin & Wilkins, 2022). Visual supports: (1) are a method of external control that some students require in order to access other environments, (2) help decrease errors, (3) promote maintenance and generalization of skills, and (4) serve as constant reminders (West, 2008). Visual supports are quite adaptable allowing students to enhance communication, understand verbal directions, teach a variety of skills, enhance academic and social skills, and reduce problematic behavior (Earles-Vollrath et al., 2018). Noting the importance of structure and visual supports, Smith Myles and Southwick (2005) encourage teachers to secure visual prompts within student notebooks, to keep backups for those students who lose them, and to teach students how to organize their materials. The challenge for educators is to provide only the support needed while transferring that to more naturalistic methods.

Reinforcement in High School

It can be assumed that a student is positively reinforced when the behavior increased following reinforcement (e.g., tokens, praise, break) (Scheuermann et al., 2022). Yet, for reinforcement to be effective educators must: (1) reinforce correct behaviors/responses, (2) vary the tone with delivery, (3) stay positive and upbeat, (4) deliver quickly with enthusiasm, and (5) plan to fade (Storey & Post, 2017). Due to the varied interests of students with ASD, it is important that high school teachers be thoughtful when selecting reinforcers. Reinforcement is more effective when it is highly favored. Since students may have particular interests,

---

Sample Hidden Curriculum Items

- Treat all authority figures with respect (e.g., police, firefighters). You would not address a police officer like you would your brother.
- Not all people you are unfamiliar with are strangers you cannot trust. You may not know your bus driver or your police officer, but these are people who help you.
- What may be acceptable at your house may not be acceptable at a friend's house. For example, although it is acceptable to put your feet up on the table at home, your friend's mom may be upset if you do that in their home.
- People do not always want to know the honest truth even when they ask. Your best friend does not want to hear that she looks fat in a new dress she bought for the high school dance.
- Teachers do not have all the same rules. One teacher may allow chewing gum in the classroom, while another gives out fines for chewing gum.
- Teachers assume certain expectations for their students. For example, students are expected to greet the teachers, sit down when the bell ringers, and listen quietly to announcements.
- When a teacher gives you a warning, it means that she wants a given behavior to stop and that most likely there will be a consequence if the behavior continues or occurs again.
- It is impolite to interrupt someone talking, unless it is an emergency.
- Acceptable slag that may be used with your peers (e.g., dawg, phat) may not be acceptable when interacting with adults.
- When the teacher is scolding another student, it is not the best time to ask the teacher a question.
- When a teacher tells another student to stop talking, it is not an appropriate time for you to start talking to your neighbor.

Figure 13.1 Sample Hidden Curriculum.

From *Asperger Syndrome and Difficult Moments* (p. 89), by B. Smith Myles and J. Southwick, 2005, Shawnee, KS: Autism Asperger Publishing Co. Copyright (2015) by Kirsten McBride. Reprinted with permission.

such as computer time, class time to discuss sports scores, gaming, designing, movies, music or time to be alone, effective educators conduct reinforcement assessments. Perner and Delano (2013) note procedures educators can utilize for students with ASD who have limited communication (See Figure 13.1).

Behavior Reduction Techniques

Alberto et al. (2022) describe a behavior reduction procedural model. Included in Level 1 of their alternatives is Reinforcement-based strategies such as differential reinforcement or non-contingent reinforcement; Level 2, Extinction; Level 3 Removal of the desired stimuli (i.e., time-out, response cost); and Level 4, Presentation of an aversive. Even so, punishment is never a first option. Only when a child's safety is in question or for serious behaviors, may physical or other aversive consequences be acceptable (Alberto et al., 2022). Limitations to behavior reduction options include parent/administrator/guardian consent, a detailed description of the plan (e.g., who will interact with the student, what will be done) and when the team will reconvene to examine the data (Simpson & Otten, 2005). High school teachers of students with ASD should use positive alternatives to decrease or eliminate inappropriate behavior. While teachers may feel students who exhibit inappropriate behavior should not be given choices, as it will increase the behavior, students can and do benefit from choice-making opportunities (White et al., 2022).

In the middle school, Mathias chooses where he wants to sit in the classroom and the method for completing an assignment (i.e., computer, paper and pencil, orally). Mr. Dominguez believes that Mathias will benefit from continued choice opportunities in high school. For example, he can choose when he wants a sensory break (i.e., brief activity break) and how he completes group assignments (e.g., working one on one with a peer; working in a small group).

Choice-making

Researchers identified choice-making as one of the components of self-determined behavior (Brown et al., 2020; Schwartz et al., 2020; Shogren & Wehmeyer, 2018). The literature supports teaching students with ASD to engage in choice-making opportunities (Brown et al., 2020; Shevin & Klein, 2004; Watanabe & Sturmey, 2003). Choice-making opportunities can begin by pointing, through the use of facial expressions or gestures, labeling an item, and through the use of oral communication (Brown et al., 2020). Students with ASD can be taught a choice-making framework within the instructional setting, home environment, and community (Schwartz et al., 2020; Shevin & Klein, 2004; Shogren et al., 2004). Educators can encourage high school students to choose where they want to sit in the classroom, how they would like to complete a classroom assignment or activity, or evaluate routines that occur naturally within their daily environment (Shevin & Klein, 2004; Wehmeyer et al., 2010; White et al., 2022).

Hidden Curriculum

In particular, the hidden curriculum is challenging for adolescents with ASD (McKeithan & Sabornie, 2020). The hidden curriculum refers to the unwritten principles, norms, rules, or ethics adopted by most individuals and which are not specifically taught (Lee, 2011). An adolescent with ASD may inadvertently break an unwritten rule and suffer the negative consequences (Smith Myles et al., 2013). Lack of knowledge of socially expected behaviors can impacts the youth's social acceptance by same

---

**Steps to Conducting a Reinforcer Preference Assessment for Students
With ASD With Limited Verbal Skills**

---

1. Start with a pool of items that may be reinforcing for the student. It is often easiest to observe the student to determine the sensory input she enjoys. For example if she seeks visual input, work with the OT to identify visually-based items that may serve as reinforcers. Identify 10 to 20 objects in this category.
2. Organize two containers: (a) one for items selected and (b) one for items not selected. If an object will not fit into a container, place a picture in the container.
3. While sitting with the student, show her two items and give the direction, "Pick one."
4. Provide adequate wait time for the student to select an item using her form of communication (e.g., visual orientation, reach, point, switch). Allow the student to interact with the item for a brief time period (i.e., 30 seconds using a visual/auditory timer to indicate start and end time).
5. Place items in the appropriate container (selected/not selected)
6. Continue the selection process until all items are presented to the student and placed in the proper container.
7. Place the container near the student's work area for reinforcement as appropriate.

Figure 13.2 Reinforcer Preference Assessment.

From *A Guide to Teaching Students with Autism Spectrum Disorders* (p. 14), by D. Perner and M. E. Delano, 2013, Arlington, VA: Division on Autism and Developmental Disabilities of the Council for Exceptional Children. Copyright (2015) by Darlene Perner. Reprinted with permission.

age peers (Smith Myles et al., 2013). For example, a high school age student with ASD may not grasp that there are different rules that apply at home, at lunch, in the classroom and with friends. Thus, professionals play a critical role in identifying teachable moments when the hidden curriculum can/should be taught. The direct teaching of these unwritten rules is important at every grade level as it can impact students' quality of life outside of school and beyond graduation (Smith Myles & Southwick, 2005). (See Figure 13.2.)

Social Skills Training

The importance of social skills training for secondary students with ASD cannot be overstated. High school students with ASD may experience difficulties forming or maintaining friendships, resulting in social rejection or limited social interaction. They often become even more isolated since they have not established positive reciprocal friendships, the byproducts from the mutual interchanges among friends (Laugeson et al., 2009). Social modeling, scripts, and stories can be effective ways to support students with ASD, allowing them to visually demonstrate behaviors, thoughts and feelings, and help to reduce fears and judgement in social situations (Bellini & Merrill, 2017; Peck-Stichter & Conroy, 2018).

Social skills instruction, as with the hidden curriculum, requires direct instruction since students with ASD do not learn these competencies through incidental observation (Cihak & Smith, 2017). A few research and/or evidence-based strategies that help promote students' social skills include: *Program for the Education and Enrichment of Relational Skills* (Laugeson et al., 2009); comic strip conversations and social stories (Earles et al., 2018), power cards (Boutot et al., 2017; Cihak & Smith, 2017), and *Building Social Relationships 2* (Bellini, 2016). It is recommended that educators take time every day to teach social skills and assess opportunities that lend themselves to instruction (e.g., those natural occurring situations) (Boutot et al., 2017).

Social Communication

One major factor affecting youth with ASD in achieving positive peer social relationships is poor social communicative behaviors. Research suggests Pivotal Response Treatment (PRT) can support and enhance diverse students' communication skills (Kim & Trainor, 2020; Koegel & Koegel, 2012; Wong et al., 2013). For example, students with ASD may struggle with several pivotal behaviors (e.g., motivation, social initiation, self-management) that impact communication. However, the teaching of pivotal behaviors can improve high school-age students with ASD skills in other areas (e.g., social, affect, perseveration, academics) (Koegel & Koegel, 2012).

Technology-Aided Instruction

There is strong consensus that technology-aided instruction (TAI) is effective as a teaching tool for students' with ASD academics, communication, and social skills (Odom et al., 2010; Wood et al., 2017). The overall purpose of technology is to facilitate a student's learning, not to be the primary teacher (Ayres & Whiteside, 2018). A variety of studies have involved the use of various forms of TAI (e.g., iPad, portable electronic devices). For instance, adolescents with autism solved mathematical problems using video self-monitoring (VSM) and the iPad (Burton et al., 2013). Data suggest (Mechling et al., 2009; Mechling & Savidge, 2011) that middle and high school age students with ASD can perform tasks independently with the support of technological devices (e.g., iPad, PDA, video). TAI can be beneficial in that the device prompts responses and the level of prompt can be changed for the learner (e.g., visual, visual and audio, video) (Mechling & Savidge, 2011). Mechling et al. (2009) brings importance to teachers utilizing technology to assist students when first learning a task, to facilitate reaching criterion level and to assess for maintenance. TAI appears to be a natural addition when teaching behavioral and academic skills to students with ASD (Kouo & Visco, 2021;

Odom et al., 2010; Steinbrenner et al., 2020; Velez-Coto, 2017; Wong et al., 2013; Wood et al., 2017).

Cognitive Behavioral Modification Strategies

Cognitive behavioral interventions have proven helpful in enabling students with autism to regulate their emotions (e.g., anger, anxiety, frustrations) (Crutchfield & Wood, 2018). Cognitive behavioral interventions, such as self-determination, problem solving, social stories, cartooning, self-management, goal setting, self-instruction, self-evaluation, and self-reinforcement can support students in managing their behaviors (Alberto et al., 2022; Scheuermann et al., 2022; Simpson & Otten, 2005). One goal of a cognitive behavioral approach is to empower a student with ASD to understand feelings and how they affect the body (Sofronoff et al., 2007). Teachers can take advantage of cognitive behavioral methods to improve students' performance in (a) self-determination, (b) problem solving, (c) goal setting, (d) self-reinforcement, and (e) self-advocacy. They are presented in the following section.

Self-Determination

Self-determination plays a critical role in the education of students with disabilities (Shogren & Wehmeyer, 2018; Stang et al., 2009; Wehmeyer, 2005). Self-determination is a set of necessary component skills (e.g., decision making, goal setting) that individuals need to learn in order to exercise control over their lives (Raley et al., 2018). Students who are self-determined express wants and needs and make good or bad decisions as the causal agent in their lives (Wehmeyer, 2005). Therefore, self-determination is an important quality for a student with ASD to possess. Providing opportunities for students to learn to self-advocate, necessitates that they be provided with chances to exercise the skills that lead to self-determination (Boutot & Myles, 2011; Stansberry Brusnahan et al., 2018). Students with ASD must have equal access to and participate in the same activities as their typical peers. This means being encouraged to make decisions about one's own life, welfare, living arrangements, and job preference. Thus, there is reason for students with ASD to utilize self-determined behaviors in everyday life situations (Zager & Wehmeyer, 2017). During instruction, it is important to provide students opportunities for role-play, self-advocacy, and personal preference (Thoma & Getzel, 2005).

Problem Solving

Students with disabilities need support in meeting/attaining their goals. Without the ability to problem solve, goals may become unattainable

(Gagné,1959). Nevertheless, for students with ASD this process can be extremely difficult (Simpson & Myles, 2016). There is some evidence to support the use of teaching problem-solving skills to students with ASD to increase appropriate behaviors, and to facilitate meeting individualized education plan (IEP) goals (Wehmeyer & Shogren, 2017). Problem-solving skills need to be taught specifically to students with ASD, modeled, and practice needs to be ongoing (Diamond, 2018). In order to increase self-awareness and acquisition of personal efficacy, students with ASD need to be taught to recognize the supports and resources available in helping them to navigate and achieve goals. When students learn to find and locate answers to their own questions, they become more independent. Researchers suggest that educators and families provide occasions for developing problem-solving skills, and encouraging students to develop their own thinking (Diamond, 2018; Simpson & Myles, 2016).

Goal Setting

Students with autism struggle with setting goals, another component of self-determination (Simpson & Myles 2016). Often, students with ASD have difficulty attending to multiple goals that contain complex steps. Research has shown the benefits of the Self-Determination Model of Learning Instruction (SDMLI) in teaching middle school and high students with autism to identify, set, and achieve goals (Shogren & Wehmeyer, 2018; Wehmeyer & Shogren, 2017). Goals need to be broken into smaller chunks or steps, making the goal attainable and not overwhelming the student with ASD (Simpson & Myles, 2016). More importantly goal setting enables a student with ASD to be an active participant in preparing for the future (Zager & Wehmeyer, 2017).

Self-Management

Self-management, another EBP, has come to be closely associated with increasing or reducing behavior and improving social, adaptive, and communication skills in students with ASD (Simpson & Otten, 2005; Wong et al., 2013). Students with ASD can be taught how to independently regulate their own behavior (Crutchfield & Wood, 2018; Steinbrenner et al., 2020). A step-by-step framework for implementing self-management is as follows: (a) instruct students on how to monitor behavior, (b) teach students to record behavior (e.g., outburst, talking out, participation, social interaction), (c) show students ways to self-evaluate behavior and performance, and (d) determine a reward system for when meeting criterion (Neitzel & Busick, 2009; Sulaimani & Bagadood, 2020). The goal of teaching self-management to students with ASD is for them to learn to self-regulate, to be aware and accountable for their behavior (Lee et al., 2007). Not surprisingly, research has shown the benefits of self-management to be successful when implemented properly with students with ASD across age levels (i.e., pre-school, elementary, middle school, secondary) (Newman et al.,1996; Newman et al, 1995; Odom et al., 2010; Soares et al., 2009; Stahmer & Schreibman, 1992; Steinbrenner et al., 2020; Wong et al., 2013). The outcome of teaching students to self-manage is to enhance their overall quality of life (Crutchfield & Wood, 2018; Sulaimani & Bagadood, 2020).

Self-Advocacy

In order to display self-advocacy, students must be taught and given opportunities to communicate basic needs and wants (Burke et al., 2018). Additionally, they must have an understanding of those basic needs and wants and how to use that knowledge in an appropriate manner (Schreiner, 2007; Zager & Dreyfus, 2017). Researchers identified a self-advocacy conceptual framework as knowledge of oneself and rights, and the ability to effectively communicate those needs or rights (Shogren & Wehmeyer, 2018; Test et al., 2014). Students can participate in their IEP using self-advocacy and leadership skills (Cook & Odom, 2013; Lee et al., 2011, Test et al., 2014; Van Reusen et al., 2007; Zager & Dreyfus, 2017). Some of the resources listed in Table 13.2 are designed to aid student self-advocacy.

Mr. Dominguez and the team utilize PBS strategies that are research-based and/or EBP in the classroom and at the school site. Mathias has made significant improvements across all areas (i.e., social, academic, behavioral) in middle school. The IEP team wants to ensure that Mathias maintains the skills in high school, therefore, a plan is developed for the various activities and subjects (Henry & Smith Myles, 2013).

Comprehensive Autism Planning (CAPS)

Due to the dynamics of school change, teachers and parents are rightly concerned when children with ASD transfer to secondary settings. Based on EBP for students with ASD the *Comprehensive Autism Planning System* (CAPS) was designed to support student success and facilitate smooth transitions from preschool into elementary, middle and high school (Henry & Smith Myles, 2013). CAPS is a systematic model that multidisciplinary team members in addition to the IEP can use to support students with ASD throughout their school day (e.g., sensory strategies, reinforcement). Teachers of students with ASD have found CAPS a meaningful support throughout different times/periods of the

Table 13.2 Self-Advocacy Resources

Self-Advocacy Strategies, Curriculum, and Resources
http://project10.info/DPage.php?ID=185

Self-Advocacy Strategy Student (Manual and CD)
www.edgeenterprisesinc.com/product/self-advocacy-strategy-student-manual-cd/

Whose Future Is It Anyway? (36 lesson sessions)
www.ou.edu/education/centers-and-partnerships/zarrow/transition-education-
materials/whos-future-is-it-anyway

A Curriculum for Self-Advocates (resource guide)
https://autisticadvocacy.org/wp-content/uploads/2015/02/
CurriculumForSelfAdvocates_r7.pdf

It's My Choice (individual transition plan resource)
https://mn.gov/mnddc/extra/publications/Its-My-Choice.pdf

ME! Lessons for Teaching Self-Awareness and Self-Advocacy (lesson plans)
www.ou.edu/education/centers-and-partnerships/zarrow/transition-education-
materials/me-lessons-for-teaching-self-awareness-and-self-advocacy

Stepping Forward: A Self-Advocacy Guide for Middle and High School Students
(self-advocacy resource)
https://cpacinc.org/docs/SteppingForward_-Interactive_062117.pdf

day and when planning and setting goals (Smith Myles et al., 2009). A student's schedule can be matched to the components of CAPS: (a) time, (b) activity, (c) targeted skills to teach, (d) structure/ modifications, (e) reinforcement, (f) sensory strategies, (g) communication/social skills, (h) data collection, and (i) generalization (Henry & Myles, 2013; Smith Myles et al., 2009).

Mr. Dominguez and the related service providers collaborate to complete the CAPS (Henry & Myles, 2013) in preparation for Mathias's transition. The team review the high school schedule, the periods throughout the day, Mathias's IEP goals, and the type of structure or modifications he needs. Mr. Dominguez identifies activities of concern such as transitions and or social interactions, identifies the skills to teach, and lists possible reinforcers consistent with the activity.

Modified Comprehensive Autism Planning (M-CAPS)

Middle and high school teachers may find the *Modified Comprehensive Autism Planning System* (M-CAPS) helpful in the transition (Smith Myles et al., 2007). M-CAPS focuses on individualizing specific activities for students with ASD such as: (a) independent work, (b) group work, (c) tests, (d) lectures, and (e) homework (Smith Myles et al., 2007). This resource can be useful in providing documentation and just the right support students need as they transfer to various educational programs. (See Figure 13.3.)

Teacher, Parent and Community Roles in the PBS Learning Environment

Teachers, parents, and community members all play a vital role in providing students with ASD positive behavior supports. Families of children with ASD go through many adjustments. First, they have the everyday stressors that families typically face during child rearing as they go through the many transitions: birth to elementary school, elementary to middle school, middle school to high school, and high school to adulthood (Cappe et al., 2021). Additionally, families of students with ASD have additional issues regarding the health and overall wellbeing of their children (Boutot & Smith Myles, 2011; Boutot & Walberg, 2017). It is important to bear in mind both student and family needs while aware of the transitions all members of the family will face on graduation (Burke et al., 2018).

Culturally and Linguistically Diverse (CLD) Behavioral Support

Attention must be given to the appreciation and respect of/for *all* students in the classrooms (Zirpoli, 2016). There is no question that family value systems, language, and culture must be taken into account when discussing student behavior. The increasing numbers of students from culturally and linguistically diverse backgrounds necessitates that school cultures adapt to meet the needs of all (Boutot & Smith Myles, 2011; Pillay et al., 2021, Simpson & Otten, 2005). It is critical for high school teachers to help students recognize their interests, yet, consider parent views and perceptions within the family unit (Gadd & Butler, 2020; Ruiz & Scott, 2021). In order to support diverse families, it is important to take into account their cultural identity, values, and use a family centered approach (Papoudi et al., 2021; Tincani et al., 2010). Teachers may support students in a culturally responsive manner by: (a) becoming knowledgeable of other cultures (i.e., characteristics, belief system, level of acculturation, individualistic/collectivistic views), (b) researching one's own culture, (c) identifying cultural differences, (d) increasing cultural relevance, (e) ensuring culturally valid measures are used, (f) prioritizing critical consciousnesses methods, (g) engaging in ongoing reflective culturally sustaining practices, and (h) promoting cultural justice (Lindo, 2020; Ruiz & Scott, 2021; Vincent et al., 2011). Essentially important is to be sensitive to CLD students' feelings of alienation, to value all family members, to establish positive collaborative relationships between the school and family, and to maintain high expectations (Zirpoli, 2016). Indeed, culturally responsive PBS involves data collection as evidence of the methods teachers, schools, districts, and IEP teams use to improve cultural responsiveness (e.g., surveys, culturally responsive practices trainings, critical reflection and action, parent/community involvement,

M-CAPS
Michael Thomas

Activity	Skills/STO	Structure/Modifications	Reinforcement	Sensory Strategies	Social Skills Communication	Data Collection	Generalization
Independent Work	Task completion	-Task organizer -Organization calendar -Peer buddies	-Completing homework/ in-class work (from menu)	-Coping cards -Ear plugs -Stress thermometer	-Asking for help	-Task organizer -Organization calendar	-Homework completion
Group Work	Conversational rules	-Task organizer -Organization calendar -Peer buddies	-Completing homework/ in-class work (from menu)	-Relaxation techniques	-Cues for commenting and asking questions -Social Stories™ about group work	-Task organizer	-Lunch conversation
Tests	Task completion	-Task organizer -Organization calendar	-Calming skills -Test completion (from menu)	-Relaxation techniques -Stress thermometer	-Cues for commenting and asking questions		-Turning in assignments
Lectures	Attention to task	-Task organizer -Organization calendar	-Appropriate conversation (from menu)	-Coping cards -Stress thermometer	-Conversational cues -Cues for commenting and asking questions	-Organization calendar	-Listening during group work
Homework	-Task completion -Materials and supplies needed	-Homework checklist (double-check with student)	-Homework turned in (from menu)	-Relaxation techniques -Stress thermometer	NA	-Homework turned in complete	-Turning in classwork

Figure 13.3 Sample M-CAPS.

From *Planning a Comprehensive Program for Students with Autism Spectrum Disorders Using Evidence-Based Practices*, by B. Smith Myles, B. Grossman, R. Aspy, S. Henry, and A. B. Coffin, 2007, *Education and Training in Developmental Disabilities*, 42, p. 407. Copyright (2015) by Stanley Zucker. Reprinted with permission.

assessment for underrepresented groups, adaptations/modifications made to resources) (Ruiz & Scott, 2021; Vincent et al., 2011).

Summary

It is important for educators and families to recognize that students with ASD go through many transitions throughout their lifetime. There are a variety of EBP strategies and resources described in detail throughout this chapter to support students with ASD at the secondary level. See *Table 13.3* for a list of websites and professional organizations.

Using the evidence-based tools and resources provided will help educators and families as students with ASD transition into secondary school settings. Using a culturally responsive framework with students with ASD helps cultivate a climate of respect, inclusiveness and equitableness (Batemen & Wilson, 2021; Lindo, 2020; Ruiz & Scott, 2021). A PBS approach emphasizes the supports needed to prepare adolescents for life's transitions. When comprehensive positive behavior supports are in place, adolescents with ASD are much better prepared to experience life to the fullest while offering support to family members throughout major life transitions.

Table 13.3 Websites and Professional Organizations

Websites and Professional Organizations
Autism Focuses Intervention Resources and Modules https://afirm.fpg.unc.edu/afirm-modules
Autism Internet Modules www.autisminternetmodules.org
Council for Exceptional Children www.cec.sped.org
Division on Autism and Developmental Disabilities http://daddcec.org
IRIS Center https://iris.peabody.vanderbilt.edu/
National Autism Association https://nationalautismassociation.org
Positive Behavioral Interventions and Supports www.pbis.org
PBIS World www.pbisworld.com
The National Clearinghouse on Autism Evidence and Practice https://ncaep.fpg.unc.edu
The National Professional Development Center on Autism Spectrum Disorders http://autismpdc.fpg.unc.edu
What Works Clearinghouse http://ies.ed.gov/ncee/wwc/

References

Alberto, P. A., Troutman, A. C., & Axe, J. (2022). *Applied behavior analysis for teachers* (10th ed.). Upper Saddle, NJ: Merrill Pearson Education, Inc.

Andzik, N., Cannella-Malone, H., & Sigafoos, J. (2016). Practitioner-implemented functional communication training: A review of the literature. *Research and Practice for Persons with Severe Disabilities*, 4(2) 79–89. https://doi.org/10.1177/1540796916633874

Ayres, K., & Whiteside, E. (2018). *Assistive and instructional technology* (2nd ed.). Austin, Texas, Pro Ed. Publishing.

Bambara, L., Janney, R., & Snell (2015). *Behavior support* (3rd ed.). Baltimore, MD: Paul H. Brookes Publishing Co.

Bateman, K., & Wilson, E. (2021). Supporting diverse learners with autism through a culturally responsive visual communication intervention. *Intervention in School and Clinic*, 56(5) 301–307. https://doi.org/10.1177/1053451220963090

Becker-Cottrill, B., McFarland, J., & Anderson, V. (2003). A model of positive behavioral support for individuals with autism and their families: The family focus process. *Focus on Autism and Other Developmental Disabilities, 18*(2), 110–120. https://doi.org/10.1177/108835760301800205

Bellini, S. (2016). *Building social relationships 2-A systematic approach to teaching socialinteraction skills to children and adolescents on the autism spectrum* (2nd ed.). Shawnee Mission, KS: Autism Asperger Publishing Co.

Bellini, S., & Merrill, A., J. (2017). *Social challenges of children and youth with autism spectrum disorders*. In E. Amanda Boutot (2nd ed.). *Autism Spectrum Disorders: Foundations, Characteristics, and Effective Strategies* (123–140), Pearson Education, Inc.

Boutot, E. A., Ramey, D., & Pullen, N. (2017). *Managing appropriate behaviors*. In D. Zager, D. Cihak, & A. Stone-Macdonald (4th ed.). *Autism Spectrum Disorders: Identification, Education, and Treatment* (187–210), NY and London: Routledge: Taylor & Francis Group.

Boutot, E. A., & Smith Myles, B. (2011). *Autism spectrum disorders: Foundations, characteristics, and effective strategies* (1st ed.). Upper Saddle River, NJ: Pearson/Prentice Hall.

Boutot, E. A & Walberg, J. (2017). *Working with families of children with autism*. In E. Amanda Boutot (2nd ed.). *Autism Spectrum Disorders: Foundations, Characteristics, and Effective Strategies* (40–58), Pearson Education, Inc.

Brown, F., McDonnell, J., & Snell, M. (2020). *Instruction of students with severe disabilities* (9th ed.). Boston, MA: Pearson Education, Inc.

Bryant, D., Bryant, B., & Smith, D. (2020). *Teaching students with special needs in inclusive classrooms* (1st ed.). SAGE Publications, Thousand Oaks, CA.

Burke, K., Shogren, K., & Wehmeyer, M. (2018). Transition focused program plans. In L. Lynn Stansburry Brusnahan, R. Stodden, & S. Zucker (Volume 11). *Transition to adulthood: Work, community, and educational success* (35–48), Council for Exceptional Children.

Burton, C. E., Anderson, D. H., Prater, M. A., & Dyches, T. T. (2013). Video self- modeling on an iPad to teach functional math skills to adolescents with autism and intellectual disability. *Focus on Autism and Other Developmental Disabilities, 28*(2), 76–77. https://doi.org/10.1177/1088357613478829

Cappe, E., Downes, N., Albert-Benaroya, S., Ech-Chouikh, J. A., & Gaulmyn, A., Luperto, L., Caron, V., Roussel, E., Taton, R., & Sankey, C. (2021). Preliminary results of the effects of a psychoeducational program on stress and quality of life among french parents of an child with autism. *Focus on Autism and Other Developmental Disabilities, 36*(3), 176–186. https://doi.org/10.1177/1088357620986946

Carr, E. G., & Horner, R. H. (2007). The expanding vision of positive behavior support: Research perspectives on happiness, helpfulness, hopefulness. *Journal of Positive Behavior Interventions, 9*(1), 3–14. https://doi.org/10.1177/10983007070090010201

Carr, M. E., Moore, D. W., & Anderson, A. (2014). Self-management interventions on students with autism: A meta-analysis of single subject research. *Exceptional Children, 81*(1), 28–44. https://doi.org/10.1177/0014402914532235

Carter, E. W., Harvey, M. N., Taylor, J. L., & Gotham, K. (2013). Connecting youth and young adults with autism spectrum disorders to community life. *Psychology in the Schools, 50*(9), 888–898. https://doi.org/10.1002/pits.21716

Center on Positive Behavioral Intervention and Supports (2021). Retrieved September 16, 2021, from www.pbis.org

Chandler, L. K., & Dahlquist, C. M. (2015). *Functional assessment strategies to prevent and remediate challenging behavior in school settings* (4th ed.). Upper Saddle River, NJ: Pearson Education, Inc.

Cihak, D. F., & Smith, C. C. (2017). *Developing social interaction competence.* In D. Zager, D. Cihak, & A. Stone-Macdonald (4th ed.). Autism Spectrum Disorders: Identification, Education, and Treatment (242–263), NY and London: Routledge: Taylor & Francis Group.

Cook, B. G., & Odom, S. L. (2013). Evidence-based practices and implementation science in special education. *Exceptional Children, 79*,135–144. https://doi.org/10.1177/001440291307900201

Cook, B. G., Tankersley, M., & Harjusola-Webb, S. (2008). Evidence-based special education and professional wisdom: Putting it all together. *Intervention in School and Clinic, 44*(2), 105–111. https://doi.org/10.1177/1053451208321566

Cooper, J. O., Heron, T. E., & Heward, W. L. (2007). *Applied behavior analysis* (2nd ed.). Upper Saddle, NJ: Pearson Education, Inc.

Council for Exceptional Children (2015). Code of Ethics. Retrieved September 16, 2021, from https://exceptionalchildren.org/sites/default/files/2020-07/Code%20of%20Ethics.pdf

Crutchfield, S., & Wood, L. (2018). *Self-management and cognitive behavior Interventions* (2nd ed.). Austin, Texas. Pro-Ed Publishing.

de Boer, S. (2018). *Discrete trial training.* (2nd ed.). Austin, Texas. Pro-Ed Publishing.

Diamond, L. (2018). Problem solving using visual support for young children with autism. *Intervention in School and Clinic, 54*(2), 106–110. https://doi.org/10.1177/1053451218765234

Earles-Vollrath, T., Tapscott Cook, K., Kemper, T., & Ganz, J. (2018). *Visual supports* (2nd ed.). Austin, Texas. Pro-Ed Publishing.

Flannery, K. B., Sugai, G., & Anderson, C. M. (2009). School-wide positive behaviors support in high school. *Journal of Positive Behavior Interventions, 11*(3), 177–185. https://doi.org/10.1177/1098300708316257

Franzone, E., & Collet-Klingenberg, L. (2008). Overview of video modeling. Madison, WI: The National Professional Development Center on Autism Spectrum Disorders, Waisman Center, University of Wisconsin. Retrieved from: https://csesa.fpg.unc.edu/sites/csesa.fpg.unc.edu/files/ebpbriefs/VideoModeling_Overview_1.pdf

Gadd, S., & Butler, B. R. (2020). *Culturally responsive practices and positive behavioral interventions and supports (PBIS)* National Technical Assistance Center on Transition. Retrieved October 29, 2021, from: https://files.eric.ed.gov/fulltext/ED605917.pdf

Gagne, R. M. (1959). Problem solving and thinking. *Annual Review of Psychology, 10,* 147–172. Retrieved from: www.annualreviews.org/doi/abs/10.1146/annurev.ps.10.020159.001051

Gongola, L. C., & Daddario, R. (2010). A practitioner's guide to implementing a differential reinforcement of other behaviors procedure. *Teaching Exceptional Children, 42*(6), 14–20. https://doi.org/10.1177/004005991004200602

Gonzalez, K., Cassel, T., Durocher, J., & Lee, A. (2017). Overview of autism spectrum disorders. In E. Amanda Boutot (2nd ed.). *Autism Spectrum Disorders: Foundations, Characteristics, and Effective Strategies* (1–20), Pearson Education, Inc.

Henry, S., & Smith Myles, B. (2013). *The comprehensive autism planning system (CAPS) for individuals with autism spectrum disorder and related disabilities: Integrating evidence-based practice throughout the student's day* (2nd ed.). Shawnee Mission, KS: Autism Asperger Publishing Company.

Huaqing, C., Barton, E., Collier, M., & Lin, Y. (2018). A systematic review of single-case research studies on using video modeling interventions to improve social communication skills for individuals with autism spectrum disorder. *Focus on Autism and Other Developmental Disabilities, 33*(4), 249–257. https://doi.org/10.1177/1088357617741282

Individuals with Disabilities Education Act. (1997). 20 U.S.C. § 1400 et seq.

Jones, V., & Jones, L. (2021). *Comprehensive classroom management* (12th ed). Upper Saddle River, NJ: Pearson Education, Inc.

Kern, L., Gallagher, P., Starosta, K., Hickman, W. & George, M. (2006). Longitudinal outcomes of functional behavioral assessment-based intervention. *Journal of Positive Behavior Interventions, 8*(2), 67–78. https://doi.org/10.1177/10983007060080020501

Kim, S. Y., Crowley, S., & Lee, Y. (2022). A scoping review of technology-based vocational interventions for individuals with autism. *Career Development and Transition For Exceptional Individuals, 45*(1), 44–56. https://doi.org/10.1177/21651434211041608

Kim, S. & Trainor, A. (2020). Applicability and feasibility of pivotal response treatment with Korean American children with autism. *Education and Training in Autism and Developmental Disabilities, 55*(1), 75–88.

Kirby, A., Bagatell, N., & Baranek, G. (2020). The formation of postsecondary expectations among parents of youth with autism spectrum disorder. *Focus on Autism and Other Developmental Disabilities*, 35(20), 118–128. https://doi.org/10.1177/1088357619881221

Koegel, R. L., & Koegel, L. K. (2012). *The PRT pocket guide*. Baltimore, MD: Paul H. Brookes Publishing Co.

Kouo, J., & Visco, C. (2021). Technology-aided instruction and intervention in teaching students with autism to make inferences. *Focus on Autism and Other Developmental Disabilities*, 36(3), 148–155. https://doi.org/10.1177/108835 76211012597

Laugeson, E. A., Frankel, F., Mogil, C., & Dillon, A. R. (2009). Parent-assisted social skills training to improve friendships in teens with autism spectrum disorders. *Journal of Autism and Developmental Disorders*, 39(4), 596–606. https://doi.org/10.1007/s10803-008-0664-5

LeBlanc, L., Raetz, P., Sellers, T., & Carr, J. (2016). A proposed model for selecting measurement procedures for the assessment and treatment of problem behavior. Behavior Analysis Practice, 9(1), 77–83. https://doi.org/10.1007/s40 617-015-0063-2

Lee, H. J. (2011). Cultural factors related to the hidden curriculum for students with autism and related curriculum. *Intervention in School and Clinic*, 46(3), 141–149. https://doi.org/10.1177/1053451210378162

Lee, G. K., & Carter, E. W. (2012). Preparing transition-age students with high functioning autism spectrum disorders for meaningful work. *Psychology in the Schools*, 49(10), 988–1000. https://doi.org/10.1002/pits.21651

Lee, S. H., Simpson, R. L., & Shogren, K. A. (2007). Effects and implications of self-management for students with autism: A meta-analysis. *Focus on Autism and Other Developmental Disabilities*, 22(1), 2–13. https://doi.org/10.1177/ 10883576070220010101

Lee, Y., Wehmeyer, M. L., Palmer, S. B., Williams-Diehm, K., Davies, D. K., & Stock, S. E. (2011). The effect of student- directed transition planning using a computer-based reading support program on the self- determination of students with disabilities. *The Journal of Special Education*, 45(2), 104–117. https://doi.org/10.1177/0022466909358916

Lindo, E. J. (2020). Committed to advancing cultural competence and culturally sustaining pedagogy. *Teaching Exceptional Children*, 53(1), 10–11. https://doi.org/10.1177/0040059920945644

Martin, R., & Wilkins, J. (2022). Creating visually appropriate classroom environments for students with autism spectrum disorder. *Intervention in School and Clinic*, 57(3), 176–181. https://doi.org/10.1177/10534512211014882

McKeithan, G., & Sabornie, E. (2020). Social behavioral interventions for secondary level students with high functioning autism in public school settings: A meta analysis. *Focus on Autism and Other Developmental Disorders*, 35(3), 165–175. https://doi.org/10.1177/1088357619890312

Mechling, L. C., Gast, D. L., & Seid, N. H. (2009). Using a personal digital assistant to increase independent task completion by students with autism spectrum disorder. *Journal of Autism and Developmental Disorders*, 39, 1420–1434. https://doi.org/10.1007/s10803-009-0761-0

Mechling, L. C., & Savidge, E. J. (2011). Using a personal digital assistant to increase completion of novel tasks and independent transitioning by students with autism spectrum disorder. *Journal of Autism and Developmental Disorders*, 41, 687–704. https://doi.org/10.1007/s10803-010-1088-6

Monaco, S. D., & Wolfe, P. (2018). Comparison of individualized and non-specific video-prompts to teach daily living skills to students with autism spectrum disorders. *Education and Training in Autism and Developmental Disabilities*, 53(4), 378–392. Retrieved from: www.jstor.org/stable/26563480

Neitzel, J., & Busick, M. (2009). *Overview of self-management*. Chapel Hill, NC: National Professional Development Center on Autism Spectrum Disorders. Frank Porter Graham Child Development Institute, The University of North Carolina. Retrieved from: https://autismpdc.fpg.unc.edu/sites/autismpdc.fpg.unc.edu/files/SelfManagement_Overview.pdf

Newman, B., Buffington, D. M., & Hemmes, N. S. (1996). Self-reinforcement used to increase the appropriate conversation of autistic teenagers. *Education and Training in Mental Retardation and Developmental Disabilities*, 31(4), 304–309. Retrieved from: www.jstor.org/stable/23879105

Newman, B., Buffington, D. M., O'Grady, M. A., McDonald, M. E., Poulson, C. L., & Hemmes, N. S. (1995). Self-management of schedule following in three teenagers with autism. *Behavioral Disorders*, 20(3), 190–196. Retrieved from: www.jstor.org/stable/23887574

Odom, S. L., Collet-Klingenberg, L., Rogers, S. J., & Hatton, D. D. (2010). Evidence-based practices in interventions for children and youth with autism spectrum disorders. *Preventing School Failure*, 54(4), 275–282. https://doi.org/10.1080/10459881003785506

Ogilvie, C. R. (2011). Step by step: Social skills instruction for students with autism spectrum disorder using video models and peers mentors. *Teaching Exceptional Children*, 43(6), 20–26. https://doi.org/10.1177/004005991104300602

Olive, M., Boutot, E. A., & Tarbox, J. (2017). *Teaching students with autism using the principles of applied behavior analysis*. In E. Amanda Boutot (2nd ed.). Autism Spectrum Disorders: Foundations, Characteristics, and Effective Strategies (79–95), Pearson Education, Inc.

O'Neill, R. E., Albin, R. W., Storey, K., Horner, R. H., & Sprague, J. R. (2015). *Functional assessment and program development for problem behavior* (3rd ed.). Belmont, CA: Cengage.

Papoudi, D., Jorgensen, C. R., Guldberg, K., & Meadan, H., (2021). Perceptions, experiences, and needs of parents of culturally and linguistically diverse children with autism: A scoping review. *Review Journal of Autism and Developmental Disorders*, 8, 195–212 https://doi.org/10.1007/s40489-020-00210-1

Peck-Stitcher, J., & Conroy, M. (2018). *Social skills and social interactions* (2nd ed). Austin, Texas. Pro-Ed Publishing.

Perner, D. E., & Delano, M. E. (2013). *A guide to teaching students with autism spectrum disorders* (Volume 7). Arlington, VA: Division on Autism and Developmental Disabilities of the Council for Exceptional Children.

Pillay, Y., Brownlow, C., & March, S. (2021). Transition services for young adults on the autism spectrum in Australia. *Education and Training in Autism and Developmental Disabilities*, 56(1), 101–111. Retrieved from: www.dadd cec.com/uploads/2/5/2/0/2520220/etadd_march_56_1_2021.pdf

Raley, S., Shogren, K. A., Mumbardo-Adam, C., Simo-Pinatella, D., & Gine, C. (2018). Curricula to teach skills associated with self-determination: A review of existing research. *Education and Training in Autism and Developmental Disabilities*, 53(4), 353–362. Retrieved from: www.jstor.org/stable/26563478

Robinson, J., Gershwin, T., & London, D. (2019). Maintaining safety and facilitating inclusion: Using applied behavior analysis to address self-injurious behaviors within general education classrooms. *Beyond Behavior*, 28(3), 154–167. https://doi.org/10.1177/1074295619870473

Ruiz, A. B., & Scott, L. A. (2021). Guiding questions for a culturally responsive framework during preemployment transition services. *Teaching Exceptional Children*, 53(5), 369–375. https://doi.org/10.1177/0040059920982312

Rusby, J. C., Crowley, R., Sprague, J., & Biglan, A. (2011). Observations of the middle school environment: The context for student behavior beyond the classroom. *Psychology in the Schools*, 48(40), 400–415. https://doi.org/10.1002/pits.20562

Savage, M. N., & AFIRM Team. (2017). *Differential reinforcement*. Chapel Hill, NC: National Professional Development Center on Autism Spectrum Disorder, FPG Child Development Center, University of North Carolina. Retrieved October 15, 2021, from: https://afirm.fpg.unc.edu/differential-reinforcement

Sayeski, K. L., & Brown, M. R. (2014). Developing a classroom management plan using a tiered approach. *Teaching Exceptional Children*, 47(2), 119–127. https://doi.org/10.1177/0040059914553208

Scheuermann, B. K., Billingsley, G., & Hall, J. A. (2022). *Positive behavioral supports for the classroom*. (4th Edition). Upper Saddle River, NJ: Pearson Education, Inc.

Schreiner, M. B. (2007). Effective self-advocacy: What students and special educator need to know. *Intervention in School and Clinic*, 42(5), 300–304. https://doi.org/10.1177/10534512070420050701

Schwartz, R. J., Robertson, R. E., & Westerfield, S. (2020). Increasing the provision of choices within an adult transition program. *Education and Training in Autism and Developmental Disabilities*, 55(3), 348–361. Retrieved from: www.daddcec.com/uploads/2/5/2/0/2520220/etadd__september_55_3_2020.pdf

Shea, T. M., & Bauer, A. M. (2012). *Behavior management a practical approach for educators* (10th ed.). Upper Saddle River, NJ: Pearson Education, Inc.

Shevin, M., & Klein, N. (2004). The importance of choice-making skills with students with severe disabilities. *Research & Practice for Persons with Severe Disabilities*, 29(3), 161–168. https://doi.org/10.2511/rpsd.29.3.161

Shogren, K. A., Fagella-Luby, M., Bae, Sung J., & Wehmeyer, M. L. (2004). The effect of choice-making as an intervention for problem behavior: A meta-analysis. *Journal of Positive Behavior Interventions*, 6(4), 228–237. https://doi.org/10.1177/10983007040060040401

Shogren, K. A., & Wehmeyer, M. L. (2018). *Self-determination* (2nd ed.). Austin, Texas. Pro-Ed Publishing.

Simpson, R. L., & Smith Myles, B. (2016) *Educating children and youth with autism: Strategies for effective practices* (3rd ed.). Austin, TX: Pro Ed.

Simpson, R. L., & Otten, K. (2005). *Structuring behavior management strategies and building social competence* (3rd ed.). In Dianne Zager (Ed.), *Autism Spectrum Disorders* (pp. 367–394). New York, NY: Routledge.

Smith Myles, B., Grossman, B. G., Aspy, R., & Henry. S. A. (2009). Planning a comprehensive program for young children with autism spectrum disorder. *International Journal of Early Childhood and Special Education, 1*(2), 164–180. https://doi.org/10.20489/intjecse.107984

Smith Myles, B., Grossman, B. G., Aspy, R., Henry. S. A., & Coffin, A. B. (2007). Planning a comprehensive program for students with autism spectrum disorder using evidence-based practices. *Education and Training in Developmental Disabilities 42*(4), 398–409. Retrieved from: www.texasautism.com/Worksh opFiles/PlanningAComprehensiveInterventionETDD.pdf

Smith Myles, B., & Southwick, J. (2005). *Asperger syndrome and difficult moments practical solutions for tantrums, rage, and meltdowns* (2nd ed.). Shawnee Mission, KS: Autism Asperger Publishing Co.

Smith Myles, B., Trautman, M. L., & Schelvan, R. L. (2013). *The hidden curriculum for understanding the unstated rules in social situations for adolescents and young adults*. Shawnee Mission, KS: Autism Asperger Publishing Co.

Smith, S. W., & Yell, M. L. (2013). *A teacher's guide to preventing behavior problems in the elementary classroom* (1st ed.). Upper Saddle, NJ: Pearson Education, Inc.

Soares, D., Vannest, K., & Harrison, J. (2009). Computer aided self-monitoring to increase academic production and reduce self-injurious behavior in a child with autism. *Behavioral Interventions, 24*(3), 171–183. https://doi.org/10.1002/bin.283

Sofronoff, K., Attwood, T., Hinton, S., & Levin, I. (2007). A randomized controlled trial of a cognitive behavioural intervention for anger management in children diagnosed with Asperger syndrome. *Journal of Autism and Developmental Disorders, 37*(7), 1203–1214. https://doi.org/10.1007/s10 803-006-0262-3

Stahmer, A. C., & Schreibman, L. (1992). Teaching children with autism appropriate play in unsupervised environments using a self-management treatment package. *Journal of Applied Behavior Analysis, 25*(2), 447–459. https://doi.org/10.1901/jaba.1992.25-447

Stang, K., Carter, E., Lane, K., & Pierson, M. (2009). Perspectives of general and special educators on fostering self-determination in elementary and middle school. *Journal of Special Education, 43*(2), 94–106. https://doi.org/10.1177/0022466907313452

Stansberry Brusnahan, L. L., Sparks, S., Cote, D., & Vandercook, T. (2018). *Person-centered planning, summary of performance, and guardianship*. In L. Lynn Stansburry Brusnahan, R. Stodden, & S. Zucker (Volume 11). Transition to adulthood: Work, community, and educational success (49–66), Council for Exceptional Children.

Steinbrenner, J. R., Hume, K., Odom, S. L., Morin, K. L., Nowell, S. W., Tomaszewski, B., Szendrey, S., McIntyre, N. S., Yücesoy-Özkan, S., & Savage, M. N. (2020). *Evidence-based practices for children, youth, and young adults with Autism*. The University of North Carolina at Chapel Hill, Frank Porter Graham Child Development Institute, National Clearinghouse on Autism

Evidence and Practice Review Team. Retrieved from: https://fpg.unc.edu/publi cations/evidence-based-practices-children-youth-and-young-adults-autism-spectrum-disorder-1

Storey, K., & Post, M. (2017). *Positive behavior supports in classrooms and schools* (2nd ed.). Springfield, IL: Charles C Thomas, LT.

Sugai, G., Horner, R. H., Dunlap, G., Hieneman, M., Lewis, T., Nelson, C. M., Scott, T., Liauspin, C., Sailor, W., Turnbull, A., Turnbull, H., Wickham, D., Wilcox, B., & Ruef, M. (2000). Applying positive behavior support and functional behavioral assessment in schools. *Journal of Positive Behavior Interventions*, 2(3), 131–143. https://doi.org/10.1177/109830070 000200302

Sulaimani, M. F., & Bagadood, N. H. (2020). Self-management as an evidence-based practice for students with autism spectrum disorder الإدارة الذاتية كممارسة قائمة على الأدلة للطلاب ذوى اضطراب طيف التوحد. *Journal of Special Education and Rehabilitation*, 11(39), 1–25. Retrieved from: https:// sero.journ als.ekb.eg/article_126444_1001c172744a2c69542e7cb2a07674f1.pdf

Sullivan, L., & Bogin, J. (2010a). *Overview of extinction.* Sacramento: CA. National Professional Development Center on Autism Spectrum Disorders, M.I.N.D. Institute. University of California at Davis Medical School. Retrieved from: https://csesa.fpg.unc.edu/sites/csesa.fpg.unc.edu/files/ebpbriefs/Extinction_ Overview_0.pdf

Sullivan, L., & Bogin, J. (2010b). *Steps for implementation: Extinction.* Sacramento, CA: The National Professional Development Center on Autism Spectrum Disorders, M.I.N.D Institute, University of California at Davis School of Medicine. Retrieved from: https://csesa.fpg.unc.edu/sites/csesa.fpg. unc.edu/files/ebpbriefs/Extinction_Steps_0.pdf

Test, D. W., Coyle, J., Rusher, D., Carter, E., Seaman-Tullis, R., & Odom, S. (2020). Secondary transition of students with autism spectrum disorder: Recommendations for researchers. *Education and Training in Autism and Developmental Disabilities*, 55(3), 247–263. Retrieved from: www.dadd cec.com/uploads/2/5/2/0/2520220/etadd__september_55_3_2020.pdf

Test, D. W., Smith, L. E., & Carter, E. W. (2014). Equipping youth with autism spectrum disorders for adulthood: Promoting rigor, relevance, and relation-ships. *Remedial and Special Education*, 35(2), 80–90. https://doi.org/10.1177/ 0741932513514857

The IRIS Center. (2005). *Addressing disruptive and noncompliant behaviors (part 2): Behavioral interventions.* Retrieved from http://iris.peabody.vanderb ilt.edu/module/bi2/#content

Thoma, C., & Getzel, E. (2005). Self-determination is what it's all about: What post-secondary students with disabilities tell us are important considerations for success. *Education and Training in Developmental Disabilities*, 40(3), 234–242. www.jstor.org/stable/23879718

Tincani, M., Lorah, E., & Dowdy, A. (2018). *Functional behavioral assessment* (2nd ed.) Austin, Texas. Pro-Ed Publishing.

Tincani, M., Travers, J., & Boutot, A. (2010). Race, culture, and autism spectrum disorder: Understanding the role of diversity in successful educational interven-tions. *Research & Practice for Persons with Severe Disabilities*, 34(3), 81–90. https://doi.org/10.2511/rpsd.34.3-4.81

Travers, J., & Nunez, L. (2017). *Environmental arrangement to pre-vent contextually inappropriate behavior* (2nd ed.). Autism Spectrum Disorders: Foundations, Characteristics, and Effective Strategies (59–78), Pearson Education, Inc.

Turnbull, A., Edmonson, H., Griggs, P., Wickham, D., Sailor, W., Freeman, R., Guess, D., Lassen, S., McCart, A., Park, J., Riffel, L., Turnbull, R., & Warren, J. (2002). A blueprint for schoolwide positive behavior support: Implementation of three components. *Exceptional Children, 68*(3), 377–402. https://doi.org/10.1177/001440290206800306

Van Reusen, A. K., Bos, C. S., Schumaker, J. B., & Deshler, D. D. (2007). Self-Advocacy Strategy Student. Retrieved October 29, 2021 from: https://kucrl.ku.edu/self-advocacy-strategy

Velez-Coto, M., Rodriguez-Fortiz, M. J., Rodriguez-Almendros, M. L., Cabrera-Cuevas, M., Rodriguez-Dominguez, C., Ruiz-Lopez, T., Burgos-Pulido, A., Garrido-Jimenez, I., & Martos-Perez, J. (2017). SIGUEME: Technology-based intervention for low-functioning autism to train skills to work with visual signifiers and concepts. *Research in Developmental Disabilities, 64*, 25–36. https://doi.org/10.1016/j.ridd.2017.02.008

Viezel, K., Williams, E., & Dotson, W. (2020). College based support programs for students with autism. *Focus on Autism and Other Developmental Disorders, 35*(4) 234–245. https://doi.org/10.1177/1088357620954369

Vincent, C. G., Randall, C., Cartledge, G., Tobin, T. J., & Swain-Bradway, J. (2011). Toward a conceptual integration of cultural responsiveness and schoolwide positive behavior support. *Journal of Positive Behavior Interventions, 13*(4), 219–229. https://doi.org/10.1177/1098300711399765

Watanabe, M., & Sturmey, P. (2003). The effect of choice making opportunities during activity schedules on task engagement of adults with autism. *Journal of Autism and Developmental Disabilities, 33*(5), 535–538. https://doi.org/10.1023/A:1025835729718

Wehmeyer, M. L. (2005). Self-determination and individuals with severe disabilities: Re-examining meanings and misinterpretations. *The Association for Persons with Severe Disabilities, 30*(3), 113–120. https://doi.org/10.2511/rpsd.30.3.113

Wehmeyer, M. L., & Shogren, K. A. (2017). *Self-determination for school and community.* In D. Zager, D. Cihak, & A. Stone-Macdonald (4th ed.). *Autism Spectrum Disorders: Identification, Education, and Treatment* (264–284), NY and London: Routledge: Taylor & Francis Group.

Wehmeyer, M. L., & Shogren, K. A., Zager, D., Smith, T., & Simpson, R. (2010). Research- based principles and practices for educating students with autism: Self-determination and social interactions. *Education and Training in Autism and Developmental Disabilities, 45*(4), 475–486. Retrieved from www.jstor.org/stable/23879754

West, E. A. (2008). Effects of verbal cues versus pictorial cues on the transfer of stimulus control for children with autism. *Focus on Autism and Other Developmental Disabilities, 23*(4), 229–241. https://doi.org/10.1177/10883 57608324715

Wheeler, J. J., & Richey, D. D. (2019). *Behavior management: Principles and practices of positive behavior supports* (4th ed.). Upper Saddle, NJ: Pearson Education, Inc.

White, A. N., Oteto, N. E., & Brodhead, M. T. (2022). Providing choice making opportunities to students with autism during instruction. *Teaching Exceptional Children*, January 2022 https://doi.org/10.1177/00400599211068386

Wong, C., Odom, S. L., Hume, K., Cox, A. W., Fettig, A., Kucharczyk, S., Brock, M., Plavnick, J., Fleury, V., & Schultz, T. R. (2013). *Evidence-based practices for children, youth, and young adults with autism spectrum disorder.* Chapel Hill: The University of North Carolina, Frank Porter Graham Child Development Institute, Autism Evidence-Based Practice Review Group. Retrieved from: https://cidd.unc.edu/Registry/Research/Docs/31.pdf

Wood, L., Thompson, J. L., & Root, J. (2017). *Development of academic skills in childhood.* In D. Zager, D. Cihak, & A. Stone-Macdonald (4th ed.). *Autism Spectrum Disorders: Identification, Education, and Treatment* (211–241), NY and London: Routledge: Taylor & Francis Group.

Zager, D., & Dreyfus, F. L. (2017). *Promoting integrated employment options.* In D. Zager, D. Cihak, & A. Stone-Macdonald (4th ed.). *Autism Spectrum Disorders: Identification, Education, and Treatment* (376–413), NY and London: Routledge: Taylor & Francis Group.

Zager, D., & Wehmeyer, M. (2017). *Transition to postsecondary environments for students with autism spectrums disorder* (2nd ed.). Autism Spectrum Disorders: Foundations, Characteristics, and Effective Strategies (217–232), Pearson Education Inc.

Zirpoli, T. J. (2016). *Behavior management: Positive applications for teachers.* (7th ed.). Upper Saddle, NJ: Pearson Education, Inc.

Chapter 14

Services and Supports for Transition from High School to Higher Education

L. Lynn Stansberry Brusnahan,[1] Marc Ellison,[2] and Dedra Hafner[3]
[1]School of Education, University of St. Thomas
[2]Marshall University
[3]Innovations Now

By establishing that separate educational facilities are inherently unequal, the United States Supreme Court in Brown v Topeka Kansas Board of Education (1954) contributed to the enactment of a series of laws that provide access and opportunities for inclusive education for individuals with disabilities who were previously segregated from society. The Individuals with Disabilities Education Act with reauthorizations (IDEA, 1990, 1997; IDEIA, 2004) ensures students with disabilities in K-12 settings have the right to access a free appropriate public education (FAPE) that prepares them for postsecondary options including employment, independent living, and further education. When students with disabilities transition to higher education environments, they are no longer covered by the IDEA mandates but still have civil rights protections. When meeting with a postsecondary disability office, a K-12 Section 504 or Individualized Education Program (IEP) plan can be a useful tool as these plans document the student's disability and previous accommodations (RISE, Respond, Innovate, Succeed, and Empower Act of 2021).

Section 504 of the Rehabilitation Act (1973), the Americans with Disabilities Act with Amendments (ADA, 1990; ADAAA, 2008), along with the Higher Education Opportunity Act (HEOA, 2008; originally HEA, 1965 PL 89-329), provides protections for individuals with disabilities against discrimination in higher education settings that receive federal aid. HEOA improves access to students with disabilities who wish to continue their education after high school. Section 504 and ADA protects students with disabilities by requiring access to reasonable accommodations. Institutes of Higher Education (IHEs) need to make modifications as long as they don't alter fundamental requirements of an academic course. The Workforce Innovation and Opportunity Act (WIOA, 2014) expects individuals who receive vocational rehabilitation

DOI: 10.4324/9781003255147-17

funds to participate in competitive integrated employment and requires vocational rehabilitation agencies to provide counseling on opportunities for enrollment in comprehensive transition or PSE programs at IHEs for students between the ages of 14 and 24 (Think College, 2021).

Inclusive PSE can be defined as *all learning options* available to students following high school (Think College, 2021). PSE includes degree, certificate, or non-degree programs at IHEs designed to support students with disabilities who are seeking to continue academic, career and technical, and independent living instruction to obtain competitive integrated employment (Think College, 2021). In this chapter, the focus is on individuals on the autism spectrum with and without co-occurring intellectual disabilities (ID) and/or mental health challenges. Autism has been clearly defined in other chapters within this text. HEOA defines ID as a student who currently or formerly was eligible for a FAPE under the IDEA with a cognitive impairment, characterized by significant limitations in (a) intellectual and cognitive functioning; and (b) adaptive behavior as expressed in conceptual, social, and practical adaptive skills. As colleges and universities open their doors wider to students with a broader array of disabilities, these individuals are experiencing substantially greater participation and better outcomes in employment, community living, and social engagement (Scheef, et al., 2020).

Since access to and full participation in PSE was identified as one of the key challenges in the future of secondary education and transition for students with disabilities, the development and expansion of inclusive postsecondary education programs in the past decade has been extraordinary (National Center on Secondary Education and Transition, 2004; Grigal, 2021). PSE has been linked to increased earning potential for youth who continue their education after high school, even for those who have not earned a degree (U.S. Bureau of Labor Statistics, 2018). Previously, low expectations coupled with minimal opportunities have prevented many students with disabilities from receiving the opportunity to acquire an education post high school contributing to poor outcomes. For example, over one in three young adults on the autism spectrum do not transition into either education or employment after high school (Roux et al., 2015).

Typically, individuals with ID including those on the autism spectrum have had difficulty being accepted through the standard college admission procedures and accessing services in PSE (Grigal et al., 2021). With support from the Office of Postsecondary Education, Transition and Postsecondary Programs for Students with Intellectual Disability (TPSIDs) have been created at some IHEs so that previously excluded individuals with disabilities can think about college. With many individuals on the autism spectrum having the academic ability to meet entrance criteria and initiatives to open higher education campuses to individuals with ID, increasing numbers of students with disabilities are present at colleges and universities (Grigal, 2021; Cox et al., 2017).

Each year, roughly 49,000 students on the autism spectrum complete high school and approximately 16,000 of those students will subsequently pursue higher education (Wei et al., 2015). This chapter highlights evidence-based practices for preparation for students on the autism spectrum to choose to continue their education after high school (Steinbrenner et al., 2020). We then describe the benefits of continued education and a variety of higher education models of services and supports for these students. We also provide checklists for individualized decision-making for college selection, benchmarks for campus readiness, along with challenges to success at both the institutional and autism level.

Effective Practices in High School

Research to date suggests many students with disabilities lack PSE success because educational programs fail to offer comprehensive transition programming to help them succeed (Lee & Taylor, 2022; Nietupski et al., 2001). Identification of factors that play a role in PSE success is essential to inform educational practices and interventions prior to high school graduation. When examining the secondary to postsecondary transition within the lens of practices that contribute to success and perseverance, factors that have been identified as critical include: (a) focusing on PSE during transition planning; (b) utilizing universal design for transition (UDT) principles; (c) creating a summary of performance (SoP); and (d) enhancing self-determination skills.

Focus on Transition Planning for Higher Education

For many years, public school educational programs have primarily focused on preparing individuals with disabilities for postsecondary transition to employment (Domin et al., 2020). Statistics reveal very few (~12 %) students with autism and ID have a high school transition goal for preparation for PSE in the IEP (Grigal et al., 2021; Newman et al., 2011). The mindset that a student with a disability will not attend or succeed in higher education can ultimately set up barriers to future employment. Thus, educators should create goals focused on PSE for students with disabilities who wish to continue their education to provide them the same opportunities as their peers.

Transition services begin at age 16 or younger and consist of a coordinated set of activities focused on improving academic and functional achievement to facilitate movement from high school to life after high school, including PSE (IDEA, 2004). Educators are required to develop postsecondary goals based upon transition assessments related to training, education, employment, and independent living skills when appropriate. From the beginning of the discussion on transition in high school, transition goals and activities that will prepare a student for PSE should be part of the conversation.

Ensuring opportunities for success in PSE requires planning to assure that coursework, support, and accommodations are provided (Mazzotti et al., 2021; Whirley et al., 2020). A person-centered planning process can identify individual goals and help students, families, and professionals create plans that support students as they strive to achieve their dreams. According to the National Center on Secondary and Education and Transition (NCSET), the person-centered planning process can strengthen the transition to postsecondary activities by:

- enhancing quality of assessments and planning;
- fostering positive collaborations, connections, and working relationships between student, families, school professionals, and outside agencies;
- providing better coordination of services and ensuring support for the student's goals; and
- identifying and cultivating natural supports.

Many states start transition planning at age 14 to assure students can PSE goals. When planning a student's course of study, it is important not to waive high school courses that are needed in PSE because this could limit access to higher education (Shaw et al., 2010). In addition to ensuring full academic access to high school courses, educators should teach independence, social, and interpersonal skills (Berg, et al., 2017; Shaw et al., 2010).

Utilize Universal Design for Transition (UDT)

As mentioned in previous chapters, universal design for learning (UDL) provides a framework to address instructional design and delivery to meet academic standards. Universal design for transition (UDT) addresses preparing students for a successful transition to adult life adding transition domains to UDL to link academic standards to transition domains (Scott et al., 2019). Planning should additionally involve: (a) transition domains, (b) transition assessments, (c) self-determination, and (d) transition resources (Thoma et al., 2009).

Create a Summary of Performance (SoP)

Over a student's K-12 experience, schools accumulate a wealth of information including: (a) functional and academic strengths, (b) needed accommodations, (c) successful strategies, and (d) preferences. To ensure important information transitions with the student, schools create a summary of performance (SoP), which is an exit from secondary school document focused on meeting the needs of a student in their post high school environment (IDEIA, 2004). This exit document includes: (a) background information, (b) postsecondary goals, and (c) a summary of academic achievement and functional performance along with recommendations on how to meet PSE goals. Table 14.1 highlights suggested contents of the SoP (National Transition Documentation Summit, 2005).

To capture a student's functional performance, it is important to conduct dynamic and collaborative transition assessments to assess the individual's strengths, interests, and preferences (Stansberry Brusnahan et al., 2018). Schools should utilize direct and indirect methods of assessment to gather information such as: (a) interviews, (b) observations, (c) standardized tests, (d) curriculum-based assessments, (e) performance samples, and (f) situational assessments (Koehler, 2013). When planning assessments for the student who will be attending PSE, it is helpful to determine postsecondary education support needs in areas such as: (a) academics, (b) independent living skills, (c) socialization, (d) safety, (e) sexuality, (f) stress, and (g) self-determination.

The SoP is viewed as a powerful tool that can provide a seamless transition and bridge the gap as students shift from the secondary to postsecondary environment (Sopko, 2008; Shaw et al., 2012). Local education agencies (LEAs) are required to create a SoP when a student's special education eligibility terminates due to exceeding the state's maximum age eligibility for a FAPE or due to graduation with a high school diploma or certificate. The SoP is to be completed no later than the final year of a student's high school education. The intent of the SoP is to

Table 14.1 Summary of Performance Contents

Background Information
• Student name, birth date, graduation date
• Disability information
• Individualized education program (IEP) or Section 504 plan information
• Most recent copy of diagnostic and functional assessments

Postsecondary Goals
• Goal (s) focused on the postsecondary environment(s) the student intends to transition to upon completion of high school

Summary of Performance
• Academic, cognitive, and functional levels of performance
• Adaptations (e.g., accommodations, modifications, assistive technology) utilized to assist the student in achieving progress
• Recommendations to assist the student in meeting postsecondary goals

Source: National Transition Documentation Summit, 2005.

provide information to those who may assist the individual in the future, thus providing that information when it is most timely makes the most sense. Some LEAs wait until spring of a student's final year to provide the most up to date performance information. LEAs could choose to prepare an SOP earlier for students who are meeting with a college disability services coordinator.

The SoP can be linked with the IEP transition planning process and information contained in the IEP, but it should be a separate document which condenses, summarizes, and organizes key information to provide the student's next location with information to help them get to know the individual. The document should be written in a clear non-jargon manner so that personnel without backgrounds in disability can interpret the information and to assure that the student understands the contents. The SoP should include information about life goals. Educators should ensure student involvement in the development of the SoP to facilitate a deeper understanding of their disability as the greater the involvement, the greater the likelihood of the individual understanding their disability and corresponding needs (Kochhar-Bryant & Izzo, 2006). In IHEs, students must be able to self-disclose their disability to receive accommodations.

Enhance Self-determination Skills

A powerful predictor of positive postsecondary outcomes is self-determination skills (Shogren et al., 2018). Self-determination skills enable individuals to problem-solve, self-advocate, self-manage, set goals, and make choices and decisions that impact their lives (Rowe et al., 2015). Teaching self-determination is important because as students transition from high school to PSE, the responsibility for advocacy shifts from relying on accommodations to be arranged by school personnel or parents directly to the individual with the disability. To contribute to more positive PSE outcomes, schools should focus transition planning on the development of key self-determination skills (Burke et al., 2018). Self-determination skills are critical, yet it is estimated that only half of public schools implement curricula to teach these skills to secondary students with disabilities (Kochhar-Bryant & Izzo, 2006). Recommendations to ensure students graduate high school with self-determination skills include: (a) embed self-determination skills in IEP goals; (b) teach self-determination skills; and (c) teach self-advocacy and goal setting skills.

Embed Skills in IEP Goals

Schools should embed self-determination in student's IEP goals as there is a positive correlation between the degree of self-determination and quality of life for individuals with disabilities (Wehmeyer et al., 2010). Research suggests educators know the importance of providing instruction in self-determination, yet few address these skills in IEP goals (Wehmeyer et al., 2011). Educators play a vital role in promoting the acquisition of self-determined behaviors and must work collaboratively with students, families, and the community to find opportunities to expose and support students in instruction that facilitates growth of self-determination skills (Rowe et al., 2015; Burke et al., 2018). Embedding self-determination in IEP goals promotes educators working on teaching these important life skills.

Teach Self-disclosure Skills

Schools should help students understand their disability and rights to self-disclosure. Students who are unable to articulate their disability or needs may be unable to initiate or request needed adaptations. Thus, transition programming should provide students an understanding of their disability, including its effect on the individual and schoolwork. Students should leave high school knowing how, when, and where to request needed adaptations.

In PSE settings, students with disabilities must disclose or inform the disability services on campus of their disability. Disclosure can be defined as the individual telling the college, university or an individual professor about a documented disability and requesting accommodations. Educators should teach a student their rights and best ways in which to self-advocate for assistance and disclose disability. Educators should teach students to access, accept, and use individually needed supports. Students with disabilities can first begin to apply their self-advocacy skills within the context of high school IEP meetings when the multi-disciplinary team discusses the student's educational program (Field & Hoffman, 2007). The individual with a disability is required to be invited to attend the IEP team meeting if a purpose of the meeting will be the consideration of the postsecondary goals and the transition services needed to assist in reaching those goals (IDEIA, 2004). Students' participation in the development of the SoP is another opportunity for students to practice self-advocacy and decision-making skills as well as better understand their disability (Kochhar-Bryant & Izzo, 2006).

Teach Self-advocacy and Goal-setting Skills

It is important for students with disabilities to develop self-determination skills for the transition to postsecondary settings so they can self-advocate for the supports and services they need for success (Koehler, 2013). Once a student understands their disability and rights, educators should teach them strategies to solve problems and reach goals (Wehmeyer et al.,

2010). Individuals with disabilities who possess self-determination skills can self-advocate for their needs (Test et al., 2005).

Higher Education Benefits for Individuals with Disabilities

The College Board (Baum et al., 2013) reports PSE benefits include higher quality of life such as increased health, longevity, and happiness. IHEs offer coursework and subjects that individuals with disabilities may not have access to in high school (Grigal et al., 2021) allowing an individual to gain additional knowledge and skills (Hartz, 2014; Uditsky & Hughson, 2012). This section highlights benefits of participation in higher education for individuals with disabilities which include: (a) economic and employment, (b) inclusive and social, (c) self-determination, and (d) independent living.

Economic and Employment Benefits

Higher education can lead to financial benefits, such as a successful career path and enhanced lifetime earnings (Carnevale et al., 2011). More specifically, postsecondary education benefits include more stable and meaningful employment and greater job satisfaction (Baum et al., 2013). Statistics reveal education results in higher earnings (U.S. Bureau of Labor Statistics, 2018). Many of today's jobs require training and PSE can prepare individuals for high growth employment opportunities. Approximately 90% of the fastest growing job areas require PSE (U.S. Department of Education, 2019). Since 2000, there has been a pattern of higher unemployment rates corresponding with lower levels of educational attainment (U.S. Department of Education, 2013). The median annual earnings of individuals' ages 25–34 years with an associate or bachelor's degree are greater than individuals who only complete high school (U.S. Department of Education, 2013). Even with some college but no degree, individuals earn 14% more than high school graduates working full time (Baum et al., 2013). When comparing peers with and without disabilities, youth with disabilities have significantly lower PSE, lower earnings, limited employment options, higher rates of poverty, and are disproportionately represented in low-skilled jobs (Hart et al., 2005).

One predictor of a greater likelihood of employment for students with disabilities is having a PSE transition goal (Grigal et al., 2021). Access to opportunities afforded by PSE can make a difference in employability of individuals with disabilities (Gilmore et al., 2001). Youth with disabilities who complete PSE are more likely to have more opportunities and be competitively employed and obtain higher earnings than peers who do not further their education (Lindstrom et al., 2011). Findings show that individuals with disabilities who have taken even some amount of PSE are employed at double the rate of those with just a high school diploma (Gilmore et al., 2001). As a result of employment outcomes, vocational agencies recognize PSE as a path to employment for students with disabilities (Thacker & Sheppard-Jones, 2011). In this increasingly competitive workforce, individuals need every bit of education and training they can get especially with the positive relationships found between level of education, employment, and disability (Wehman, 2002).

Inclusive and Social Benefits

There are many advantages to higher education inclusion including numerous social benefits for students with disabilities. In addition to PSE providing the opportunity to develop as lifelong learners (Hart et al., 2005), it provides a unique opportunity for young adults with disabilities to develop a sense of community and belonging (Hafner, 2008). Participating in higher education can improve integration and provide increased opportunities for socialization and friendships with typical peers (Uditsky & Hughson, 2012; Nasr et al., 2015). The college campus provides students with disabilities opportunities to have contact with socially appropriate role models that they can observe and imitate (Hartz, 2014). Through social interactions, individuals can build their social communication skills (Alper, 2003). IHEs provide an individual with a disability a social outlet through campus organizations such as fraternities, sororities, clubs, and athletics. These outlets provide access for individuals with disabilities to engage in nonacademic activities (Grigal et al., 2021) and can expand social networks and involvement with people without disabilities (Hart et al., 2005). This involvement increases the probability that students with disabilities will continue to participate in a variety of integrated settings throughout their lives (Alper, 2003).

Self-Determination Benefits

As previously discussed, self-determination is an important element of special education and transition services for youth with disabilities (Hartz, 2014). There is evidence to support the importance and impact of promoting self-determination in the lives of students with disabilities (Cobb et al., 2009; Wehmeyer et al., 2011). The demands of living and learning on campus create an ideal place to gain self-advocacy skills (Lindstrom et al., 2011). Participating in higher education allows an individual to build self-confidence (Hartz, 2014; Uditsky & Hughson, 2012). PSE provides a unique opportunity for young adults with disabilities to develop a sense of identity (Hafner, 2008). Students with disabilities report acting and viewing themselves differently after the opportunity to learn in an inclusive PSE setting (Folk et al., 2012). In addition, students report that PSE at an IHE influenced them to learn more, reach their own potential, and show other people what they could do (Folk et al., 2012).

Independent Living Skills Benefits

Going to college or a university provides independent living skill development, which is an important part of learning for both PSE students with and without disabilities (Hartz, 2014). Leaving home and moving to a campus can increase critical life skills that contribute to the successful, independent functioning of an individual in adulthood (Alwell & Cobb, 2009). To be successful after high school, students with disabilities are likely to have better adult outcomes if they master functional independent living skills (Bouck, 2010). Thus, it is important to provide students with opportunities to develop and learn life skills, which may require repeated instruction in different settings (Carothers & Taylor, 2004). The demands of living and learning on campus create an ideal place to gain independence (Lindstrom et al., 2011). When students with disabilities live in integrated settings, it can contribute to positive outcomes and enhance their academic performance, personal, and social development (De Araujo & Murray, 2010). From typical peers, students with disabilities can learn about responsibility, self-discipline, and increased independence by becoming part of the college community (Hafner & Moffatt, 2012).

The College Search

The College search can be one of the most important aspects in determining which IHE to attend. While students on the autism spectrum are still in high school, the act of visiting several colleges needs to be part of their self-determination planning process. There is a saying, "If you have seen one college, you have seen one college", meaning that each IHE has their own culture and climate. Through college visits, students on the autism spectrum can talk with peers about their experiences on campus. The following section highlights interviews with students with autism and intellectual disabilities to determine how they selected which college they attended (Hafner, 2019).

Location and Size of the College

One student described how she wanted a college where she would feel most comfortable while being away from home, saying: "I knew that being away from my family would be hard." This student decided to go to a college that was near her home as opposed to a college further away and chose to live in campus housing. Another student stated, "The size of the college campus and number of people were important to me. I went to a big high school. I don't like big groups. I feel shy, nervous, and don't feel connected with classmates. I chose a smaller college. I don't feel as nervous." While a third student described his choices, "I wanted to go to a big college because I knew they would have more options. It is peaceful to be surrounded by others, but be on my own" (Hafner, 2019).

Being Included

In interviews, students also spoke about how being included was important to them. They wanted to go to a college where they would be just like all the other students. They found that their choice of a college was based on how students with disabilities were included in campus life. When visiting their top college choices, they liked the colleges best where they would be included (Hafner, 2019). One student stated "Inclusion means that I get to be in the same classes with other students and not being separated because of disabilities. Inclusion is very important to me and being accepted for who I am." "I looked at how students with disabilities are included on campus. It was a turn-off for me when there was a lack of inclusion by separating students apart from others. Some colleges had programs that put students with disabilities into the same classes. They moved together as a group. I didn't want to be separated from my friends." Another student said, "I did a week-long stay at one college where students with disabilities were kept away from regular campus life. We couldn't take the same courses that other college students could take, and we were limited to certain subjects. For the meals, we had to cook one group meal and if you didn't like it, that was too bad. I didn't get to choose what I wanted to eat so I didn't eat at all". One student shared, "I went to the open house for this college. I knew that I wanted to go to this college because it was inclusive to everyone! I heard the students speak about their experiences in college. This experience was a lot different from the other colleges that I looked at".

Social Opportunities and Fitting-In

One student shared his experience as a freshman, living away from home in the residence hall. He said, "I am very reserved. I don't go out of my way to fit in, I wait for others to approach me. During my freshman year, I got scared and spent a lot of time in my dorm room." He knew that he had to be brave and put himself out there. "When people get to know me, they know that I have charisma and a sarcastic wit. It took a while to fit in. I had to learn how to break out of my shell. I did this by going door-to-door in my resident hall seeing if I could join in. I hooked up with other students who were interested in gaming. I just had to throw myself

Table 14.2 College Visit Questions

Can I take the same courses as other students?
Can I take courses for non-degree, credit, or audit?
Can I participate in athletics?
Can I live on campus in the residence halls?
Can I participate in clubs and activities on campus?
Can I work in paid jobs on campus?
Can I choose internships that fit my career goals?
What does the college do to make sure that I feel like I belong here?
Will I be able to participate in the university commencement events?

Note: Use with permission: Hafner, 2019.

out there, otherwise I wouldn't have done it." Some colleges have peer mentors to help new students get connected. A peer mentor is an experienced college student who can provide social or academic support. For example, when going to the fitness center together, the peer mentor may invite a friend to come along to expand the number of people on campus that an individual gets to know. One student stated that she liked having peer mentors help her connect with other students. She stated, "It's hard for me to meet and connect to new people. I feel more comfortable when I have peer mentors around me who will introduce me to their friends and then I get to know them better without having to be the first one to start the introduction".

Table 14.2 can be used by individuals visiting a college to ask the staff about non-degree, certificate-seeking, or degree-seeking options. Using the collected data, students with autism can create a "pros and cons list" of the options available for each college to use in their decision-making process.

Higher Education Participation

Inclusion in higher education is a term with varying definitions, both in the literature and in descriptions of inclusive programs. This section highlights different higher education service delivery approaches for the inclusion of students with disabilities on the college or university campus and their distinguishing features along with case studies. Identified approaches include: (a) traditional disability services; (b) dual enrollment while in high school; (c) inclusive individual; (d) substantially separate; and (e) mixed hybrid (Hart et al., 2006). Table 14.3 provides an overview of these models.

Disability Support Services Model

The disability supports services model relies on the college or university disability services office, by law, to provide equal access and

Table 14.3 Higher Education Participation for Individuals with Disabilities

Models	Student Participation	Admission
Traditional disability support services	Students participate in courses, certificate programs, and degree programs using disability support services for qualified individuals with disabilities (Graham-Smith & LaFayette, 2004)	Traditional enrollment with qualified disability
Dual enrollment: Transition partnership	Students participate in courses, certificate programs, and degree programs through high school transition partnerships with school districts using dual enrollment (Moon, et al., 2001).	Alternative enrollment Students still in high school or an 18-21 year old transition program and may or may not officially be a college or university student.
Inclusive individual	Students participate in courses, certificate programs, and degree programs and receive individual services and support guided by their personal vision and career goals (Hart et al., 2006).	Traditional enrollment
Substantially separate	Students participate in courses primarily designed for students with disabilities. They may participate in social activities on campus and have employment experiences.	Alternative enrollment
Mixed hybrid	Students participate in academic courses and/or social activities with peers with and without disabilities. Programs offer person-centered planning that includes internships and paid employment.	Traditional enrollment or Alternative enrollment

Source: Grigal & Hart, 2010; Hart et al., 2006.

reasonable accommodations to qualified individuals with disabilities (Duffy & Gugerty, 2005). The student is responsible to self-disclose and provide disability documentation. Students can then request accommodations to be made for their disability that provides equal access to academic programs (Schutz, 2002). Research has found that students who frequently use available disability support services have better self-advocacy skills and higher grade point averages compared to the students who use the supports infrequently (Getzel et al., 2004).

Common characteristics of this model include (Graham-Smith & LaFayette, 2004):

- Tutoring and academic services (e.g. Student Learning Center).
- Test accommodations (e.g. extended test-taking time, separate room, alternative formats).
- Early semester course registration and pre-college summer orientations.
- Training on executive function skills (e.g. time management, schedule study times).
- Auxiliary aids, and access to campus technology and assistive technology (e.g. dictation, auditory books, note-taking tools, and alternative format textbooks).

Case Study: Emmanuel is graduating from high school this year and has completed the required course requisites for attending college. Emmanuel and his family signed up for a college visit. After the presentation, he arranged to meet with the director of the Accessibility and Disability Services office. He disclosed that he is autistic. The director described to Emmanuel and his family, the types of services and accommodations that have worked well for other college students on the autism spectrum. Emmanuel applied to the college through the traditional enrollment process and signed up for a precollege summer student orientation, along with a weekly meeting with his disability services advisor.

Dual Enrollment: Transition Partnership Model

The dual enrollment or transition partnership program model *bridges* the transition from high school to PSE. This process begins with transition goals, designed through person-centered planning, to meet the needs, preferences, and interests of an individual student (Grigal et al., 2021). Through the high school IEP transition planning process, students set their own PSE goals. While taking college courses, when they are still in high school, the students are supported by "partners" (e.g. high school staff, adult service providers, and natural community support) (Whetstone & Browning, 2002). For example, students may receive transition services through a local school district while taking courses, as well as participating in activities on an IHE campus. For students with disabilities between the ages of 18–21, attending a college or university provides them with an age-appropriate environment. Students can enroll as a non-degree student such as "Limited Status" or "Early College Credit

Program" status. Students can take inclusive college courses for audit or credit and participate in integrated course experiences and campus activities. Common characteristics of this model include:

- Dual enrollment in the K-12 educational system and PSE for students between the ages of 18–21 with disabilities.
- Blended funding approach using a variety of resources: the local public school districts, legislative state funds, vocational rehabilitation programs, and community service providers (Neubert et al., 2002).

Case Study: After four years in high school, Maria, a student on the autism spectrum, is about to attend a transition program for students between the ages of 18–21 years. The school district has a postsecondary program that is located within their 2-year community college. While Maria still has an active IEP, she plans on taking two college courses: "Introduction to Writing" and "Success in College." Maria has enrolled as a "Limited Status" student where she plans on taking one course for credit and the second course for audit. Maria will be supported by teachers from the high school who have their offices located at the community college. Her high school teachers assist her in learning academic, functional, and foundational skills. Two days a week, Maria will be doing an internship at an animal hospital that is supported through the state vocational rehabilitation agency. This internship was chosen for Maria based on her love for animals.

Inclusive Individual Model

The inclusive individual support model strives to meet the true intent of full-inclusion and offers a menu of areas of study and activities as well as individual services and adequate support (e.g., educational and natural) (Hart et al., 2006). This model incorporates a person-centered approach, and a plan of study is created and guided by the student's personal vision and career goals. Students can audit or take classes for credit working towards a possible certificate, internship, or degree (Stodden & Whelley, 2004). In this model, academic classes and non-academic activities are not separate so there are no special programs or specially designated classes for the students with disabilities. Value is placed on the beneficial experience of inclusion to the students with disabilities and to the greater community. These inclusive programs try to reflect natural proportions.

This type of model provides opportunities to engage in extracurricular activities and facilitates relationships through natural activities and interests and does not seek out students to volunteer to be *buddies* in prearranged relationships (Greenholtz et al., 2005). In this model, students might engage in meaningful paid employment. Common characteristics of this model include:

- A person-centered planning focus, which might include support services based on student choices and preferences.
- A student-centered program of inclusion where the student's disability is not their defining characteristic.
- Individualized services, accommodations, and supports to ensure access and participation.
- An inclusive environment that mirrors a typical undergraduate IHE experience to students with disabilities.
- Socially valued roles through participation in the same activities and environments as peers providing students with disabilities opportunities to establish friendships and relationships.
- Education extends beyond the classroom and does not limit a student's education to just classroom learning.
- A natural transition and pathway to the world of work and community involvement.
- Job training and/or opportunities for internships.
- Matriculate to work toward completion of a course of study resulting in employment.
- Blended funding through a collaboration by the college, local public school districts, and families.

Case Study: Ruby is Native American and on the autism spectrum. She has maintained a high grade point average in her classes in high school and wants to go on to college to learn more about sustainable energy, like wind turbines. She has enrolled at the local tribal community college where her cousins attend. She has anxiety when meeting new people and has asked her cousins to support her as study-partners. She plans on volunteering time at the science lab.

Substantially Separate Model

The substantially separate model provides individuals with disabilities a college-like experience that may take place on an IHE campus in a separate self-contained academic program from the traditional college students. In this model, students participate in life skills and transition courses on a college campus with other students with disabilities and do not generally have the option of taking standard college courses with peers who do not have disabilities. PSE programs with separate programs tend to serve a larger number of students than the mixed/hybrid or independently inclusive programs (Hart et al., 2005). This model's curriculum generally emphasizes vocational training, independent living, developmental growth, and leisure time activities. This model may provide opportunities for students with disabilities to participate in generic social activities on campus and employment experiences through pre-established employment slots (Hart et al., 2006). In this model, students may have access to campus cafeterias, unions, libraries, and exercise facilities. Common characteristics of this model include:

- Separate courses as opposed to courses for typical undergraduate students.
- Housing in separate dorm-like settings or congregate settings.
- A schedule that does not follow a typical college semester sequence.
- Participation may not result in recognized certificates, licenses, or degrees.
- Limited or no sustained interaction with peers without disabilities.
- Focus on life skills curriculum and job training.
- Instruction is provided by special education teachers and adult service providers, not by college faculty.
- Funding through the local public education school districts and families.

There are also programs offering life skills or transition programs that utilize the term "college" in their name or description of their program, but they are not actually based on or linked in any way to an IHE campus.

Case Study: Neoki is on the autism spectrum and experiences some mental health challenges. He attends the same high school as his twin brother. Neoki wants to attend college, like his brother. He likes listening to class discussion, but he is not interested in reading or doing coursework. In college, Neoki wants to take a couple of life enrichment courses with other students with disabilities. Neoki is looking forward to sitting in the student section at football games where he can cheer with the crowd. He plans to seek a paid job such as setting up the audio/visual equipment for lecture rooms in buildings on campus.

Mixed and Hybrid Model

The mixed or hybrid program model incorporates a combination of integrated campus courses of study as well as separate life skills programs on the IHE campus (Stodden & Whelley, 2004). In a review of inclusion in PSE, more than half of the programs use a mixed or hybrid combination of inclusive and non-inclusive features with a combination of separate settings or segregated classrooms (National Survey on Postsecondary Programs for Youth with Intellectual Disabilities, 2005). In this model, students are supported in taking inclusive academic courses, participating in campus-wide social activities while also taking separate life skill courses that focus on functional life skills. These programs are designed to admit a small number of students per year that are naturally proportioned to student enrollment. An "inclusive program of study" refers to the courses, expectations, and requirements needed for program completion. Inclusive programs typically provide an individualized, student-centered plan of study that might include objectives in areas such as: (a) general studies, (b) vocational development, (c) independent life, and (d) socialization. Students may work to possibly earn a certificate or matriculate into an accredited degree program. Programs utilizing this model might provide students with trained college peer mentors who assist in tutoring and social inclusion. These programs might provide on-campus residency meaning students are housed on campus. This model provides interaction with the general student body through campus events. Common characteristics of this model include:

- College academic courses (e.g., audit or modified courses).
- Separate classes (e.g., life skills or transition classes).
- Social activities with students with and without disabilities.
- Employment experiences on and off campus.
- Blended funding through the college (e.g., scholarships and work-study), local public school districts, and families.

> *Case Study:* After high school, Cory tried completing courses at a community college on his own. At that time, he chose not to disclose to the college that he was on the autism spectrum. Cory struggled with attending classes and executive functioning skills. Even though his first attempt in college wasn't successful, Cory applied to a mixed-hybrid program through an alternative admissions process at a private 4-year college. While Cory was able to take inclusive college courses, the program also offered a series of first-year college preparation courses that covered topics, such as: effective study strategies, time-management, test preparation, and writing and proofing

college essays. In these courses, Cory gained strategies that he could apply in all his courses. Through the support of peer mentors, Cory chose to live in inclusive housing on campus in the resident halls. By his third year in the program, Cory applied to be a Resident Hall Orientation Advisor for the freshman in the resident hall. Cory successfully completed a four-year certificate in web-site development.

Challenges in Higher Education for Students on the Autism Spectrum

While academics are anticipated by many to be the primary challenge for college students, nonacademic social and independent living needs are important to address when assisting students on the autism spectrum (Ellison et al., 2013). Research suggests that effectively meeting the challenges related to the PSE of students on the autism spectrum requires a combination of services and supports such as those embedded in the models discussed in this chapter. In addition to an array of evidence-based strategies being necessary to meet the needs of students with disabilities, holistic supports that address all areas of campus living including mental health may be necessary.

Case Study: James graduated near the top of his class in high school. During high school, his teachers primarily focused on academics and did little to prepare James for the social rigors of college. James is challenged by social communication and social interaction. James typically interprets verbal communication literally, has significant difficulties reading body language, and is often uncertain about how to interact with others. As a result, James lives with a great deal of anxiety. Like others in his family, James is expected to attend college. James and his family feel his success will depend on choosing a school that provides *more* than traditional academic support. James will need social and independent living supports too.

Ellison et al., (2013) employed a Delphi survey of experts on autism in higher education to identify the support needs of IHE students on the autism spectrum. These findings inform the following needed services to support the positive college experience for this student population.

- *Finances and resources* dedicated to non-academic needs, such as needs associated with social and independent living skill challenges common to autism, are important to success.

- Assistance with so*cial interaction, independent living,* and *cognitive organization* needs are potentially more important for this student population than *academic* support. Resources dedicated to *social challenges* are integral to successful outcomes for students with autism. In addition to challenges with day-to-day social interaction, social and emotional challenges related to sexual orientation and gender identity may add physical and psychological distress to college students diagnosed with autism who identify as lesbian, gay, bisexual, transgender, queer, or questioning+ (LGBTQ+) (Hall et al, 2020; Lewis et al., 2021).
- *Campus-based knowledge about autism* is integral to the provision of successful support services. Dedicated staff with specialized autism training, a campus community that is well-informed about the autism spectrum, and a well-staffed support program that employs autism specialists foster success. This knowledge can influence positive *faculty and staff attitudes* about autism, which may be fundamental to success for IHE students with autism.

Barriers to PSE Success

Unfortunately, some faculty and staff within higher education do not understand the characteristics of autism spectrum. Recognizing and understanding autism can be difficult for college personnel because of the continuum of how individual students experience characteristics, which may range from mild to profound (Farrell, 2004; VanBergeijk et al., 2008). As a result, faculty may be unsure how to recognize challenges in the classroom, and disability service staff may be unsure how to design appropriate services. Understanding challenges related to autism as well as overcoming institutional barriers appears integral to proper support (Ellison et al., 2013). Campus readiness, institutional attitudes, and characteristics of autism can all serve as barriers that prevent students on the autism spectrum from experiencing success on a college campus.

Campus Readiness

The checklist provided in Table 14.2 provides an initial screening for narrowing the college choices. As a secondary level of scrutiny, students can utilize the Benchmarks of Effective Supports for Higher Education for Autism Spectrum for a more in-depth analysis of the supports available in higher education for potential students to assess if a college is ready to meet their needs. This is an assessment tool with which to determine the readiness of specific institutions of higher learning to support the academic, social, and independent living needs of students on the autism spectrum (Ellison, et al., 2013). These 18 benchmarks listed in

Table 14.4, when fully in place, can meet the holistic needs of college students on the autism spectrum. The checklist and benchmark tools can help narrow down a list of universities that will meet the needs of the student, but it is important for individuals to consider which college would be the right fit for their individual needs. A secondary use of the provided benchmarks list is it could be used by college administrators to gauge campus readiness for this student population.

Institutional Barriers

There are many institutional barriers that can stand in the way of an individual on the autism spectrum experiencing success in the PSE setting. These barriers include breaking down the perception of who the higher education student is and the attitudinal bias that accompanies this historical perspective. Another institutional barrier includes a lack of holistic support.

History and Tradition. Higher education is noted for having a long, historical resistance to change. Change appears to be especially difficult when it involves the enrollment of what was once considered *nontraditional students*. Wechsler (2007) wrote:

> The arrival of a new constituency on a college campus has rarely been an occasion for unmitigated joy. Perhaps such students brought with them much needed tuition dollars. In that case, their presence was accepted and tolerated. Yet higher education officials, and often students from traditional constituencies, usually perceived the arrival of new groups not as a time for rejoicing, but as a problem: a threat to an institution's stated mission (official fear) or to its social life (student fear).
>
> (p.442)

In 1973, fewer than 3%of all college students in the United States disclosed a disability (Madaus, 2011). Psychological or psychiatric disorders are currently the most common disorders disclosed by IHE students (Madaus, 2011). The ADA offers only broad instructions on the delivery of support services within higher education (Dillon, 2007). Terms fundamental to the federal act, such as reasonable accommodations, are not well defined (Hughes, 2009). As a result, there are various interpretations as to how disability support services within higher education must be carried out.

Attitudinal Bias. Research to date suggests that on-campus attitudinal bias may play an integral role in the effective support of students with autism. Ellison and colleagues (2013) concluded from their survey of experts:

Table 14.4 Benchmarks of Effective Supports for Higher Education for Autism

Directions: Place an "X" in the column that best describes the availability of each specific support listed. Use the last column to list specific items or needs necessary for making supports fully available.

Supports					
Campus Living Supports	N/A to Needs	Not Available	Partially Available	Fully in Place	Specific Items or Needs to Make Supports Fully Available
Dedicated finances and on-campus resources for supporting students on the autism spectrum.					
On-campus expertise regarding autism and the supports necessary for an effective college experience.					
Professionals who assist with the development of on-campus social networks.					
Professionals who assess and teach independent living skills.					
Mentoring services that support organizational needs, such as: goal setting, meeting deadlines, completing assignments, and planning.					
Mentoring services that assist students in recognizing a need for self-advocacy, and to support skill development for carrying out the activity.					
Professionals who facilitate social learning and skill development.					

Academic Supports

Access to basic academic adjustments and reasonable accommodations (e.g., extended time on tests, note taking services) necessary for success in the classroom.					
Professionals available to provide information, support, and assistance to faculty and academic staff.					

(continued)

Table 14.4 Cont.

Supports

Directions: Place an "X" in the column that best describes the availability of each specific support listed. Use the last column to list specific items or needs necessary for making supports fully available.

Campus Living Supports	N/A to Needs	Not Available	Partially Available	Fully in Place	Specific Items or Needs to Make Supports Fully Available
Existing systems dedicated to teaching self-advocacy and disclosure skills necessary for positive academic outcomes.					
Professionals available to provide assistance with academic organization, guidance, and mentoring.					
Existing systems that provide specialized assistance to educators, staff, and other college personnel to aid or improve academic outcomes.					
An on-campus support program that provides traditional academic accommodations but recognizes the importance of delivering supports for identified non-academic needs.					

Non-Academic Supports

Professionals available to teach skills necessary for social networking.					
Professionals available to teach and mentor the development of social communication skills.					
Professionals available to provide assistance with identifying available on-campus and off-campus resources.					
Professionals available to provide assistance with learning or improving independent living skills.					
Mental health professionals trained to provide assessment, counseling, and other therapeutic services to students on the autism spectrum.					

Note: Use with permission: Ellison et al., 2013.

The tradition within higher education is to admit, instruct, and support students who exhibit the academic and social leadership skills necessary to transition into the workforce. Panel members in this study suggest [students with AS] may suffer an on-campus attitudinal bias: attitudes about the disorder may create unwillingness to provide intensive support, and a general lack of understanding about the disorder may lead to the development of a deeper bias.

(p.70)

Lack of Holistic Support. PSE students on the autism spectrum typically require specialized assistance to have what is considered by many to be a full IHE experience – living in campus housing, developing and maintaining social networks, utilizing self-advocacy skills, interacting effectively with faculty, and using independent living skills on a day-to-day basis. Research suggests holistic services are needed to effectively meet the needs of PSE students with autism (Ellison et al., 2013). Campus disability services are traditionally focused on academic support and generally lack the expertise and financial resources necessary to holistically support this student population (Ellison et al., 2013).

Supports to address the social and independent living needs of PSE students on the autism spectrum are as essential as the academic supports traditionally provided (Ellison et al., 2013). Still, those supports appear to be lacking within higher education. In a survey of public colleges and universities in the United States, only 4.8% of institutions which responded to the survey item related to *independent living skills* (n = 186) employ staff fully dedicated to assisting students on the autism spectrum in learning about, and improving upon, their independent living skills (Ellison, 2013). Nearly one-third of those responding to the survey item related to social-related services (n = 187) reported no staff were employed to teach skills related to *social networking* (32.1%) and *social communication* needs (32.1%). Findings from the survey suggest that if those services are provided on IHE campuses to students on the autism spectrum, they are carried out only through traditional disability service programs (Ellison, 2013).

Autism Specific Barriers

Other barriers to PSE success for students are related specifically to autism characteristics. Although individuals on the autism spectrum experience characteristics of the disorder to varying degrees of difficulty, each presents with clinically significant challenges in social communication, social interaction, and restricted interests or repetitive patterns of behavior (American Psychiatric Association, 2014). Characteristics such as theory of mind (ToM), comorbidity, executive function, and sexuality can impact a student's PSE success. Most IHEs require students to meet minimum academic achievement prior to admission unless they are participating in a non-matriculated program. Success in higher education requires more than intellectual ability. Social networking, planning for and carrying out self-advocacy, personal flexibility, and the ability to structure free time are all important skills needed for college success. A well-formed plan should be developed to address individual characteristics and assist with the transition from high school to PSE (Wolf et al. 2009). An assessment can be used to help determine an individual with autism's college readiness and identify areas of need. The assessment outlined in Table 14.5 considers seven domains of campus living. Individuals with autism, family members, and professionals supporting students while attending or preparing individuals for college can score each criterion on a scale to identify areas that the individual can work on to prepare or be successful while in college.

Theory of Mind. Challenges related to theory of mind (ToM) may present one of the most pervasive needs for intensive supports for college students with autism (Ellison, 2022). The development of a ToM allows humans to predict the behavior of others and is a skill necessary for social communication and understanding (Colle et al., 2007). ToM helps one recognize and understand that others have thoughts, feelings, and beliefs different from one's own. A poorly developed ToM may create significant difficulties related to social communication and social networking such as social interest in sharing observations and events with other people, joint attention skills, and the ability to connect emotionally with others.

Comorbidity. Research to date suggests that in addition to diagnostic criteria, some individuals identified on the autism spectrum may also experience comorbid conditions (de Bruin et al., 2007). Individuals with autism can experience ADHD, co-existing developmental disorders not related to autism, and psychiatric disorders (Lord et al., 2018; Bailey & Ellison, 2019). Anxiety disorders appear common to the autism spectrum (Tureck et al., 2014). This comorbidity often results in "reduced functioning and quality of life" (Selles & Storch, 2013, p. 410). The characteristics associated with autism, combined with common comorbid psychiatric conditions, may create significant challenges to a successful transition from high school to PSE. Research on the transition for first year IHE students with autism found those who live with higher levels of internalizing symptoms (e.g., anxiety, depression) make poorer adjustments in PSE (Emmons et al., 2010).

Executive Dysfunction. While some students with autism have the cognitive ability to achieve academically, difficulties related to executive functioning may create academic challenges (Gibbons & Goins, 2008). Difficulties related to regulating emotions, remembering classroom etiquette, solving problems, and coping with the transitions that occur in a

Table 14.5 Assessment

Directions: *Rate the ability to complete the skills in the following college domains by identifying the level of needed support using the following rubric.*
0 No Support 1 Infrequent Support 2 Some Support 3 Frequent Support 4 Constant Support

Domain 1. Academics	Level
Attends class or tutoring sessions regularly.	
Alerts course instructors (e.g., professors or tutors) if absence is necessary.	
Listens, participates, and learns in the classroom.	
Engages in commonly understood and appropriate classroom etiquette.	
Reads educational texts carefully, understands key concepts, and rephrases those concepts into his or her own words.	
Captures notes while listening to a class lecture.	
Completes all assigned homework and out-of-class assignments.	
Understands and practices appropriate classroom behavior.	
Respects debate and the opinions of others while still being able to express individual opinions.	
Accepts academic evaluations from professors and tutors.	
Possesses study habits that can contribute to academic success.	
Possesses a high level of academic curiosity.	

Domain 2. Independent Living

Leads efforts to plan for and carry out his or her educational experience.
Expresses his or her need for additional academic help to professors, tutors or to other students.
Manages his or her time effectively.
Recognizes when reasonable accommodations are needed and alerts an authority to that need.
Manages small amounts of money on a day-to-day basis.
Manages large amounts of money (i.e., regular bills) on a periodic and routine basis.
Plans and follows a personal menu that meets dietary needs or identified dietary restrictions.
Manages medications, including self-medicating and refilling prescriptions.
Travels independently through the local community, including planning for and using public transportation.
Seeks out and participates in activities that promote career or vocational exploration.

Domain 3. Socialization

Joins and attends campus-based groups, clubs, and other recreational activities.
Joins and attends community-based social and recreational activities.
Plans social activities, including making appropriate accommodations and preparations.
Enjoys the company of others and seeks out friendships.
Possesses wide and varied interests.

(continued)

Table 14.5 Cont.

Directions: *Rate the ability to complete the skills in the following college domains by identifying the level of needed support using the following rubric.*
0 No Support 1 Infrequent Support 2 Some Support 3 Frequent Support 4 Constant Support

Domain 4. Safety

Recognizes when he or she is being taken advantage of by others.
Walks safely through traffic and crosses public streets of all designs.
Recognizes personal illness or injury that will require medical treatment
and alerts an authority to that need.
Recognizes situations that are of an urgent, emergency or crisis level and
takes appropriate action.
Engages in activities that promotes physical, emotional, and psychological
wellness.

Domain 5. Sexuality and Gender Identity

Demonstrates a mature understanding of his or her sexual values and
gender identity.
Possesses a mature understanding of sexuality, including sexual
intercourse, sexually transmitted diseases, birth control, consent, and
the practice of safe sex.
Respects the views of others regarding sexuality and gender identity.
Recognizes the private nature of sexual interest and activity.
Distinguishes between friendship and romance.

Domain 6. Stress

Recognizes distress and adjusts to alleviate symptoms.
Participates in activities designed to reduce stress in a healthy
manner, including activities such as: physical exercise, improved time
management, relaxation techniques, and other wellness activities.
Responds calmly and is resilient in a crisis, urgent situation, or personal
setback.
Accepts assistance from others and values collaborative teamwork.
Responds well in competitive environments and situations.

Domain 7. Self – Determination

Sets personal goals and designs a plan to reach those goals.
Chooses a field of study or major.
Seeks out new and challenging experiences.
Accommodates when sudden change occurs and remains flexible.
Accepts a high level of personal responsibility.
Articulates knowledge of his or her specific disability.

Note: Used with permission: West Virginia Autism Training Center at Marshall University.

school setting can create significant challenges for the education of individuals with autism. Difficulty predicting and integrating sensory based information such as light, sound, and smells commonly creates challenges in the classroom for students with autism. These cognitive difficulties can create significant challenges in the classroom.

Sexuality and Gender Diversity. The prevalence of autism and associated traits may be elevated among gender-diverse individuals (Warrier et al., 2020). Individuals with autism who identify as gender-diverse and part of the LGBTQ+ community experience more mental, physical, and behavioral health issues than do heterosexual or straight adults diagnosed with autism (Hall et al., 2020; Ellison, 2021). "LGBQ+ students with diagnosed disabilities agreed less with feeling comfortable being themselves, feeling valued by their institutions, or feeling like part of their campus communities than their LGBQ+ peers without diagnosed disabilities" (BrckaLorenz et al., 2020, p. 85). One significant reason for this may be the fact that individuals are members of intersectional marginalized social identities. Support should be in place to prepare individuals for experiences they may face from their dual identities. IHEs must work proactively, not reactively, to ensure institutional culture and climate is well prepared to include this student population (Nachman et al., 2020). Campus-based residence life programs should lead this transformation of campus climate (BrckaLorenz et al., 2020). The mental health needs for this student population may best be served by creating communal living environments that promote awareness and acceptance, and by developing coalitions with mental health professionals and LGBTQ+ advocates.

Effective Practices in Higher Education

Many of the PSE students with autism have the intellectual ability to succeed in a college classroom (Ellison et al., 2013). Experts agree, however, that faculty and staff must understand how best to prepare the environment and provide support for the academic, social, and independent living needs of this student population. The strategies discussed in this section include: (a) universal design, (b) academic supports, and (c) social and independent living supports, and (d) employment preparation.

Universal Design for Learning

As mentioned in other chapters in this text, universal design involves designing environments in higher education that can be accessed readily by the widest possible range of individuals anticipating in advance the need for alternatives, options, and adaptations to meet the challenge of diversity (Rose et al., 2006). Universal Design for Transition (UDT) adds transition domains to the UDL framework to link academic standards to transition domains.

Academic Supports

It is known that specialized classroom instruction is most useful for students on the autism spectrum (Donaldson & Zager, 2010; Simpson et al., 2010). Research recommends that academic supports be designed to meet the individualized needs of IHE students with autism (Dillon, 2007). The most effective support occurs when educators understand characteristics associated with autism (Smith, 2007) and modify their instructional style (Hughes, 2009). Effective support may include non-traditional classroom support and the use of technology.

Non-traditional classroom support. While traditional disability services within higher education – such as extended testing time, note-taking assistance, and alternative test formats – can help, evidence shows the needs of students on the autism spectrum may extend beyond the scope of traditional disability services (Hughes, 2009; Ellison et al., 2013). Because individuals with autism experience characteristics to varying degrees, it is considered best practice to design academic supports to meet the unique needs of each student (Dillon, 2007). Research suggests faculty be thoughtful of their instructional style to accommodate the needs of students with autism. Suggestions for educators include: (a) provide detailed instructions; (b) provide clear deadlines for assignments; (c) offer students a summary of key lecture points at the start and conclusion of each class; (d) share visual forms of information (e.g., PowerPoints); (e) break down assignments into smaller, manageable chunks; and (f) use peer mentors to clarify assignments and answer basic questions for students on the autism spectrum (Hughes, 2009).

Technology. Technology may provide for effective academic supports for IHE students with autism. Assistive technology (AT) increases access and support by limiting or overcoming barriers in the environment for individuals with disabilities. Relatively "low-tech" (e.g., written scripts) to "high-tech" (e.g., computer technology) AT can provide an impact on PSE experiences for students with disabilities. Students can compensate for organizational challenges, caused by executive dysfunction, by using simple tools such as online calendars and technology with alarms (Dillon, 2007). Laptop computers or other electronic devices may help students overcome motor challenges that otherwise may impede note- and test-taking (Hughes, 2009).

Social and Independent Living Supports

Services designed to support social needs are essential to success for students with autism in higher education. Research suggests social supports may be even more critical for postsecondary success than academic supports, as students with autism admitted into a matriculated college program are generally "intellectually capable of performing in the classroom but struggle with the social and organizational aspects of the college lifestyle" (Ellison et al., 2013, p. 70). Traditional disability services, due to a lack of resources and expertise, may be lacking in the ability to support the social needs of this student population (Ellison et al., 2013). Some areas in which support may be necessary include: (a) campus housing, (b) social skills, (c) independent living, and (d) mental health.

Campus Housing Support. Navigating the community that is a college or university campus may be daunting to students on the autism spectrum (Dillon, 2007; Ellison et al., 2013). The social networking inherent within campus housing may pose significant challenges for this student population (Hughes, 2009). Research suggests that challenges related to social skills and social communication may prevent students from fully advocating for their on-campus needs, including making appropriate and timely decisions regarding self-disclosure (Ellison et al., 2013). A well-informed community appears important to the social support of this student population.

Social Support. Anticipating social needs of students with autism affords disability service professionals the opportunity to develop basic systemic supports that may reduce social anxiety, such as providing students with an early and detailed schedule of orientation, and identifying quiet, less populated cafeteria space in which students with autism may eat meals (Hughes, 2009). Research highlights the importance of assessing social skill challenges of students with autism, and formalizing individual and group activities that promote the development of social skills training to meet identified needs (Ellison et al. 2013). The use of peer mentors can facilitate the development of social relationships while providing advice and support for organizational needs (Dillon, 2007).

Independent Living Support. Research suggests college students with autism are often challenged by having under-developed independent living skills (Ellison et al., 2013). Students within this population tend to struggle with transition, flexibility, free time, and self-advocacy (Wolf et al, 2009). A college campus is a complex society with rules, protocols, and customs that can overwhelm a student with autism (VanBergeijk et al., 2008). Regularly scheduled psychoeducational meetings may be beneficial to students with autism to improve social and independent living skills and provide an opportunity for social networking. Table 14.6 illustrates possible topics (Kiss, 2015) discussed during a semester in group or individual meetings.

Mental Health Support. Access to appropriate on-campus mental health services appears important to the success of PSE students with autism. The mental health of students on the autism spectrum must be carefully considered when designing non-academic disability services (VanBergeijk et al., 2008). Comorbidity is common. Students with autism may experience symptoms of anxiety disorders, obsessive compulsive

Table 14.6 Session Topics Examples

Topic	Points for Discussion
Orientation	• Conduct introductions. • Create group rules and expectations. • Identify topics to explore, understand or learn more about. • Learn about self and explore likes, beliefs, and personal values.
Developing time management skills and goals	• Learn executive functioning skills, including planning, time management, scheduling, organizing, and prioritizing. • Budget time for academic and social success. • Set goals for academic and social success utilizing a step-by-step approach.
Developing social communication skills	• Identify communication style. • Learn when and how to approach someone to start, maintain, repair, and end a conversation. • Read body language during a conversation. • Practice reading body language and learn what subtle movements and expressions really mean. • Engage in small talk to learn how it's done. • Discuss the difference between talking (monolog) and having a conversation (dialog). • Learn about under sharing versus over sharing and finding the balance.
Building healthy relationships	• Discuss theory of mind and how people have their own thoughts, motivations, and intentions. • Learn how to find out about others and how to build relationships. • Identify what the early phases of relationship building look like. • Learn how shared interests can impact relationships. • Identify what a healthy relationship looks like. • Identify cues to tell if someone is interested in you. • Learn next steps if you are interested in building a relationship with someone.
Building a positive reputation	• Define and discuss reputations. • Learn the influence of actions and words on how you're perceived. • Learn the difference between how you talk to professors versus talking to friends.
Making decisions and resolving conflicts	• Identify questions to ask before making an important decision. • Engage in independent decision making. • Experience consequences of a right and wrong decision. • Learn to analyze conflict situations to understand the other party involved. • Learn how to disagree and tell someone you think they're wrong and not get into an argument doing it.
Coping with stress and anxiety	• Identify what it feels and looks like to be stressed. • Learn to recognize personal triggers. • Assess sensory sensitivity and stress and learn possible links. • Learn prevention strategies and how to cope with stress.
Managing anger	• Learn ways to appropriately express frustration and have control over thoughts and feelings. • Learn to take criticism but avoid being hurt. • Practice recognizing and understanding your own feeling.

Note: Used with permission: West Virginia Autism Training Center at Marshall University.

disorder (OCD), and depressive disorders (VanBergeijk et al., 2008). Due to challenges related to executive dysfunction, ToM, and social communication, students with autism who need mental health services may not attempt to access them, highlighting the need for a campus community well-informed about autism (Ellison et al., 2013). Students with autism may need to rely on faculty, staff, and peers to provide unsolicited advice about seeking mental health services. The rate of suicidal ideation has been found to be three times higher for those diagnosed with autism than the general population (Kõlves et al., 2021). For some individuals a delay in accurate autism diagnoses, which happens frequently especially in females, may have exacerbated their mental health challenges (Bargiela et al., 2016).

There is concern that on-campus mental health services may be generally ineffective in meeting the needs of this student population. For example, insight development as a goal of traditional psychotherapy may be ineffective due to the communication and cognitive challenges common to the autism spectrum (VanBergeilk et al., 2008). The micro-counseling skills used traditionally by therapists to establish rapport, assess progress, and guide therapy may be less helpful with this population due to challenges specific to social communication, ToM, and speech pragmatics (Ellison et al., 2013). Researchers agree that a more directive, psychoeducational approach that emphasizes skill building is most helpful to individuals with autism involved in mental health counseling (Vanbergeijk et al., 2008; Ellison et al., 2013).

Post-College Employment

Once individuals with autism have completed their PSE, many individuals struggle with the transition to a career despite having the skill sets and expertise to excel in the workplace. Many students with autism have learned to manage within the structure of higher education, such as: to manage their study time, be on time for class, and seek out professors during office hours. However, once that college routine is done, some young adults will struggle with the shift into the adult world. It is important while individuals are receiving their PSE that IHEs ensure they are preparing them for the transition to adulthood and success in their employment endeavors.

Summary

In this chapter, we have highlighted effective practices for preparation of students with autism transitioning from high school to PSE. We described the benefits of participation in higher education for students with disabilities. We presented a variety of higher education models and programs of services and supports to facilitate inclusion of students with disabilities.

Checklists and benchmarks of readiness for success in higher education were discussed. Challenges both institutional and directly related to autism characteristics were addressed. Most important, we highlighted effective practices at the PSE level to meet the needs of students with autism.

Discussion Questions

- Teaching self-determination is important because as students transition from high school to PSE, the responsibility for advocacy shifts from relying on accommodations to be arranged by school personnel or parents directly to the individual with the disability. Describe an activity that a teacher can utilize to provide students with autism the opportunity to practice the self-advocacy skills they will need to get their needs met at a college or university.
- Describe a transition aged student with autism's characteristics and determine which of the variety of higher education models' services and supports would best meet the needs of this student.
- Describe how you could utilize the checklist and benchmarks tools to assist a student seeking a college campus that is prepared to meet the needs of students with autism and would be a good fit for the individual student.
- Describe psychoeducational meetings that may be beneficial to students with autism to improve their social and independent living skills and provide an opportunity for social networking.

References

Alper, S. (2003). The relationship between inclusion and other trends in education. In D. Ryndak, & S. Alper (Eds.), *Curriculum and instruction for students with significant disabilities in inclusive setting* (2nd ed.), 13–30. Boston, MA: Allyn and Bacon.

Alwell, M., & Cobb, B. (2009). Functional life skills curricular interventions for youth with disabilities: A systematic review. *Career Development for Exceptional Individuals*, 32(2), 82–93.

American Psychiatric Association. (2013). *Diagnostic and statistical manual of mental disorders* (5th ed.). Washington, DC: Author.

Americans with Disabilities Act of 1990 (ADA). (1990). Public Law No. 101-336, 42 U.S.C. 12101 et seq. Retrieved from www.ada.gov/pubs/ada.htm

Americans with Disabilities Act Amendments Act of 2008 (ADAAA). (2008). Public Law No. 110-325, 42 U.S.C. 12101 et seq. Retrieved from www.ada.gov/pubs/ada.htm

Bailey, C. G., & Ellison, M. (2019) *Diagnostic Assessment and Treatment Plan Development for Clients with Autism Spectrum Disorder*. [Seminar] Continuing Education Alliance, Huntington, WV.

Bargiela, S., Steward, R., & Mandy, W. (2016). The experiences of late-diagnosed women with autism spectrum conditions: an investigation of the female autism phenotype. *Journal of Autism and Developmental Disorders, 46*(10), 3281–3294.

Baum, S., Ma, J., & Payea, K. (2013). Education pays: The benefits of higher education for individuals and society. *College Board*. Retrieved from: https://trends.collegeboard.org/sites/default/files/education-pays-2013-full-report.pdf

Berg, L. A., Jirikowic, T., & Haerling, K. (2017). Navigating the hidden curriculum of higher education for postsecondary students with intellectual disabilities. *American Journal of Occupational Therapy, 71*(3), 1–9.

Bouck, E. C. (2010). Reports of life skill training for students with intellectual disabilities in and out of school. *Journal of Intellectual Disability Research 54*, 1093–1103.

BrckaLorenz, A., Fassett, K. T., Hurtado, S. S. (2020). Supporting LGBQ+ students with disabilities: Exploring the experiences of students living on campus. *Journal of College and University Student Housing, 46* (3) 78–91.

Brown v. Board of Education, 347 U.S. 483 (1954).

Burke, K. M., Shogren, K. A., & Wehmeyer, M. L (2018). Transition-focused program plans. In L. L. Stansberry Brusnahan, R. A. Stodden, R. A. & S. H. Zucker (Eds.), Transition to adulthood: Work, community, and educational success (pp. 49–66). Council for Exceptional Children)

Carnevale, A. P., Rose, S. J. & Cheah, B. (2011). The college payoff: Education, occupations, lifetime earnings. The Georgetown University Center on Education and the Workforce.

Carothers, D. E., & Taylor, R. L. (2004). How teachers and parents can work together to teach independent living skills to children with autism. *Focus on Autism and Other Developmental Disabilities, 19*(2), 102–104.

Cobb, B., Lehmann, J., Newman-Gonchar, R., & Alwell, M. (2009). Self-determination for students with disabilities: A narrative metasynthesis. Career Development and Transition for Exceptional individuals, 32(2). 108–114.

Colle, L., Baron-Cohen, S., & Hill, J. (2007). Do children with autism have a theory of mind? A non-verbal test of autism vs. specific language impairment. *Journal of Autism and Developmental Disorders, 37*(4), 716–723.

Cox, B. E., Thompson, K., Anderson, A., Mintz, A., Locks, T. Morgan, L., Edelstein, J., & Wolz, A. (2017). College experiences for students with autism spectrum disorder (ASD): Personal identity, public disclosure, and institutional support. *Journal of College Student Development, 58*(1), 71–87.

De Araujo, P. & Murray, J. M. (2010). Channels for improved performance – From living on campus. *American Journal of Business Education 3*(12), 57–64.

de Bruin, E. I., Ferdinand, R. F., Meester, S., de Nijs, P. A., & Verheij, F. (2007). High rates of psychiatric co-morbidity in PDD-NOS. *Journal of Autism and Developmental Disorders, 37*(5), 877–886.

Dillon, M. R. (2007). Creating supports for college students with Asperger syndrome through collaboration. *College Student Journal, 41*(2), 499–504.

Domin, D., Taylor, A. B., Haines, K. A., Papay, C. K., & Grigal, M. (2020). "'It's not just about a paycheck': Perspectives on employment preparation of students with intellectual disability in federally funded higher education programs." *Intellectual and Developmental Disabilities* 58.4 (2020): 328–347.

Donaldson, J. B., & Zager, D. (2010). Mathematics interventions for students with high functioning autism/Asperger's syndrome. *Teaching Exceptional Children, 42(6)*, 40–46.

Duffy, J. T., & Guerty, J. (2005). The role of disability support services. In E. E. Getzel and P. Wehman (Eds.)., Going to College: Expanding Opportunities for People with Disabilities, 89–115. Baltimore, MN: Brookes Publishing.

Ellison, L. M. (2013). Assessing the readiness of higher education to instruct and support students with Asperger's Disorder. Theses, Dissertations and Capstones. Paper 428.

Ellison, M. (2021). *Seeing Through the Camouflage: Recognizing Autism in Females* [Conference] Autism Across the Lifespan, Huntington, WV.

Ellison, M. (2022) *Developing Relationships with Customers Diagnosed with Autism Spectrum Disorder*. University of North Texas Workplace Inclusion and Sustainable Employment [Seminar], Huntington, WV.

Ellison, M., Clark, J., Cunningham, M. & Hansen, R. (2013). *Academic and Campus Accommodations that Foster Success for College Students with Asperger's Disorder*. Southern Regional Council on Educational Administration.

Ellison, M., Hovatter, P., & Nelson, A. (2013). Asperger's disorder: Developing a therapeutic relationship. Autism Society of America session, Pittsburgh, PA.

Emmons, J., McCurry, S., Ellison, M., Klinger, M. R., & Klinger, L. G. (2010). College programs for students with ASD: Predictors of successful college transition. International Meeting for Research Poster session, Philadelphia, PA.

Farrell, E. F. (2004). Asperger's confounds colleges. *Chronicle of Higher Education, 51(7)*, 35–36.

Field, S., & Hoffman, A. (2007). Self-determination in secondary transition assessment. *Assessment for Effective Instruction, 32(3)*, 181–190.

Folk, E. D. R., Yamamoto, K. K., & Stodden, R. A. (2012). Implementing inclusion and collaborative teaming in a model program of postsecondary education for young adults with intellectual disabilities. *Journal of Policy and Practice in Intellectual Disabilities, 9(4)*, 257–269.

Getzel, E. E., McManus, S., & Briel, L. W. (2004). An effective model for college students with learning disabilities and attention deficit hyperactivity disorders. *Research to Practice, 3(1)*.

Gibbons, M. M., & Goins, S. (2008). Getting to know the child with Asperger syndrome. *Professional School Counseling, 11(5)*, 347–352.

Gilmore, S., Bose, J., & Hart, D. (2001). Postsecondary education as a critical step toward meaningful employment: Vocational rehabilitation's role. *Research to Practice, 7(4)*, 1–4.

Graham-Smith, S. & LaFayette, S. (2004). Quality disability support for promoting belonging and academic success within the college community. *College Student Journal, 38(1)*, 90–99.

Greenholtz, J., Mosoff, J., & Hurtado, T. (2005). STEPS forward: Inclusive post-secondary education for young adults with intellectual disabilities. *Society for Research into Higher Education,* December.

Grigal, M., & Hart, D. (2010). *Think college! Postsecondary education options for students with intellectual disabilities.* Baltimore, MD: Paul H. Brookes Publishing Company.

Grigal, M., Hart, D., & Migliore, A. (2011). Comparing transition planning, postsecondary education, and employment outcomes of students with intellectual disabilities. *Career Development for Exceptional Individuals, 34*(1), 4.

Grigal, M. (2021). *Building on a Decade of Progress. Inside Think College.* https://thinkcollege.net/ blog/building-on-a-decade-of-progress

Grigal, M., Hart, D., Papay, C., Wu, X., Lazo, R., Smith, F., & Domin, D. (2021). *Annual Report of the Cohort 2 TPSID Model Demonstration Projects (Year Five 2019–2020).* Boston, MA: University of Massachusetts Boston, Institute for Community Inclusion.

Hafner, D. (2008). Inclusion in postsecondary education: Phenomenological study on identifying and addressing barriers to inclusion of individuals with significant disabilities as a four-year liberal arts college. Doctoral Dissertation, Edgewood College.

Hafner, D., & Moffatt, C. (2012). *Cutting-Edge Report 2007-2012,* Edgewood College.

Hafner, D. (2019). Voices of Experience: Students Share College Search Advice. *How To Think College,* 6. Boston, MA: University of Massachusetts Boston, Institute for Community Inclusion.

Hall, J. P., Batza, K., Streed, C. G. Jr., Boyd, B., & Kurth, N. K. (2020). Health disparities among sexual and gender minorities with autism spectrum disorder. *Journal of Autism and Developmental Disorders* 50, 3071–3077.

Hart, D., Grigal, M., Sax, C., Martinez, D., & Will, M. (2006). Postsecondary education options for students with intellectual disabilities. *Research to Practice-Issue* 45.

Hart, D., Zimbrich, K., & Parker, D. (2005). Dual enrollment as a postsecondary education option for students with intellectual disabilities. In E. Getzel & P. Wehman (Eds.), *Going To College: Expanding Opportunities For People With Disabilities,* 253–266, Baltimore, MD: Paul Brookes Publishing Co.

Hartz, E. J. (2014). *Outcomes of inclusive postsecondary education for students with intellectual disabilities at Edgewood College* (No. 3623549). [Doctoral dissertation]. ProQuest Dissertations and Theses.

Higher Education Opportunity Act of 2008 (HEOA). (2008). Public Law No. 110–315 § 122 Stat. 3078 (August 14, 2008).

Hughes, J. (2009). Higher education and Asperger's syndrome. *Chronicle of Higher Education, 55*(40), 21.

Individuals with Disabilities Act 20 U.S.C. § 1400. (1990). Public Law No. 101–476.

Individuals with Disabilities Act 20 U.S.C. § 1400. (1997). Public Law No. 105-17.

Individuals with Disabilities Education Act, 20 U.S.C. § 1400. (2004). Public Law No. 108-446.

Kiss, E. (2015) Skill building group topic examples. West Virginia Autism Training Center: Marshall University, WV.

Kochhar-Bryant, C., & Izzo, M. (2006). Access to post-high school services: Transition assessment and the summary of performance. *Career Development for Exceptional Individuals*, 29, 70–89.

Koehler, J. L. (2013). Predictors of postsecondary education attendance for youth with learning disabilities. Dissertation.

Kõlves, K., Fitzgerald, C., Nordentoft, M., Wood, S. J., Erlangsen, A. (2021). Assessment of suicidal behaviors among individuals with autism spectrum disorder in Denmark. *JAMA Netw Open*. 4(1).

Lee, C. E., & Taylor, J. L. (2022). A Review of the Benefits and Barriers to Postsecondary Education for Students With Intellectual and Developmental Disabilities. *The Journal of Special Education*, 55(4) 234–245.

Lewis, L. F., Ward, C., Jarvis, N. & Crawley, E. (2021). "Straight sex is complicated enough!": The lived experiences of autistics who are gay, lesbian, bisexual, asexual, or other sexual orientations. *Journal of Autism and Developmental Disorders*, 51(7), 2324–2337.

Lindstrom, L., Doren, B., & Miesch, J. (2011). Waging a living: Career development and long term employment outcomes for young adults with disabilities. *Exceptional Children*, 77(4), 423–434.

Lord, C., Elsabbagh, M., Baird, G., & Veenstra-Vanderweele, J. (2018). Autism spectrum disorder. *Lancet*, 392, London: England.

Madaus, J. W. (2011). The history of disability services in higher education. *New Directions for Higher Education*, 154, 5–15.

Mazzotti, V. L., Rowe, D. A., Kwiatek, S., Voggt, A., Chang, W., Fowler, C. H., & Test, D. W. (2021). Secondary transition predictors of postschool success: An update to the research base. *Career Development and Transition for Exceptional Individuals*, 44(1), 47–64.

Moon, M.S., Grigal, M., & Neubert, D. (2001). High school and beyond. *The Exceptional Parent*, 31(7), 52–57.

Nachman, B. R., Miller, R. A., Vallejo Peña, E. (2020). "Whose liability is it anyway?" Cultivating an inclusive college climate for autistic LGBTQ students. *Journal of Cases in Educational Leadership*. 23(2), 98–111.

Nasr, M., Cranston-Gingras, A., & Jang, S. E. (2015). Friendship experiences of participants in a university based transition program. *International Journal of Whole Schooling*, 11, 1–15.

National Center on Secondary and Education and Transition (NCSET). (2004). Person-centered planning: A tool for transition. Retrieved from www.ncset. org/publications/viewdesc.asp?id=1431

National Survey on Postsecondary Programs for Youth with Intellectual Disabilities (2005).

National Transition Documentation Summit. (2005). Summary of performance model template. Council for Exceptional Children. Council for Educational Diagnostic Services. Retrieved from: http://community.cec.sped.org/ceds/home

Neubert, D. A., Moon, M. S., Grigal, M., & Redd, V. (2002). Post-secondary education and transition services for students age 18–21 with significant disabilities. *Focus on Exceptional Children*, 34(8), 1–11.

Newman, L., Wagner, M., Huang, T., Shaver, D., Knokey, A.-M., Yu, J., Contreras, E., Ferguson, K., Greene, S., Nagle, K., & Cameto, R. (2011). Secondary school programs and performance of students with disabilities. A special topic report of findings from the National Longitudinal Transition Study-2 (NLTS2) (NCSER 2012-3000). *U.S. Department of Education. Washington, DC: National Center for Special Education Research.* Menlo Park, CA: SRI International.

Nietupski, J., McQuillen, D., Berg, D., Daughtery, V., & Hamre-Nietupski, S. (2001). Preparing students with mild disabilities for careers in technology: A process and recommendations from Iowa's high school high tech program. *Journal of Vocational Rehabilitation, 16,* 179–188.

Respond, Innovate, Succeed, and Empower Act (RISE) (2021).

Rose, D. H., Harbour, W. S., Johnston, C. S., Daley, S. G., & Abarbanell, L. (2006). Universal design for learning in postsecondary education: Reflections on principles and their application. *Journal of Postsecondary Education and Disability, 19*(2), 135–151.

Roux, A. M., Shattuck, P. T., Rast, J. E., Rava, J. A., & Anderson, K. A. (2015). National Autism Indicators Report: Transition into Young Adulthood. Philadelphia, PA: Life Course Outcomes Research Program, A.J. Drexel Autism Institute, Drexel University,

Rowe, D., Mazzotti, V., & Sinclair, J. (2015). Strategies for teaching self-determination skills in conjunction with the common core. *Intervention in School and Clinic, 5*(3), 131–141.

Scheef, A., Hollingshead, A., Barrio, B. (2020). Supporting Students With Intellectual and Developmental Disability in Postsecondary Education. Journal of College Student Development, 61(4), 528–531.

Schutz, P. F. (2002). Transition from secondary to postsecondary education for students with disabilities: An exploration of the phenomenon. *Journal of College Reading and Learning, 33* (1).

Scott, L., Bruno, L., Gokita, T., & Thoma, C. A. (2019) Teacher candidates' abilities to develop universal design for learning and universal design for transition lesson plans, *International Journal of Inclusive Education.*

Section 504 of the Rehabilitation Act of 1973. (1973). Public Law No. 93–112, 29 U.S.C. § 701 et seq.

Selles, R., & Storch, E. (2013). Translation of anxiety treatment to youth with autism spectrum disorders. *Journal of Child & Family Studies, 22*(3), 405–413.

Shaw, S. F., Dukes, L. L., & Madaus, J. W. (2012). Beyond compliance: Using the summary of performance to enhance transition planning. *Teaching Exceptional Children, 44*(5), 6–12.

Shaw, S. F., Madaus, J. W., & Dukes, L. L. (2010). *Preparing students with disabilities for college success: a practical guide for transition planning.* Baltimore: Brookes.

Shogren, K. A., Wehmeyer, M. L., Shaw, L. A., Grigal, M., Hart, D., Smith, F. A, & Khamsi, S. (2018). Predictors of Self-Determination in Postsecondary Education for Students with Intellectual and Developmental Disabilities. *Education and training in autism and developmental disabilities, 53*(2), 146–159.

Simpson, C. G., Gaus, M. D., Biggs, M., & Williams Jr., J. (2010). Physical education and implications for students with Asperger's syndrome. *Teaching Exceptional Children, 42*(6), 48–56.

Smith, C. P. (2007). Support services for students with Asperger's syndrome in higher education. *College Student Journal, 41*(3), 515–531.

Sopko, K. (2008). Summary of performance. Project Forum at NASDSE. In forum Brief Policy Analysis. Retrieved from www.nasdse.org/Portals/0/Summa ryofPerformance.pdf

Stansberry Brusnahan, L. L., Sparks, S. L., Cote, D. L. & Vandercook, T. (2018). Person-centered planning, summary of performance, and guardianship. In L. L. Stansberry Brusnahan, R. A. Stodden, R. A. & S. H. Zucker (Eds.), Transition to adulthood: Work, community, and educational success (pp. 49–66). Council for Exceptional Children.

Steinbrenner, J. R., Hume, K., Odom, S. L., Morin, K. L., Nowell, S. W., Tomaszewski, B., Szendrey, S., McIntyre, N. S., Yücesoy-Özkan, S., & Savage, M. N. (2020). Evidence-based practices for children, youth, and young adults with Autism. The University of North Carolina at Chapel Hill, Frank Porter Graham Child Development Institute, National Clearinghouse on Autism Evidence and Practice Review Team.

Stodden, R. A., & Whelley, T. (2004). Postsecondary education and persons with intellectual disabilities: An introduction. *Education and Training in Developmental Disabilities, 39*(1), 6–15.

Test, D., Fowler, C., Wood, W., Brewer, D., & Eddy, S. (2005). A conceptual framework of self-advocacy for students with disabilities. *Remedial and Special Education, 26*(1), 43–54.

Thacker, J., & Sheppard-Jones, K. (2011). Research brief: Higher education for students with intellectual disabilities. A study of KY OVR counselors. Lexington, KY: University of Kentucky, Human Development Institute.

Think College (n.d.). Differences between high school and college. Retrieved from www.thinkcollege.net/topics/highschool-college-differences

Think College National Coordinating Center Accreditation Workgroup (2021). *Report on Model Accreditation Standards for Higher Education Programs for Students with Intellectual Disability: Progress on the Path to Education, Employment, and Community Living.* Boston, MA: University of Massachusetts Boston, Institute for Community Inclusion.

Thoma, C. A., Bartholomew, C. C., & Scott, L. A. (2009). *Universal design for transition: A roadmap for planning and instruction.* Baltimore, MD: Brookes Publishing.

Tureck, K., Matson, J., May, A., Whiting, S., & Davis, T. (2014). Comorbid symptoms in children with anxiety disorders compared to children with autism spectrum disorders. *Journal of Developmental & Physical Disabilities, 26*(1), 23–33.

Uditsky, B., & Hughson, E. (2012). Inclusive postsecondary education -an evidence-based moral imperative. *Journal of Policy and Practice in Intellectual Disabilities, 9*(4), 298–302.

U.S. Department of Education. (2019). Increasing Postsecondary Opportunities and Success for Students and Youth with Disabilities. www2.ed.gov/policy/spe ced/guid/increasing-postsecondaryopportunities-and-success-09-17-2019.pdf

U.S. Department of Education, National Center for Education Statistics. (2013). The Condition of Education 2013 (NCES 2013–037), Annual Earnings of Young Adults. Retrieved from: http://nces.ed.gov/fastfacts/display.asp?id=77

U.S. Department of Education, Office of Special Education and Rehabilitative Services. (2020). A Transition Guide to Postsecondary Education and Employment for Students and Youth with Disabilities, Revised. Washington, D.C.

U.S. Bureau of Labor Statistics. (2018). Unemployment rates and earnings by educational attainment. Retrieved from www.bls.gov/emp/chart-unemployment-earnings-education.htm

VanBergeijk, E., Klin, A., & Volkmar, F. (2008). Supporting more able students on the autism spectrum: College and beyond. *Journal of Autism and Developmental Disorders*, 38(7), 1359–1370.

Warrier, V., Greenberg, D., Weir. E., Buckingham, C., Smith, P., Meng-Chuan, L., Allison, C., & Baron-Cohen, S. (2020) Elevated rates of autism, other neurodevelopmental and psychiatric diagnoses, and autistic traits in transgender and gender-diverse individuals. *Nature Communications*.

Wechsler, H. (2007). An academic Gresham's Law: Group repulsion as a theme in American higher education. In L. Foster (Ed.), *The History of Higher Education*, 442–456. Boston, Mass: Pearson Custom Publishing.

Wehman, P. (2002). Testimony to President's Commission on Excellence in Special Education Transition Task Force Meeting. Retrieved from www.beachcenter.org/Books%5CFullPublications%5CPDF%5CPresidentReport.pdf.

Wehmeyer, M. L., Abery, B., Zhang, D., Ward, K., Willis, D., Amin, W. H., Balcazar, F., Ball, A., Bacon, A., Calkins, C., Heller, T., Goode, T., Jesien, G., McVeigh, T., Nygren, M., Palmer, S., & Walker, H. (2011). Personal self-determination and moderating variables that impact efforts to promote self-determination. *Exceptionality*, 19, 19–30.

Wehmeyer, M., Shogren, K., Smith, T., Zager, D., & Simpson, R. (2010). Research-based principles and practices for educating students with autism: Self-determination and social interactions. *Education and Training in Autism and Developmental Disabilities*, 45(4) 475–486.

Wei, X., Wagner, M., Hudson, L., Yu, J., & Javitz, H. (2015). The Effect of Transition Planning Participation and Goal-Setting on College Enrollment Among Youth With Autism Spectrum Disorders. *Remedial and Special Education*. 37.

West Virginia Autism Training Center. (2015). Higher Education Readiness Assessment Marshal University.

Whetstone, M., & Browning, P. (2002). Transition: A frame of reference. *Alabama Federation on Council for Exceptional Children On-Line Journal*, 1. Retrieved from www.afcec.org/pubs/journal/vol1/02F_definition1.pdf

Whirley, M. L., Gilson, C. B., & Gushanas, C. M. (2020). Postsecondary Education Programs on College Campuses Supporting Adults With Intellectual and Developmental Disabilities in the Literature: A Scoping Review. *Career Development and Transition for Exceptional Individuals*, 43(4) 195–208.

Wolf, L., Brown, J., & Bork Kuikiela, R. (2009). *Students with Asperger syndrome: A guide for college personnel*. Shawnee Mission, KS: Autism Asperger Publishing Company.

Workforce Innovation and Opportunity Act. (WIOA) (2014). Public Law No. 113–128, 128 Stat. 1425, 29 U.S.C. §§3101 et seq.

Chapter 15

Promoting Integrated Employment Options

Dianne Zager
Consulting LLC, Westchester, New York

Case Vignette: Introducing Sangit

Sangit, in Hindi written as संगीत, is 17-years-old and attends a large public high school. His parents immigrated to the U.S. when Sangit was 10-years-old. When Sangit arrived in the U.S. he spoke Hindi and some Tamil, as his parents were raised in different sections of India. In addition to being fluent in the two languages of his parents, he has mastered English. Sangit has a mild intellectual disability and autism level 2 (i.e., requiring substantial support). He has been doing well in general education classes with differentiated modified assignments. In his classes, he receives support from a special education teacher and paraprofessional, both of whom also work with other students in the classes. Academically, Sangit is reading on a fourth-grade level and is able to perform basic math operations. His favorite class is science, where he enjoys participating in group work to conduct experiments. Sangit exhibits stereotypic hand flapping, especially when anxious, and tends to like to calm himself by making a low humming noise. He functions best in a quiet environment with a regular routine. Environments and situations, such as lunchtime in the cafeteria are overstimulating to Sangit, with their loud noise levels, food odors, and random movement of other students. He prefers a quiet corner in the cafeteria where he usually has lunch with one friend. Noting Sangit's strengths, preferences and challenges, his teachers have begun to help him and his parents prepare for a successful transition to a career of his choice. We will revisit Sangit throughout this chapter.

DOI: 10.4324/9781003255147-18

Historical Perspectives on Employment for People with ASD

The first edition of this text appeared in 1992. Since that date, in the ensuing three decades, there have been advances in legislation and funding initiatives. Schools increasingly have begun to offer meaningful transition preparation, scattered programs of excellence have developed, and various new options for integrated employment have emerged. Yet, today competitive employment outcomes for adults with ASD still remain poor. Despite decades of U.S. federal regulations mandating the implementation of transition services, successful competitive employment outcomes for people with autism are not yet widespread. Employment outcomes for individuals with autism on the international level are also disappointing (Black et al., 2019). This is a global situation, not limited to the United States, as evidenced in reports from countries, such as Italy (Cappa et al., 2020), Australia (Hayward et al., 2019) and Ireland (Stack et al., 2021). Adults with autism spectrum disorder continue to struggle with unemployment or underemployment issues, which remain at a high rate and which were amplified world-wide during the coronavirus (COVID) pandemic.

Employment Data

In an exploratory study representing seven continents (Bury et al., 2021), employees on the autism spectrum (N = 29) and supervisors (N = 15) were asked to provide written examples of workplace-based challenges, their interpretation, consequences and resolution. Information garnered from this study highlighted the universality of low employment success for persons with autism. Statistics from Great Britain, specifically, show a dismal picture with just 21.7% of autistic people successfully engaged in employment. The Labour Force Survey from the Office for National statistics employment statistics reported that approximately half of people with disabilities (52.1%) aged 16 to 64 years in the UK were employed in 2020 compared with 8 in 10 (81.3%) of non-disabled people. This analysis used estimates from the year 2019–2020, which did not reflect the impact of coronavirus on outcomes of people with disabilities.

In the U.S., approximately 75% of the 5.6 million adults on the autism spectrum are unemployed or underemployed. Fifty percent of 25-year-olds with autism have never held a paying job, in spite of their skill level or potential to succeed in employment (Palumbo, 2021). Although U.S. policy and resultant interventions have attempted to promote school programs for transition from school to work, low employment rates continue to exist. This is worthy of note, especially in light of the need for workers throughout many sectors of the labor force. A survey by the National Federation of Independent Business found that 42% of small business owners in the U.S. had job openings that could not be filled, a record high. Ninety-one percent of those hiring or trying to hire reported few or no qualified applicants (Fox, 2021) for the positions they were trying to fill. Findings from the 2017 U.S. National Autism Indicators Report (Alverson & Yamamoto, 2018), show only 14% of autistic adults were employed and paid for their work at an integrated job site, while 54% were unpaid for their work in segregated settings. Twenty-seven percent of adults with ASD reported no participation in work.

The above figures point to the pressing need to improve employment options for people with ASD. The problem of underemployment often is not due to an inability to perform jobs. It has been demonstrated that when students have received intentional delivery of job-related services, such as job search, job placement, and ongoing support, their rates of employment success have risen to reflect the benefit of appropriate education in this domain (Roux et al., 2021). In large measure, the answer to positive employment outcomes for persons with significant disabilities lies in preparation for work, employer education, and ongoing support.

Analysis of Employment Outcomes

The majority of earlier studies on outcomes of adults with ASD originated from follow-up studies and analyses of data from the National Longitudinal Transition Study-2 (NLTS2) conducted in the United States from 2001 to 2009, including 11,000 individuals with disabilities. Specifically, the NLTS2 data included 922 youth and adults with ASD from 13 to 26 years old (Burgess & Cimera, 2014). Shattuck et al. (2011), in analyzing the NTLS2 data, reported that in the eight years after exiting high school, only 53% of individuals with autism had worked for pay and only 6% of young adults were employed in competitive jobs. Similarly, in reviewing the NTLS2 data, Roux et al. (2013) found that only 53% of adults with ASD aged 21–25 had ever worked for a salary outside of the home, the lowest rate among all the disability groups. Shattuck et al. (2012) reported that the employment outcomes, for 500 individuals with ASD were poor particularly in the first two years after leaving high school; young adults with ASD were not working or attending school. Studies analyzing the NTLS2 data reported that individuals with ASD from lower-income families and those individuals with more significant functional impairments were more likely to be disengaged from employment (Chiang et al., 2013; Roux et al., 2013; Shattuck et al. 2012).

Several studies of employment outcomes revealed limited opportunities for adults with ASD. Howlin et al. (2004) studied the employment outcomes for 68 adults (21–48 years old) in the United Kingdom;

approximately 34% of the adults were employed and approximately 13% were in competitive employment. Taylor and Seltzer (2011) conducted a longitudinal ten-year study of 66 adults (19–26 years old), who graduated from high school between 2004 and 2008; 6% were in competitive employment, 12% in supported employment, a majority of the young adults (56%) were in sheltered workshops or day center (adult habilitation) activities, and 12% did not participate regularly in any activities in adulthood.

Due to their cognitive ability, it is assumed that adults with higher functioning autism and Asperger's syndrome would have more success in being employed and sustaining employment; however, existing studies do not support this conclusion (Chen et al., 2014). Although, a number of adults with higher functioning autism and Asperger's syndrome were employed, from 11 to 55% (Farley et al. 2009; Howlin, 2000; Hurlbutt & Chalmers, 2004; Mawhood & Howlin, 1999), generally individuals were underemployed. Adults with Asperger's syndrome and higher functioning autism who had completed high school and attended postsecondary education (and also obtained college degrees) were employed in unskilled jobs, paid below the minimum wage, and often unemployed for extended periods (Chen et al., 2014; Hurlbutt & Chalmers, 2004; Wilczynski et al., 2013).

According to self-reports from individuals with ASD, maintaining employment and professional success were related to social interaction and communication skills rather than their specific job responsibilities (Barnhill, 2007; Bury et al., 2021; Hurlbutt & Chalmers, 2004). Shattuck et al. (2012) reported that youth with ASD have the highest risk of being disengaged from employment; the risk was greater than 50% for the first two years following high school graduation. Burgess and Cimera (2014) studied the employment outcomes of 34,501 transition-aged young adults from 2002 to 2011 throughout the United States who were served by vocational rehabilitation services. Of the 34,413 individuals receiving transition services, more than 20,000 individuals did not achieve successful employment. Further, youth with ASD who were employed were underemployed; they worked fewer hours (17–30 hours per week) and their overall yearly wages were below the poverty level for a single wage earner (Burgess & Cimera, 2014).

In reviewing the scientific interventions and practices for young adults with ASD, Chen et al. (2014) found a scarcity of empirical research to identify specific models to promote successful employment outcomes. Most research that has been conducted consists of experimental designs with small numbers of participants or qualitative studies (Chen et al., 2014). As a result, there has been an emphasis on utilizing correlation research to identify evidence-based predictors associated with employment outcomes (Gerhardt & Lainer, 2011; Test et al., 2009; Wehman et al., 2014). The growing awareness of the need to provide instruction and experiences to help students with autism spectrum disorder (ASD) transition to employment has led to investigation on the types of support needed to prepare students for employment (Wong et al., 2021).

One transition model was found to be especially effective by Schall et al. (2020). They conducted a review of interventions for competitive employment for individuals with autism spectrum disorder and found strong empirical support for a transition-to-work program called Project SEARCH Plus ASD Supports (PS+ASD). The SEARCH model has been so successful that it has grown from its original site in Cincinnati to more than 200 sites in the United States and Canada, England, Scotland, and Australia (Wehman et al., 2020).

Transition Preparation

Based on a correlational review of the literature and several studies, the National Secondary Transition Technical Assistance Center (NSTTAC) has identified transition planning as an evidenced-based practice for increasing the probability of young adults with ASD securing competitive employment. Roux et al. (2015), using the NTLS2 data, found that only 58%of youth with ASD had a transition plan developed by the age of 14, the federally required age. Furthermore, according to Wagner et al. (2007) in their survey of young adults with ASD, transition plans included 20% of goals for competitive employment, 25% of goals for supported employment, and 15% for sheltered workshop, and approximately 40% looked forward to some form of postsecondary education. Typically, transition plans do not include paid employment during high school in preparation for competitive employment. Roux et al. (2015) reported that only 58%of young adults worked for a salary between high school and their early twenties, a significantly lower rate than young adults with other disabilities.

Generally, studies focusing on transition planning have made broad-based suggestions for improving the transition process (Landmark, Ju & Zhang, 2010; Papay & Bambara, 2014; Van Schalkwyk & Volkmar, 2017; Wehman et al., 2014). Using NLTS2 data, Shogren & Plotner (2012) reported that young adults with ASD were assigned a lower number of transition goals leading to competitive employment as compared to other disability groups. The study indicated that the majority of students with ASD did not assume a key role in designing their transition education. They also found that students with ASD required a higher level of postsecondary support services. According to Hagner et al. (2012), poor adult outcomes for individuals with ASD were heightened by their experiences in a transition process that was professionally controlled without encouraging participation by the student or family.

Transition Legislation and Federal Initiatives

The term *transition services* refers to a coordinated set of activities for students with disabilities designed as a results-oriented process that is focused on improving academic and functional achievement to facilitate movement from school to postschool activities, including post-secondary education, vocational education, employment, independent living, and community participation. Planning should take into account individual strengths, preferences, and interests. Education and related services should be directed toward development of employment and other postschool adult living skills. More specifically, the Individuals with Disabilities Act (2004) defined the process of transition planning as a coordinated array of activities to ensure that every student with a disability has individualized goals on their IEP in the areas of postsecondary options, including employment or vocational training and community living. For high school students with ASD, it is critical that the IEP detail a course of study linked to transition goals.

Congress reauthorized the IDEA in 2004 and amended the IDEA through Public Law 114-95, the Every Student Succeeds Act, in December 2015. According to the Individuals with Disabilities Education Improvement Act (IDEIA, 2004), postsecondary goals indicated on the student's IEP should frame the trajectory of skills that students need to learn to function as adults, including career and vocational skills (Hendricks & Wehman, 2009).

Since the 1980s, the need for comprehensive transition education has been a major focus of disability regulations encompassing, employment, adult services, and independent living options. Federal initiatives were created to improve transition services for youth with disabilities based on their needs, preferences, and abilities (Morningstar & Liss, 2008). Transition services were mandated with the Individuals with Disabilities Education Act of 1990, the subsequent re-authorization of the Act in 1997, and the last re-authorization entitled the Individuals with Disabilities Education Improvement Act, IDEIA (2004). The Americans with Disabilities Act (1990) required schools to prepare students with disabilities to transition to postschool options by including a statement of services needed into the student's Individualized Education Program (IEP) by the age of 16 and to update the IEP annually. According to IDEA, postschool activities may include postsecondary education, vocational training, integrated (including supported) employment, adult education and services, and independent living and community participation (Morningstar & Liss, 2008). The last revision of IDEIA mandated that schools must address the transition needs and services for the student not later than the first IEP to be in effect when the child turns 16, or younger if determined appropriate by the IEP Team; however, states may choose to continue beginning the IEP transition requirement at age 14. [34 CFR 300.320(b) and (c)] [20 U.S.C. 1414 (d)(1)(A)(i)(VIII)]. According to IDEIA, transition goals must be measurable and results oriented, based on an age-appropriate transition assessment, and include areas related to postsecondary goals such as training, education, employment, and, if appropriate, independent living skills (Etscheidt, 2006; Morningstar & Liss, 2008; Wehman, 2013).

In 1990, The Americans with Disabilities Act (ADA) banned discrimination in employment for individuals with disabilities and ensured accessibility to workplaces, public services, and accommodations. The School-To-Work Opportunities Act of 1994 (Public Law 103-239) was similar to IDEA in its purpose to create result-oriented, performance-based education and training programs statewide to prepare all youth for competitive employment. The regulation addressed opportunities for students to participate in career exploration and counseling, work experiences during high school, and standards-based instruction that focused on achievement in occupational and academic skills. The Workforce Investment Act (1998) created federally funded demonstration projects for job training and employment services. This Act included mandates for state and local governments to include accommodations for the needs of individuals with disabilities (Hardman & Dawson, 2010).

Key Components of Transition Preparation for Competitive Employment

The Workforce Innovation and Opportunity Act (WIOA) defines *competitive integrated employment* as work that is performed on a full-time or part-time basis for which an individual is: (a) compensated at or above minimum wage and comparable to the customary rate paid by the employer to employees without disabilities performing similar duties and with similar training and experience; (b) receiving the same level of benefits provided to other employees without disabilities in similar positions; (c) at a location where the employee interacts with other individuals without disabilities; and (d) presented opportunities for advancement similar to other employees without disabilities in similar positions. Supported employment refers to competitive employment in an integrated setting with ongoing support services for individuals with significant disabilities limiting their independent functioning.

Self-Determination and Self-Advocacy. Self-determination involves individuals assuming an active, self-directed role in changing their life by making plans, implementing, and adjusting those plans as necessary. Self-determination is built upon skills in choice-making, decision-making, problem-solving, goal-setting, and self-evaluation skills, independence, self-awareness skills, and self-advocacy and leadership skills (Wehman et al., 2014; Wehmeyer et al., 2010). Importantly, teaching high school students with ASD to participate in transition planning is a strategy to enhance their self-advocacy and self-determination skills (Test et al., 2014).

Research studies have identified evidence-based practices in transition planning for young adults with ASD. Test et al. (2009), using the National Secondary Transition Technical Assistance Center (NSTTAC) database, concluded that student participation in the transition process is critical to adult success, citing specifically teaching students self-advocacy and self-determination skills as evidence-based practices.

Person-Centered Planning. Participation in the transition process should be designed to teach students to recognize their own strengths, self-advocate based on realistic career preferences in the context of a community-based environment, participate in career exploration to collect information, and make choices and decisions (Hagner et al., 2012). For adolescents and young adults with ASD, person-centered planning is an essential process to effectively prepare for adult life. The plan focuses on the desires, hopes, concerns, and needs of individuals and their families (Martin & Williams-Diehm, 2013). It includes a long-term vision and descriptive statement of the desired outcomes for the young adult in three to five years and is the blueprint for learning experiences, supports, and services for the individual and the family (Meadan et al., 2010). Talents, interests and preferences are key factors in designing programs for students with autism. Personal interests, as well as challenges and educational needs, change over time as individuals with ASD progress through different stages of development (Zager et al., 2013).

It is critical that school staff consider student and family values in transition planning. The message that the student's voice is heard and respected can create enjoyable, less stressful meetings and enhance the planning process (Hagner et al., 2012). When educators value students' and parents' input, collaborative planning is strengthened.

Family Involvement. Family involvement is particularly important to achieving postschool success for young adults with autism. Given the important role of family involvement in providing support to a young adult with ASD, including advocacy, linkages with the community and service providers, and developing postsecondary supports, family participation in the transition process is a critical predictor of positive postsecondary outcomes (Landmark et al., 2010; Schall et al., 2012).

Despite the obvious and clear need for family involvement, and mandates for family involvement, school-home partnerships remain elusive. This is particularly true for low-income and culturally and linguistically diverse families (Hirano et al., 2018). Barriers to school-home collaboration may be due to issues and obstacles within the family, school, and/or adult service agency. Family barriers may be related to limited resources, lack of cultural capital, and low perceptions of self-efficacy. Parents often experience multiple stressors that impact their time and emotional resources.

Utilizing the NLTS2 data, including 830 youth with ASD, Shogren and Plotner (2012) found that only 67%of families received information about postsecondary services. Transition programs that have resulted in positive outcomes have consistently involved families throughout a student's years in school (Schall et al., 2012). A study conducted by Hagner et al. (2012) focused on families with young adults with ASD, 16–19 years old, who participated in training on strategies for person-centered planning and utilized adult service options to create postsecondary opportunities. As a result, the families reported higher student and family expectations for the future, improvement in the young adults' self-determination skills, and appropriate future career decision-making plans.

Vocational Rehabilitation Services. The Rehabilitation Act of 1973, as amended and re-authorized in 1998 under the Workforce Investment Act of 1998, provides federal grants to states to coordinate transition planning and vocational rehabilitation (VR) services to individuals. Services for individuals can include: assessments to determine eligibility of services, counseling, job placement, supported employment, and vocational training. Although the VR system is a core resource for individuals with disabilities, it has not been prepared to meet the needs of youth and adults with ASD (Chen et al., 2014; Hendricks, 2010). Lawer et al. (2009) examined the experiences of individuals with ASD in the VR system. The subjects included 382,221 adults ages 18–65 served by VR, whose cases were closed in 2005; 1,707 of these were adults with ASD. The study revealed that adults with ASD were more likely than adults with other disabilities to be denied services due to the severity of their disability. Furthermore, VR services did not provide job coaching or on-site supports that met the unique needs of individuals.

From 2002 to 2011, the numbers of adults with ASD seeking VR services increased dramatically (Burgess & Cimera, 2014). Schaller and Yang (2005), analyzing the employment outcomes of 1,323 adults with ASD, found that 62% received VR services for supportive or competitive employment services and, as a result, 66% were successfully employed. The costs of providing VR services for individuals with ASD are costly compared to other disability groups (Cimera & Cowan, 2009). However, it is less cost effective to support adults with ASD who leave VR services and earn lower wages and work fewer hours.

The Workforce Innovation and Opportunity Act of 2014 placed new requirements on state VR agencies transitioning youth with significant disabilities to employment options. This act mandates that VR services increase their role in transition through coordination between VR and other agencies (Hoff, 2014), extending services for VR in supported employment from 18 to 24 months, and also modifying eligibility to promote access to individuals with the most significant disabilities.

Special educators and vocational rehabilitation counselors play critical roles in preparing students with ASD to obtain employment and live within their community. Lack of educators' knowledge about transition programming, as well as about support service systems, has contributed to inadequate career development and the resulting underemployment of people with autism and developmental disabilities (Müller et al., 2003; Standifer, 2009). Effective secondary education to prepare students with ASD for employment that builds skills to enable all individuals to live, work, and recreate within their communities has the potential to improve the current low rates of unemployment (Chiang et al., 2013) and to help individuals succeed in integrated community living. Unfortunately, although federal policy has focused on transition to employment initiatives for people with disabilities for over two decades (Luecking & Luecking, 2015), a clear effective pathway to successful employment has yet to be proven.

At the recent IEP meeting, Sangit's teacher had suggested that an additional meeting be held to begin discussing Sangit's postsecondary options and to identify specific goals and strategies to prepare and support him in transitioning to adulthood. Although his IEP had included broad transition goals, Sangit's plans for after he turned 21 hadn't been formalized. She told his parents that the meeting would include herself, the speech-language therapist, transition specialist, representative from the local vocational rehabilitation office, advocate, if the parents wished, and most importantly, Sangit. Sangit's parents were anxious before their meeting with the transition-team but were appreciative that the teacher had reached out to them to begin planning for the future. They hadn't thought about what Sangit would be doing after high school, as they had felt that this was far into the future. The teacher had encouraged them to attend this next meeting so that they could work as a team to begin making plans in earnest.

Implicit Challenges in Autism Spectrum Disorders

Inherent characteristics of autism, as they affect behavior and learning for *each individual* should influence educational planning. By respecting underlying characteristics of autism and building on student strengths while accommodating cognitive, sensory and social challenges, practitioners can improve transition outcomes. Limited employment opportunities for people with ASD are related to a lack of understanding of their unique cognitive, communication, and behavior challenges, which may result in difficulty navigating work situations (Hendricks & Wehman, 2009; Walsh et al., 2014). Stereotypic behaviors, which can include unusual motor movements and vocalizations, along with insistence on rigidity and sameness, and sensory issues may interfere with performance of work (Schall & McDonough, 2010; Taylor & Seltzer, 2011). Such behaviors may be unsettling to those unfamiliar with autism.

Demands in work environments and ability to comprehend communication and materials used by employers (e.g., verbal directions, written handbooks, and facial expressions) present challenges that frustrate supervisors, other employees, as well as the individual with ASD. Adapting to social and cultural norms of workplace environments tends to be difficult, as well. These challenges have been cited as factors that play a role in preventing individuals with autism from attaining and succeeding at work (Chiang et al., 2013; Schall & McDonough, 2010; Shattuck et al., 2012; Walsh et al., 2013).

Reports provided by international stakeholders support the need to understand individuals with ASD in a broader perspective, extending beyond diagnostic criteria into many areas of functioning and environmental domains (Mahdi, 2018). Service delivery has been fraught with widespread lack of understanding of the employment support needs of this population delivery (Schall et al., 2013). Yet, on a positive note, as surveys and research studies (e.g., Carter et al., 2012; Shattuck et al., 2012), continue to draw attention to the inadequacy of prevailing secondary education programs (Kucharczyk et al., 2015), there has been growing momentum in the field to improve transition programs.

Individuals with autism have markedly different service needs than individuals with other disabilities. Cimera and Cowan (2009) reported that adults with autism were likely to be denied services because of the magnitude of their needs, which often require intensive services. Lack of knowledge of characteristics of autism spectrum disorders, especially unfamiliarity with strengths and abilities that may exist in individuals on the spectrum, has contributed heavily to this problem. While it is true that communication, cognitive, behavioral, sensory, and social characteristics inherent in this disorder may necessitate ongoing services (Chiang et al., 2013), appropriate supports can increase success rates and enable individuals with autism to make significant contributions to the workplace and their communities.

Increased understanding within special education and vocational rehabilitation of the needs of individuals with autism in adulthood, along with knowledge about available options to accommodate and support them (McEathron et al., 2013), can impact employment outcomes (Müller et al., 2003; Standifer, 2009). The juxtaposition of evidence that people with autism can successfully sustain employment when provided with adequate support and reports showing the inadequacy of employment support, points directly to a need for improved systems that will enable individuals with autism to be employed (Zager et al., 2014). The following section discusses three key areas of difficulty (interpersonal interaction, executive functioning, and sensory processing), each of which is an implicit challenge in autism that may significantly impact employment and community living outcomes.

Interpersonal Interaction Differences

Success in the workplace is dependent, in large measure, on the ability to navigate the social terrain of the job site. Social communication and interpersonal interaction can be difficult for people with autism, affecting transition to new environments. Problems understanding the behaviors and feelings of others, referred to as *Theory of Mind* can result in verbal, as well as behavioral responses that may be deemed inappropriate (BaronCohen et al., 1985). In short, interacting appropriately with co-workers, employers, and patrons is critical to maintaining employment. While people with autism may lose their job due to problems in productivity or accuracy (Smith & Philippen, 2005), jobs are more likely to be lost because of behaviors that do not fit in the workplace (Gorenstein, et al., 2020). An employee may be expected to solve problems, work collaboratively, and comply with appropriate etiquette and varied other non-work skills referred to as soft skills. According to the U.S. Department of Labor's Office of Disability Employment Policy, some key skills needed on the job are: (a) communicating effectively, (b) managing time, (c) taking initiative, (d) responding to the needs of others, (e) maintaining a positive attitude, (f) participating on collaborative teams, and (g) thinking critically to solve problems (Zager et al., 2013). A lack of proficiency in these soft skills, which are particularly challenging for individuals on the spectrum, is more likely to cause job loss, than is difficulty with specific job-related skills.

Executive Functioning Challenges

Executive functions serve to enable individuals to manage themselves, engage in activities, and complete tasks in order to reach their goals. These abilities have been compared to a Global Positioning System that guides the brain to keep individuals focused and headed in the right direction during tasks (Azano & Tuckwiller, 2011). Executive function is neurologically based and serves to control emotions and self-regulatory behavior. The numerous definitions of executive functioning have a basic commonality in that they describe a set of skills needed to accomplish everyday tasks, such as planning, organizing, prioritizing, and multitasking (Hughes et al., 1994; Russell et al., 1999). Executive functions are critical in goal-directed behavior and for directing one's performance, especially guiding the planning processes required in task completion, organizing, strategizing, sustaining attention to and remembering details, along with management of time and space.

Executive dysfunction may interfere with an individual's work performance in a variety of ways. Some examples of challenges related to executive dysfunction include following multi-step instructions, coordinating sets of activities, and attending to pertinent details in assigned tasks Such abilities are necessary to be able to follow a morning routine to get to work on time, or to complete tasks according to a designated time frame (Zager et al., 2013).

The degree of executive competence individuals possess in organization and management affects their behavior. As anxiety resulting from problems caused by executive dysfunction escalates and individuals feel overwhelmed by task complexity, self-regulation of behavior becomes increasingly difficult. The good news is that executive function relies on modifiable and teachable skills (Thoma et al., 2013). Special educators, vocational counselors, and family members can be instrumental in fostering the development of employment-related and independent living skills that will lead to improved executive functioning. By providing concrete literal instruction in relevant real-life training opportunities (Zager & Feinman, 2013), it is possible to improve job-related skills, as well as executive functioning.

Sensory Integration Issues

Sensory integration refers to the ability to process external and internal stimuli simultaneously. Humans are continually confronted with oncoming stimuli, which our senses are expected to perceive and interpret, leading to some form of response. Intact sensory processing enables people to adapt their behavior in order to participate in community life. For instance, in a loud bar, people tend to raise their voices to be heard; or while driving in the city, drivers must be responsive to oncoming traffic from different directions, traffic signals, pedestrians, and weather conditions.

People with autism may be hyper- or hypo-sensitive to stimuli, either over-reacting or under-reacting to visual, tactile, or auditory stimuli. Some individuals find themselves unsure as to where another person's space begins and ends. When external stimuli are coming from more than one source—such as smell, sound, and touch—a person with ASD may become overwhelmed (Miller & Lane, 2000). It is much easier to avoid or prepare for overwhelming situations than it is to rectify the resultant issues and behaviors. Some ways to prepare for situations are to desensitize the individual to a particular environment, step by step building tolerance. Other possibilities include accommodations, such as headphones to block noise. Needed supports should be determined on an individual basis and should be situation specific.

Considerations in Educational Planning for Transition

The goal of education for all individuals is to expand their knowledge and skills so that they can achieve personal independence and assume adult responsibilities upon graduation from school (Hendricks & Wehman, 2009; Hendricks, 2010; Wehman et al., 2014). The transition from school to postsecondary education and paid employment should improve the possibility that individuals will become independent, productive, and participating members of their community.

Transition Approaches for Secondary and Postsecondary Students

Approaches for instructing students with ASD have received varying degrees of empirical support. It is useful to consider how approaches might be adapted and combined on an individual basis to facilitate the transition process. During the childhood years education for students with autism is often provided through approaches, such as Applied Behavior Analysis (ABA), the TEACCH model of structured teaching (Treatment and Education of Autistic and Related Communication-Handicapped Children), and relationship-based models like the Developmental Individual Difference Relationship Model (DIR/FloorTime). Secondary school programs tend to place more emphasis on development of functional academics, independence and self-determination, with attention directed to longitudinal goal setting and life-long planning.

The research and literature base in the field of autism have shown that instructional effectiveness is improved through application of behavioral techniques (e.g., providing and fading prompts and utilizing positive reinforcement techniques) (see, for example, Baer et al., 1968; Hundert, 2009; Iovannone et al., 2003). There is also abundant research and written material promoting the TEACCH method (Marcus et al., 1978; Mesibov et al., 2002; Mesibov & Shea, 2010). Regardless of the level of functioning of students on the spectrum, these techniques provide a framework for learning. In addition, the DIR Model, has gained support (Greenspan, 1999; Greenspan & Wieder, 2006; Mahoney & Perales, 2005; Wieder & Greenspan, 2003).

For adolescents and young adults who have benefited from years of behavioral intervention, transition instruction should be presented through a broader behavioral framework. Behavioral programming can increase age-appropriate behaviors required in inclusive community settings, where naturally occurring reinforcement is a powerful tool. Relating new concepts to actual experiences can enhance meaning and facilitate learning new knowledge. Because individuals with ASD and other developmental disabilities often have difficulty generalizing learned information to new situations, it is incumbent upon teachers at the secondary level to conduct a large portion of instruction in settings beyond their classroom walls, utilizing community-based learning strategies for transition. Research studies (e.g., Schall, 2010; Wacker et al., 1985) have noted the importance of generalization and community-based instruction in the preparation of youth with autism and other severe disabilities. In selecting transition preparation settings, environmental factors should be considered. Noise, lighting, smells, crowds, animals, etc. may pose sensory discomfort for individuals with ASD. By taking into account these considerations, agitation and maladaptive behaviors may be reduced, therein increasing the likelihood of successful transition. Instructional approaches to prepare students with autism to be successful in work and adult living should focus on (a) building on strengths and interests, rather than on a deficit-based model; (b) presenting opportunities to learn in varied ways to accommodate challenges associated with autism, such as sensory issues (e.g., hyper-sensitivity to noise, smell, or touch), distractibility, restricted interests, repetitive behaviors; and (c) turning behaviors that could be perceived negatively into work-related assets (e.g., over-attention to detail, persistent attraction to specific activities).

Universal Design for Transition

The promotion of integrated community-based work for people with ASD requires creation of effective sustainable models of employment intervention. One model that has been shown to be effective in transition programming for secondary school students with intellectual disabilities and that shows promise for students with ASD is Universal Design for Transition (UDT) (Thoma et al., 2009). Universal Design for Transition offers evidence-based practices for preparing adults with autism for employment. Universal Design for Transition practices have been demonstrated to be highly effective in preparing persons for disabilities for the transition to work, by providing the framework for employment preparation and serving as a guide to move individuals toward attainment of their goals.

This model is founded on the principles of Universal Design for Learning: (1) multiple means of representation, (2) multiple means of expression, and (3) multiple means of participation and engagement. Universal Design for Learning (UDL) builds on individuals' strengths and interests rather than using a deficit-based model. As with UDL, the goal of UDT is to enable all individuals to sustain competitive/supported employment by ensuring maneuverable and accessible work environments. In UDT, tasks are scaffolded into sequential segments, permitting participants to enter the task at their level. Assistive technology is utilized to provide options for information presentation and task completion. Knowledge and skills are presented concretely, aligned with individual talents and interests, and taught in a meaningful way through real-life experiences. For example, a person who wants to work in a restaurant would benefit from experiential instruction on-site in a restaurant or simulated restaurant. Skills taught might include sorting silverware and dishes, setting tables, following directions for job tasks, and conversing with co-workers and patrons.

Self-Determination Competence in UDT. Self-determination is a critical component of UDT employment training. A clear connection between self-determination competence and improved outcomes in employment has been demonstrated (Wehmeyer & Shogren, 2014). Self-determination instruction utilizes person-centered planning and is based on a problem-solving approach that encourages individuals to bridge the gap between current situations and targeted goals. Instruction should guide learning through a series of questions that help steer future planning, and interface with person-centered planning to include (a) goal setting, (b) constructing learning plans, and (c) adjusting behaviors. Utilization of UDT with emphasis on self-determination competence has been shown to enhance work-related learning (Thoma et al., 2009) leading to improved employment outcomes.

Multiple avenues for service delivery are helpful in identifying and using strengths to meet employment goals. Essential elements in successful programming are: (a) varied work experiences in multiple settings that take into account students' strengths as well as challenges associated with autism, such as executive dysfunction, concrete thinking, rigidity, sensory issues, and social communication challenges; (b) self-determination competence instruction that considers special talents and skills that have been developed and honed to high levels through over-selective interests in specific topics; (c) multiple representations of learning tasks, such as modeling and video presentations, that accommodate unique learning and behavior characteristics associated with autism (e.g., difficulty with abstract concepts, trouble with fast-paced language, preference for well-organized visual presentation); (d) multiple engagement in varied work activities, such as individual work, cooperative tasks, and technology driven activities to afford opportunities to circumvent learning and behavior challenges (e.g., difficulty with generalization of learned information to new situations, desire to have friends but inability to take initiative or act reciprocally, difficulty understanding expectations in cooperative group situations); (e) multiple expressions of knowledge such as role playing, drawing, and writing that utilize skills and strengths that can be used to demonstrate competence; and (f) reflection and evaluation of learned knowledge through self-assessment, involving the need to look objectively at consequences of one's actions and considering response to one's acts by others.

Employment intervention should include (a) work experiences in settings that consider the learner's strengths as well as challenges (e.g., sensory issues, rigidity social communication issues); (b) person-centered planning that focuses on development of self-determination competence; (c) modeling, role playing, and videos to illustrate critical job components; (d) technology-assisted instruction that accommodates unique learner characteristics; (e) participation in cooperative activities as appropriate; (f) self-assessment and reflection to look at the consequences of one's actions, understand the response of others to these actions, and proactively plan more appropriate actions.

Role of Educators

It is the responsibility of educators to deliver transition curriculum that incorporates person-centered planning, targeted academic instruction for job readiness, real-life work experiences, family involvement, and employer support into their transition programs. Educators involved in transition programs need to be familiar with their state agencies and systems in order to help families obtain services and make a seamless transition to adult services.

Family involvement is essential to successful employment outcomes. Engaging and supporting parents/families in the employment process involves ongoing communication. Family members may need assistance in accessing necessary services, resolving obstacles to job attainment, and navigating agency bureaucracy. It is essential that educators listen to concerns of students and their families, to help them obtain needed services, navigate agencies' bureaucracies, and resolve problems and obstacles. It is also critical to include work supervisors who will be interacting with individuals with ASD at the jobsite. Supervisors will benefit from information about the core challenges associated with autism, such as the difficulty that persons with autism have in understanding abstract language and concepts (Zager & Alpern, 2010). As supervision responsibilities are transferred from the job coach to on-site personnel, communication channels between key stakeholders should remain open so that difficult situations that arise may be handled swiftly and seamlessly.

It is the educator's job to deliver evidence-based instructional activities that utilize strategies that enable all students to progress. As with all instruction, transition programs should provide appropriate accommodations and supports, including technology to meet specific needs associated with autism (e.g., communication difficulty, sensory issues, restricted interests, repetitive behaviors). They should utilize ongoing assessment to evaluate program effectiveness, reflect on progress, adapt and modify programs as necessary, manage pertinent data, and communicate with other stakeholders in the employment support process. Programs should build on individuals' strengths and interests rather than using a deficit-based model. A major focus should center on enhancing self-determination for employment, including identifying employment goals, working toward goals, and adjusting plans or goals as needed (Wehmeyer & Shogren, 2014). Teachers need to engage in person-centered planning to facilitate choice-making, goal setting, and self-advocacy. This will lead to channeling students' behaviors that could be perceived negatively, such as over-attention to detail and persistent attraction to specific activities, into work-related assets.

Instructional strategies should build on strengths, respect individual interests and preferences, and accommodate challenges inherent in autism. During the school years, students should be guided to identify jobs that utilize their abilities and talents and maximize their potential. Generic skills and behaviors vital for success in community-based employment settings should be taught, such as helping students plan and implement strategies to self-regulate, attend to and complete tasks, follow directions, organize activities, manage time efficiently, and work cooperatively with others. Students should learn how to request assistance, appropriately converse with co-workers, be active listeners, and engage in appropriate social etiquette. Challenging behaviors should be handled in a manner that can be generalized to the workplace, incorporating behavior management strategies, positive behavior supports, and relationship-based approaches for building positive behavior and resolving behavior issues in community-based settings. Curricula must address living skills related to job success, guiding students as they learn to manage tasks related to bill paying, financial budgeting, laundry, personal hygiene, time management, meal preparation, getting to work on time, and home cleanliness.

Collaborating with Vocational Rehabilitation

Individuals with autism may require accommodations and supports to be successful in employment. The type and amount of support available for adults typically are not as comprehensive as the services they may have received in school and may vary depending on the employment setting and employers' understanding of disabilities.

A potential source of support for young adults with autism can be found through Vocational Rehabilitation (VR). VR funded employment services in the United States for people with disabilities including autism are usually administered by states using a combination of federal and state funds, and delivered through local VR offices, in order to assist in the preparation and engagement in competitive integrated employment. By communicating and collaborating with VR representatives, educators can enhance job placement and maintenance (Kaya et al., 2016), leading to higher likelihood of sustained employment for individuals with autism.

Integrated Supported Employment Options

Employment First, enacted in 2012, is based on the premise that all citizens, including youth and adults with significant disabilities, are capable of full inclusion in integrated employment and community life, and that individuals with disabilities secure employment that offers at least minimum or customary benefits and wages (U.S. Department of Labor, Office of Disability Employment Policy, n.d.). Subsequently, in July 2014, the federal government re-authorized the Workforce Investment Act of 1998, now titled the Workforce Innovation and Opportunity Act (WIOA). The Act defines supported employment as integrated competitive employment including ongoing support services for individuals with the most severe disabilities for whom competitive employment has not occurred or has been intermittent due to a severe disability. Supported employment is a viable option for individuals who need intensive supported services due to the severity of their disabilities and extended services. For young adults with ASD, in relation to their needs for support in behavioral, job-related skills, and social communication skills, supported employment is a critical phase in the transition to competitive employment. Competitive integrated employment includes supported and customized employment, or employment in an integrated work setting in which an individual with a significant disability is working toward competitive integrated employment that is individualized and customized, and that is consistent with the strengths, abilities, interests, and informed choice of the individual, with ongoing support services for individuals with significant disabilities.

Individuals with ASD have the same rights to competitive employment as their neurotypical peers and peers with other disabilities (Chen et al., 2014; Walsh et al., 2014). A key component in achieving employment equality may be focusing on changing employers' and co-workers' attitudes regarding employability of individuals with ASD (Chappel & Sommers, 2010; Gerhardt & Lainer, 2011; Hendricks, 2010; Morgan & Alexander, 2005). Studies focused on employers' attitudes indicate that lack of understanding of autism spectrum disorders is the most significant challenge to successful employment for individuals with ASD (Chen et al., 2014; Hendricks, 2010; Morgan & Alexander, 2005; Nesbitt, 2000; Wilczynski et al., 2013). Studies identifying advantages to employing individuals with ASD included consistent attendance and high productivity, as well as employers' compliance with workforce diversity policies (Hagner & Cooney, 2005; Henderson & Cone, 2014; Morgan & Alexander, 2005).

To identify workplace accommodations that can contribute to obtaining or maintaining employment for adults with autism spectrum disorder, a review was undertaken by Khalifa et al., (2020) of articles published between January 1987 and March 2018. Inclusion criteria for selected studies included adults with autism participants of 18 years of age or older with intervention studies that described support for securing or maintaining employment/skills training, and education for employee/employers to support adults with autism. Of the 25 selected studies, most focused on types of job coaching using different strategies. Technology was also noted as an essential form of support. Workplace strategies for individuals with autism spectrum disorder that were demonstrated to be helpful included minimizing distractions, reducing noise, and predictable job duties. Support for employers and co-workers was highlighted, as well.

At the initial transition planning meeting, Sangit, his parents, his special education teacher, the speech-language therapist, the transition specialist, and a representative from the local vocational rehabilitation office were present. The teacher had invited the speech therapist to join the meeting so that they could work collaboratively toward building Sangit's self-determination and self-advocacy competence. Prior to the meeting the transition specialist had met with Sangit to assess his strengths, interests and challenges, as well as to identify his hopes for a career. At this first transition meeting, the group reviewed Sangit's assessment, and Sangit had an opportunity to share his hopes and his interests.

Supported Employment

According to Griffin et al. (2014), enrollment in sheltered workshops increased during the 1990s, despite one of the strongest economies in the history of the United States. Historically, employment options for individuals with ASD have been sheltered workshops, in which individuals with disabilities have been paid less than minimum wages, or participated in voluntary, unpaid work experiences (Hendricks, 2010; Nicholas et al., 2015). Community-based competitive employment options that offer work for a minimum wage remain limited for individuals with ASD. Müller and Cannon (2014) conducted research focusing on the quality of life for 22 young adults with ASD and cognitive impairments. The study revealed that only 26% were employed in competitive employment while the majority of individuals, 65%, were volunteers in an organization.

Supported employment is an option that recognizes the capacity of an individual to be employed while ongoing supports are provided (Gerhardt & Lainer, 2011). Supported employment includes support services that are necessary for an individual to gain and maintain paid employment in an integrative environment (Nicholas et al., 2015). Hendricks (2010) examined the research focusing on successful supported employment programs and case studies of adults with ASD. Vocational supports for individuals with ASD may be grouped into five areas: job placement, supervisors and co-workers, on-the-job training, workplace modification, and long-term support. The range of supports includes (a) job assessment based on the individual's goals and interests; (b) job development in relation to career searches and job site training when the individual finds employment, (c) support strategies including the use of technology, and (d) long-term supports to ensure job retention (Wehman et al., 2012; Wilczynski et al., 2013). Westbrook et al. (2012), identified additional effective supports for individuals with ASD, including functional behavioral assessments, positive reinforcement, social skills training, task analyses for facilitating training in specific job duties, and task preference assessments.

Job-site training facilitated by a job coach is often necessary for individuals with ASD to learn job-specific tasks and assimilate successfully into the culture of the workplace. Specifically, the job coach assists the employee to identify the workplace's natural supports (including identifying supports from co-workers and supervisors), compensatory strategies, self-management skills, and specific instruction in job skills (Nicholas et al., 2015; Wehman et al., 2014; Wilczynski et al., 2013). Holmes (2007) concluded that failure to adequately assess and provide necessary supports resulted in continual job loss for individuals with ASD. Although there has been limited research conducted focusing on teaching skills to individuals with ASD in workplace environments (Hendricks, 2010), supported work programs that included on the-job training by a job coach and with effective supports have been shown to result in increased employment rates, wages, and job retention rates for individuals with ASD.

Westbrook et al. (2012) identified two quasi-experimental studies conducted by Mawhood and Howlin (1999) and Garcia-Villamisar et al. (2000) that demonstrated the advantages of supported employment work programs. The Mawhood and Howlin two-year study compared employment outcomes of 50 individuals with Asperger's syndrome. The experimental group of 30 adults received assistance from a job coach, compared to a control group of 20 individuals matched by age, intellectual ability, and education who did not receive this support. During the two-year period more participants in the experimental group found paid employment, worked for longer periods of time, earned higher wages, and were employed in higher-level jobs (e.g., technical and administrative positions), as compared to the individuals in the control group.

A study conducted by Garcia-Villamisar, Ross and Wehman (2000) has significant implications for individuals with ASD participating in supportive employment. The study compared employment outcomes of 51 young adults with ASD who participated in supported and sheltered employment groups in relation to the clinical symptomology of autism, demonstrating that individuals in the sheltered workshop group exhibited increased symptoms and a deterioration of their skills, while subjects in the supported employment group showed fewer symptoms than the other group and were more likely to maintain employment.

Hillier et al. (2007) evaluated the impact of a vocational support program that provided on-site job coaching and other workplace supports for high school students and recent high school graduates with ASD. At the conclusion of the program, the majority of participants had retained their initial job placements, and their income increased. A study by Wehman, et al. (2012) of adults with ASD enrolled in a supported employment program who worked individually with an on-site employment specialist, showed the importance of implementing individualized supports, including long-term supports to foster job retention. Wehman et al. (2013) documented the results of a randomized clinical trial of Project SEARCH (an intensive internship program for high school-age students) providing vocational training and supports (e.g., specialized structure and schedules, intensive social skills instruction). Of the 24 young adults who were 18–21 years old in the treatment group, 21 acquired employment with higher than minimum wages. Of the 16 participants in the control group, only one participant gained employment. These qualitative studies indicate the efficacy of supported employment in increasing employment, wages, and the ability of individuals with ASD to retain employment. For individuals who were employed for longer periods of time and received higher wages, the quality of their life substantially improved (Westbrook et al., 2012). For adults with ASD who were employed for at least six months, there were significant improvements in their behavior in relation to independent functioning and socialization skills with coworkers.

Additionally, supported employment may be correlated with increased cognitive performance of individuals with ASD. Garcia-Villamisar and Hughes (2007) studied 44 adults with ASD engaged in supported employment and a group of adults who were unemployed. Adults in the supported employment program scored significantly higher on executive functioning skills, such as working memory and problem solving, in comparison to the unemployed groups who exhibited no change in cognitive functioning.

Customized Employment

Customized employment is defined as individualizing the relationship between an individual job seeker and an employer in a way that meets the needs of both (Citron et al., 2008; U.S. Department of Labor, Office of Disability Employment Policy, 2005). According to the National Center on Workforce and Disability (n.d.), customized employment results in jobs designed for the individual and have the potential for advancement for individuals with significant disabilities who have been chronically unemployed or underemployed.

According to Griffin et al. (2014), the success in individuals acquiring community-based employment was the result of a paradigm shift that focused on an economic development approach to creating job opportunities for individuals with significant disabilities. Compared to supported employment, which generally matches individuals to existing jobs, customized employment focuses on creating an individualized job for the employee through employer negotiations resulting in a highly customized job description (Gerhardt & Lainer, 2011). It may include other employment strategies such as supported employment, supported entrepreneurial initiatives, and individualized job development, or other strategies that result in job responsibilities customized to meet the needs of an individual with ASD.

Customized employment begins with an exploration process in collaboration with a personal representative to identify individual interests, strengths, and need for supports. Generally, the personal representative is a vocational rehabilitation specialist or other public or private disability service providers. The representative identifies potential employers and approaches them with the possibility of creating and negotiating a specific job description to meet the unique skills of the job seeker and the employer's business needs. The negotiation process addresses areas such as job duties and terms of employment. Other components in this process are creating a system of job supports, if necessary (e.g., job coaching, technology, transportation) that is individualized and meets the needs of the job applicant. The applicant confers with the employer and if the job description and responsibilities mutually meet the needs of both, the applicant is hired.

In conjunction with the process and principles of customized and supportive employment Condon and Callahan (2008) advocate for implementation of the Individualized Career Planning Model for adolescents attending high school (14–21 years old) to plan for transition to competitive employment, including self-employment options. Key steps in this model include working with the individual to identify interests, strengths, and support needs included in a Vocational Profile, creating a representational portfolio to negotiate a job with an employer, and utilization of

Social Security Work Incentives and linkages to promote collaborative funding and choices of services.

Self-Employment

According to Griffin et al. (2014), there are an estimated 700,000 new businesses launched annually. The self-employment rate is increasing by more than 20% annually, with microenterprises (businesses employing one to five employees) generating 64% of all new jobs in the United States. Traditionally, self-employment was not an option for individuals with ASD and it is now an employment model that is evolving into a viable reality. As of 2013, with the implementation of the Employment First legislation (Griffin et al., 2014), self-employment and business ownership are recognized in revised state VR policies and through policies of the U.S. Department of Labor's Office of Disability Employment Policy.

The Rehabilitation Act of 1973 and the Workforce Investment Act of 1998 (WIA) require vocational rehabilitation programs to assist individuals with disabilities to purchase equipment, training, and access supports. Griffin et al. (2007), advocate for individuals with disabilities to develop resource ownership (i.e., a skill or resource) that the individual can provide or perform. The resource belongs to the individual (e.g., repairing computers) and may provide the trajectory of employment opportunities from customized employment to self-employment and, possibly, business ownership.

Business Partnership Models

As a result of federal legislation to initiate equal opportunities for youth and adults with ASD to engage in competitive employment opportunities, business partnerships have expanded. The legislation and resultant partnerships are enabling more individuals to enter the workforce (Carter et al., 2009; Henderson & Cone, 2014). Sustaining business partnerships has been critical in supporting individuals as they enter the labor force. Several large business corporations have been promoting employment of individuals with disabilities. For example, the Marriott Bridges School to Work program, established in 1990, has assisted more than 15,000 young adults, 17–22 years old with disabilities including autism, to successfully transition to customized employment (Marriott Foundation for People with Disabilities, 2013). The Bridges program is a 15–24-month internship program for young adults and includes the components of skill assessment, career planning, job development, job placement, evaluation, and follow-up. According to the Bridges from School to Work Progress report, during 2012, 813 young adults with disabilities were placed in employment and 539 remained employed for at least 180 days in 358 participating businesses. The National Secondary Transition Technical Assistance Center identified students' completion of the Bridges from School to Work Program as a moderate, evidenced-based indicator in predicting post-school employment for transition-age youth with disabilities, including individuals with ASD.

Similarly, Walgreens, the retail pharmacy chain, has been at the forefront of creating inclusive work environments and embedded job supports for individuals with ASD. In 2007, Walgreens pioneered hiring individuals with ASD in its distribution center located in South Carolina and it has extended this hiring practice throughout its facilities with the intention of hiring 20 percent of its workforce from people with disabilities (Walgreens, 2011). Walgreens provides accommodations using assistive technology for employees with ASD. Visual prompting systems use pictures to provide instructions to employees for task completion, along with computers with icon-based touch screens. Additionally, to assist individuals with ASD with sensory challenges, Walgreens has equipped some facilities with special chairs and other materials to appropriately meet their employees' needs in the workplace.

A unique business partnership concept that was launched in 2013 involved Specialisterne U.S.A, and its collaboration with Computer Aid, Inc. (CAI). Computer Aid, Inc. hires individuals with ASD, in collaboration with Specialisterne for information technology projects with the intent of hiring individuals with ASD (to constitute 3% of its workforce) throughout the United States (Autism Speaks, 2012). Specialisterne was originally founded in Denmark in 2004 to create jobs for individuals with high-functioning ASD and Asperger syndrome thorough entrepreneurships and customized employment models in technology; specifically in the areas of software management, testing and registration, and data logistics (Ozretic, 2013). Specialisterne provides assessment of the individual's abilities and needs for supports as well as training in software testing, data handling, and social interaction skills such as working with colleagues.

Employer and Co-worker Supports. Employees with ASD may need extended support to prevent deterioration of acquired job and interpersonal skills that may occur if support services are removed, and which then can result in loss of employment (Hendricks, 2010). Personal accounts from adults with ASD highlight the need for long-term supports to assist them mediate the daily challenges they experience at work (Hurlbutt & Chalmers, 2004; Müller et al., 2003). On the other hand, models that rely on individualized on-site job training and sustained coaching are costly to maintain. Further, this intensive level of support may be detrimental to the individual with ASD in assimilating into the work culture and maintaining adherence to routines and job responsibilities (Autism Speaks, 2012; Targett & Wehman, 2009).

As on-site support from the job coach fades and is ultimately eliminated, relationships and support strategies are transferred to supervisors and co-workers to sustain and continue to provide support in the workplace. Existing support structures in businesses may be utilized and include human resource personnel and employee assistance programs, and trade associations (Wilczynski et al., 2013). According to Hagner and Cooney (2004), the key components of supervising employees with ASD are ensuring that communication is direct, assisting the individual to comprehend social communication cues in the workplace, and explaining changes and supporting the individual to cope with them (e.g., schedule). Similarly, co-workers can function as mentors and trainers of employees of ASD and provide supports that include prompting and modeling job responsibilities, performance feedback, and social interactions. Wilczynski concluded that the support of co-workers is critical in assisting employees with ASD to cope with their communication challenges and increase social interactions.

Assistive Technology Supports. In relation to implementing supports for employees with ASD in the workplace, research suggests the use of strategies that include applied behavior analysis, video modeling, structured reward systems, errorless learning, prompt systems and the use of computers and hand held personal digital assistant devices (PDAs) (Chen et al., 2014; Nicholas et al., 2015; Test et al., 2014; Wilczynski et al., 2013; Walsh et al., 2014). Technology is an evidence-based practice that is effective in teaching work-related skills and increasing the ability for employees with ADS to perform job tasks independently (Odom et al., 2010). Over the past several decades, technologies such as video modeling, audio cueing, video prompting, computer instruction, and virtual reality have been utilized for different training purposes with individuals with ASD.

Allen et al. (2010) investigated the efficacy of using video modeling and positive behavior reinforcement with three young adults with ASD. The study focused on the employees who received video instruction that presented demonstrations of skills necessary to promote products in a retail environment. Employees were observed during a four-month period before and after watching a video. The participants were able to correctly implement the skills modeled in the video in the workplace.

Similarly, Van Laarhoven et al. (2012) demonstrated the effectiveness of the use of video modeling on the maintenance of vocational tasks with six young adults with ASD and developmental disabilities. Two tasks were assigned to each individual. Their independence in completing the task was measured before and after a two-week period. One group was assigned to the video modeling intervention and the other was a control group. The video-modeling intervention group reviewed the videos during the two-week period. As a result of viewing the videos, the students increased their independence with both tasks. Both of these studies indicated that by modeling behaviors on videotape, students were able to learn, memorize, and generalize the behaviors effectively in the workplace. Studies have determined that video modeling resulted in expediting the rate of skill acquisition for individuals with ASD. Additionally, videos can be used repeatedly and ensure that training is delivered in a standardized manner (Chaffee, et al., 2018; Kellems & Morningstar, 2012).

Other studies have reported on young adults with ASD being trained to use iPhones and Apple video iPods, and PDA devices to prompt the completion of tasks. Burke, et al. (2010) designed a prompt system using an adapted iPhone application to teach six young adults work-related, social-vocational skills. The young adults were employed to assist in conducting a fire safety training session and to complete 63 scripted behaviors necessary to facilitate the training. One study focused on the participant completing the company's training program and using the iPhone and the performance cue system to meet performance criteria. The other study involved different participants who used only the iPhone to learn the same work behaviors. The results of the study indicated that five of the six participants attained the task criteria only after using the iPhone and the performance cue system. The iPhone technology was effective in providing prompts to enable individuals to learn and execute complex tasks. Similarly, Kellems and Morningstar (2012) evaluated the efficacy of using video modeling through an Apple video iPod to teach job-related tasks (e.g., facility maintenance skills, recycling materials, and refilling vending machines and inventory) to four young adults, aged 20–22, in community workplaces. Observational data revealed that the participants improved the percentage of steps they independently completed in each task using the iPod. The study also indicated, based on informal participant interviews, that the use of the iPod was beneficial in that the participants enjoyed using the device, and it was socially acceptable to use the iPod at work.

Another technological intervention, the use of virtual reality, is promising for facilitating the development of work-related social skills that are relevant to acquiring and maintaining employment. Strickland et al. (2013) developed an internet-based training program with an embedded virtual reality environment to teach young adults with high functioning ASD job interview skills. The study revealed that the young adults who completed the training sessions using virtual reality practice demonstrated more effective interview skills.

Another promising use of virtual technology, specifically Google Glass, is its potential to assist individuals with ASD to identify the emotions of others (Autism Speaks, 2013). Google Glass, an eye-glass wearable computer, displays information in a smartphone prototype hands-free format and permits the user to communicate with the internet using voice commands (Fichten et al., 2014). Applications for Google Glass have been developed to teach individuals with ASD social interaction skills, including improving eye contact and understanding non-verbal social cues. Specifically for individuals with ASD who, due to the nature of the disorder, are challenged by social interactions and interpersonal communication, using Google Glass could significantly assist them in learning these essential work-related skills.

Sangit has had transition goals included in his IEP since he was 14 years old. When he reached the age of 17, his teacher, along with his transition team and his parents, began to work more intensely to plan and implement a specific goal-oriented transition program. Goals were determined with Sangit's input as a major participant. Through collaborative planning utilizing universal design for transition (UDT), it was possible to infuse his academic curriculum with work-related skills.

Sangit had determined that he wanted to work in a hospital setting. For two years of high school, he spent 2 hours twice weekly at the local hospital. He learned how to clean and store laboratory equipment, read thermometers and blood pressure monitors. He worked in the hospital cafeteria serving food and heating frozen entrees. In addition, he worked at the main reception desk.

Sangit's academic program was aligned with his internship experiences. Math, language arts, and speech/communication sessions were designed to teach and reinforce necessary job-related skills. Upon graduation, he was hired by the hospital to work in maintenance, taking care of storage areas that housed medical supplies. In Hindi, Sangit's name means symphony. It is clear that his teacher orchestrated the team to work in concert and create a symphony, leading to his eventual employment success.

Conclusion

While the last decade has witnessed increased transition programs in schools and employment preparation is a more familiar concept than it was years ago, employment outcomes for people with autism remain poor. The dilemma remains that transition programming requires funds to hire staff and provide community-based instruction. A lack of knowledge pertaining to transition curriculum and strategies prevails. However, studies have demonstrated that effective employment intervention can enable and empower individuals with autism to use their unique talents and interests to attain and sustain employment through building on their strengths; recognizing and accommodating cognitive, sensory, and social challenges; and respecting preferences and interests. Ideally, transition preparation should begin in the primary school years, continuing in the secondary school years to prepare adolescents to move on to postsecondary education or employment, so that they may live, work, and recreate within their community.

Through research-based knowledge combined with person-centered planning, it is possible to create instructional models that will improve the chances that people with autism and related disabilities can attain and succeed in employment. Preparation of students for work through the use of strategies based on principles of Universal Design for Transition, in combination with broadly based principles of applied behavior analysis, structured teaching and relationship-based models, will significantly enhance the effectiveness of secondary and postsecondary programs. Further, by infusing this intervention with strategies that have been designed to build self-determination competence, educators will be able to identify, target, and meet employment goals that they develop with their students.

In order to utilize diverse talents and strengths of individuals with ASD, varied employment models may be necessary. Supported employment and customized employment are widely used models. Employer and co-worker supports, along with assistive technology, can significantly enhance success in the workplace. These options recognize the capacity of individuals with significant disabilities to be gainfully employed when they are provided with ongoing supports, and when job descriptions are tailored to enable them to succeed in the workplace.

Author Note

This revised chapter includes new, as well as updated, content from the previous edition written with Francis Dreyfus, Ed.D. Appreciation to Dr. Dreyfus is noted for her work on the fourth edition.

References

Allen, K.D., Wallace, D.P., Renes, D., Bowen S.L., & Burke, R.V. (2010). Use of video modeling to teach vocational skills to adolescent with autism spectrum disorders. *Education and Treatment of Children, 33*(3), 339–349.

Alverson, C.Y., Yamamoto, S.H. (2018). Employment outcomes for individuals with autism spectrum disorders: A decade in the making. *Journal of Autism and Developmental Disorders, 48*(1), 151–162. doi: 10.1007/s10803-017-3308-9.

Americans With Disabilities Act of 1990, Pub. L. No. 101-336, 104 Stat. 328 (1990).

Autism Speaks. (2012). Employment think tank report. Retrieved March 1, 2015, from www.autismspeaks.org/sites/default/files/as_think_tank_exec_

Autism Speaks. (2013, Oct. 23). Google Glass shows promise improving lives of people with autism. Retrieved from http://autismspeaks.org/news-item-goo gle- glass-shows-promise-improving-lives

Azano, A., & Tuckwiller, E.D. (2011). GPS for the English classroom: Understanding executive dysfunction in secondary students. *Teaching Exceptional Children, 43,* 38–44.

Baer, D.M., Wolf, M.M., & Risley, T.R. (1968). Some current dimensions of applied behavior analysis, *Journal of Applied Behavior Analysis, 1*(1), 91–97.

Barnhill, G.P. (2007). Outcomes in adults with Asperger syndrome. *Focus on Autism and other Developmental Disabilities, 22*(2), 116–126.

Baron-Cohen, S., Leslie, A.M., & Frith, U. (1985). Does the autistic child have a theory of mind? *Cognition, 21,* 37–46.

Black, M.H., Mahdi, S., Milbourn, B., Thompson, C., D'Angelo, A., Ström, E., Falkmer, M., Falkmer, T., Lerner, M., Halladay, A., Gerber, A., Esposito, C., Girdler., S., & Bölte, S. (2019). Perspectives of key stakeholders on employment of autistic adults across the United States, Australia, and Sweden, *Autism Research, 12*(11), 1648–1662. doi: 10.1002/aur.2167

Burgess, S., & Cimera, R.E. (2014). Employment outcomes of transition-aged adults with autism spectrum disorders: A state of the states report. *American Journal of Intellectual and Developmental Disabilities, 119*(1), 63–84. doi: 10.1352/1944-7558-119.1.64

Burke, R.V., Anderson, M.N., Bowen, S.L., Howard, M.R., & Allen, K.D. (2010). Evaluation of two instruction methods to increase employment options for young adults with autism spectrum disorders. *Research in Developmental Disabilities, 31*(6), 1223–1233.

Bury, R.L., Flower, R., Zulla, D.B., Nicholas, D.H. (2021). Workplace social challenges experienced by employees on the autism spectrum: An international exploratory study examining employee and supervisor. Journal *on Autism Developmental Disorders,* 51, 1614–1627. https://doi.org/10.1007/s10803-020-04662-6

Cappa, C., Figoli, & M., & Rossi, P. (2020). Network of services facilitating and supporting job placement for people with autism spectrum disorders. The experience of the ASL Piacenza, Italy, *Ann Ist Super Sanità, 56*(2), 241–246. doi: 10.4415/ANN_20_02_14. PMID: 32567574

Carter, E. W., Owens, L., Trainor, A. A., Sun,Y., & Swedeen, B. (2009). Self-determination skills and opportunities of adolescents with severe intellectual and developmental disabilities. American Journal on Intellectual and Developmental Disabilities, 114, 179Y192. doi:10.1352/1944-7558-114.3.179

Carter, E. W., Austin, D., & Trainor, A. A. (2012). Predictors of postschool employment outcomes for young adults with severe disabilities. *Journal of disability policy studies, 23*(1), 50–63.

Chaffee, E., Ho, T., & Ng, K. (2018). Pilot Study: Assistive Technology as a Vocational Support for Individuals with Autism Spectrum Disorder. Graduate Master's Thesis. https://doi.org/10.33015/dominican.edu/2018.OT.03

Chappel, S.L. & Somers, B.C. (2010). Employing persons with autism spectrum disorders: A collaborative effort. *Journal of Vocational Rehabilitation, 32,* 117–124. doi: 10.3233/JVR-2010-0501

Chen, J.L., Leader, G., Sung, C., & Leahy, M. (2014). Trends in employment for individuals with autism spectrum disorder: A review of the research literature. *Review Journal of Autism and Developmental Disorders*. Retrieved from http://link.spinger.com/article/10.1007/s40489-014-0041-6

Chiang, H.M., Cheung, Y.K., Li, H., & Tsai, L.Y. (2013). Factors associated with participation in employment for high school leavers with autism. *Journal of Autism and Developmental Disorders*, 43, 1832–1842. doi: 10.1007/s10803-012-1734-2

Cimera, R.E., & Cowan, R.J. (2009). The costs of services and employment outcomes achieved by adults with autism in the US. *Autism*, 13(3), 285–302. doi: 10.1177/1362361309103791

Citron, T., Brooks-Lane, N., Crandell, D., Brady, K., Cooper, M., & Revell, G. (2008). A revolution in the employment process of individuals with disabilities: Customized employment as the catalyst for system change. *Journal of Vocational Rehabilitation*, 28(3), 169–179.

Condon, E. & Callahan, M. (2008). Individualized career planning for students with significant support needs utilizing the discovery and vocational profile process, cross-agency collaboration funding and Social Security work incentives. *Journal of Vocational Rehabilitation*, 28, 85–96.

Etscheidt, S. (2006). Issues in transition planning: Legal decisions. *Career Development for Exceptional Individuals*, 29(1), 28–47.

Farley, M. A., McMahon, W. M., Fombonne, E., Jenson, W. R., Miller, J., Gardner, M., ... & Coon, H. (2009). Twenty-year outcome for individuals with autism and average or near-average cognitive abilities. *Autism Research*, 2(2), 109–118.

Fichten, C. S., Asuncion, J., & Scapin, R. (2014). Digital technology, learning, and postsecondary students with disabilities: Where we've been and where we're going. *Journal of Postsecondary Education and Disability*, 27(4), 369–379.

Fox, M. (2021, May 6), As small businesses recover from the pandemic, they face a new obstacle: finding workers {online news post]. www.cnbc.com/2021/05/06/small-businesses-struggle-to-find-workers-as-pandemic-eases.html

Garcia-Villamisar, D., & Hughes, C. (2007). Supported employment improves cognitive performance in adults with autism. *Journal of Intellectual Disability Research*, 51(2), 142–150. doi: 10/1111/j.1365-2788.2006.00854.x

Garcia-Villamisar, D., Ross, D., & Wehman, P. (2000). Clinical differential analysis of persons with autism: A follow-up study. *Journal of Vocational Rehabilitation*, 14, 183–185.

Gerhardt, P. F., & Lainer, I. (2011). Addressing the need of adolescents and adults with autism: A crisis on the horizon. *Journal of Contemporary Psychotherapy*, 41, 37–45. doi: 10.1007/s10879-010-9160-2

Gorenstein, M., Giserman-Kiss, I., Feldman, E., Isenstein, E. L., Donnelly, L., Wang, A. T., & Foss-Feig, J. H. (2020). A job-based social skills program (JOBSS) for adults with autism spectrum disorder: A pilot randomized controlled trial. *Journal of Autism and Developmental Disorders*, 50(12), 4527–4534. doi: 10.1007/s10803-020-04482-8. PMID: 32297122

Greenspan, S. (1999). *Building healthy minds: The six experiences that create emotional growth in babies and young children.* Cambridge, MA: Perseus Books.

Greenspan, S. I., & Wieder, S. (2006). *Engaging autism: Using the Floortime approach to help children relate, communicate, and think.* Cambridge, MA: DaCapo.

Griffin, C., Brookes-Lane, N., Hammis D. C., & Crandell, D. (2007). Self-employment: Owning the American dream. In P. Wehman, K.J. Inge, W.G. Revell Jr., & V. A. Brooks (Eds.), *Real Work for Real Pay: Inclusive Employment for People with Disabilities* (pp. 215–235). Baltimore, MD: Paul H. Brookes Publishing Co.

Griffin, C., Hammis, D., Keeton, B., & Sullivan, M. (2014). *Making self employment work for people with disabilities* (2nd ed.) Baltimore, MD: Paul H. Brooks Publishing.

Hagner, D., & Cooney, B.F. (2005). "I do that for everybody": Supervising employees with autism. *Focus on Autism and Other Disabilities, 20*(2), 91–97.

Hagner, D., Kurtz, A., Cloutier, H., Arakelian, C., Brucker, D.L., May, J. (2012). Outcomes of a family-centered transition process for students with autism spectrum disorders. *Focus on Autism and Other Developmental Disabilities, 27*(1), 43–50. doi: 10.1177/1088357611430841

Hardman, M. L., & Dawson, S. A. (2010). *Historical and legislative foundations.* Thousand Oaks, CA: Sage Publications, Inc.

Hayward, S. M., McVilly, K. R., & Stokes, M. A. (2019), Autism and employment: What works, *Research in Autism, 60,* 48–58.

Henderson, L., & Cone, A. A. (2014). Answering employers' questions about hiring people with significant disabilities. *TASH Connections, 40*(1), 35–40.

Hendricks, D. (2010). Employment and adults with autism spectrum disorders: Challenges and strategies for success. *Journal of Vocational Rehabilitation, 32,* 125–134. doi: 10.3233/JVR-2010-0502

Hendricks, D., & Wehman, P. (2009). Transition from school to adulthood for youth with autism spectrum disorders: Review and recommendations. *Focus on Autism and Other Developmental Disabilities, 24*(2), 77–88.

Hillier, A., Campbell, H., Mastriani, K., Izzo, M.V., Tucker-Kool, A.K., Cherry, A., & Beversdorf, D. Q. (2007). Two-year evaluation of a vocational support program for adults on the autism spectrum. *Career Development for Exceptional Individuals, 30*(1), 35–47.

Hirano, K. A., Rowe, D., Lindstrom, L., & Chan, P. (2018). Systemic barriers to family involvement in transition planning for youth with disabilities: A qualitative metasynthesis. *Journal of Child and Family Studies, 27,* 3440–3456. https://doi.org/10.1007/s10826-018-1189-y

Hoff, D. (2014). WIA is now WIOA: What the new bill means for people with disabilities. *Institute for Community Inclusion.* Retrieved March 1, 2015 from www.communityinclusion.org.

Holmes, D. (2007). When the school bus stops coming: The employment dilemma for adults with autism. *Autism Advocate, 46*(1), 16–21.

Howlin, P. (2000). Outcome in adult life for more able individuals or Asperger syndrome. *Autism, 4*(1), 63–81.

Howlin, P., Alcock, J. & Burkin, C. (2005). An 8-year follow-up of a specialist supported employment service for high-ability adults with autism or Asperger syndrome. *Autism, 9*(5), 533–549.

Howlin, P., Goode, S., Hutton, J., & Rutter, M. (2004). Adult outcomes for children with autism. *Journal of Child Psychology and Psychiatry, 45*(2), 212–229.

Hughes, C., Russell, J., & Robbins, T.W. (1994). Evidence for executive dysfunction in autism. *Neuropsychologia, 32*(4), 477–492.

Hundert, J. (2009). *Inclusion of students with autism: Using ABA-based supports in general education.* Austin, TX: Pro-Ed.

Hurlbutt, K., & Chalmers, L. (2005). Employment and adults with Asperger syndrome. *Focus on Autism and other Developmental Disorders, 19(4),* 215–222.

Individuals with Disabilities Education Improvement Act (2004). Pub. L. 108–466.

Iovannone, R., Dunlap, G., Huber, H., & Kincaid, D. (2003). Effective educational practices for students with autism spectrum disorder. *Focus on Autism and Other Developmental Disabilities, 18*(3), 150–165.

Kaya, C., Chan, F., Rumrill, P., Hartman, E..Wehman, P., Iwanaga, K., Pai, C., Avellone, L. (2016). Vocational rehabilitation services and competitive employment for transition-age youth with autism spectrum disorders, *Journal of Vocational Rehabilitation, 45*(1), 73–83.

Kellems, R.O., & Morningstar, M.E. (2012). Using video modeling delivered through iPods to teach vocational tasks to young adults with autism spectrum disorders. *Career Development and Transition for Exceptional Individuals, 35*(3), 155–167. doi: 10.1177/0885728812443082

Khalifa, G., Sharif, Z., Sultan, M., & DiRezze, B.. (2020). Workplace accommodations for adults with autism spectrum disorder: a scoping review. *Disabilities Rehabilitation, 42*(9):1316–1331. doi: 10.1080/09638288.2018.1527952. Epub 2019 Feb 3. PMID: 30714420.

Kucharczyk, S., Reutebuch, C.K., Carter, E.W., Hedges, S.E.L., Zein, F., Fan, H., . . . Gustafson, J.R. (2015). Addressing the needs of adolescents with autism spectrum disorder: Considerations and complexities for high school interventions, *Exceptional Children, 8*(3), 329–349.

Landmark, L.J., Ju, S., & Zhang, D. (2010). Substantiated best practices in transition: Fifteen plus years later. *Career Development for Exceptional Individuals, 3,* 165–176.

Lawer, L., Brusilovkiy, E., Salzer, M.S., Mandell, D.S. (2009). Use of vocational rehabilitative services among adults with autism. *Journal of Autism and Developmental Disorders, 39*(3), 487–494.

Lee, G.K., Curtiss, S.L., Kuo, H.J., Chun, J., Lee, H., & Nimako, D.D. (2021). The role of acceptance in the transition to adulthood: A multi-informant comparison of practitioners, families, and youth with autism. *Journal of Autism and Developmental Disorders.* doi: 10.1007/s10803-021-05037-1

Luecking, D.M., & Luecking, R.G. (2015). Translating research into a seamless transition model. *Career Development and Transition for Exceptional Individuals, 38*(1), 4–13.

Mahdi, S., Viljoen, M., Yee, T., Selb, M., Singhal, N., Almodayfer, O., Granlund, M., deVries, P.J., Zwaigenbaum, L., & Bölte., S. (2018). An international qualitative study of functioning in autism spectrum disorder using the World Health Organization international classification of functioning, disability and health framework. *Autism Research, 11*(3), 463–475. doi: 10.1002/aur.1905

Mahoney, G., & Perales, E. (2005). A comparison of the impact of relationshipfocused intervention on young children with pervasive developmental disorders and other disabilities. *Journal of Developmental and Behavioral Pediatrics*, 26, 77–85.

Marcus, L.M., Lansing, M., Andrews, C.E., & Schopler, E. (1978). Improvement of teaching effectiveness in parents of autistic children. *Journal of the American Academy of Child Psychiatry*, 17, 625–639.

Marriott Foundation for People with Disabilities. (2013). *Bridges from School to Work Progress Report*. Retrieved on March 25, 2015, from www.bridge sto work.org.

Martin, J. E., & Williams-Diehm, K. (2013). Student engagement and leadership of the transition planning process. *Career Development and Transition for Exceptional Individuals*, 36(1), 43–50.

Mawhood, L., & Howlin, P. (1999). The outcome of a supported employment scheme for high functioning adults with autism or Asperger syndrome. *Autism*, 3(3), 229–254. doi: 10.1177/1362361399003003003

McEathron, M.A., Beuhring, T., Maynard, A., & Mavis, A. (2013). Understanding the diversity: A taxonomy for postsecondary education programs and services for students with intellectual and developmental disabilities. *Journal of Postsecondary Education and Disability*, 26(40), 303–320.

Meadan, H., Shelden, D.L., Appel, K., & DeGrazia, R.L. (2010). Developing a long-term vision: A road map for students' futures. *Exceptional Children*, 43(2), 8–13.

Mesibov, G.B., Browder, D.M., & Kirkland, C. (2002). Using individual schedules as a component of positive behavioral support for students with developmental disabilities, *Journal of Positive Behavioral Interventions*, 4, 73–79.

Mesibov, G.B., & Shea, V. (2010). The TEACCH program in the era of evidence-based practice. *Journal of Autism and Developmental Disorders*, 40(5), 570–579.

Miller, E.K., & Lane, S.(2000). Toward consensus in terminology in sensory integration theory and practice. Part 1: Taxonomy of neuropsychological processes. *Sensory Integration Special Interest Section*, 23(1), 1–4.

Morgan, R.L., & Alexander, M. (2005). The employer's perception: Employment of individuals with developmental disabilities. *Journal of Vocational Rehabilitation*, 23, 39–49.

Morningstar, M.E., & Liss, J.M. (2008). A preliminary investigation of how states are responding to the transition assessment requirements under IDEIA 2004. *Career Development for Exceptional Individuals*, 31(1), 48–55. doi: 10.1177/0885728807313776

Müller, E., & Cannon, L. (2014). Parent perspectives on outcomes and satisfaction levels of young adults with autism and cognitive impairments. *Focus on Autism and Other Developmental Disabilities*, 1–12. doi: 10.1177/1088357614528800

Müller, E., Schuler, A., Burton, B.A., & Yates, G.B. (2003). Meeting the vocational support needs of individuals with Asperger syndrome and other autism spectrum disabilities, *Journal of Vocational Rehabilitation*, 18(3), 163–175.

National Center on Workforce and Disability (n.d.). *Customized Employment: Principles and Indicators*. Retrieved on February 17, 2015, from www.onestops.info/article.php?article_id=254&subcat_id=101

Nesbitt, S. (2000). Why and why not? Factors influencing employment for individuals with Asperger syndrome, *Autism, 4*, 357–369.

Nicholas, D.B., Attridge, M., Zwaigenbaum, & Clarke, M. (2015). Vocational support approaches in autism spectrum disorder: A synthesis review of the literature. *Autism, 19*(2), 235–245. doi: 10.1177/1362361313516548

Odom, S.L., Collet-Klingenberg, L., Rodgers, S.J. & Hatton, D.D. (2010). Evidence-based practices in intervention for children and youth for children and youth with autism spectrum disorders. *Preventing School Failure, 54*, 275–282. doi: 10.1080/10459881003785506

Ozretic, A. (2013, Oct. 22). Creating great employees (who happen to be autistic). *Techonomy Exclusive*. Retrieved on March 30, 2015 from http://techonomy. com/2013/10/creating-great-employees-happen-autistic/.

Palumbo, J. (2021, April 27.) Why Autism Speaks Is Encouraging Companies to Hire Those on The Autistic Spectrum. Forbes Magazine. www.forbes.com/sites/jenniferpalumbo/2021/04/27/why-autism-speaks-is-encouraging-companies-to-hire-those-on-the-autistic-spectrum/?sh=7fdeba5152a2

Papay, C.K., & Bambara, L.M. (2014). Best practices in transition to adult life for youth with intellectual disabilities. *Career Development and Transition for Exceptional Individuals, 37*(3), 136–148.

Roux, A.M., Rast, J.E., Anderson, K.A., Garfield, T., Shattuck, P.T. (2021). Vocational rehabilitation service utilization and employment outcomes among secondary students on the autism spectrum. *Journal of Autism and Developmental Disabilities, 51*(1), 212–226. doi:10.1007/s10803-020-04533-0

Roux, A.M., Shattuck, P.T., Cooper, B.P., Anderson, K.A., Wagner, M., & Narendorf, S.C. (2013). Postsecondary employment experiences among young adults with autism with an autism spectrum disorder RH: Employment in young adults with autism. *Journal of the American Academy of Child and Adolescent Psychiatry, 52*(9), 931–939. doi: 10.1016/jaac.2013.05.019

Roux, A.M., Shattuck, P.T., Rast, J.E., Rava, J.A., & Anderson, K.A. (2015). *National autism indicators report: Transition into young adulthood.* Life Course Outcomes Research Program, A.J. Drexel Autism Institute. Philadelphia: PA. Retrieved on March 1, 2015 from Drexel.edu/autisminstitute/researchprojects/research/ResearchPrograminLifeCourseOutcomes

Russell, J., Jarrold, C., & Hood, B. (1999). Two intact executive functions in autism: Implications for the nature of the disorder. *Journal of Autism and Developmental Disorders, 29*, 103–285.

Schall, C. M. (2010). Positive behavior support: Supporting adults with autism spectrum disorders in the workplace. *Journal of Vocational Rehabilitation, 32*, 109–115. doi: 10.3233/JVR-2010-0500&

Schall, C. M. & McDonough,T. J. (2010). Autism spectrum disorders in adolescence and early adulthood: Characteristics and issues. *Journal of Vocational Rehabilitation, 32*, 81–88. doi: 10.3233/JVR-2010-0503

Schall, C., Targett, P., & Wehman, P. (2013). Applications for youth with autism spectrum disorders. In P. Wehman (Ed.), *Life beyond the classroom*, 5th ed. (pp. 447–472). Baltimore, MD: Paul H. Brookes Publishing.

Schall, C., Wehman, P. & McDonough, J. L. (2012). Transition from school to work for students with autism spectrum disorders: Understanding the process and achieving better outcomes. *Pediatric Clinics, 59*(1), 189–202. doi: http://dx.org/10.1016/j.pcl.2011.10.009

Schall, C., Wehman, P., Avellone, L., & Taylor, J.P. (2020). Competitive integrated employment for youth and adults with autism: Findings from a scoping review. *Child and Adolescent Psychiatry Clinics of North America, 2,* 373–397. doi: 10.1016/j.chc.2019.12.001

Schaller, J., & Yang, N. K. (2005). Competitive employment for people with autism: Correlates of successful closure in competitive and supported employment. *Rehabilitation Counseling Bulletin, 49*(1), 4–16. doi: 10.1177/003435520504 90010201

Shattuck, P. T., Narendorf, S. C., Cooper, B., Sterzing, P. R., Wagner, M., & Taylor, J. L. (2012). Postsecondary education and employment among youth with an autism spectrum disorder. *Pediatrics, 129*(2), 1042–1049. doi: 10.1542/peds.2011-2864

Shattuck, P.T., Wagner, M., Narendorf, S., Sterzing, P., & Hensley, M. (2011). Post high school service use among young adults with autism spectrum disorder. *Archives of Pediatric Medicine, 165*(2), 141–146. doi: 10.1001archpediatrics.2010.279

Shogren, K. A. & Plotner, A. J. (2012). Transition planning for students with intellectual disability, autism, or other disabilities: Data from the national longitudinal transition study-2. *Intellectual and Developmental Disabilities, 50*(1), 16–30. doi: 10.1352/1934-9556-50.1.16

Smith, M. D., & Philippen, L. R. (2005). Community integration and supported employment. In D. Zager (Ed.). *Autism spectrum disorders: Identification, education, and treatment (3rd ed.),* (pp. 493–5140. Mahwah, NJ: Lawrence Erlbaum Associates.

Stack, K., Symonds, J. E., & Kinsella, W. (2021). The perspectives of students with Autism Spectrum Disorder on the transition from primary to secondary school: A systematic literature review, *Research in Autism Spectrum Disorders,* 84, 101782, 101782, ISSN 1750-9467, https://doi.org/10.1016/j.rasd.2021.10178

Standifer, S. (2009). *Adult autism and employment: A guide for vocational rehabilitation professionals.* Disability Policy Studies, School of Health Professions, University of Missouri. Retrieved February 10, 2014, www.dps.missouri.edu/ Autism/Adults

Strickland, D. C., Coles, C. D., & Southern, L. B. (2014) JobTIPS: A transition to employment program for individuals with autism spectrum disorders. *Journal of Autism and Developmental Disorders, 43*(10), 2472–2483. doi: 10.1007/s10803-013-1800-4

Targett, P. S., & Wehman, P. (2009). Integrated Employment. In P. Wehman, M. D., & C. Schall (Eds.), *Autism & the transition to adulthood: Success beyond the classroom.* Baltimore, MD: Paul H. Brooks Publishing Co.

Taylor, J. L. & Seltzer, M. M. (2011). Employment and post-secondary educational activities for young adults with autism spectrum disorders during the transition to adulthood. *Journal of Autism and Developmental Disorders, 41*(5), 566–574. doi: 10.1007/s10803-010-1070-3

Test, D.W., Fowler, C.H., Richter, S.M., White, J., Mazzotti, Walker, A.R., . . . Kortering, L. (2009). Evidence-based practice in secondary transition. *Career Development for Exceptional Individuals, 32*(2), 115–128.

Test, D. W., Smith, L. E. & Carter, E. W. (2014). Equipping youth with autism spectrum disorders for adulthood: Promoting rigor, relevance, and relationships. *Remedial and Special Education, 35*(2), 80–90.

Thoma, C. A., Bartholomew, C. C., & Scott, L. A. (2009). *Universal design for transition: A roadmap for planning and instruction.* Baltimore: Paul H. Brookes Publishing Co.

Thoma, C. A., Gentry, R., Boyd, K., & Streagle, K. (2013). Academic assessment in transition planning in C. A. Thoma & R. Tamura (Eds.). *Demystifying transition assessment.* Baltimore: Paul H. Brookes.

U.S. Department of Education (November, 2009). *State of the science conference on postsecondary education for students with intellectual disabilities.* Fairfax, VA.

U.S. Department of Labor, Office of Disability Employment Policy. (2005). *Customized employment: Practical solutions for employment success.* Retrieved March 10, 2015, from www.dol.gov/odep/categories/workforce/Cus tomized Employment

U.S. Department of Labor, Office of Disability Employment Policy. (n.d.). *Employment First.* Retrieved January 20, 2015 from www.dol.gov/odep/topics/EmploymentFirst

Van Schalkwyk, G. I., & Volkmar, F. R. (2017). Autism spectrum disorders: Challenges and opportunities for transition to adulthood. Child and Adolescent Psychiatry Clinics of North America, 26(2), 329–339. doi: 10.1016/j.chc.2016.12.013

Van Laarhoven, T., Winiarskii, L., Blood, E., & Chan, J. M. (2012), Maintaining vocational skill of individuals with autism an developmental disabilities through video modeling. *Education and Training in Autism and Developmental Disabilities, 47*(4), 447–461.

Wacker, D. P., Berg, W. K., Berrie, P., & Swatta, P. (1985). Generalization and maintenance of complex skills by severely handicapped adolescents following picture prompt training. *Journal of Applied Behavior Analysis, 18*, 329–336.

Wagner, M., Newman, L., Cameto, R., Levine, P., & Marder, C. (2007). *Perceptions of youth with disabilities: A special topic report of findings with the National Longitudinal Transition Study-2 (NTLS)* (NSCER 2007–3006). Menlo Park: CA SRI International. Retrieved March 1, 2015 from http://eri ced.gov/?id=ED498185

Walgreens. *Aim Hire* (2011, October). Retrieved February 28, 2015 from, www.walgreens.com/topic/sr/sr_disabiity_inclusions_awards_recognition

Walsh, L., Lyndon, S., & Healy, O. (2014). Employment and vocational skill among individuals with autism spectrum disorder: Predictors, impact, and interventions. *Review Journal of Autism and Developmental Disorders, 1*, 266–275. Retrieved from http://link.springer.com/article 10.1007/s40489014-0024-7

Wehman, P. (2013). Transition from school to work: Where are we and where do we need to go? *Career Development and Transition for Exceptional Individuals, 36*(1), 58–66. doi: 10.1177/2165143413483137

Wehman, P., Lau, S., Molinelli, A., Brooke, V., Thompson, K., Moore, C., & West, M. (2012). Supported employment for young adults with autism spectrum disorder: Preliminary data. *Research and Practice for Persons with Severe Disabilities, 37*(3), 160–169.

Wehman, P., Schall, C., Carr, S., Targett, P., West, T. & Cifu, G. (2014). Transition from school to adulthood for youth with autism spectrum disorder: What we know and what we need to know. *Journal of Disability Policy Studies, 25*(1), 30–40. doi: 10.1177/1044207313518071

Wehman, P., Schall, C. M., McDonough, J., Kregel, J., Brooke, V., Molinelli, A., Ham, W., . . . Thiss, W. (2013b). Competitive employment for youth with autism spectrum disorders: Early results from a randomized clinical trial. *Journal of Autism and Developmental Disorders, 44*(3), 487–500. doi: 10.1177/1098300712459760

Wehman, P., Schall, C., McDonough, J., Sima, A., Brooke, A., Ham, W., Whittenburg, H., Brooke, V., Avellone, L., & Riehle, E. (2020). Competitive Employment for Transition-Aged Youth with Significant Impact from Autism: A Multi-site Randomized Clinical Trial. *Journal of Autism and Developmental Disorders, 50*(6), 1882–1897. https://doi.org/10.1007/s10803-019-03940-2

Wehmeyer, M. L., & Shogren, K. (2014, January). *Evidence-based practices to promote self-determination on postschool outcomes.* Paper presented at conference of the Division on Autism and Developmental Disabilities, Clearwater, FL.

Wehmeyer, M., Shogren, K. A., Smith, T. E. C., Zager, D., & Simpson, R. (2010). Research-based principals and practices for educating students with autism: Self-determination and social interactions. *Education and Training in Autism and Developmental Disabilities, 45*(4), 475–486.

Westbrook, J. D., Nye, C., Fong, C.J., Wan, J. T., Cortopassi, T., & Martin, F. H. (2012). Adult employment assistance services for persons with autism spectrum disorders: Effects on employment outcomes. *Campbell Systematic Reviews.* Retrieved from http://ideas.repec.org/p/mpr/mprres/7398.html

Whitney, S. (2021, December). What Do the Laws Say About Transition Plans, Goals, Services and Timelines? www.wrightslaw.com/heath/transition.work.htm

Wieder, S., & Greenspan, S. (2003). Climbing the symbolic ladder in the DIR model through floortime/interactive play, *Autism, 7,* 425–436.

Wilczynski, S. M., Trammell, B. & Clarke, L. S. (2013). Improving employment outcomes among adolescents and adults on the autism spectrum. *Psychology in the Schools, 50*(9), 876–887. doi: 10.1002/pits.21718

Wong, J., Coster, W. J., Cohn, E. S., & Orsmond, G. I. (2021). Identifying school-based factors that predict employment outcomes for transition-age youth with autism spectrum disorder. *Journal of Autism and Developmental Disorders,1,* 60–74. doi: 10.1007/s10803-020-04515-2. PMID: 32356081

Zager, D., Alpern, C., McKeon, B., Maxam, S., & Mulvey, J. (2013). *Educating college students with autism spectrum disorders.* New York: Routledge.

Zager, D., & Feinman, S. (2013, Winter). Employing evidence-based practices in high school to enhance accessibility to learning and to build executive competence. *Autism Spectrum News, 5*(3), 8, 34.

Zager, D., Thoma, C. A., & Fleisher, S. M. (2014, Spring). Employment for persons on the autism spectrum: Examination of the state of the field and the path to pursue. *Autism Spectrum News, (6)*4, 1, 18, 42.

Chapter 16

Collaboration and Interdisciplinary Practice in Education and Transition

Emily C. Bouck,[1] Jordan Shurr,[2] Holly Long,[1] and Allison White[1]

[1]Department of Counseling, Educational Psychology, and Special Education, Michigan State University

[2]Faculty of Education, Queens University

Case Vignette: Introduction

Jan and Raul are two high school students with autism. Jan, who is 17 years old, lives in a rural county and enjoys being outdoors and caring for the animals on her family's small farm. In school, Jan works on academic skills with a functional focus in the general education classroom, and resource room, as well as occasionally in the community through a community-based vocational instruction (CBVI) work-skills program. Jan hopes to work with animals as a career after high school and is interested in learning more about animals, making friends with similar interests, and living in an apartment on her own. Raul, who is 15 years old, lives in a suburban area down the street from a large shopping center with several bus stops. In his spare time, Raul enjoys drawing and reading manga style comics. Raul is working on grade-level academics in the general education classroom with consultative support and a one-hour study skills course with the special education teacher. He is not sure what he wants to do after high school but is interested in learning more about graphic design.

Collaboration and Students with ASD

Interdisciplinary collaboration is an important component in the education of students with disabilities (Friend & Cook, 2017). Although collaboration can mean different things to different individuals, for the purposes of this chapter, we subscribed to Friend and Cook's (2017) definition of collaboration as "a style for direct interaction between at least two coequal parties voluntarily engaged in shared decision-making as they work toward a common goal" (p. 5). In other words, those engaged in collaboration need to agree to collaborate, have equal voice within the collaborative decision-making, understand they are striving for at least

DOI: 10.4324/9781003255147-19

one mutual goal, and share in the responsibility for the outcome of the decision (Friend & Cook, 2017).

While collaboration is an essential ingredient in the education of all children, it is especially important in the education of students with autism spectrum disorders (ASD). Given that ASD is characterized by challenges in communication, social interaction, and restricted interests that impact a child's educational attainment, it seems intuitive that an interdisciplinary method is the best way to approach the education of students with ASD (Donaldson & Stahmer, 2014; Gargiulo & Bouck, 2020; Individuals with Disabilities Education Act [IDEA], 2004; Simpson et al., 2011). Positive and effective interdisciplinary collaboration—meaning multiple service providers and/or other individuals (e.g., parents) working and making decisions together—improves the education and life outcomes of students with ASD (Kelly & Tincani, 2013; Simpson et al., 2011).

In special education, interdisciplinary collaboration occurs through formal (e.g., multidisciplinary evaluation teams [MET] and individualized education program [IEP] teams) and informal opportunities (Kelly & Tincani, 2013). Interdisciplinary collaboration among educators who are providing direct and related services or supplementary services is essential (Gargiulo & Bouck, 2020; Simpson et al., 2011). Aside from general and special education teachers, other professionals collaborating to provide services to students with ASD include—but are not limited to—audiologists, interpreters, medical providers (e.g., school nurses), occupational therapists, orientation and mobility specialists, physical therapists, counselors, social workers, school psychologists, recreational therapists (e.g., music or art therapists), speech-language pathologists, behavioral specialists or analysts, transition specialists, and assistive technology specialists (Gargiulo & Bouck, 2020; see Table 16.1 for information regarding different service providers and their roles). Paraprofessionals (i.e., aides working one-on-one or with multiple students in a classroom) also collaborate with service providers. In addition, parents are key collaborators with all service providers and educational teams in the education of students with disabilities, including students with ASD (Taber-Doughty & Bouck, 2012).

Collaboration During the Adolescent School Years

Collaboration during the adolescent school years should build upon a strong foundation of collaboration established during the early and middle years of education for students with ASD. Typically, collaboration during the secondary school years continues to involve many of the same individuals who fill the same roles as during early and middle childhood special education (e.g., teachers, speech-language pathologists, occupational therapists, social workers, behavioral therapists), with add-itional new collaborations emerging to support students with transition to post-school life. However, the nature of services received by students with ASD during the adolescent school years may vary depending on their age, as well as the severity and unique characteristics of their disability (Wei et al., 2014). Kucharczyk et al. (2015) reported a large range of col-laborators supporting the education of secondary students with autism, from families to school staff and adult service providers. Kucharczyk et al. also noted the lack of attention in interventions to support adoles-cents with autism that consider the interdisciplinary collaborations and multiple stakeholders involved in supporting students.

Wei et al. (2014) reported a variety of related services received by stu-dents with ASD across different grade spans. For secondary students with ASD, the most frequently received related service was speech and language therapy (66.8%), followed by special transportation (54%), adaptive physical education (50.9%), and behavioral support (34.6%). Other services received by students with ASD included adaptive phys-ical education, social work services, and counseling to the family. Given that students with ASD in secondary schools received, on average, 3.9 services, a lot of collaboration is—or should be—occurring around the education of students with ASD (Wei et al., 2014). A more recent study by Ishler et al. (2021) examined the services received by adolescents and young adults with ASD, finding that, on average, adolescents and young adults with ASD typically receive six school services including medical, mental health, employment support, case management, and educational supports.

Key Collaborators

As noted, students with ASD receive services from various professionals, and often these are similar across elementary and secondary education (refer to Table 16.1). While all of the collaborators contribute to the edu-cation of adolescents students with ASD, we highlight the following key players: parents, paraprofessionals, and behavior specialists or analysts.

Parents. During all years of a child's education, collaboration with parents is key. In fact, parental advocacy and engagement was the impetus for the special education law in the United States and remains one of the six main mandates of the Individuals with Disabilities Education Act (IDEA, 2004). Parents must be given notice and consent to both their child's evaluation and special education services as well as receive reports on their child's progress on IEP goals (Yell, 2019). In addition, parents are invited to be active members of the IEP development, including pro-viding input on goals and services (Yell, 2019).

Researchers examining parent-teacher collaboration regarding stu-dents with ASD emphasized the dual need to both acknowledge a

Table 16.1 Service Providers Involved in Interdisciplinary Collaboration and Their Roles

Role	Information
General education teacher	• Provides instruction in general education setting
	• Provides or supports instruction in special education setting
Special education teacher	• Consults, collaborates, or co-teaches with general education teachers
	• Provides case management services
Speech-language pathologist	• Identifies students with speech or language impairments
	• Provides speech and language services
Occupational therapist	• Provides therapy to promote independent functioning, in areas including motor skills, play, and perceptual abilities
Physical therapist	• Provides physical therapy relative to movement or other gross motor functions
Social worker	• Assesses students for special education eligibility
	• Provides individual or group counseling and support to students
Behavior analyst	• Provides applied behavior analysis (ABA) therapy
	• Consults with teachers regarding behavior strategies
School psychologist	• Assesses students for special education eligibility
	• Consults or manages counseling services for families
Recreational therapist	• Provides recreational therapy, such as music or art therapy
Assistive technology specialist	• Assesses students for assistive technology needs
	• Provides assistive technology services and maintains assistive technology devices
Transition specialist	• Provides or supports transition services (i.e., coordinated activities to promote post-school success)
Rehabilitation counselor	• Provides services focused on employment, community integration, and/or independence
Counseling services	• Provides parent counseling or training
Paraprofessional	• Provides one-on-one or group support to students in a variety of settings
Audiologist	• Identifies students with hearing loss
	• Provides audiology services to eligible students
	• Consults with other educators regarding educational programming
Interpreter	• Provides interpretation services, such as sign language transliteration or oral transliteration
Medical provider (e.g., school nurse)	• Provides medical services as needed for student to receive a free appropriate public education (FAPE)
Orientation and mobility specialist	• Provides services to help students with visual impairments orient and move within their environments

Note: Adapted from Roles of related services personnel in inclusive schools. In R. Villa & J. Thousand (Eds.), *Restructuring for caring and effective education: Piecing the puzzle together* (2nd ed.) by M. F. Giangreco, P. Prelock, R. Reid, R. Dennis, and S. Edelman (pp. 360–388). Copyright 2000 by Paul H. Brookes. Adapted from *The law and special education* (5th ed.) by M. Yell, 2019. Adapted from the Individuals with Disabilities Education Improvement Act. Copyright 2004.

range of parent involvement, from over- to under-involved, while also supporting parent advocacy efforts on behalf of their children (Schultz et al., 2016). Others (e.g., Anthony & Campbell, 2020) have detailed how teachers can encourage collaboration and engagement with parents, through an emphasis on providing frequent communication opportunities between both parties. The importance of transition-related processes and activities for adolescent students cannot be underestimated, and collaboration between parents and educators in this endeavor is essential. Josilowski & Morris (2019) found secondary students with collaborative teacher-parent teams experienced positive results, such as favorable ease of transition and high rates of student engagement and adjustment into post-school roles and responsibilities.

Paraprofessionals. Paraprofessionals are aides that work to support students with disabilities and their teachers through instruction-oriented duties such as supporting students learning in one-on-one or group settings as well as preparing educational materials. In all cases, paraprofessionals receive supervision from a licensed teacher (IDEA, 2004). Researchers reported paraprofessionals play an important role in educating and supporting students with ASD, including at the secondary level, and are also increasingly being used to do so (Biggs et al., 2019). Paraprofessionals can perform a variety of roles but recent data suggest both the nature and fidelity of these activities can vary widely from school to school and training is needed to ensure effective practices (Mason et al., 2021). Besides the general concern with paraprofessionals in the education of students with autism at the secondary level (e.g., individuals with the least amount of education, often working with students who need the most intensive services; Brock & Carter, 2013), additional issues regarding paraprofessionals include the potential for social stigmatization and a reduction of positive peer interactions (Carter et al., 2015). Recent attention has been paid to how paraprofessionals supporting secondary students with disabilities, like ASD, can facilitate peer support and decrease the dependence on adult aids (Scheef et al., 2018).

Behavior specialists. While behavior support can arise from multiple individuals (e.g., school social workers, classroom teachers), behavior specialists are professionals whose primary function is to provide such support to students with disabilities. One type of behavioral support is referred to as applied behavior analysis (ABA). ABA techniques and behavioral interventions (i.e., antecedent based interventions, differential reinforcement, time delay) are supported by research and are classified as evidence based (Steinbrenner et al., 2020). These interventions can be used to teach students with ASD critical skills, including communication, social interaction, play, task engagement, self-help skills, and regulation of problem behavior (Padilla et al., 2020; Steinbrenner et al., 2020).

Behavior specialists can have a variety of certifications including board certified behavior analyst (BCBA), board certified assistant behavior analyst (BCaBA), or registered behavior technician (RBT). This team of behavior specialists collaborate with one another as well as others including parents, classroom teachers, social workers, paraprofessionals, and other behavior interventionists to establish goals and implement interventions to support students with ASD across settings (Padilla et al., 2020; Slim & Reuter-Yuill, 2021). Often behavior analysts provide ABA therapy in homes, clinics, centers, or private schools; however, they can collaborate on behavioral interventions for students with ASD in traditional school settings (Slim & Reuter-Yuill, 2021). Behavior analysts are increasingly collaborating with school professionals to support students with ASD (Padilla et al., 2020), and such collaboration and inclusion of ABA in school settings benefits students.

Collaboration During Transition and Beyond

Along with the service personnel involved in the education of students with ASD during the secondary school years, transition specialists and vocational rehabilitation counselors may (or should) play a major role during a student's transition from school to adult life. Given the complexity of transition services, it is imperative that personnel from diverse agencies and organizations are involved in transition planning to help students achieve their post-school goals (Snell-Rood et al., 2020). Such involvement and collaboration is also mandated by special education law, which defines transition services as a "coordinated set of activities for a child with a disability..." ([34 CFR 300.43 (a)] [20 U.S.C. 1401(34)]). In other words, planning and providing transition services is a multi-faceted process involving teachers, related services personnel from the school district, the student, family members, and adult service agencies (Cihak et al., 2019; Plotner et al., 2020). A student's transition from school to life postschool is not exclusively the school's responsibility but requires involvement from adult agencies and organizations to support students during this process by providing funding and/or services. In fact, the National Technical Assistance Center on Transition (2016) determined interagency collaboration to be an evidence-based predictor for successful employment and post-secondary education experiences for students with disabilities.

Research and Practice Issues

Fundamental differences exist between services students receive during high school and those they receive after leaving school, including a lack of a single point of service coordination as well as the change from services provided by entitlement under IDEA to those determined by eligibility under Section 504 of the 1973 Rehabilitation Act or the Americans with Disabilities Act Amendments Act of 2008 (Brooke et al., 2013; Getzel & Briel, 2013; Yell, 2019). Students and their families must navigate through a maze of unfamiliar agencies and service providers to learn about the services available and to obtain those necessary (Brooke et al, 2013). The transition from a school system to the adult service system is often accompanied by decreased services and limited support for accessing such services (Lubetsky et al., 2014). Given the challenges in obtaining postschool services that meet the unique and varied needs of students with ASD, Test et al. (2014) recommended natural community supports of family, friends, and the local community be considered as part of their comprehensive transition planning. These natural community supports are in addition to formalized interagency relationships (Plotner et al., 2020).

The need for increased attention to interagency collaboration regarding transition for all students—including students with ASD—exists. Data from the National Transition Longitudinal Study (NTLS and NTLS2) suggest there has been a decrease in the percentage of students with ASD who meet with school staff to develop their transition plans. However, while still in the low range, the data also show an increase in the percentage of students with ASD who gave input on their transition plans (41%; Liu et al., 2018), indicating both a concerning trend and hope for increased student-school collaboration. Further, students with ASD experience more negative post-school outcomes than other students, indicating the need for direct and intentional interagency collaboration in planning for successful transitions. From the National Longitudinal Transition Study 2 (NLTS2), researchers found the employment rate for adults within two years of leaving high school to be under 25% (Bouck & Park, 2018). And while employment rates for students with ASD who attended post-secondary education improved slightly, compared to those who did not, the rates of post-secondary attendance were less than one-third of the general population. Finally, it was found that less than 25% of adults with ASD were living independently within four years of leaving school (Bouck & Park, 2018).

Based on the unique and diverse characteristics of students with ASD, interagency collaboration is beneficial throughout the transition process—assessment, training, provision of specific supports and services as well as follow-up (Westbrook et al., 2015). In practice, however, external agency participation and collaboration in transition planning has been historically limited for students with ASD, resulting in low rates of necessary support services upon exiting school (Plotner & Dymond, 2017; Shattuck et al., 2011; Shogren & Plotner, 2012).

Key Collaborators

Students with ASD require thorough and personalized transition planning given their unique characteristics including strengths, needs, and desired post-school outcomes (Test et al., 2014). Needless to say, such transition programming requires the involvement of a variety of service providers at the school, district, and the community level (Plotner et al., 2020; Test et al., 2014;). While several collaborators contribute to the transition of students with ASD, we highlight the following: transition specialists, vocational rehabilitation counselors, and college support programs or disability service offices (Please see Table 16.2 for a non-exhaustive list of external agency service providers).

Transition specialist. The Council for Exceptional Children's Division on Career Development and Transition defined a transition specialist as "...an individual who plans, coordinates, delivers, and evaluates transition education and services at the school or system level, in conjunction with other educators, families, students, and representatives of community organizations" (Council for Exceptional Children, 2000, p.1). A transition specialist is a school or district employee responsible for service coordination, as well as assembling transition teams, executing activities identified by the team, and ensuring effective functioning of the team (Test et al., 2006). Transition specialists also play the role of a liaison between various stakeholders in the transition process such as students, parents, and staff to connect transition goals with educational programming (Morningstar & Claveanna-Deane, 2014). Although all schools may not have a dedicated transition specialist position, often times several staff members, such as guidance counselors, work-study coordinators, special education teachers, and supervisors may jointly perform the role (Baer & Flexer, 2013).

Vocational rehabilitation. Vocational rehabilitation (VR) is a cooperative program between state and federal governments that provides a variety of resources and supports focused on employment, as well as other services such as assessment, vocational counseling, training, personal assistant services, rehabilitation technology services, job exploration, work readiness, self-advocacy, job placement, and supported employment services (Revell & Miller, 2009; U.S. Department of Education [U.S. DOE], 2016). While VR counselors typically engage with individuals post-high school, these individuals can and often do work with students prior to exiting school to support the transition process (Neubert et al., 2018). In fact, researchers suggested almost one-third of caseloads for vocational rehabilitation counselors can be youth with disabilities who have yet to exit school (Honeycutt et al., 2015). Despite the importance of VR in adult services as well as transition, researchers suggested collaborating with schools and school personnel regarding transition and individualized

Table 16.2 External Agency Service Providers Involved in Transition Collaboration

Agency	Role
Developmental Disability Administration	Provide wide range of services such as vocational service programs, housing, and social services
Social Security Administration	Provide financial support through programs such as Supplemental Security Income (SSI), Medicaid and Medicare
Community Rehabilitation Programs	Assist in providing assessments, job placement, and follow-up services
Centers for Independent Living	Provide information on community resources and provide training in such areas as socialization, financial management, and other aspects of independent living
One Stop Career Centers	Provide information and referral services to available community resources, job listings for potential opportunities, career guidance, and competitive employment services including skills training, placement, and follow-up
Community Colleges and Vocational-technical institutions	Provide support and information on applications, financial aid, and accessibility
Disability support services at Institutions of Higher Education	Determine eligibility to receive services and address specialized support or accommodation requests such as scribes, extra time on tests, distraction free testing environment, and organizational help

Note: Adapted from Postsecondary options for students with autism. In P. Wehman, M. D. Smith, & C. Schall (Eds.), *Autism and the transition to adulthood: Success beyond the classroom* by L. W. Briel and E. E. Getzel, p. 189–207. Copyright 2008 by Paul H. Brookes. Adapted from Transition planning and community resources: Bringing it all together. In P. Wehman (Ed.), *Life beyond classroom: Transition strategies for young people with disabilities* by V. Brooke, W. G. Revell, J. McDonnough, and H. Green, p. 143–171. Copyright 2013 by Paul H. Brookes. Adapted from Pursuing postsecondary education opportunities for individuals with disabilities. In P. Wehman (Ed.), *Life beyond classroom: Transition strategies for young people with disabilities* by E. E. Getzel and L. W. Briel, p. 363–376. Copyright 2013 by Paul H. Brookes. Adapted from Navigating the world of adult services and benefits planning. In P. Wehman, M. D. Smith, & C. Schall (Eds.), *Autism and transition to adulthood: Success beyond the classroom* by G. Revell and L. A. Miller, p. 139–162. Copyright 2009 by Paul H. Brookes. Adapted from *Growing up: Transition for adult life for students with disabilities* by D. E. Steere, E. Rose, and D. Cavaiuolo. Copyright 2007 by Allyn and Bacon. Adapted from Supporting more able students on the autism spectrum: College and beyond by E. VanBergeijk, A. Klin, and F. Volkmar, 2008, *Journal of Autism and Developmental Disorders, 38*, p. 1379. Copyright 2008 by Springer. Adapted from Educational supports for high functioning youth with ASD: The postsecondary pathway to college, by S. M. Zeedyk, L. A. Tipton, and J. Blacher, 2014, *Focus on Autism and Other Developmental Disabilities*, Advanced Online Publication. Copyright 2014 by Sage.

education programs (IEPs) is viewed as less important work by VR counselors (Neubert et al., 2018).

College programs. Increasingly, programs are existing on college campuses to explicitly support students with intellectual disability and/or

ASD to attend post-secondary education at institutions of higher education (ThinkCollege, 2021). While historically institutions of higher education supported the educational needs of students with disabilities through the disability services office—and continue to do so, other options have emerged regarding Transition and Postsecondary Programs for Students with Intellectual Disability (TPSID) or comprehensive transition programs (CTP; Briel & Getzel, 2009; Getzel & Briel, 2013; Think College, 2019; Whirley et al., 2020). These specialized programs range from substantially separate entities to truly immersive and inclusive programs (Briel & Getzel, 2009; Getzel & Briel, 2013; Wehmeyer & Patton, 2012). From the 2019 report on programs from Think College, students with ASD and intellectual disability comprise 32% of the population attending at TPSID program. Data from TPSID program completers suggested 64% of those who responded to a survey were employed one year after existing the program and 33% were living without family. Further, almost all reported social life satisfaction (Think College, 2019).

Case Vignette: Connection

Jan and Raul have clear interests, passions, and/or some hopes for the future. Since Jan is 17, her transition plan was designed the previous year. Raul's family and teacher have begun discussions to start his plan next year. Throughout the school week, Jan receives support from a special education teacher, several general education teachers, members of the community (in the CBVI program), a school bus driver, speech language therapist, behavioral specialist, occupational therapist, several school staff members, and occasional check-ins by the school psychologist. In addition to knowing Jan as a person, each member of this broad team, including Jan's family, need to be on the same page in order to best support Jan both on a daily basis and more generally to help her achieve transition and post-school goals. For instance, Jan is working to increase her skills in caring for animals through collaboration between a local veterinary clinic, her teacher, and her family by frequent opportunities to practice related skills. The veterinary clinic partners have suggested that Jan could enroll in courses with the local University-Extension agricultural program after high school to gain additional experience and practical skills related to her career interests.

In addition to beginning to plan for transition, Raul's educational team has been working collaboratively on providing consistent behavioral supports and cues. He has been having some trouble interacting with peers in a few of his classes. After some meetings between the behavior specialist, the general and special education teachers, his family, and the school psychologist, a clear behavior plan including a strategy for instruction and support of improved peer interaction was created. All members of the team were then able to support Raul both effectively and consistently across settings.

Important Changes Since 2016 and Remaining Gaps in Literature

Since 2016 there have been many notable changes surrounding collaboration to support students with ASD. One such development involves the increasing number of individuals with ASD are enrolling is post-secondary education (Hu & Chandrasekhar, 2021; Nachman, 2020). Although post-secondary education programs existed prior to 2015, it has recently taken on greater attention. Many colleges and universities have developed their own Autism-Specific College Support Programs (ASPs; Nachman et al., 2021). ASPs are designed to support students with ASD in college by providing supports that target their specific needs. ASPs typically provide a combination of the services, including: testing accommodations, curriculum planning accommodations, tutoring services, specialized orientation or transition services, parent involvement, social skills training, life skills training/support, mental health support/ therapy, accommodations for class activities, and peer mentors (Nachman et al., 2022).

As the number of students with ASD attending college increases, colleges are tasked with creating an infrastructure to support these students. Although students without disabilities face challenges while attending college, these can be exacerbated for students with ASD. Difficulties faced by students with ASD in colleges include: adapting to reduced structure and unexpected transitions, attending new social situations, building relationships, managing time independently, navigating academic demands, and attending to mental health needs (Hu & Chandrasekhar, 2021). University and college counseling centers (UCCCs) are often responsible for providing mental health resources to students facing challenges, including individual and group counseling and psychiatric care. A recent study by Hu & Chandrasekhar (2021) found over two-thirds (69.7%) of students with ASD request mental health services while in college. As a result of the increase in need for students with ASD, UCCCs are now making more formal collaborations with disability services or campus organizations aimed to advocate for individuals with disabilities (Hu & Chandrasekhar, 2021).

Aside from the increase attention in research and practice to postsecondary education for students with ASD, a few other small changes to issues of collaboration in school and community settings have occurred. One such issue involves the importance of community and for educators to consider and involve community and community stakeholders within the secondary education and transition process for students, particularly when considering more rural communities (Carter et al., 2021; Eastman et al., 2021). One such means to do this is through community conversations, which are dialogues within the community with stakeholders to potential solutions or strategies for individuals with disabilities. One outcome of community conversations noted by Carter et al. (2021) was increased community and collaboration with parents. Use of community conversations or investment or engagement of stakeholders in the community in the secondary education, transition, and post-secondary lives of students with disabilities can lead to positive outcomes.

While some small changes have occurred since 2016 relative to issues of collaboration and the consideration of secondary education, transition and post-school lives of students with ASD, there are still some unanswered questions and research areas that need addressing. Despite historic attention to the active involvement of parents in IEPs and the educational experiences and decision-making of students, more work is needed to support teachers in learning to effectively communicate with parents and encourage active involvement in educational decisions (Kurth et al., 2020). Further, more can be done to support parents with resources on their rights as well as how to advocate for themselves and their child when making educational decisions. Beyond parents, students themselves should be active in discussions and decisions relative to secondary education, transition, and post-secondary life (Chandroo et al., 2018). Future research should seek to explore ways to support student involvement when making educational decisions and to encourage students with ASD to become stronger self-advocates (Chandroo et al., 2018).

Conclusion

Collaborative problem solving is key to addressing the educational needs and planning of all students, including students with ASD. Collaboration among different educators, with families, and with other agencies is providing the best educational and transition programming for students with ASD and delivering programs that will improve their educational and post-school outcomes. To fully embrace collaborative problem solving, we need to ensure that all key players have the training and resources to engage in a collaboration (Blacher et al., 2015).

Case Vignette: Conclusion

While the path to success post-high school has not been completely set in stone, both Jan and Raul have made considerable progress toward achieving their future goals. Through Jan's large support team of various education professionals as well as family and community members, she has been able to increase her knowledge, skills, and comfort in caring for animals. And, importantly, she will be able to use this early career-oriented exposure in high school as a stepping stone to direct and support her continued education, employment, and independent living goals.

Additionally, through the collaborative work and support of Raul's educational team, he will have the time and opportunity to practice essential social and behavioral skills that will help him access and make the most of learning opportunities and experiences both in and out of school. This support, in addition to specific transition planning developed and reinforced by his educational team, will help to tailor Raul's education with an eye toward his preferred future of work, further education, and independent living.

Recommendations for Educators and Practitioners Related to the Topic

Collaboration is essential to the education of all students, regardless of age. The education, transition, and post-school lives of individuals with ASD improve when collaboration and interdisciplinary practice occurs in both K-12 education as well as the transition planning and experience. As such, educators and other practitioners should plan early for collaboration and seek to get multiple individuals and perspectives involved when both planning for the education of students with ASD (e.g., IEP or transition planning) or implementing educational practices. To achieve collaboration and interdisciplinary practice, educators and other practitioners can engage in the following:

- Invite a range of individuals to IEP and Transition IEP meetings, including—but not limited to—parents or other families members, transition specialists, related service providers, general education educators, special education teachers, employers and/or job coaches, the student themselves, peers, college disability specialists, vocational rehabilitation, volunteer supervisors, and adults that engage the student in extracurriculars (e.g., coaches, religious clubs, band)
- Engage in regular communication and connection among invested collaborators in the student's life, not just during the IEP
- Create networks of support in and out of school for the students with ASD

Additional Important Resources Related to the Topic (websites, books, journals, etc.)

- IRIS Module on <u>Family Engagement: Collaborating with Families of Students with Disabilities</u>

- IRIS Module on <u>School Counselors: Facilitating Transitions for Students with Disabilities from High School to Post-School Settings</u>
- IRIS Module on <u>Secondary Transition: Interagency Collaboration</u>
- <u>Collaboration</u> (High-Leverage Practice)
- Autism Internet Modules: <u>Preparing Individuals for Employment</u>
- Autism Internet Modules: <u>Social Supports for Transition-Aged Individuals</u>
- College Autism Network: https://collegeautismnetwork.org/

References

Americans with Disabilities Act Amendments Act (ADAAA) of 2008, Pub. L. No. 110–325, 42 U.S.C. §§ 12101 et seq.

Anthony, N., & Campbell, E. (2020). Promoting collaboration among special educators, social workers, and families impacted by autism spectrum disorders. *Advances in Neurodevelopmental Disorders, 4*(2020), 319–324. https://doi.org/10.1007/s41252-020-00171-w

Baer, R., & Flexer, R. (2013). Coordinating transition services. In R. W. Flexer, R. M. Baer, P. Luft, & T. J. Simmons (Eds.), *Transition planning for secondary students with disabilities* (pp. 227–250). Pearson.

Biggs, E. E., Gilson, C. B., & Carter, E. W. (2019). "Developing that balance": Preparing and supporting special education teachers to work with paraprofessionals. *Teacher Education and Special Education, 42*, 117–131. https://doi.org/10.1177/0888406418765611

Blacher, J., Linn, R. H., & Zeedyk, S. M. (2015). The role of graduates schools of education in training autism professionals to work with diverse families. In D. E. Mitchell, & R. K. Reem (Eds.), *Professional responsibility: The fundamental issue in education and health care reform* (pp. 231–246). https://doi.org/10.1007/978-3-319-02603-0_14

Bouck, E. C., & Park, J. (2018). Exploring post-school outcomes across time out of school for students with autism spectrum disorder. *Education and Training in Autism and Developmental Disabilities, 53*(3), 253–263.

Briel, L. W., & Getzel, E. E. (2009). Postsecondary options for students with autism. In P. Wehman, M. D. Smith, & C. Schall (Eds.), *Autism and the transition to adulthood: Success beyond the classroom* (pp. 189–207). Brookes.

Brock, M. E., & Carter, E. W. (2013). A systematic review of paraprofessional-delivered educational practices to improve outcomes for students with intellectual and developmental disabilities. *Research and Practice for Persons with Severe Disabilities, 38*, 211–221. https://doi.org/10.1177/154079691303800401

Brooke, V., Revell, W. G., McDonnough, J., & Green, H. (2013). Transition planning and community resources: Bringing it all together. In P. Wehman (Ed.), *Life beyond classroom: Transition strategies for young people with disabilities* (pp. 143–171). Paul H. Brookes Publishing Co.

Carter, E. W., Moss, C. K., Asmus, J., Fesperman, E., Cooney, M., Brock, M. E., Lyons, G., Huber, H. B., & Vincent, L. B. (2015). Promoting inclusion, social connections, and learning through peer support arrangements.

Teaching Exceptional Children, 48(1), 9–18. https://doi.org/ 10.1177/ 0040059915594784

Carter, E. W., Schutz, M. A., Gajjar, S. A., Maves E. A., Bumble, J. L., & McMillan, E. D. (2021). Using community conversations to inform transition education in rural communities. *The Journal of Special Education, 55*(3), 131–142. https://doi.org/10.1177/0022466920950331

Chandroo, R., Strnadova, I., & Cumming, T. M. (2018). A systematic review of the involvement of students with autism spectrum disorder in the transition planning process: Need for voice and empowerment. *Research in Developmental Disabilities, 83*(1), 8–17. https://doi.org/10.1016/j.ridd.2018.07.011

Cihak, D. F., O'Reilly, C. L., Krile, M. J., & Eshbaugh, J. (2019). Vocational education and training. In E. C. Bouck, B. Jimenez, & J. Shurr (Eds.), *Educating students with intellectual disability and autism spectrum disorder: Book 4 Academics, life skills, and transition* (pp. 49–74). Council for Exceptional Children.

Council for Exceptional Children, Division on Career Development and Transition. (2000). *Transition Specialist Competencies (Fact Sheet)*. Retrieved from www.nsttac.org/sites/default/files/assets/pdf/DCDTFactSheeCompentenc ies.pdf

Donaldson, A. L., & Stahmer, A. C. (2014). Team collaboration: The use of behavior principles for serving students with ASD. *Language, Speech, and Hearing Services in Schools, 45*, 261–276.

Eastman, K., Zahn. G., Ahnupkana, W., & Havumaki, B. (2021). Small town transition services model: Postsecondary planning for students with autism spectrum disorder. *Rural Special Education Quarterly, 40*(3), 157–166. https:// doi.org/10.1177/87568705211027978

Friend, M. & Cook, L. (2017). *Interactions: Collaboration skills for school professionals.* (8th ed.). Pearson.

Gargiulo, R., & Bouck, E. C. (2015). *Special education in contemporary society: An introduction to exceptionality* (7th ed.). Sage.

Getzel, E. E., & Briel, L.W. (2013). Pursuing postsecondary education opportunities for individuals with disabilities. In P. Wehman (Ed.), *Life beyond classroom: Transition strategies for young people with disabilities* (pp. 363–376). Paul H. Brookes Publishing Co.

Giangreco, M.F., Prelock, P., Reid, R., Dennis, R., & Edelman, S. (2000). Roles of related services personnel in inclusive schools. In R. Villa & J. Thousand (Eds.), *Restructuring for caring and effective education: Piecing the puzzle together* (2nd ed.) (pp. 360–388). Paul H. Brookes.

Honeycutt, T., Thompkins, A., Bardos, M., & Stern, S. (2015). State differences in the vocational rehabilitation experiences of transition-age youth with disabilities. *Journal of Vocational Rehabilitation, 42*(1), 17–30.

Hu, Q., & Chandrasekhar, T. (2021). Meeting the mental health needs of college students with ASD: A survey of university and college counseling center directors. *Journal of Autism and Developmental Disorders, 51*(2021), 341–345. https://doi.org/10.1007/s10803-020-04530-3

Individuals with Disabilities Education Improvement Act of 2004, Pub. L. No. 108–446, 20 U.S.C. §§ 1400 *et seq.*

Ishler, K. J., Biegel, D. E., Wang, F., Olgac, T., Lytle, S., Miner, S., Edguer, M., & Kaplan, R. (2021). Service use among transition-aged youth with autism spectrum disorder. *Journal of Autism and Developmental Disorders.* [Advanced Online Publication] https://doi.org/10.1007/s10803-021-04999-6

Josilowski, C. S., & Morris, W. A. (2019). A qualitative exploration of teachers' experiences with students with autism spectrum disorders transitioning and adjusting to inclusion: Impacts of the home and school collaboration. *The Qualitative Report, 24*(6), 1275–1286.

Kelly, A., & Tincani, M. (2013). Collaborative training and practice among applied behavior analysts who support individuals with autism spectrum disorder. *Education and Training in Autism and Developmental Disabilities, 48,* 120–131.

Kurth, J. A., Love, H., & Pirtle, J. (2020). Parent perspectives of their involvement in IEP development for children with autism. *Focus on Autism and Other Developmental Disabilities, 35*(1), 36–46. https://doi.org/10.1177/108835761 9842858

Kucharczyk, S., Reutebuch, C. K., Carter, E. W., Hedges, S., Zein, F. W., Fan, H., & Gustafson, J. R. (2015). Addressing the needs of adolescents with autism spectrum disorder: Considerations and complexities for high school intervention. *Exceptional Children, 81*(3), 329–349. https://doi.org/10.1177/0014 42914563703

Liu, A. Y., Lacoe, J., Lipscomb, S., Haimson, J., Johnson, D. R., & Thurlow, M. L. (2018). *Preparing for life after high school: The characteristics and experiences of youth in special education. Findings from the National Longitudinal Transition Study 2012. Volume 3: Comparisons over time (Full report)* (NCEE 2018–4007). U.S. Department of Education, Institute of Education Sciences, National Center for Education Evaluation and Regional Assistance

Lubetsky, M. J., Handen, B. L., Lubetsky, M., & McGonigle, J. J. (2014). Systems of care for individuals with autism spectrum disorder and serious behavioral disturbance through the lifespan. *Child and Adolescent Psychiatric Clinics of North America, 23,* 97–110. https://doi.org/10.1016/j.chc.2013.08.004

Mason, R. A., Gunersel, A. B., Irvin, D. W., Wills, H. P., Gregori, E., An, Z. G., & Ingram, P. B. (2021). From the frontlines: Perceptions of paraprofessionals' roles and responsibilities. *Teacher Education and Special Education, 44*(2), 97–116. https://doi.org/10.1177/088840641986627

Morningstar, M. E., & Clavenna-Deane, B. (2014). Preparing secondary special educators and transition specialists. In P. T. Sindelar, E. D., McCray, M. T. Brownell, & B. Lignugaris/Kraft (Eds.), *Handbook of research on special education teacher preparation* (pp. 405–419). Routledge.

Nachman, B. R., McDermott, C. T., & Cox, B. E. (2022). Brief report: Autism-specific college support programs: Differences across geography and institutional type. *Journal of Autism and Developmental Disorders, 52*(2), 863-870.

Nachman, B. R. (2020). Enhancing transition programming for college students with autism: A systematic literature review. *Journal of Postsecondary Education and Disability, 33*(1), 81–95. https://eric.ed.gov/?id=EJ1273654

National Technical Assistance Center on Transition (2016). *Evidence-based practices and predictors in secondary transition: What we know and what we still need to know*. Authors. Retrieved from: https://transitionta.org/wp-content/uploads/docs/EBPP_Exec_Summary_2016_12-13.pdf

Neubert, D. A., Luecking, R. G., & Fabian, E.S. (2018). Transition practices of vocational rehabilitation counselors serving students and youth with disabilities. *Rehabilitation Research, Policy, and Education, 32*(1), 54–65. http://doi.org/10.1891/2168-6653.32.1.54

Padilla, K., Akers, J. S., & Kirkpatrick, M. (2020). Coordinating ABA services. In McClain M., Shahidullah J., Mezher K. (eds.) Interprofessional care coordination for pediatric autism spectrum disorder. Springer, Cham. https://doi.org/10/.1007/978-3-030-46295-6_15

Plotner, A. J., & Dymond, S. K. (2017). How vocational rehabilitation transition specialists influence curricula for students with severe disabilities. *Rehabilitation Counseling Bulletin, 60*(2), 88-97.

Plotner, A. J., Mazzotti, V. L., Rose, C. A., & Teasley. K. (2020). Perceptions of interagency collaboration: Relationships between secondary transition roles, communication, and collaboration. *Remedial and Special Education, 4*(1), 28–39. https://doi.org/10.1177/0741932518778029

Rehabilitation Act of 1973, Pub. L. 93–112, Section 504, 29 U.S.C. §§ 794 *et seq.*

Scheef, A. R., Hollingshead, A., & Voss, C. S. (2018). Peer support arrangements to promote positive postschool outcomes. *Intervention in School and Clinic, 54*(1), 219–224. https://doi.org/10.1177/1053451218782430

Schultz, T. R., Able, J., Sreckovic, M. A., & White, T. (2016). Parent-teacher collaboration: Teacher perceptions of what is needed to support students with ASD in the inclusive classroom. *Education and Training in Autism and Developmental Disabilities, 51*(4), 344–354.

Shattuck, P. T., Wagner, M., Narendorf, S., Sterzing, P., & Hensley, M. (2011). Post-high school service usage among young adults with an autism spectrum disorder. *Archives of Pediatrics and Adolescent Medicine, 165*, 141–146. https://doi.org/10.1001/archpediatrics.2010.279

Shogren, K. A., & Plotner, A. J. (2012). Transition planning for students with intellectual disability, autism, and other disabilities: Data from the National Longitudinal Transition Study -2. *Intellectual and Developmental Disabilities, 50*, 16–30. https://doi.org/10.1352/1934-9556-50.1.16

Simpson, R. L., Mundschenk, N. A., & Heflin, L J. (2011). Issues, policies, and recommendations for improving the education of learners with autism spectrum disorders. *Journal of Disability Policy Studies, 22*, 3–17. https://doi.org/10.1177/1044207310394850

Slim, L., & Reuter-Yuill, L. M. (2021). A behavior-analytic perspective on interprofessional collaboration. *Behavior Analysis in Practice* (Advance Online Publication). https://doi.org/10.1007/s40617-021-00652-x

Snell-Rood, C., Ruble, L., Kleinert, H., McGrew, J. H., Adams, M., Rodgers, A., Odom, J., Wong, W. H., & Yu, Y. (2020). Stakeholder perspectives on transition planning, implementation, and outcomes for students with autism spectrum disorder, *Autism, 24*(5), 1164–1176. https://doi.org/10.1177/1362361319894827

Steere, D. E., Rose, E., & Cavaiuolo, D. (2007). *Growing up: Transition for adult life for students with disabilities*. Allyn and Bacon.

Steinbrenner, J. R., Hume, K., Odom, S. L., Morin, K. L., Nowell, S. W., Tomaszewski, B., Szendrey, S., McIntyre, N. S., Yücesoy-Özkan, S., & Savage, M. N. (2020). Evidence-based practices for children, youth, and young adults with Autism. The University of North Carolina at Chapel Hill, Frank Porter Graham Child Development Institute, National Clearinghouse on Autism Evidence and Practice Review Team.

Taber-Doughty, T., & Bouck, E. C. (2012). Family support and involvement throughout the school years. In D. Zager, M. Wehmeyer, & R. Simpson (Eds.), *Educating students with autism spectrum disorders: Research-based principles and practices* (pp. 262–277). Routledge.

Test, D. W., Aspel, N. P., & Everson, J. M. (2006). *Transition methods for youth with disabilities.* Pearson Education, Inc.

Test, D. W., Smith, L. E., Carter, E. W. (2014). Equipping youth with autism spectrum disorders for adulthood: Promoting rigor, relevance, and relationships. *Remedial and Special Education, 35,* 80–90. https://doi.org/10.1177/07419 32513514857

Think College. (2019). Year four annual report of the TPSID model demonstration projects (2018-20119). Authors. Retrieved from, https://files.eric.ed.gov/fulltext/ED611254.pdf

Think College (2021). https://thinkcollege.net/

United States Department of Education. (2016). Final rule, 34 CFR parts 361, 363, and 397: State vocational rehabilitation services program; state supported employment services program; limitations on use of subminimum wage. *Federal Register, 81*(161), 55630–55789.

VanBergeijk, E., Klin, A., & Volkmar, F. (2008). Supporting more able students on the autism spectrum: College and beyond. *Journal of Autism and Developmental Disorders, 38,* 1359–1370. https://doi.org/10.1007/s10 803-007-0524-8

Wei, X., Wagner, M., Christiano, E. R. A., Shattuck, P., & Yu, J. W. (2014). Special education services received by students with autism spectrum disorders from preschool through high school. *The Journal of Special Education, 48,* 167–179. https://doi.org/10.1177/0022466913483576

Wehmeyer, M. L., & Patton, J. R. D. (2012). Transition to postsecondary education, employment, and adult living. In D. Zager, M. L. Wehmeyer, & R. L. Simpson (Eds.), *Educating students with autism spectrum disorder: Research-based principles and practices.* Routledge.

Westbrook, J. D., Fong, C. J., Nye, C., Williams, A., Wendt, O., & Cortopassi, T. (2015). Transition services for youth with autism: A systematic review. *Research on Social Work Practice, 25,* 10–20, https://doi.org/10.1177/10497 31514524836

Whirley, M. L., Gilson, C. B., & Gushanas, C. M. (2020). Postsecondary education programs on college campuses supporting adults with intellectual and developmental disabilities in the literature: A scoping review. *Career Development and Transition for Exceptional Individuals, 43*(4), 195–208. http://doi.org/10.1177/2165143420929655

Yell, M. (2019). *The law and special education* (5th ed.). Pearson.

Zeedyk, S. M., Tipton, L. A., & Blacher, J. (2014). Educational supports for high functioning youth with ASD: The postsecondary pathway to college. *Focus on Autism and Other Developmental Disabilities* [Advanced Online Publication]. Table https://doi.org/10.1177/1088357614525435

Section IV

Cross-cutting Themes in the Field of Autism

Chapter 17

Trauma and Autism in Childhood

Jonathan B. Bystrynski[1,2]
[1]Department of Pediatrics, University of California, Davis
[2]UC Davis MIND Institute, University of California, Davis

Introduction

Resma Menakem once said, "Trauma decontextualized in a person looks like personality." As someone who has spent time working at the intersection of trauma and neurodevelopmental differences, I would add that trauma decontextualized in an autistic person looks like autism. This is not to make the absurd assertion that autism describes a personality style, but rather to emphasize how trauma-related distress interacts with facets of autism while often eluding being recognized as such.

The complexity of the phenomena of autism and trauma results in understanding their interactions to be a formidable task. Children on the spectrum are vulnerable to having adults misattributing trauma-related distress to autism because of the variability of both. To illustrate this intricacy, imagine a girl on the spectrum who had struggled with tolerating riding in cars, a difficulty for many children with autism. She gets into a car accident while riding with her family, and she finds the resulting chaos overwhelming. Riding in cars now causes fear of another accident, and she tantrums when having to go into the family's new car. The adults in her life may exclusively attribute these spikes in distress to her difficulty with transitions and the sensory aspects of car rides, which are common in autism. Those components may be true, but not attending to the trauma-related distress is not only a disservice to the child that may limit her growth while reenforcing adults' overfocus on autism as the primary explanation of her behavior. Although adults should consider how autism could frame an experience for a child on the spectrum, caregivers and professionals need to actively combat the reflex to frame behaviors exclusively through an autism lens, and trauma is an area where this skill is essential.

This chapter is designed to strengthen the knowledge of trauma among individuals who support children on the spectrum. It is essential to emphasize that research on this topic has historically gone neglected in the imbalanced field of autism research (Kerns et al., 2015; Leveto, 2018;

DOI: 10.4324/9781003255147-21

Levy & Perry, 2011; Loveland, 2001). This means there are more questions than answers and the need to combat harmful myths such as autism being caused by trauma (Mayes et al., 2019). However, this review of what is known will hopefully direct practitioners and researchers to their next step.

To help facilitate learning, a case study has been woven into this chapter. Fallon is an adorable 9-year-old girl with autism. She lives with her parents, Blake and Alexis, her younger brother Steven, and their two dogs. Fallon currently attends a public elementary school in a general education classroom led by Mr. Colby. She is served by an IEP that gives her social skills training and access to the school's sensory room. Over the past months, Blake, Fallon's father, experienced serious deterioration in his health. Fallon repeatedly saw her father have health crises that included seeing him pass out as well as being taken to the hospital in an ambulance. Major changes in daily life came along with Blake's health difficulties. Initially thought to be diabetes, her father was eventually diagnosed with pancreatic cancer. Case studies cannot present an exhaustive understanding a phenomenon, but Fallon's experiences will highlight the common challenges of children on the spectrum who experience trauma.

Literature Review

Literature provides us with the first glimpses of the phenomenon that we describe as trauma with ancient texts describing soldiers' unseen wounds of war (Lasiuk & Hegadoren, 2006). Within the field of psychology, combat was also the source for early work focused on trauma (Benedek & Ursano, 2009). Over time, the field acknowledged how traumatic stress does not exclusively manifest under extreme circumstances such as war, and research emphasized that an expansion of understanding was required (Davison & Foa, 1991). This broadening of the definition can be seen in the criterion for what events can be considered contributing to posttraumatic stress disorder (PTSD). The DSM-III defined a traumatic experience as something that would "evoke significant symptoms of distress in almost everyone" (APA, 1980, p. 238). Three decades later, under the DSM-5, the description of a traumatic event expanded to include witnessing or learning about an event (APA, 2013). Still, the DSM-5 emphasizes "exposure to actual or threatened death, serious injury, or sexual violence" as the measure of what makes an event qualify as an antecedent for posttraumatic stress disorder (APA, 2013, p. 271). This is a more limited set of events that can evoke trauma-related distress especially amongst people on the spectrum (Rumball et al., 2020). It is essential to note that, amongst the cavalcade of problems related to the diagnostic text, the DSM-5 is likely best understood as a lagging indicator of what is known about psychopathology.

Those definitions of a traumatic event are within the context of PTSD, which is only one of the ways that trauma presents. Still, they illuminate an important tension: what should be considered a trauma? This question has become more salient given the rapid adoption of the adverse childhood experiences (ACEs) scale and its misuse as a measure of trauma (Anda et al., 2020). The ACEs scale is a retrospective questionnaire compiled by taking items from empirically developed measures in order to understand physical health in adults (Chapman et al., 2004). Children on the spectrum often have higher scores on the ACEs scale (Kerns & Lee, 2015), but this type of research is appropriate to identify population needs rather than understanding individual trauma. The measure's simplicity is part of its appeal, but it also results in deep limitations for its utility at the individual level. This results in harmful consequences when used incorrectly (Anda et al., 2020; Racine, Killam, & Madigan, 2020). Although often confused as such, the ACEs scale does not measure an individual's experience with trauma. Trauma is more than just the count of one's experiences with adversity.

So how can we understand trauma in a way that takes into account more than just the number of challenges faced by a person? Luckily, there is a framework that can handle the intricate nature of trauma even in the context of autism. SAMHSA's concept of trauma was developed out of their Trauma and Justice Strategic Initiative, and the framework is flexible enough to be used across settings and disciplines (SAMHSA, 2014). Specifically, it describes that:

> Individual trauma results from an event, series of events, or set of circumstances that is experienced by an individual as physically or emotionally harmful or life threatening and that has lasting adverse effects on the individual's functioning and mental, physical, social, emotional, or spiritual well-being.
>
> (SAMHSA, 2014, p. 7)

This Event-Experience-Effect framework allows for flexibility without loss of meaning, and it is a particularly effective tool for discussing autism and trauma. Events deemed traumatic are not from a preordained list but are the results of the individual's appraisal of an event. This focus on individual experience makes space for the differences in interpretation common in autism; that is, it does not rely on potentially ableist boundaries about what counts as a trauma. Additionally, this definition casts a wide net regarding the negative effects while maintaining that effects must be long-lasting. Given the likely interactive relationship between autism and trauma (Kerns et al., 2015), this is an effective way to capture unique autism-specific trauma responses without losing the need for negative effects to be more than just ephemeral. Thus, this framework from SAMHSA will be used to organize a review of trauma and autism.

Events

Exposure to a potentially traumatic event (PTE) is incredibly common for all children in the United States with about two in three being exposed to multiple before their eighteenth birthday (Turner et al., 2010). Overall, children with disabilities are at elevated risk for experiencing physical and sexual abuse (Jones et al., 2012). There is less known about children with autism specifically, but children on the spectrum are certainly not exempt from the PTEs that are common in childhood.

Much of the limited research available has been to capture prevalence rates, and there are theories that people on the spectrum are exposed to some PTEs at different rates due to facets of autism and how autistic people are treated by others (Edelson, 2010; Kerns et al., 2015). Some differences in PTE rates may be accounted for by other factors such as sex differences in autism interacting with gendered forms of PTE like sexual abuse. The following is meant to highlight what is known and is far from an exhaustive list of PTEs.

Physical Abuse. Since social isolation and family stress contribute to risk of physical violence on children (Seng & Prinz, 2008; Stith et al., 2009), children with autism are potentially more vulnerable to this type of abuse given that their families experience higher rates of isolation and stress (Hayes & Watson, 2013). This elevated risk appears to play out in the data with children with autism experiencing higher rates of physical abuse within population samples (McDonnell et al., 2019; Hall-Lande et al., 2015). This type of abuse is even more common among children on the spectrum who also have an intellectual disability (McDonnell et al., 2019). Still, other studies suggest no clear difference among those with and without ASD (Spencer et al., 2005; Sullivan & Knutson, 2000).

It is important to stress that harsh, coercive, erratic parenting styles are harmful for all children, and physical discipline is damaging to children even when experienced in a cultural context that normalizes it (Chang et al., 2003; Lansford et al., 2005; Pinquart, 2017). There is no debate – spanking is harmful with outcomes similar to physical abuse and does not result in target behaviors (Gershoff & Grogan-Kaylor, 2016). These forms of abuse may be particularly harmful for autistic children given their differences in social communication and need for predictability (APA, 2013), and they likely compound harm when experienced by a child already handling trauma-related distress.

Sexual Abuse. Children on the spectrum are also sexually abused (Mandell et al., 2005). Girls on the spectrum may be at elevated risk for coercive sexual abuse (Gotby et al., 2018), but the study reported lower rates for child sexual abuse overall relative to the world more broadly (Barth et al., 2013), so caution is appropriate. Social communication differences likely make children on the spectrum vulnerable to this form of violence and exploitation. Sexual predators may target children on the spectrum especially those who are nonspeaking. Edelson (2010) melds research from criminology and disability studies to suggest that communication limitations make people on the spectrum targets to manipulate and intimidate into sexual assault. However, social discomfort common in autism possibly contributes to less sexual assault victimization due reduced exposure to offenders (Bystrynski, 2021).

Peer Victimization. Peer victimization (i.e., bullying) has historically dominated the field over other PTEs (Hoover, 2015). This attention is appropriate given that children on the spectrum report roughly three times as much peer victimization compared to their peers who are not on the spectrum (Maïano et al., 2016). There are many sources for vulnerability, and many exist outside of the child's social ability (Hebron et al., 2017). Children who are bullied are at risk for perpetrating peer victimization themselves, and this appears true for children on the spectrum; however, rates of perpetration among children on the spectrum are likely better accounted for by other co-morbid disorders (Hwang et al., 2018).

Accidental Injury. Children on the spectrum are at higher risk for experiencing accidental injury relative to children without developmental differences. The National Survey of Children's Health identified children on the spectrum as being about twice as likely to be injured in a way that required medical attention (Lee et al., 2008). One study identified children with autism and other developmental disorders as being over seven times more likely to experience a poisoning (McDermott et al., 2008).

COVID-19. The COVID-19 pandemic changed many aspects of daily life while creating a milieu of uncertainty. These changes, particularly quarantining, altered many individuals' risk for experiencing violence and other PTEs (Rieger et al., 2022). There is some evidence that physical abuse on children has increased during lockdown (Kovler et al., 2021). For some children on the spectrum, the pandemic brought about symptoms resembling trauma-related distress (Mutluer et al., 2020). Many children and parents reported disruptions in mood, increased worry, and the feeling of loss (Asbury et al., 2021). Research is only beginning to understand the consequences of the pandemic on children, and children on the spectrum faced unique challenges during this time.

PTEs Related to Facets of Identity. In addition to the pains of ongoing stigma for being on the spectrum (Botha et al., 2020; Mitter et al., 2019; Nicolaidis et al., 2015), autistic children experience PTEs related to other facets of their identity. The neurodiversity paradigm is compatible with many values related to intersectionality (Strand, 2017), and these connections emphasize how the wellbeing of one oppressed group is tied directly to others. For example, unsupportive environments contribute to transgender individuals experiencing elevated distress (Valentine & Shipherd, 2018), and these harmful experiences are equally relevant for trans children on the spectrum (Murphy et al., 2020). Having autism does not remove the relevance of these identity-based PTEs; rather, they become more salient as an individual begins to connect the interlocking mechanisms of oppression that are related to neurodiversity and other components of identity (Botha & Gillespie-Lynch, 2022). As children on the spectrum step into understanding facets of their identity, there is a risk for experiencing trauma-related distress as they face the ongoing oppression of marginalized individuals (Botha & Frost, 2020).

Sources of Vulnerability for Experiencing PTEs. There is some evidence to suspect increased risk of PTEs for children on the spectrum due to facets of autism and how autistic children are treated.

The ability to detect and respond to coercive interpersonal tactics is limited among some people on the spectrum, and this may leave individuals at risk for victimization when in unsupportive environments (Baron-Cohen, Jolliffe, Mortimore, & Robertson, 1997, Murray et al., 2017). In addition, evidence suggests that people on the spectrum may have less social protection than people with other disabilities; relative to children with other disabilities, those with autism have lower risk awareness, lower social protection from peers, and higher perceived vulnerability. (Fisher, Moskowitz, & Hodapp, 2013). This lack of a social buffer may increase their risk of experiencing victimization, and it worsens when autistic children are overtaught compliance. Weiss and Fardella (2018) did not find that social communication ability was tied to victimization experiences among those with autism; however, their small sample (45 adults) were almost all college graduates and had other demographic idiosyncrasies that suggest this question is unresolved especially since autistic children with intellectual disabilities are at higher risks of victimization (McDonnell et al., 2019).

There are also contextual factors that contribute to people on the spectrum's risk particularly as it relates to sexual victimization. Children on the autism spectrum receive less sex education through formal and informal sources (Dewinter et al., 2013; Gilmour et al., 2012; Koller, 2000). This is likely the result of multiple issues including parents' hesitancy to discuss sexual safety (Ballan, 2012) and the false belief that people on the spectrum are asexual and thus do not require such education (George & Stokes, 2018). There is some evidence that this knowledge of sexual education is particularly important in buffering the risk of sexual victimization into adulthood (Brown-Lavoie et al., 2014), and this emphasizes the need for active education rather than harmful avoidance.

PTEs Connected to Components of Autism. Individuals on the spectrum report many traumatic experiences that would not typically be captured on trauma measures (Rumball et al., 2020). There are everyday experiences that may be overwhelming for those on the spectrum. For example, think of the sensory components of getting a haircut. The sharp snips of the metal scissors, the piercing buzz of clippers, the tight choke of a barber cape. Tolerating these experiences can be extremely overwhelming for a child on the spectrum. Still, a seemingly mundane experience like getting a haircut would not be captured on many existing trauma checklists. Higher quality measures for trauma (e.g., the Early Childhood Traumatic Stress Screen) include catch-all questions, but caregivers might not frame these everyday experiences as potentially traumatic despite being overwhelming to the child. Many trauma measures start with experiences and then ask about trauma symptoms (e.g., the UCLA PTSD Reaction Index for DSM-5), but professionals may want to return to the question of experiences after discussing symptoms to capture overlooked experiences that may be sources of trauma-related distress.

Some readers may be relieved or disappointed that applied behavioral analysis (ABA) has not been identified as a source of trauma. Discussions about ABA are too complex to unpack in this chapter, but avoiding the topic would be unwise. ABA describes an array of interventions and thus requires specificity for meaningful debate. High quality, evidence-based interventions derived from ABA principles are not inherently traumatic. Still, adults have abused children within the context of ABA services including physical and psychological abuse. High-quality interventions often have built-in components that can reduce risk of abuse on a child. For example, the Early Start Denver Model emphasizes following the child's interests while using the caregiver-child relationship as the context to provide the intervention rather than separating them (Rogers et al., 2012). These are components that reflect trauma-informed practices (Burdick & Corr, 2021), but they are far from universal experiences for families involved in other interventions services. The door for abuse gets opened when vigilance is reduced, an adult's stress increases, and a child's autonomy is not respected. Within ABA-based early interventions, this may occur when providers do not use evidence-based interventions to fidelity, when interventions do not include caregivers, when compliance is valued more than autonomy, when providers do not receive proper support, and when companies utilize practices that encourage high turnover. The discussion of ABA and trauma is far from over, but efforts to infuse trauma-informed care into these services have begun (e.g., Rajaraman et al., 2022).

Fallon's Events. This period of high stress was difficult for Fallon, and witnessing her father's symptoms was often overwhelming. She saw him repeatedly faint, vomit, be doubled over in pain, and experience other serious symptoms. Previously, Fallon found her father getting a haircut difficult; Fallon now had to contend with his weight loss, fatigue, and at times yellowed skin. Fallon's loss of this predictability contributed to her feelings of distress. In addition, her uncle moved in with the family to help with daily life, but his limited understanding of Fallon's needs often exacerbated her stress level. The changes in routine, while difficult for many kids, were particularly painful for Fallon given that they served as both disorienting in the moment, as well as reminders of her father's absence and potential death.

Experience

Experiencing an event encompasses both the physiological response as well as how the event is contextualized by the person. This appraisal is deeply personal and intertwined with one's environment, history, temperament, and identity. A child's understanding of what has occurred plays a major role in how they respond following a PTE. For children, their awareness and ability to contextualize events varies across development, and thus a child's appraisal of the same event would vary based on their developmental stage when it occurs (NCTSN, 2012). As a result, the timing of PTEs during development results in different patterns of trauma responses in children (Grasso et al., 2016). In addition to broad differences in baseline sensitivity to stressors, the effects of previous PTEs play a role in how even very young children respond to stressors (Bruce et al., 2013; Grasso et al., 2013).

For children on the spectrum, their experience with a potentially traumatic event will be impacted by how they see and interact with the world. This is how facets of autism can influence the potential for trauma-related distress. There are many hypothesized sources of vulnerability for autistic children to experience PTEs as overwhelming and more likely to experience enduring distress. These include differences in physiology, cognitive style, social-emotional ability, and sensory experiences.

Differences in Arousal. There are potentially neurobiological correlates between ASD and PTSD that suggest similar patterns of connectivity; this has resulted in researchers suggesting that people on the spectrum are more prone to experiencing PTEs as distressing (Mazefsky et al., 2014). The relationship among cortisol and stressors in autistic children is complex and distinct from other children; it may explain heightened stress responses in some children with autism (Corbett et al., 2009; Spratt et al., 2012). These differences may influence the immediate response to a PTE and contribute to ongoing distress after.

Social-Emotional Ability. Many PTEs occur within a social context (e.g., sexual abuse, peer victimization), and one's social knowledge underlies interpretation of these events. Children on the spectrum can have difficulty with accurately identifying the emotions of others (Harms et al.,

2010; Wieckowski et al., 2020), and positive or benign interactions can become interpreted as hostile or unfair. Despite originating from a misinterpretation, these events can be experienced as genuinely distressing.

Children with autism typically have a hard time regulating their emotions (Jones et al., 2011), and problems with identifying their own emotions is common (Kinnaird et al., 2019). This is particularly worrisome as emotional awareness and clarity play a meaningful role in a person's experience with worry and ability to cope (Eckland & Berenbaum, 2021). These difficulties with emotion regulation can result in more distress for this population during a PTE (Mazefsky et al., 2014).

Additionally, shame can play a powerful role in the development of posttraumatic stress (Schoenleber et al., 2022). Researchers are still working to understand the ways autistic individuals experience shame (Gaziel-Guttman et al., 2022), but autistic children who experience elevated rates of shame engage in more disruptive behaviors (Davidson et al., 2018; Gaziel-Guttman et al., 2022). Alleviating shame can play an important role in reducing risk of trauma-related distress in children on the spectrum.

Cognitive Style. Autistic individuals are potentially predisposed for experiencing anxiety for many reasons (see Wood & Gadow, 2010 for a thoughtful discussion), but one of the most relevant facets is repetitive thinking common in autism (APA, 2013). This perseverative-iterative style describes a cognitive approach wherein an individual focuses on thoughts longer regardless of whether it is experienced as pleasant or unpleasant (Berenbaum, 2010; Davey & Levy, 1998). Although repetitive behaviors and thoughts can be calming for some folks on the spectrum, this style also contributes to worry and the potential to experience psychopathology (Berenbaum, 2010). Successful suppressions of unpleasant thoughts, wherein a person does not return to the distressing memory, is associated with fewer PTSD symptoms following a PTE (Shipherd & Beck, 2005). This may be difficult for those on the spectrum who cannot terminate worry. Simultaneously, autistic individuals are more likely to engage in strategies that incorporate avoidance when attempting to handle difficult experiences (Mazefsky & White, 2014). Although effective in the short-term, avoidance contributes to the development of term trauma-related distress (Hetzel-Riggin & Meads 2016).

Sensory Processing. Differences in sensory experiences are a very common facet of autism (APA, 2013), and this can play a role as the processing of sensory information contributes to the development of PTSD (Harricharan et al., 2021). Individuals with PTSD have been found to have differences in their ability to filter out sensory information (Stewart & White, 2008), and this may place children on the spectrum with sensory differences at greater risk for adverse reactions. Much more research is required to fully understand the complexities involved with sensory processing of PTEs by people on the spectrum.

Fallon's Experience. It is undeniably stressful to see a loved one become sick, and Fallon's rigidity, difficulty with identifying facial expressions, and sensory needs likely contributed to the harm felt by Fallon. When Blake was at the hospital or an appointment, Fallon struggled to shift off focusing on when he would return. She would repetitively ask questions about the schedule and whether different routines would still take place. Fallon started to believe her father's interactions with the healthcare system were the source of his health getting worse. Fallon's parents attempted to explain her father's illness as a method of demystifying her father's symptoms. Because of her age, Fallon was able to understand some of the concepts, but the hospital's COVID-19 policies meant she could not visit her father to help her understand. Additionally, specific incidents contributed to this distressing belief. For example, Fallon's father collapsed while the two were shopping. The ambulance was overwhelming due to the sound and lights, and Fallon interpreted the EMTs' focused demeaners as hostility towards her father. When she learned he was going to be taken to the hospital, Fallon became inconsolable until her mother arrived much later. Facets of autism intensified the way in which she experienced these stressful events.

Effects

While the effects of a trauma are often unique to a person and the event, there are patterns detectable among the ways children respond. Psychopathology, academic disengagement, and other changes often occur following exposure to a PTE (Copeland et al., 2007; Goodman et al., 2012). Not all children have an adverse response immediately, and some never do. The experience of a PTE does not occur in a vacuum, and past experiences of PTEs can culminate into increased distress for children (Finkelhor et al., 2009). The theoretical model proposed by Kerns and colleagues (2015) suggests that facets of autism and trauma shape each other; specifically, that autism may create unique trauma symptomatology that in turn can also shift a child's presentation of autism (Kerns et al., 2015). There is too little known about this interaction to make strong conclusions, but it is likely important to identify clinically significant distress and/or dysfunction through a lens that extends beyond the boundaries of traditional diagnostic frameworks for trauma. Adults need to understand behavior as a form of communication to more accurately identify when a child is struggling.

Posttraumatic Stress Disorder (PTSD) describes a specific pattern of response following a potentially traumatic event. Although often used colloquially to describe all trauma-related distress, PTSD only accounts for a percentage of outcomes for youth following a PTE (McLaughlin et al., 2012). Components of PTSD include intrusive symptoms of the event, avoidance of reminders, changes in one's mood and cognitions, and changes in arousal (APA, 2013). A recent review demonstrated that those on the spectrum experience PTSD at or above the same rate of children not on the spectrum (Rumball, 2019). Abused children with autism who receive a diagnosis of PTSD are more likely to demonstrate externalizing behaviors as well (Brenner et al., 2018). Intrusive thoughts, anhedonia, and difficulties with regulation are still common amongst the abused children who do not meet the threshold for PTSD (Brenner et al.). Other forms of psychopathology are common following exposures to PTEs (Copeland et al., 2007; McLaughlin et al., 2012), and this appears to be similar among adolescents with autism (Taylor & Gotham, 2016).

Difficulty concentrating is common for traumatized children (DePrince et al., 2009), and these children exert substantial cognitive effort to regulate themselves when stressed (McLaughlin et al., 2015). Since children on the spectrum often already experience differences in their executive functioning (Kenworthy et al., 2008), the added experience of a PTE makes executive functioning more tenuous (Havuti-Lamdan et al., 2018). Aggression is common in children who are overtaxed and unable to utilize other strategies. Some have speculated that traumatic experiences may contribute to autistic people engaging in aggressive behaviors due to the sensitization of their neural networks (Im, 2016), but this work is very limited. Still, there is evidence that abused children on the spectrum often engage in aggressive behaviors including sexually abused children engaging in problematic sexual behaviors (Mandell et al., 2005).

Child trauma contributes to later suicide risk (Zatti et al., 2017), and this includes children on the spectrum (Mandell et al., 2005). Research in this area is urgent but embarrassingly slow (Hedley & Uljarević, 2018; South et al., 2021). Many risk factors are the result of how autistic people are treated rather than autism itself. Health systems are ill prepared to work with autistic individuals, and those on the spectrum often feel misunderstood by informal supports (Calleja et al., 2020; Orsmond et al., 2004). Bullying, a contributor to suicide risk for teens, is common for autistic youth and likely contributes to risk (Klomek et al., 2010).

In addition to psychological distress, a traumatic event can contribute to a cascade of challenges within academic settings. Broadly, exposure to a PTE is associated with many negative experiences including disruptive behaviors in the classroom, difficulty with attention when learning, academic disengagement, and slowed academic achievement (Perfect et al., 2016). Running away from home is common for traumatized youth on the spectrum (Mandell et al., 2005), and this can negatively impact their learning while increasing their vulnerability to experience additional PTEs.

Case Study. Following her father's diagnosis, Fallon became more irritable and tearful, and her frustration to changes in routines increased greatly. She struggled to get along with others, and she began engaging in aggressive behaviors towards his brother. Fallon's ability to focus on schoolwork decreased, and she had difficulty falling and staying asleep. She became more socially withdrawn, and her leisure interests waned to playing on her tablet and bouncing on a trampoline. She would often pace in her room at the end of each day. Flashing lights would result in physical reactions as they served as reminders of the times her father had been taken by ambulance. Her parents noticed that Fallon would occasionally stare off reminded of her father's illness. Taken together, Fallon was demonstrating symptoms that reflected posttraumatic stress disorder.

Interventions for Trauma

Given the breadth of the impact of trauma on children, attention is required across contexts and systems. Even distal factors, such as laws and societal norms about disability, play a role in an autistic child's experiences following a PTE. Perpetrators of violence should always be accountable for their behaviors, but all stakeholders must also be responsible for reducing victimization and improving response to trauma-related distress. Transforming systems so they appropriately attend to trauma and disability will be essential for large-scale meaningful progress to be made (Corr & Santos, 2017; Liles et al., 2016).

The trauma-informed care (TIC) framework recognizes this opportunity to provide the needed trauma supports across settings. TIC describes the integration of practices and values that understand the impact of trauma, responds to the needs of traumatized individuals, and works to reduce future trauma (SAMHSA, 2014). In this framework, children do not need to be identified as having trauma-related distress to receive services that is sensitive to their trauma history. This framework can be applied across settings, and it avoids the harmful expectation that children report a PTE before receiving care. Universal application does not mean one-size-fits-all, and TIC interventions can be tailored to the needs of youth on the spectrum (e.g., Berger et al., 2021). Avoidance of all PTEs is impossible; however, developing an environment which reduces their impact with empathetic adults is an achievable (and necessary) goal.

Educational Settings

Schools can play a major role in a child's risk for and response to a potentially traumatic event. Children with trauma-related distress have their learning impacted as they often experience lower grades, emotional distress, impairing somatic symptoms, and hyperarousal (NCTSN, 2008). Unfortunately, schools are prone to frame these behaviors as defiance, and teachers struggle with responding even when they know how trauma is playing a role. (Alisic, 2012; Burdick & Corr, 2021; NCTSN, 2008; Wiest-Stevenson & Lee, 2016). Still, schools are often safe havens for children who have turbulent home lives, and teachers equipped with knowledge about abuse and neglect can play a powerful role in helping children receive supports (Goebbels et al., 2008). Taking a trauma-informed care approach in the classroom can radically transform how traumatized children, including those on the spectrum, experience school (Berger, 2019; Berger et al., 2021).

Teachers should promote healthy attachments to enhance students' sense of safety and reduce their likelihood of using aggression (Burdick & Corr, 2021; Little & Kobak, 2003; Spilt et al., 2016). For children on the spectrum, this requires clear teaching of these boundaries that enriches the child's social knowledge. This explicit articulation of what is expected, combined with the teacher's consistency, will make children on the spectrum feel safer.

Encouraging self-regulation skills and a sense of belonging in children can be transformative for students (Franzen, 2019), and these practices can mitigate the impact of even ongoing trauma (Nuttman-Shwartz, 2019). Recognizing that regulation is a skill to be built rather than just a choice can meaningly shift educational spaces (Burdick & Corr, 2021). Strategies rooted in cognitive behavior therapy (e.g., cognitive reframing, relaxation strategies) are effective and appropriate for children on the autism spectrum (Lang et al., 2010; Storch et al., 2013). Approaches from acceptance and commitment therapy are also possible options for students on the spectrum (Byrne & O'Mahony, 2020). Using clear, consistent language and visual cues will enhance the child's adoption of these strategies. Schools can help children on the spectrum enhance their use of sensory interests also, as possible sources for emotion regulation strategies.

Clinical Interventions

No parenting approach can eliminate the risk of a child experiencing trauma-related distress, but different parenting styles can reduce or increase the intensity of distress. Interventions like parent-child interaction therapy (PCIT) and parent-child care (PC-CARE) provide families with autistic children the skills to prevent or alleviate trauma-related distress (Hawk & Timmer, 2018; Scudder et al., 2019; Solomon et al., 2008). These interventions are powerful in helping families adapt strategies that will safely reduce disruptive behaviors while strengthening the bonds of a family. Focusing on the dyad, these interventions reduce trauma symptoms in children even without directly focusing on the event (Timmer et al., 2021). Parent-Child Care (PC-CARE) can be used preventatively when children are likely to experience stressors like being placed with a foster family (Hawk et al., 2020). Both are appropriate for children on the spectrum, and they address the externalizing behaviors are common in autistic youth with PTSD (Brenner et al., 2018).

Trauma-focused cognitive behavioral therapy (TF-CBT) is a powerful intervention that focuses on processing trauma, and it can be adapted to children with autism (Stack & Lucyshyn, 2019). TF-CBT helps by providing psychoeducation, regulation strategies, emotion education, and cognitive restructuring tools that eventually culminate in reprocessing the traumatic experiences. TF-CBT typically utilizes trusted adults to help process the trauma and respond to the distortions in the child's understanding of the world (Peterson et al., 2019). The flexibility within TF-CBT is powerful and makes it an asset for helping children on the spectrum with a range of communication approaches and ways of expressing themselves. As with all interventions with autistic individuals, therapy should be focused on enhancing the fit between the person and their environment and not focused on "treating" autism.

Fallon's Interventions

Many of Fallon's behaviors, although potentially framed as disruptive, play a key role in helping Fallon regulate herself. Pacing, bouncing on the trampoline, insisting on routines, and using her tablet are all ways she regulated her emotions and felt safer. It is established that repetitive behaviors are connected to emotion regulation in autistic children (Samson et al., 2013), and adults on the spectrum report that they are sources of stress relief as well (Collis et al., 2021). Distracting oneself, while not typically a helpful long-term strategy (Benotsch et al., 2000), is an essential skill, and Fallon is using her internal resources to process her experiences and emotions. It was essential that the adults in her life recognize these behaviors, and not individual problems, but rather manifestations of the need for additional supports.

Fallon's parents recognized that her father's illness was having negative effects, and they started PC-CARE with a psychologist through a community mental health service. This brief form of therapy allowed for a reduction in Fallon's disruptive behaviors while providing her with positive experiences with her parents, as well as her uncle and brother. PC-CARE gave her parents new strategies and confidence to help Fallon by setting limits and consistently applying them, even in the face of frequent changes at home. This predictability helped Fallon feel safer. Fallon required additional supports, and she started TF-CBT at the clinic. This intervention allowed her to focus on expanding her coping strategies while processing the trauma of her father's illness.

At school, Mr. Colby was able to act on her distress before she was able to vocalize it herself. Mr. Colby encouraged Fallon to use nondisruptive sensory-based strategies to help her focus and remain calm at school following a consultation with the occupational therapist. Fallon's psychologist, teacher, and parents communicated frequently, and this allowed for easier tracking of symptoms and stressors. The team's persistence in communication was transformative for reducing Fallon's trauma-related distress.

Gaps Left in the Field & Recommendations

There is a serious need for a thoughtful expansion of the research on autism and trauma. The recent popularity of this work, combined with the silo-ed nature of the two fields, places the topic at risk for poor quality research having an outsized impact. Best practices for both autism and trauma research should be integrated into future work. This area of research requires work done at multiple levels of analysis to avoid myopic, iatrogenic interventions, and it should be driven by the voices of autistic people.

The field must move beyond the ACEs scale given its limited utility and risk of harm; applied settings (e.g., classrooms, pediatricians' offices) in particular should stop given the risk of harm (Anda et al., 2020). Adults must expand what they believe might be distressing to children. Parents and professionals should listen to children's behaviors to help detect trauma-related distress. Those working with nonspeaking children need to be particularly vigilant given these children's risk for exploitation and their difficulties in reporting. Children who use augmentative or alternative communication strategies should have options to express distress and disagreement.

Professionals should incorporate components of TIC in their work. Adults must clearly model consent with children and highlight appropriate boundaries. Sexual education is essential. Refusing or delaying it for children on the spectrum contributes to their risk of being abused. Emotion regulation skills are fundamental to successful development, and children on the spectrum are not exempt to this truth. Because learning does not happen when a child (or parent) is dysregulated, these skills must be taught *prior* to their use. Finally, adults should remember that a child's trauma response, even if disruptive, is how the child is protecting themselves after seeing how unpredictable the world can be.

Resources

1. SAMHSA's Concept of Trauma and Guidance for a Trauma-Informed Approach, by SAMHSA; https://store.samhsa.gov/sites/default/files/d7/priv/sma14-4884.pdf
2. First-Hand Perspectives on Behavioral Interventions for Autistic People and People with other Developmental Disabilities, by the Autistic Self Advocacy Network; https://autisticadvocacy.org/policy/briefs/interventions/
3. Child Trauma Toolkit for Educators from the National Child Traumatic Stress Network; www.nctsn.org/resources/child-trauma-toolkit-educators
4. Information about PCIT & PC-CARE; https://pcit.ucdavis.edu/
5. Helping Teachers Understand and Mitigate Trauma in their Classrooms, by Lynn S. Burdick & Catherine Corr
6. NCTSN Child Trauma Toolkit for Educators; https://illinoisearlylearning.org/podcasts/impact-trauma1/
7. Understanding, Supporting, and Preventing Childhood Trauma Module by OneOp; https://oneop.org/trauma/

References

Alisic, E. (2012). Teachers' perspectives on providing support to children after trauma: a qualitative study. *School Psychology Quarterly*, *27*(1), 51.American Psychiatric Association. (1980). *Diagnostic and statistical manual of mental disorders* (3rd ed.).

American Psychiatric Association. (2013). *Diagnostic and statistical manual of mental disorders* (5th ed.). https://doi.org/10.1176/appi.books.9780890425596

Anda, R. F., Porter, L. E., & Brown, D. W. (2020). Inside the adverse childhood experience score: strengths, limitations, and misapplications. *American Journal of Preventive Medicine*, *59*(2), 293–295.

Asbury, K., Fox, L., Deniz, E., Code, A., & Toseeb, U. (2021). How is COVID-19 affecting the mental health of children with special educational needs and disabilities and their families?. *Journal of Autism and Developmental Disorders*, *51*(5), 1772–1780.

Ballan, M. S. (2012). Parental perspectives of communication about sexuality in families of children with autism spectrum disorders. *Journal of Autism and Developmental Disorders*, *42*(5), 676–684.

Baron-Cohen, S., Jolliffe, T., Mortimore, C., & Robertson, M. (1997). Another advanced test of theory of mind: Evidence from very high functioning adults with autism or Asperger syndrome. *Journal of Child psychology and Psychiatry*, *38*(7), 813-822.

Barth, J., Bermetz, L., Heim, E., Trelle, S., & Tonia, T. (2013). The current prevalence of child sexual abuse worldwide: a systematic review and meta-analysis. *International Journal of Public Health*, *58*(3), 469–483.

Benedek, D. M., & Ursano, R. J. (2009). Posttraumatic stress disorder: From phenomenology to clinical practice. *Focus*, *7*(2), 160–175.

Benotsch, E. G., Brailey, K., Vasterling, J. J., Uddo, M., Constans, J. I., & Sutker, P. B. (2000). War Zone stress, personal and environmental resources, and PTSD symptoms in Gulf War Veterans: A longitudinal perspective. *Journal of Abnormal Psychology*, *109*(2), 205–213. https://doi.org/10.1037/0021-843X.109.2.205

Berger, E. (2019). Multi-tiered approaches to trauma-informed care in schools: A systematic review. *School Mental Health*, *11*(4), 650–664.

Botha, M., Dibb, B., & Frost, D. M. (2020). " Autism is me": an investigation of how autistic individuals make sense of autism and stigma. *Disability & Society*, 1–27.

Botha, M., & Frost, D. M. (2020). Extending the minority stress model to understand mental health problems experienced by the autistic population. *Society and Mental Health*, *10*(1), 20–34.

Botha, M., & Gillespie-Lynch, K. (2022). Come as you are: Examining autistic identity development and the neurodiversity movement through an intersectional lens. *Human Development*.

Brenner, J., Pan, Z., Mazefsky, C., Smith, K. A., & Gabriels, R. (2018). Behavioral symptoms of reported abuse in children and adolescents with autism spectrum disorder in inpatient settings. *Journal of Autism and Developmental Disorders*, *48*(11), 3727–3735.

Brown-Lavoie, S. M., Viecili, M. A., & Weiss, J. (2014). Sexual knowledge and victimization in adults with autism spectrum disorders. *Journal of Autism and Developmental Disorders*, *44*(9), 2185–2196.

Bruce, J., Gunnar, M. R., Pears, K. C., & Fisher, P. A. (2013). Early adverse care, stress neurobiology, and prevention science: Lessons learned. *Prevention Science*, *14*(3), 247–256.

Burdick, L. S., & Corr, C. (2021). Helping Teachers Understand and Mitigate Trauma in Their Classrooms. *TEACHING Exceptional Children*, 00400599211061870.

Byrne, G., & O'Mahony, T. (2020). Acceptance and commitment therapy (ACT) for adults with intellectual disabilities and/or autism spectrum conditions (ASC): a systematic review. *Journal of Contextual Behavioral Science*, *18*, 247–255.

Bystrynski, J. (2021). *Facets of autism and university life: the relationships among autism traits and difficult experiences* (Unpublished doctoral thesis). University of Illinois at Urbana-Champaign.

Calleja, S., Islam, F. M. A., Kingsley, J., & McDonald, R. (2020). Healthcare access for autistic adults: A systematic review. *Medicine*, *99*(29).

Chang, L., Schwartz, D., Dodge, K. A., & McBride-Chang, C. (2003). Harsh parenting in relation to child emotion regulation and aggression. *Journal of Family Psychology*, *17*(4), 598.

Chapman, D. P., Whitfield, C. L., Felitti, V. J., Dube, S. R., Edwards, V. J., & Anda, R. F. (2004). Adverse childhood experiences and the risk of depressive disorders in adulthood. *Journal of Affective Disorders*, *82*(2), 217–225.

Copeland, W. E., Keeler, G., Angold, A., & Costello, E. J. (2007). Traumatic events and posttraumatic stress in childhood. *Archives of General Psychiatry*, *64*(5), 577–584.

Corbett, B. A., Schupp, C. W., Levine, S., & Mendoza, S. (2009). Comparing cortisol, stress, and sensory sensitivity in children with autism. *Autism Research*, 2(1), 39–49.

Corr, C., & Santos, R. M. (2017). "Not in the same sandbox": Cross-systems collaborations between early intervention and child welfare systems. *Child and Adolescent Social Work Journal*, 34(1), 9–22.

Davison, J, R, T, & Foa, E, B. (1991), Refining criteria for posttraumatic stress disorder. *Hospital and Community Psychiatry*, 42, 259-261.

Davidson, D., Hilvert, E., Misiunaite, I., & Giordano, M. (2018). Proneness to guilt, shame, and pride in children with Autism Spectrum Disorders and neurotypical children. *Autism Research*, 11(6), 883–892.

DePrince, A. P., Weinzierl, K. M., & Combs, M. D. (2009). Executive function performance and trauma exposure in a community sample of children. *Child Abuse & Neglect*, 33(6), 353–361.

Dewinter, J., Vermeiren, R., Vanwesenbeeck, I., & Van Nieuwenhuizen, C. (2013). Autism and normative sexual development: A narrative review. *Journal of Clinical Nursing*, 22(23–24), 3467–3483.

Eckland, N. S., & Berenbaum, H. (2021). Emotional awareness in daily life: Exploring its potential role in repetitive thinking and healthy coping. *Behavior Therapy*, 52(2), 338–349.

Edelson, M. G. (2010). Sexual abuse of children with autism: factors that increase risk and interfere with recognition of abuse. *Disability Studies Quarterly*, 30(1).

Finkelhor, D., Ormrod, R. K., & Turner, H. A. (2009). Lifetime assessment of poly-victimization in a national sample of children and youth. *Child Abuse & Neglect*, 33(7), 403–411.

Fisher, M. H., Moskowitz, A. L., & Hodapp, R. M. (2013). Differences in social vulnerability among individuals with autism spectrum disorder, Williams syndrome, and Down syndrome. *Research in Autism Spectrum Disorders*, 7(8), 931–937.

Franzen, S. M. (2019). The impact of trauma-informed strategies on self-regulation and sense of belonging in elementary students.

Gaziel-Guttman, M., Anaki, D., & Mashal, N. (2022). Social Anxiety and Shame Among Young Adults with Autism Spectrum Disorder Compared to Typical Adults. *Journal of Autism and Developmental Disorders*, 1-9.

George, R., & Stokes, M. A. (2018). Sexual orientation in autism spectrum disorder. *Autism Research*, 11(1), 133–141.

Gershoff, E. T., & Grogan-Kaylor, A. (2016). Spanking and child outcomes: Old controversies and new meta-analyses. *Journal of family psychology*, 30(4), 453.

Gilmour, L., Schalomon, P. M., & Smith, V. (2012). Sexuality in a community based sample of adults with autism spectrum disorder. *Research in Autism Spectrum Disorders*, 6(1), 313–318.

Goebbels, A. F., Nicholson, J. M., Walsh, K., & De Vries, H. (2008). Teachers' reporting of suspected child abuse and neglect: behaviour and determinants. *Health Education Research*, 23(6), 941–951.

Goodman, R. D., Miller, M. D., & West-Olatunji, C. A. (2012). Traumatic stress, socioeconomic status, and academic achievement among primary school students. *Psychological Trauma: Theory, Research, Practice, and Policy*, 4(3), 252.

Grasso, D. J., Dierkhising, C. B., Branson, C. E., Ford, J. D., & Lee, R. (2016). Developmental patterns of adverse childhood experiences and current symptoms and impairment in youth referred for trauma-specific services. *Journal of abnormal child psychology, 44*(5), 871-886.

Grasso, D. J., Ford, J. D., & Briggs-Gowan, M. J. (2013). Early life trauma exposure and stress sensitivity in young children. *Journal of Pediatric Psychology, 38*(1), 94–103.

Hall-Lande, J., Hewitt, A., Mishra, S., Piescher, K., & LaLiberte, T. (2015). Involvement of children with autism spectrum disorder (ASD) in the child protection system. *Focus on Autism and Other Developmental Disabilities, 30*(4), 237–248.

Harms, M.B., Martin, A. & Wallace, G.L. Facial Emotion Recognition in Autism Spectrum Disorders: A Review of Behavioral and Neuroimaging Studies. Neuropsychol Rev 20, 290–322 (2010). https://doi.org/10.1007/s11 065-010-9138-6

Harricharan, S., McKinnon, M. C., & Lanius, R. A. (2021). How Processing of Sensory Information From the Internal and External Worlds Shape the Perception and Engagement With the World in the Aftermath of Trauma: Implications for PTSD. *Frontiers in Neuroscience, 15*, 360.

Hawk, B. N., Timmer, S. G., Armendariz, L. A., Boys, D. K., & Urquiza, A. J. (2020). Improving behaviors and placement stability for young foster children: An open trial of Parent-Child Care (PC-CARE) in the child welfare system. *Children and Youth Services Review, 119*, 105614.

Hayes, S. A., & Watson, S. L. (2013). The impact of parenting stress: A meta-analysis of studies comparing the experience of parenting stress in parents of children with and without autism spectrum disorder. *Journal of autism and developmental disorders, 43*(3), 629-642.

Hebron, J., Oldfield, J., & Humphrey, N. (2017). Cumulative risk effects in the bullying of children and young people with autism spectrum conditions. *Autism, 21*(3), 291–300.

Hedley, D., & Uljarević, M. (2018). Systematic review of suicide in autism spectrum disorder: current trends and implications. *Current Developmental Disorders Reports, 5*(1), 65–76.

Hetzel-Riggin, M. D., & Meads, C. L. (2016). Interrelationships among three avoidant coping styles and their relationship to trauma, peritraumatic distress, and posttraumatic stress disorder. *The Journal of Nervous and Mental Disease, 204*(2), 123–131.

Hoover, D. W. (2015). The effects of psychological trauma on children with autism spectrum disorders: A research review. *Review Journal of Autism and Developmental Disorders, 2*(3), 287–299.

Hwang, S., Kim, Y. S., Koh, Y. J., & Leventhal, B. L. (2018). Autism spectrum disorder and school bullying: who is the victim? Who is the perpetrator?. *Journal of Autism and Developmental Disorders, 48*(1), 225–238.

Im, D. S. (2016). Trauma as a contributor to violence in autism spectrum disorder. *Journal of the American Academy of Psychiatry and the Law Online, 44*(2), 184–192.

Jones, L., Bellis, M. A., Wood, S., Hughes, K., McCoy, E., Eckley, L., ... & Officer, A. (2012). Prevalence and risk of violence against children with disabilities: a systematic review and meta-analysis of observational studies. *The Lancet, 380*(9845), 899–907.

Jones, C. R., Pickles, A., Falcaro, M., Marsden, A. J., Happé, F., Scott, S. K., ... & Charman, T. (2011). A multimodal approach to emotion recognition ability in autism spectrum disorders. *Journal of Child Psychology and Psychiatry, 52*(3), 275-285.

Kenworthy, L., Yerys, B. E., Anthony, L. G., & Wallace, G. L. (2008). Understanding executive control in autism spectrum disorders in the lab and in the real world. *Neuropsychology Review, 18*(4), 320–338.

Kerns, C. M., Newschaffer, C. J., & Berkowitz, S. J. (2015). Traumatic childhood events and autism spectrum disorder. *Journal of Autism and Developmental Disorders, 45*(11), 3475–3486.

Kinnaird, E., Stewart, C., & Tchanturia, K. (2019). Investigating alexithymia in autism: A systematic review and meta-analysis. *European Psychiatry, 55,* 80–89. https://doi. org/10.1016/j.eurpsy.2018.09.004

Klomek, A. B., Sourander, A., & Gould, M. (2010). The association of suicide and bullying in childhood to young adulthood: A review of cross-sectional and longitudinal research findings. *The Canadian Journal of Psychiatry, 55*(5), 282–288.

Koller, R. (2000). Sexuality and adolescents with autism. *Sexuality and Disability, 18*(2), 125–135.

Kovler, M. L., Ziegfeld, S., Ryan, L. M., Goldstein, M. A., Gardner, R., Garcia, A. V., & Nasr, I. W. (2021). Increased proportion of physical child abuse injuries at a level I pediatric trauma center during the Covid-19 pandemic. *Child Abuse & Neglect, 116,* 104756.

Lang, R., Regester, A., Lauderdale, S., Ashbaugh, K., & Haring, A. (2010). Treatment of anxiety in autism spectrum disorders using cognitive behaviour therapy: A systematic review. *Developmental Neurorehabilitation, 13*(1), 53–63.

Lansford, J. E., Chang, L., Dodge, K. A., Malone, P. S., Oburu, P., Palmérus, K., ... & Quinn, N. (2005). Physical discipline and children's adjustment: Cultural normativeness as a moderator. *Child Development, 76*(6), 1234–1246.

Lasiuk, G. C., & Hegadoren, K. M. (2006). Posttraumatic stress disorder part I: Historical development of the concept. *Perspectives in Psychiatric Care, 42*(1), 13–20.

Lee, L. C., Harrington, R. A., Chang, J. J., & Connors, S. L. (2008). Increased risk of injury in children with developmental disabilities. *Research in Developmental Disabilities, 29*(3), 247–255.

Leveto, J. A. (2018). Toward a sociology of autism and neurodiversity. *Sociology Compass, 12*(12), e12636.

Levy, A., & Perry, A. (2011). Outcomes in adolescents and adults with autism: A review of the literature. *Research in Autism Spectrum Disorders, 5*(4), 1271–1282.

Little, M., & Kobak, R. (2003). Emotional security with teachers and children's stress reactivity: A comparison of special-education and regular-education classrooms. *Journal of Clinical Child and Adolescent Psychology, 32*(1), 127–138.

Loveland, K. A. (2001). Toward an ecological theory of autism. *The development of autism: Perspectives from theory and research*, 17–37.

Maiano, C., Normand, C. L., Salvas, M. C., Moullec, G., & Aimé, A. (2016). Prevalence of school bullying among youth with autism spectrum disorders: A systematic review and meta-analysis. *Autism research*, 9(6), 601-615.

Mandell, D. S., Walrath, C. M., Manteuffel, B., Sgro, G., & Pinto-Martin, J. A. (2005). The prevalence and correlates of abuse among children with autism served in comprehensive community-based mental health settings. *Child Abuse & Neglect*, 29(12), 1359–1372.

Mayes, S. D., Breaux, R. P., Calhoun, S. L., & Whitmore, K. (2019). History of maltreatment is not associated with symptom profiles of children with autism. *Journal of Developmental and Physical Disabilities*, 31(5), 623–633.

Mazefsky, C. A., Borue, X., Day, T. N., & Minshew, N. J. (2014). Emotion regulation patterns in adolescents with high-functioning autism spectrum disorder: Comparison to typically developing adolescents and association with psychiatric symptoms. *Autism Research*, 7(3), 344–354.

McDermott, S., Zhou, L., & Mann, J. (2008). Injury treatment among children with autism or pervasive developmental disorder. *Journal of Autism and Developmental Disorders*, 38(4), 626–633.

McDonnell, C. G., Boan, A. D., Bradley, C. C., Seay, K. D., Charles, J. M., & Carpenter, L. A. (2019). Child maltreatment in autism spectrum disorder and intellectual disability: Results from a population-based sample. *Journal of Child Psychology and Psychiatry*, 60(5), 576–584.

McLaughlin, K. A., Green, J. G., Gruber, M. J., Sampson, N. A., Zaslavsky, A. M., & Kessler, R. C. (2012). Childhood adversities and first onset of psychiatric disorders in a national sample of US adolescents. *Archives of General Psychiatry*, 69(11), 1151–1160.

Mitter, N., Ali, A., & Scior, K. (2019). Stigma experienced by families of individuals with intellectual disabilities and autism: A systematic review. *Research in Developmental Disabilities*, 89, 10–21.

Murphy, J., Prentice, F., Walsh, R., Catmur, C., & Bird, G. (2020). Autism and transgender identity: Implications for depression and anxiety. *Research in Autism Spectrum Disorders*, 69, 101466.

Mutluer, T., Doenyas, C., & Aslan Genc, H. (2020). Behavioral implications of the Covid-19 process for autism spectrum disorder, and individuals' comprehension of and reactions to the pandemic conditions. *Frontiers in Psychiatry*, 1263.

Peterson, J. L., Earl, R. K., Fox, E. A., Ma, R., Haidar, G., Pepper, M., ... & Bernier, R. A. (2019). Trauma and autism spectrum disorder: Review, proposed treatment adaptations and future directions. *Journal of Child & Adolescent Trauma*, 12(4), 529–547.

Pinquart, M. (2017). Associations of parenting dimensions and styles with externalizing problems of children and adolescents: An updated meta-analysis. *Developmental Psychology*, 53(5), 873.

Racine, N., Killam, T., & Madigan, S. (2020). Trauma-informed care as a universal precaution: beyond the adverse childhood experiences questionnaire. *JAMA Pediatrics*, 174(1), 5–6.

Rajaraman, A., Austin, J. L., Gover, H. C., Cammilleri, A. P., Donnelly, D. R., & Hanley, G. P. (2022). Toward trauma-informed applications of behavior analysis. *Journal of Applied Behavior Analysis*, 55(1), 40-61.

Rieger, A., Blackburn, A. M., Bystrynski, J. B., Garthe, R. C., & Allen, N. E. (2022). The impact of the COVID-19 pandemic on gender-based violence in the United States: Framework and policy recommendations. *Psychological Trauma: Theory, Research, Practice, and Policy*, 14(3), 471.

Rogers, S. J., Estes, A., Lord, C., Vismara, L., Winter, J., Fitzpatrick, A., ... & Dawson, G. (2012). Effects of a brief Early Start Denver Model (ESDM)–based parent intervention on toddlers at risk for autism spectrum disorders: A randomized controlled trial. *Journal of the American Academy of Child & Adolescent Psychiatry*, 51(10), 1052-1065.

Rumball, F. (2019). A systematic review of the assessment and treatment of posttraumatic stress disorder in individuals with autism spectrum disorders. *Review Journal of Autism and Developmental Disorders*, 6(3), 294–324.

Rumball, F., Happé, F., & Grey, N. (2020). Experience of trauma and PTSD symptoms in autistic adults: risk of PTSD development following DSM-5 and non-DSM-5 traumatic life events. *Autism Research*, 13(12), 2122–2132.

Schoenleber, M., Collins, A., & Berenbaum, H. (2022). Proneness for and aversion to self-conscious emotion in posttraumatic stress. *Psychological Trauma: Theory, Research, Practice, and Policy*, 14(4), 680–687. https://doi.org/10.1037/tra0001020

Scudder, A., Wong, C., Ober, N., Hoffman, M., Toscolani, J., & Handen, B. L. (2019). Parent–child interaction therapy (PCIT) in young children with autism spectrum disorder. *Child & Family Behavior Therapy*, 41(4), 201–220.

Seng, A. C., & Prinz, R. J. (2008). Parents who abuse: What are they thinking?. *Clinical Child and Family Psychology Review*, 11(4), 163–175.

Shipherd, J. C., & Beck, J. G. (2005). The role of thought suppression in posttraumatic stress disorder. *Behavior Therapy*, 36(3), 277–287.

Solomon, M., Ono, M., Timmer, S., & Goodlin-Jones, B. (2008). The effectiveness of parent–child interaction therapy for families of children on the autism spectrum. *Journal of Autism and Developmental Disorders*, 38(9), 1767–1776.

South, M., Costa, A. P., & McMorris, C. (2021). Death by suicide among people with autism: beyond zebrafish. *JAMA Network Open*, 4(1), e2034018–e2034018.

Spencer, N., Devereux, E., Wallace, A., Sundrum, R., Shenoy, M., Bacchus, C., & Logan, S. (2005). Disabling conditions and registration for child abuse and neglect: a population-based study. *Pediatrics*, 116(3), 609-613.

Spratt, E. G., Nicholas, J. S., Brady, K. T., Carpenter, L. A., Hatcher, C. R., Meekins, K. A., ... & Charles, J. M. (2012). Enhanced cortisol response to stress in children in autism. *Journal of Autism and Developmental Disorders*, 42(1), 75–81.

Stack, A., & Lucyshyn, J. (2019). Autism spectrum disorder and the experience of traumatic events: review of the current literature to inform modifications to a treatment model for children with autism. *Journal of Autism and Developmental Disorders*, 49(4), 1613–1625.

Stith, S. M., Liu, T., Davies, L. C., Boykin, E. L., Alder, M. C., Harris, J. M., ... & Dees, J. E. M. E. G. (2009). Risk factors in child maltreatment: A meta-analytic review of the literature. *Aggression and violent behavior*, 14(1), 13-29.

Strand, L. R. (2017). Charting relations between intersectionality theory and the neurodiversity paradigm. *Disability Studies Quarterly, 37*(2).

Substance Abuse and Mental Health Services Administration. (2014). *SAMHSA's concept of trauma and guidance for a trauma-informed approach* (HHS Publication No. 14-4884). Retrieved from http://store.samhsa.gov/shin/cont ent/SMA14-4884/SMA14-4884.pdf

Sullivan, P. M., & Knutson, J. F. (2000). Maltreatment and disabilities: A population-based epidemiological study. *Child abuse & neglect, 24*(10), 1257-1273.

Taylor, J. L., & Gotham, K. O. (2016). Cumulative life events, traumatic experiences, and psychiatric symptomatology in transition-aged youth with autism spectrum disorder. *Journal of Neurodevelopmental Disorders, 8*(1), 1–11.

Timmer, S. G., Hawk, B., Usacheva, M., Armendariz, L., Boys, D. K., & Urquiza, A. J. (2021). The Long and the Short of It: A Comparison of the Effectiveness of Parent–Child Care (PC–CARE) and Parent–Child Interaction Therapy (PCIT). *Child Psychiatry & Human Development*, 1–11.

Turner, H. A., Finkelhor, D., & Ormrod, R. (2010). Poly-victimization in a national sample of children and youth. *American Journal of Preventive Medicine, 38*(3), 323–330.

Valentine, S. E., & Shipherd, J. C. (2018). A systematic review of social stress and mental health among transgender and gender non-conforming people in the United States. *Clinical Psychology Review, 66*, 24–38.

Weiss, J. A., & Fardella, M. A. (2018). Victimization and perpetration experiences of adults with autism. *Frontiers in Psychiatry, 9*, 203.

Wieckowski, A. T., Flynn, L. T., Richey, J. A., Gracanin, D., & White, S. W. (2020). Measuring change in facial emotion recognition in individuals with autism spectrum disorder: A systematic review. *Autism, 24*(7), 1607-1628.

Wood, J. J., & Gadow, K. D. (2010). Exploring the nature and function of anxiety in youth with autism spectrum disorders. *Clinical Psychology: Science and Practice, 17*(4), 281.

Zatti, C., Rosa, V., Barros, A., Valdivia, L., Calegaro, V. C., Freitas, L. H., ... & Schuch, F. B. (2017). Childhood trauma and suicide attempt: A meta-analysis of longitudinal studies from the last decade. *Psychiatry Research, 256*, 353–358.

Chapter 18

Current Trends and Theoretical Approaches in Autism Research

Delia Kan,[1] Kayla Malone,[1] Orla Putnam,[2] and Kara Hume[1]

[1]School of Education, University of North Carolina at Chapel Hill
[2]Division of Allied Health Sciences, School of Medicine, University of North Carolina at Chapel Hill

The prevalence rate of autism has seen general increase across the global in recent decades, although there exists high variability in prevalence estimates across different nations (Chiarotti & Venerosi, 2020). In the United States, the most recent prevalence rate is reported to be 1 in 44 children (Maenner et al., 2021), a 3.5-fold increase compared to two decades ago when the Autism and Developmental Disabilities Monitoring (ADDM) Network was first established (CDC, 2007). Increased awareness of autism, knowledge of the impact it has on individuals, families, communities all over the world, and struggles that arose with supporting the autistic community has driven rapid growth in autism related research. In the first part of this chapter, we touch on current trends in autism research with regards to publications, funding, frameworks, methodology, and theoretical approaches. The second part highlights critical gaps in autism research with suggestions on next steps the field needs to take. We round off with multiple resources that provide further details on issues highlighted in the chapter.

Part I Current Trends in Autism Research

Broad Overview of Global Autism Research Trends

The Interagency Autism Coordinating Committee (IACC) is a federal advisory committee that was first established in 2000 by the United States Congress and members include both government officials and public stakeholders, such as autistic self-advocates, parents, and researchers. The main purposes of the IACC are to give the public an idea of where research funding is allocated to, to summarize and disseminate research findings, and to establish future research directions.

In their 2012 report, the IACC analyzed autism publications from across the globe over a 30-year period (1980 to 2010) and found that there has been a 12-fold increase in research articles relating to autism published annually (from 200 to 2,400 per year). The most rapid increase

DOI: 10.4324/9781003255147-22

in autism publications began in 2000, and growth has remained steady ever since. It should be noted that while articles analyzed in this report were not restricted to publications produced from the US, research themes and trends were analyzed in the context of the seven IACC 2011 Strategic Plan critical questions and corresponding research areas, which is solely produced and decided by the IACC whose members mostly serve positions in the United States.

The IACC seven research areas are: (a) Diagnosis (When should I be concerned?), (b) Biology (How can I understand what is happening?), (c) Risk factors (What caused this to happen and can it be prevented?), (d) Treatments and Interventions (Which treatments and interventions will help?), (e) Services (Where can I turn to for services, (f) Lifespan issues, and (g) Infrastructure and surveillance (IACC, 2011). These are also the same areas included in the most recently revised strategic plan conducted in 2016–17 and hence are still relevant in today's context (IACC, 2020). The spread of publications among the seven research areas remained fairly consistent since the 1980s, where research focusing on the *Biology* topic, which investigates the biological bases of autism, accounted for the largest number of publications. There was also a rapid increase in *Biology* related publications between 2000 to 2010, rising up to an average of close to 600 publications per year. The number of publications in *Treatments and Interventions* and *Risk factors* were similar across the years, and were the next two largest publication areas after *Biology*. More than 50% of publications dedicated to risk factors investigated genetic risk factors, while behavioral intervention research was most prevalent among *Treatment and Interventions* publications. The two research areas that had the least number of publications were *Infrastructure and surveillance* and *Lifespan issues*, staying well below 100 publications per year across all 30 years of analysis. It is notable though that there was no significant difference found in growth rates of publication in research areas with smaller number of publications such as *Infrastructure and surveillance, Services,* and *Lifespan Issues* as compared to growth rates of publications in *Biology* from 2000 to 2010. These overall global trends in autism research areas are found likewise in each of the top three major producers of autism research, US, UK, and Canada, with the largest and strongest focus on the biological basis of autism (Pellicano et al., 2014; OARC, 2012, 2019, 2021).

Funding Trends in Autism Research

Funding for autism research has significantly increased over the past few decades since autism has become well known to the public. In the US, funding for autism research steadily increased 15% each year from 1997 to 2006 (Singh et al., 2009), when the Combating Autism Act of 2006 was enacted by the United States Congress. This act, named for the public's attitude towards autism at the time, drastically increased funding from the National Institute of Health (NIH) to autism research (The White House, 2006) and established the IACC. From 2008 to 2018, funding for autism research doubled from $200 million to just over $400 million (IACC, 2020). Autism research in the US is primarily funded through the federal government, with 18% of funding coming from private organization such as Autism Speaks, Autism Science Foundation, and the Simons Foundation.

Trends of autism research funding closely mirror trends of autism projects and publications. Consistently over the last 10 years, the vast majority of research funding has gone to understanding the biology and "risk" factors of autism, while research into support services and lifespan issues are consistently allocated the least funding. In their most recent strategic plan update (IACC, 2020), the IACC laid out the breakdown of autism research funding in the US: Biology projects received the most funding, taking up 32% of total funding, followed by risk factors (24%), treatments and interventions (16%), infrastructure and surveillance (10%), screening and diagnosis (8%), services (5%), and lifespan issues (2%).

Trends in Theoretical Approaches Used in Autism Research

For the past 40 years, views or models of disability have shaped research, practice, politics, and human rights for autistic people (Lawson & Beckett, 2020). Autism is most commonly understood through the medical model of disability (Pellicano & den Houting, 2021). The medical model of disability can be defined as the predominant Western approach to illness and disability, that sees the body as a complex mechanism, with illness and disability understood in terms of biological causation and treatment (Shah & Mountain, 2007). Through this lens, autism is a disability that is primarily seen as a direct consequence of an individual's biology with an emphasis on perceived deficits that require treatment (Llewellyn & Hogan, 2000). This implicitly assumes that *normal* functioning exists and the medical model positions *normality* as the "ideal state of health" (Pellicano & den Houting, 2021, p. 1).

The creation of autism as a category under the medical model has led to scientific understandings of autism. Scientific understandings of autism have increased societal awareness of autism (Happe & Frith, 2020). In fact, biological explanations of illness and disability have also been reported to reduce fear, superstition, and stigma and to increase understanding of disabled persons (Tan et al., 2020). However, there is no universal scientific truth about autism (e.g., there are no reliable genetic biomarkers of autism; Verhoeff, 2015). Leo Kanner (1943) and Hans

Asperger (1994) were the first to define the description of traits that are currently defined as autism today. As antiquated as their conceptualizations of autism are, they were informed by the medical model paradigm of their time. Today, autism is listed in both the Diagnostic and Statistical Manual of Mental Disorders (DSM-5) and the International Classification of Diseases (ICD-11) as a neurodevelopmental disorder. The DSM-5 and ICD-11 characterize the *symptoms* of autism as deficits related to social communication and interaction and restricted, repetitive, and inflexible patterns of behavior, interests, or activities (American Psychiatric Association, 2013). The diagnostic focus on deficits has material consequences for autistic stakeholders. For example, autistic students primarily receive interventions that aim to reduce *symptoms* of autism (Pellicano & den Houting, 2021). The dearth of non-diagnostic interventions (i.e., interventions that do not address diagnostic criteria) is reflective of today's medical model paradigm.

Within the last decade, there has been significant resistance to the medical model view of disability by autistic self-advocates and a push toward other strengths-based views of disability (e.g., social model, human rights model, and affirmation-model of disability; Autistic Self-Advocacy Network, 2021). The social model of disability focuses on the creation of disability through the "social, economic, political, cultural, relational and psychological exclusion" of people with impairments (Goodley, 2014, p. 244). In this view, disability and impairment are separate constructs. Disability refers to the societal, structural and environmental barriers and loss of opportunities that autistic people experience as a result of an ableist society (Lawson & Beckett, 2020). Impairment, in contrast, is an injury, illness, or congenital condition that is likely to cause a "difference or loss of physiological or psychological function" (Goodley, 2014, p. 244). Critics argue that the social model of disability fails to address the understanding of the inter-dependencies that exist between some disabled persons and their support networks and may fail to appreciate the realities of impairment for some autistic persons (Giri et al., 2021; Goodley, 2014). However, the human rights model addresses the realities of impairment by recognizing impairment as a natural part of human diversity (i.e., while centering the right to services; Lawson & Beckett, 2020). The human rights model differs from the social model by explicitly emphasizing that disabled persons are entitled to equality, dignity, and flourishing by virtue of their equal humanity, not because of their proximity to normality (Lawson & Beckett, 2020).

Models of disability can be used as tools to challenge hegemonic notions of normality (e.g., assumption that impairments are inherently negative; Lawson & Beckett, 2020). According to the affirmation model of disability, if all human beings were regarded as having "embodied differences, negative connotations attached to impairment might be avoided" (McWade et al., 2015, p. 306). In the same way that disability rights activists challenged and redefined the meaning of disability, the neurodiversity movement challenges and redefines the meaning of impairment (McWade et al., 2015).

It is important for educators and practitioners to reflect on their own understandings of normality (i.e., their idea of a *normal* or *good* student), disability (i.e., identifying barriers present in their classrooms), and belonging (e.g., reducing barriers and leveraging strengths of students in the classroom). Future research regarding models of disability and autism practice should focus on the implications of how manifestations of the models of disability impact student outcomes. For example, future research could further explore the relationship of the medical model, language, and the impact of deficit-oriented views of educators on student outcomes (Pearson et al., under review).

Budding Frameworks For Research

Neurodiversity lens. Neurodiversity is defined as a "variation in neurocognitive functioning", and the neurodiversity *movement* advocates for the rights of neurodivergent people (Hughes, 2016; Kapp, 2020, p. 2). The goal of the neurodiversity movement is to shift the frame of autism research and therapies from a *deficit* approach to a *neurodiversity-affirming* approach. This means shifting the focus of autism research from trying to eliminate autism to accepting that autism is both a difference and a disability, and we should work to support individuals' needs. It is important to note that the neurodiversity movement does not promote that autism is *not* a disability. Instead, it suggests that autism is both a difference in cognition *and* a disability, and both of these should be accepted and embraced (Kapp et al., 2013).

While the term *neurodiversity* was coined by autistic sociologist Judy Singer in the late 1990s (Singer, 1999), it has not been widely used in published academic works until very recently. Only a handful of scientific articles before 2010 was published using the word "neurodiversity", with the number of articles growing from 50 to 500 from 2010 to 2017. The last four years reflect a sharp increase in the term's popularity, with the number nearly doubling each year and nearly 4,000 articles published in 2021 (Digital Science, 2018). With this recent increase in the term's popularity in academic circles, it is the hope of many advocates that the research, treatment, and education surrounding autism will undergo meaningful change. In a recent publication, Leadbitter and colleagues (2021) have argued for professionals involved with autism intervention to work to understand and engage with neurodiversity "as a concept and movement" (p. 2). The group suggests that by moving away from the established agenda of diminishing a child's autistic traits in order to "fit in" and shifting towards the measurement of autistic-prioritized outcomes such as mental health and environmental adaptions, intervention stakeholders will better serve autistic individuals. Additional information about neurodiversity as a conceptual framework can be found in Chapter 23 of this volume "Neurodiversity and the Culture of Autism".

Community based participatory research. In traditional autism research culture, the primary role that autistic individuals play is to be passive participants in research studies that have been designed and conducted by non-autistic researchers and academics (Fletcher-Watson et al., 2019). However, the lack of involvement of autistic input during the research process has resulted in the development of interventions or solutions that are ineffective in meeting the immediate needs of the autistic community (e.g., therapeutic interventions vs programs enhancing life skills; Pellicano et al., 2014).

In the past decade, autistic advocates, activists, scholars, as well as non-autistic academics, have been speaking up to bring increasing recognition to the lack of involvement of autistic individuals in autism research (Chown et al., 2017; Pellicano et al., 2018). A guiding research framework that encourages and emphasizes equitable engagement of both autistic individuals and researchers, is community based participatory research (CBPR). CBPR is a form of action research, of which action research can be critically defined as "a pragmatic co-creation of knowing with, not on about, people" (Bradbury, 2015, p. 1). CBPR has a strong emancipatory focus on highlighting the power imbalance between research and community and works towards returning power to oppressed communities. As part of this approach, it is crucial that both academics and community partners are to be identified as co-researchers, and actively take steps to review power dynamics, equalize and share power (Nicolaidis & Raymaker, 2015). As where the research literature currently stands, there have been more common attempts to involve community stakeholders in consultative or advisory roles but rare to engage autistic individuals at the level of research coproduction (den Houting et al., 2021). All parties should be involved in all phases of the research, including planning phases of deciding on a research problem so as to ensure that the impact of the research will be on a problem that the community desires (Raymaker, 2020). Researchers have also developed communities such as AASPIRE (Nicolaidis et al., 2011) and PARC (Milton et al., 2019; see appendix) to actively investigate more appropriate and effective ways in engaging the autistic community in research and develop guidelines to aid researchers in engaging in CBPR (Cascio et al., 2020; Nicolaidis et al., 2019).

Additional Trends in Research Methodology

Beyond the increased use of CBPR methods as described above, there are a number of other shifts and emerging trends in autism intervention research methodology. Historically, the use of randomized controlled trials (RCTs) has been the gold standard of efficacy research in the autism field and beyond, with other methods deemed less credible. However, the limitations of RCTs in complex settings (e.g. schools, community), including the reliance on measuring meaningful change strictly on standardized measures, the difficulty measuring causal and support factors, and the innate challenges in randomization are pushing the field to consider both flexibility in RCT methodology and complementary methods that are rigorous, more feasible, and may lead to more informative results (Cartwright & Munro, 2010; Odom, 2021). *Process evaluations* are often used in tandem with RCTs in health care research as a means to answer questions related to implementation successes and barriers, participant perceptions, unintended consequences, and intervention diffusion to provide contextual information for interpretation of results and to make decisions about wider implementation (Lockwood et al., 2022). Only more recently used in education research, process evaluations may allow both researchers and participants to better understand what issues have potential to enhance or limit intervention impact, better interpret the results, and derive more meaningful lessons for future research (Siddiqui et al., 2018).

Design experimentation is a methodology focused on testing and refining educational interventions in the classroom setting, with an emphasis on improving the ecological validity or "fit" of educational interventions (Brown, 1992). Researchers and practitioners can work together to implement an innovation and systematically reflect and debrief around the learning pathways, environment, and real-time findings and make incremental and well-documented changes to the experiment (Cobb et al., 2003). Design-based research may also be used as an element of *implementation science*, which is the study of methods and strategies that support or inhibit the diffusion of educational interventions (Dingfelder & Mandell, 2011). While implementation science and the broader *improvement science*, which tests change ideas in rapid cycles in an effort to improve larger systems, are limited in their use as experimental approaches, they may answer important research questions in the autism field related to how systems such as schools and community-based programs work, where breakdowns occur, and what actions can be taken to improve overall performance (Lewis, 2015).

Two methods that warrant further attention moving forward, though not new to autism research and not without criticism from the field, are *single case design studies* and *mixed methods studies* (Odom, 2021), particularly those that reflect the perspectives and experiences of autistic participants. The autism field has long criticized single case design studies for limited generalizability and external validity, however high quality SCDs are now recognized by the What Works Clearinghouse as an experimental methodology that can provide evidence of efficacy, and innovative SCD designs can be used to examine outcomes of whole classrooms or whole schools—well beyond the incorrect notion that these studies include only one participant. Mixed methods studies that can experimentally examine quantitative outcomes and integrate the autistic voice in qualitative data collection and analysis can help to answer important questions in education research (Howard et al., 2019).

Current Status of Education and Intervention Realm

Recent systematic reviews and meta-analyses of the autism literature provide current data on the state of autism education and intervention research. In 2020, the National Center on Autism Evidence and Practice (NCAEP) published their third systematic review of the autism intervention literature, synthesizing data published between 1990–2017. Their review included both high quality group and single case design studies that tested behavioral or educational interventions and yielded positive effects in a number of developmental domains for children and youth ages 0-21 (Steinbrenner et al., 2020; Hume et al., 2021). Additional research groups, including Project Autism Intervention Meta-analysis (AIM) and the National Standards Project (NSP) have conducted additional reviews of the intervention literature, with AIM first examining outcomes for young children in studies using quasi-experimental and RCT designs (Sandbank et al., 2020), and the NSP reviewing the intervention literature published through 2012 targeting autistic individuals across the lifespan (National Autism Center, 2015). Findings from each review vary based on the included literature and focus of the reviews, though there are a number of areas of overlap including the identification of naturalistic, developmental behavioral interventions (or NDBIs) as an evidence-based practice with positive effects for young children and the call for improved reporting on contextual features in intervention studies.

The NCAEP report includes data from 972 high quality intervention studies and identifies 28 evidence-based practices, along with 10 manualized interventions that also met quality criteria and enough evidence of positive effects. These EBPs targeted 13 outcome areas across the age ranges, from communication and joint attention, to self-determination and vocational outcomes (see full report linked in the Resources section). The report indicates several trends and next steps in education and intervention research for the autism field. First, the proportion of studies that included autistic young adults (ages 19–22) was quite low (5% of studies), indicating a need for additional innovation and research for this age group (Hume et al., 2021). Next, there were notable increases in the number of studies that targeted academic/pre-academic, vocational and mental health outcomes since the previous review published in 2015, however studies in those areas, as well as those targeting self-determination, are critically needed. Last, there are several areas of concern related to the contextual variables analyzed in the studies published between 2012–2017. Researchers implemented more than 60% of the interventions examined in the included studies, restricting our understanding of how successfully many of these interventions could be used by the providers in the settings for which they were designed. While almost half of the studies took place in educational settings, the majority of those were conducted in 1:1 settings and delivered by research team members. This limits discussion of generalizability and the likelihood of sustainable uptake in school and community settings, a warranted limitation in much of the autism intervention literature and a barrier to closing the research to practice gap. The autism field is faced with the challenge of ensuring both methodological rigor as described previously, <u>and</u> the understanding that interventions must be designed and implemented with the end user and context in mind if ongoing implementation, meaningful change, and thoughtful interpretation of results are desired.

Part 2 Critical Gaps in Autism Research and Suggestions On Where the Field Needs To Go

In terms of where autism research currently stands in the education field, we have identified a number of critical gaps that still need to be explored in order to identify solutions to best meet the pressing needs of autistic individuals. This section serves to describe these gaps in detail, and we provided suggestions on how the field can move forward in closing these gaps.

I. Domain/instructional Outcomes in Education

Cognitive. Cognitive instructional outcomes are related to "performance on measures of intelligence, executive function, problem solving, information processing, reasoning, theory of mind, memory, creativity, or attention" (Steinbrenner et al., 2020, p. 37). Recent evidence suggests around two thirds of autistic individuals have an IQ in the average range or above (Chiarotti & Venerosi, 2020). The term *high functioning autism* has historically been used to describe individuals without ID (IQ $\geqslant$ 70), however, intelligence sometimes serves as an imprecise proxy for adaptive functioning (Alvares et al., 2019). Moreover, research has shown that gains in IQ assessment scores and increases on cognitive ability measures do not result in decreased autism *symptoms* (Johnson et al., 2021; Simonoff et al., 2020). Research has demonstrated that IQ tests have little interpretative value, meaning, it is not an accurate measure for future outcomes (e.g., employment and education; Ganuthula & Sinha, 2019). Yet, currently the use of IQ cut-offs as a surrogate for functioning levels has significant funding and service provision implications (e.g., inequitable distribution of funds for services; Alvares et al., 2019). Future research should create additional ways to characterize samples that do not have co-occurring ID. One way to characterize could be meaningful groupings that relate to the individual study (e.g., group participants by vocabulary skills for a vocabulary study). For students with co-occurring ID, future research should explore more culturally responsive measures to diagnose ID given that Black and Hispanic children are twice as likely to be diagnosed with ID (NASEM, 2015). Furthermore, educators should not rely on IQ levels to determine what services and supports a student may need, but rather should conduct more specific needs assessments to determine relevant interventions.

Joint attention. Joint attention is the shared attention of two people on the same object or objects, with both people acknowledging the others' attention to the shared object (Mundy & Newell, 2007). Joint attention is operationalized primarily through the use of gesture, speech, and eye contact (Mundy et al., 2003), and is thought to be a core component of social communication (Tomasello, 1995). Early joint attention skills have been suggested to contribute to later language skills and social development (Tomasello & Farrar, 1986), establishing it as a key target outcome for many autism interventions (Kasari et al., 2021; Rogers & Dawson, 2020).

The concept of joint attention and social engagement in the field of autism research has emerged from decades of work based around neurotypical norms of communication. With growing evidence that autistic individuals communicate well around each other using their own communication styles (Crompton et al., 2020; Rifai et al., 2021), researchers and self-advocates have argued that different eye-contact should be viewed less as a deficit that needs to be fixed and more as a cultural difference (Dekker, 1999; Hillary, 2020).

While joint attention may not be conducive to the autistic nature of social communication, there is still a need in educational settings to determine if and how a child is engaging with others in a way that fosters shared interests, experiences, and development. Current research is lacking in this area, but a good first step for families and professionals is the acknowledgement of communication differences and preferences. The autistic child may engage with a partner by talking about an object but not looking at them, or by looking away to listen as a partner talks to them. More work is needed in operationalizing what meaningful social engagement looks like to autistic people and identifying how to effectively teach skills like language learning through social interaction.

Self-determination. Self-determination is an emerging area of intervention focus as it is increasingly being recognized that autistic children and youth can and should play a greater role in establishing their own educational program (Steinbrenner et al., 2020). Researchers have also consistently identified through multiple rigorous systematic literature reviews that self-determination is a critical secondary transition predictor for improving postschool outcomes for students with disabilities (Mazzotti et al., 2021). Situated within theories of human agency, self-determination is a psychological construct that views people as causal agents who make conscious choices that make or cause things to happen in their lives (Wehmeyer, 2020).

There is currently still a clear lack of research relating to self-determination as an outcome in the autism student population (5 to 21 years old). A review by Moran and colleagues (2020) found only 18 studies that included students on the autism spectrum as part of their study sample, of which only 8 specifically targeted autistic students. Even though self-determination develops over the course of an individual's lifespan, no study has yet to examine self-determination in autistic students below the age of 12 (Moran et al., 2020). Future research studies should consider working with students on the autism spectrum in early childhood and elementary school settings, and also take steps to ensure representation in terms of race, ethnicity, and students with co-occurring conditions who may have unique support needs. Moran and colleagues (2020) also call for future studies to use validated measures of self-determination and provide greater details about context and setting for intervention studies so as to allow for greater confidence in conclusions drawn. Researchers should also work towards identifying ways to triangulate data on self-determination from multiple informants (student, parent, teacher) to provide a more comprehensive understanding of the individual's level of self-determination, as discrepancies have been found between different reporters (Tomaszewski et al., 2020), and families and autistic teens often have differing views of outcomes and the future (Kirby et al., 2021).

Vocational outcomes and the need for a lifespan view. Employment is a key endeavor in adulthood and provides multiple critical benefits to an individual. Being gainfully employed allows one to not only work towards financial independence and financial security, it also provides structure in one's life, allows one to cultivate a sense of worth and identity, and establish supportive social networks. With the right supports, work can also have positive contributions to an individual's mental health (Modini et al., 2016; Nicholas & Klag, 2020). These benefits that the general population derive from work also hold true for autistic individuals (Roux et al., 2013). However, postschool employment for transition aged autistics can be at least 30% lower than the general population in multiple parts of the world (Black et al., 2020; Bunt et al., 2020).

Given these dismal numbers, it is critical that educators and professionals know what factors are associated with optimal vocational outcomes (e.g. social skills; Nasamran et al., 2017) and which interventions and evidence-based practices are helpful for students on the autism spectrum (see NCAEP, Steinbrenner et al., 2020). Yet insufficient research is being conducted to understand how educational practices impact vocational outcomes (outcomes related to employment or employment preparation or relate to technical skills required for a specific job) for this population (Steinbrenner et al., 2020, p. 37). The National Clearinghouse on Autism Evidence and Practice (NCAEP) Review Team, found in their systematic review that between 1990 to 2017, of 972 articles reviewed, only 31 (3%) reported vocational outcomes. Further details on employment statistics in the autistic population and effective educational practices to promote competencies for employment can be found in Chapter 16 of this volume "Promoting Integrated Employment Options".

Additionally, transition planning has been recognized as an important process to guide autistic youths in determining and achieving postschool life goals (Hendricks & Wehman, 2009; Alverson et al., 2015; Test et al., 2014). Yet there is currently little research on the optimal time in a student's schooling life that transition planning should begin (U.S. Department of Health and Human Services, 2017). While countries like the United States have mandated that students should have their postsecondary goals and transition services listed out by the time they turn 16, there has been calls by multiple stakeholders in the autism community that transition planning should start much earlier, possibly even beginning at diagnosis with a lifespan approach to planning (Nicholas et al., 2017; U.S. Department of Health and Human Services, 2017), as there are other critical transition periods in a child's life as well (Marsh et al., 2017; Richter et al., 2019). More research is needed to determine whether a lifespan approach to educational planning, beyond the year-to-year goal setting taking place through individualized education plans (IEPs), will be beneficial in helping students to transit successfully to postsecondary settings and achieving their desired life goals.

II. Population Characteristics

Race and ethnicity. Most autism research uses majority-white samples (Lovelace et al., 2021; West et al., 2016). In fact, a systematic review of autism intervention research, between the years 1990 and 2017, revealed that only 25% of articles reported any data on race and ethnicity (Steinbrenner et al., 2022). The authors also found that approximately 65% of participants were White, compared to only 7.7% of participants being Black and 6.4% of participants being Asian (Steinbrenner et al., 2022). The implication that the white cis-male experience is the default experience has contributed to the disparities that autistic persons and their families from historically marginalized communities experience (Malone et al., under review). For example, Black families raising autistic children report that educators, service, and healthcare providers are unresponsive to familial needs (Dababnah et al., 2018; Pearson et al., 2021). Moreover, this highlights a critical gap in our "knowledge of desirability, feasibility, efficacy, and cultural or linguistic considerations for non-white individuals with autism, their families, and the practitioners who serve them" (Steinbrenner et al., 2022, p. 3). To address this critical gap, researchers and educators should engage in cultural reciprocity and center the voices of autistic voices of color. Educators and researchers can engage in cultural reciprocity by identifying and being transparent about their own values and beliefs and reflecting on cultural and background differences from the populations with whom they serve (Malone et al., under review). Engaging in cultural reciprocity will help to develop stronger partnerships by facilitating empowerment and support self-determination. Future research and practice should also be cautious of the generalizing results of white-majority samples to all demographics.

Gender and sexuality. There are roughly four males diagnosed with autism for every one female (Maenner et al., 2021). As a result, autistic males make up the majority of autism research participation and are also better understood compared to females. However, lower rates of autism diagnosis in females does not indicate that females are less likely to be on the autism spectrum. Qualities of autistic females may go unnoticed because they are different from those of males. Studies have found that females have different eye gaze patterns than males (looking at more social images; Harrop et al., 2018a), different repetitive behaviors (less overall, more gesture use; Knutsen et al., 2019), and less stereotypical special interests (Harrop et al., 2018b). These emerging signs of sex differences in autism suggest that females may not be as readily identified by educators, clinicians, parents, or physicians because they do not quite fit the mold of what society imagines autism to be. Until there is more concrete evidence, it is suggested that adults be considerate of these sex differences when working with young girls. Meanwhile, more studies should actively recruit and study the autistic female phenotype to better understand their needs.

Another issue that needs to be highlighted in the gender realm is the increasingly high overlap between the autistic population and identifying as LGBT (particularly transgender; Nabbijohn et al., 2019; Warrier et al., 2020). With the recognition of the relationship between autistic and LBGT identities comes a call for action in research, policy, community and education (Strang et al., 2020), given that both populations experience high rates of bullying and victimization in schools (Garaigordobil et al., 2020; Maiano et al., 2016). Professionals can assist in the comfort and understanding of LGBT autistic individuals by treating their expressions of gender with open-mindedness and dignity, and as well as promoting sexuality education in schools (Slocum et al., 2021).

III. Mental Health of Autistic Individuals

Masking and camouflaging. Camouflaging, otherwise known as "masking" or "compensation" is the act of suppressing or altering one's autistic traits in order to appear less autistic and more neurotypical (Cook et al., 2021). This often looks like the suppression of stimming behavior, forced eye contact with others, smiling more, changing one's voice to appear more cheerful, or preparing scripts of things to say in certain situations (Hull et al., 2017). Camouflaging requires a near constant self-monitoring of oneself, which may then limit one's capacity in attending to other happenings in the environment (Hull et al., 2017).

Camouflaging as a concept is relatively new, and a recent systematic review on camouflaging encapsulates much of this important work done in the last five years (Cook et al., 2021). While camouflaging can sometimes be a necessity, such as working in a job that may discriminate against autistic traits or to avoid being bullied in school, it can have incredibly negative consequences on an autistic individual. Camouflaging has been understood to take a toll on one's mental health, with a strong association with depression, anxiety, and suicidal ideations in autistic adults (Bradley et al., 2021; Hull et al., 2017). With the need to constantly be someone else and evaluate one's situation, camouflaging has a known negative impact on self-esteem, sense of relationships, and sense of identity (Bargiela et al., 2016; Tierney et al., 2016). While extra consideration should be taken for autistic individuals who are more likely to experience camouflaging, such as females, nonbinary individuals, and those with higher verbal ability (Cook et al., 2021), the biggest step in alleviating the need for individuals to camouflage is relieving *stigma* around autism traits. If a child feels comfortable around their peers, and if things like stimming are welcomed in a classroom, then children may focus less on how they are being perceived, allowing for more focused engagement with peers and the school environment.

Autistic burnout and suicide. Rates of death by suicide are seven times higher in the autistic population compared to the general population (Hirvikoski et al., 2016), with autistic children being six times more likely than other children to be at risk of making a suicide attempt (Moses, 2018). In recent years, numerous private and government agencies as well as the broader autism community have highlighted suicide prevention as an urgent need (Mandell, 2018). A large 2018 study found that 49% of autistic participants scored in the clinical range for depression and 36% reported recent suicidal ideation. They found that loneliness, social support, and autism traits predicted clinical depression scores (Hedley et al., 2018), which are themes found throughout the emerging suicide literature.

Another key risk marker for suicide in autistic individuals is burnout (Cassidy et al., 2018; Raymaker et al., 2020). Burnout is characterized by pervasive, long-term (typically 3+ months) exhaustion, loss of function, and reduced tolerance to stimulus (Raymaker et al., 2020). It is often caused by long-term camouflaging (Mandy, 2019), a lack of adequate supports, sensory overload, and overall exhaustion of navigating a neurotypical world (DeWeerdt, 2020; Raymaker et al., 2020). Phung et al. (2021) interviewed youth about their experiences with meltdown, shutdown, and burnout, and concluded that autistic children also experience burnout that is frequently misunderstood by neurotypical adults. While non-autistic burnout can usually be remediated rather quickly by taking a break from work, school, or other responsibilities, autistic burnout can be long lasting and detrimental to one's daily life (DeWeerdt, 2020).

A key protective factor found throughout examinations of suicide, burnout, and autism is social support. Multiple studies have found that adequate support, or lack thereof, was the biggest impact on an autistic adults' likelihood of having suicidal ideations (Camm-Crosbie et al., 2019; Cassidy et al., 2018). A perceived sense of *tangible* support can help alleviate depressive symptoms in autistic individuals (Hedley et al., 2017): Knowing that they have people they can go to when they feel lonely, coping tools at hand when things get overwhelming, and proper accommodations to allow them to do their job or go to school without discomfort can be lifesaving for autistic people.

Tension Within the Autism Community On Where Autism Research Should Be Heading

There is no clear consensus within the autism field on research should be headed as different stakeholders prioritize different areas of need. A recent systematic review on autism research priorities found that autistic adults would like more research to go into determining early childhood factors that can impact autistic children's developmental trajectory, as well as methods that can support greater inclusion in society. On the other hand, parents, clinicians and researchers would like more efforts to be placed on early identification of autism, and further development, improvement, and access to evidence-based services and supports (Roche et al., 2021).

Internationally, many funders have taken a clear bias towards supporting genetic studies such as understanding the causes of autism (Office of Autism Research Coordination, 2012). However, this emphasis on biology does not align well with some others in the autism community, as there have been concerns that genetic studies may encourage greater discrimination against people on the autism spectrum, and development of cures and eradication of autism (Chown et al., 2017; Hens et al., 2016). Advocates also feel that such studies do not improve the quality of life of people on the autism spectrum, and do not help to alleviate their current, urgent needs (Benevides et al., 2020; Pellicano et al., 2014). A recent example of this dispute is seen through the launch and subsequent pause of the "Spectrum 10k" study in the United Kingdom (Sanderson, 2021). Researchers aimed to collect DNA samples, as well as physical and mental health information from 10,000 autistic individuals so as to "investigate biological and environmental factors that contribute to autism and common physical and mental health conditions for autistic people" (Spectrum 10k, nd). Shortly after the study's launch, members of the autism community organized petitions and meetings to "#BoycottSpectrum10k", leading to an indefinite pause in the study while the team consults autistic individuals and their families further.

While it may not be possible to represent every voice within the autism community when determining the direction and scope of autism research, efforts should be taken to co-create research with stakeholders. These efforts may include and are not limited to involving children under the age of 18, individuals with co-occurring conditions, and individuals with intersectional needs stemming from underrepresented social categories (Cascio et al., 2020; Mallipeddi & VanDaalen, 2021). Future studies should serve and address the needs of the community with which researchers are working directly, since priorities for smaller autism communities may differ depending on the cultural context and specific challenges faced (Frazier et al., 2018).

Conclusion

The current understanding of autism, as well as the development of strategies that aid autistic individuals in meeting their needs while living in a world that has yet to fully embrace neurodiversity, would not have been made possible without the relentless pursuit in autism research. While the progress made over the past few decades is commendable, it is important to note the many urgent unmet needs still existing in the autistic population. As we strive ahead with our work in autism, we should always keep in mind that research should be conducted with, and not on, autistic people. We ought to also constantly reflect on autism research with a critical lens to reduce any personal or implicit biases in coloring how we present models, views and ideas about autism. Feedback from within autism research, as well as from partners in education and community, are key to future successes.

Author note

In respecting the diverse views of the autism community, we used both identity-first (*autistic person*) as preferred by self-advocates, and relatively neutral person-first (*person on the autism spectrum*) language throughout the chapter (Bottema-Beutel et al., 2021; Gomes, 2018; Robison, 2019).

Appendix
Resources for Educators or Practitioners

Trends in autism research (topics and funding trends)

The *Interagency Autism Coordinating Committee* (IACC) publishes multiple resources for identifying trends and advances in autism research both internationally and in the United States (https://iacc.hhs.gov/publications/). Since 2007, the committee has published yearly reports identifying research articles that discuss significant progress in the autism field (https://iacc.hhs.gov/publications/summary-of-advances/archives/).

Research frameworks

To gain a better understanding about neurodiversity, learn directly from the autistic community themselves in this book edited by Dr Steven Kapp titled '*Autistic Community and the Neurodiversity Movement- Stories from the frontline*' (https://link.springer.com/book/10.1007/978-981-13-8437-0). The book is open access, and full digital copies and individual chapters are free to download for all. For educators and practitioners, to learn more on how to help students learn about neurodiversity in the school setting, educators can review the *Learning About Neurodiversity at School (LEANS)* project by the University of Edinburgh (https://dart.ed.ac.uk/research/leans/). Their team is putting together a free classroom activity pack for mainstream primary students and teachers set for release in Spring 2022.

Educators and practitioners who are interested in conducting their own action research projects and would like to learn more about community based participatory research (CBPR) can look to the *Academic Autism Spectrum Partnership in Research and Education (AASPIRE)* for resources such as consent forms, interview guides, survey instruments, as well as inclusion guidelines (https://aaspire.org/collaboration-toolkit/). More resources and tips for inclusive and accessible autism research can also be found in *Autistica*'s research toolkit created by a team based at the UCL Institute of Education in the United Kingdom (https://www.autistica.org.uk/our-research/research-toolkit). To connect with other researchers, educators, and practitioners who are interested in CBPR, the

Participatory Autism Research Collective (PARC) is another resource (https://participatoryautismresearch.wordpress.com/).

Evidence-based Practices/Interventions

To learn more about practices that have clear evidence of positive effects on various outcomes for children, youth and young adults with autism, visit The *National Clearinghouse on Autism Evidence and Practice* (NCAEP) website for their latest report completed in 2020 (https://ncaep. fpg.unc.edu/). The NCAEP team reviewed 972 intervention research articles published between 1990 to 2017, and have identified 28 evidence-based practices with impact on 13 different outcome domains for students between the ages of 0 to 22 years.

For practitioners and families who want to learn how to plan, use, and monitor evidence-based practices (EBP) that have been identified by NCAEP, visit *Autism Focused Intervention Resource and Modules* (AFIRM) https://afirm.fpg.unc.edu/afirm-modules. All AFIRM modules are free to access for everyone, and each module consists of case examples, multimedia presentations of audio and video clips, as well as interactive assessments providing feedback as you learn. There are currently 29 EBP modules available, as well as an introductory module to autism. Another resource that educators can look to for information on interventions and recommendations on addressing challenges in their classrooms and schools is *What Works Clearinghouse* (WWC) by the Institute of Education Sciences (https://ies.ed.gov/ncee/wwc/FWW). It should be noted that resources from WWC are not specifically targeted to the autistic student population.

References

Alvares, G. A., Bebbington, K., Cleary, D., Evans, K., Glasson, E. J., Maybery, M. T., Pillar, S., Uljarević, M., Varcin, K., Wray, J., & Whitehouse, A. J. (2020). The misnomer of 'high functioning autism': Intelligence is an imprecise predictor of functional abilities at diagnosis. *Autism, 24*(1), 221–232. https://doi.org/10.1177/1362361319852831

Alverson, C. Y., Lindstrom, L. E., & Hirano, K. A. (2019). High school to college: Transition experiences of young adults with autism. *Focus on Autism and Other Developmental Disabilities, 34*(1), 52–64. https://doi.org/10.1177/1088357615611880

American Psychiatric Association (2013). *What is autism spectrum disorder?* www.psychiatry.org/patients-families/autism/what-is-autism-spectrum-disorder

Autistic Self Advocacy Network. (2021, December 9). *Functioning Labels Harm Autistic People.* https://autisticadvocacy.org/2021/12/functioning-labels-harm-autistic-people/

Bargiela, S., Steward, R., & Mandy, W. (2016). The experiences of late-diagnosed women with autism spectrum conditions: An investigation of the female autism phenotype. *Journal of Autism and Developmental Disorders, 46*(10), 3281–3294. https://doi.org/10.1007/s10803-016-2872-8

Benevides, T. W., Shore, S. M., Palmer, K., Duncan, P., Plank, A., Andresen, M.-L., Caplan, R., Cook, B., Gassner, D., Hector, B. L., Morgan, L., Nebeker, L., Purkis, Y., Rankowski, B., Wittig, K., & Coughlin, S. S. (2020). Listening to the autistic voice: Mental health priorities to guide research and practice in autism from a stakeholder-driven project. *Autism, 24*(4), 822–833. https://doi.org/10.1177/1362361320908410

Black, M. H., Mahdi, S., Milbourn, B., Scott, M., Gerber, A., Esposito, C., Falkmer, M., Lerner, M. D., Halladay, A., Ström, E., D'Angelo, A., Falkmer, T., Bölte, S., & Girdler, S. (2020). Multi-informant international perspectives on the facilitators and barriers to employment for autistic adults. *Autism Research*, 13(7), 1195–1214. https://doi.org/10.1002/aur.2288

Bottema-Beutel, K., Kapp, S. K., Lester, J. N., Sasson, N. J., & Hand, B. N. (2021). Avoiding ableist language: Suggestions for autism researchers. *Autism in Adulthood*, 3(1), 18–29. https://doi.org/10.1089/aut.2020.0014

Bradley, L., Shaw, R., Baron-Cohen, S., & Cassidy, S. (2021). Autistic adults' experiences of camouflaging and its perceived impact on mental health. *Autism in Adulthood*, 3(4), 320–329. https://doi.org/10.1089/aut.2020.0071

Bradbury, H. (2015). Introduction: How to situate and define action research. *In* Bradbury, H (Ed.), *The SAGE Handbook of Action Research*. (pp. 1–9). SAGE Publications Ltd. www.doi.org/10.4135/9781473921290

Brown, A. L. (1992). Design experiments: Theoretical and methodological challenges in creating complex interventions in classroom settings. *The Journal of the Learning Sciences, 2*, 141–178.

Bunt, D., van Kessel, R., Hoekstra, R. A., Czabanowska, K., Brayne, C., Baron-Cohen, S., & Roman-Urrestarazu, A. (2020). Quotas, and anti-discrimination policies relating to autism in the EU: Scoping review and policy mapping in Germany, France, Netherlands, United Kingdom, Slovakia, Poland, and Romania. *Autism Research*, 13(8), 1397–1417. https://doi.org/10.1002/aur.2315

Camm-Crosbie, L., Bradley, L., Shaw, R., Baron-Cohen, S., & Cassidy, S. (2019). 'People like me don't get support': Autistic adults' experiences of support and treatment for mental health difficulties, self-injury and suicidality. *Autism, 23*(6), 1431–1441. https://doi.org/10.1177/1362361318816053

Cartwright, N., & Munro, E. (2010). The limitations of randomized controlled trials in predicting effectiveness. *Journal of Evaluation in Clinical Practice*, 16(2), 260–266. https://doi.org/10.1111/j.1365-2753.2010.01382.x

Cascio, M. A., Weiss, J. A., & Racine, E. (2020). Person-oriented ethics for autism research: Creating best practices through engagement with autism and autistic communities. *Autism*, 24(7), 1676–1690. https://doi.org/10.1177/1362361320918763

Cassidy, S., Bradley, L., Shaw, R., & Baron-Cohen, S. (2018). Risk markers for suicidality in autistic adults. *Molecular Autism, 9*(1), 42. https://doi.org/10.1186/s13229-018-0226-4

Centers for Disease Control and Prevention. (2007). Prevalence of autism spectrum disorders--autism and developmental disabilities monitoring network, six sites, United States, 2000. *Morbidity and mortality weekly report. Surveillance summaries (Washington, D.C.: 2002)*, *56*(1), 1–11.

Chiarotti, F., & Venerosi, A. (2020). Epidemiology of autism spectrum disorders: A Review of worldwide prevalence estimates since 2014. *Brain Sciences*, *10*(5), 274. https://doi.org/10.3390/brainsci10050274

Chown, N., Robinson, J., Beardon, L., Downing, J., Hughes, L., Leatherland, J., Fox, K., Hickman, L., & MacGregor, D. (2017). Improving research about us, with us: A draft framework for inclusive autism research. *Disability & Society*, *32*(5), 720–734. https://doi.org/10.1080/09687599.2017.1320273

Cobb, P., Confrey, J., DiSessa, A., Lehrer, R., & Schauble, L. (2003). Design experiments in educational research. *Educational Researcher*, *32*(1), 9–13.

Cook, J., Hull, L., Crane, L., & Mandy, W. (2021). Camouflaging in autism: A systematic review. *Clinical Psychology Review*, *89*, 102080. https://doi.org/10.1016/j.cpr.2021.102080

Crompton, C. J., Ropar, D., Evans-Williams, C. V., Flynn, E. G., & Fletcher-Watson, S. (2020). Autistic peer-to-peer information transfer is highly effective. *Autism*, 1–9. https://doi.org/10.1177/1362361320919286

Dababnah, S., Shaia, W. E., Campion, K., & Nichols, H. M. (2018). "We had to keep pushing": Caregivers' perspectives on autism screening and referral practices of black children in primary care. *Intellectual and Developmental Disabilities*, *56*(5), 321–336. https://doi.org/10.1352/1934-9556-56.5.321

Dekker, M. (1999, November). *On our own terms: Emerging autistic culture*. Autscape. www.autscape.org/2015/programme/handouts/Autistic-Culture-07-Oct-1999.pdf

den Houting, J., Higgins, J., Isaacs, K., Mahony, J., & Pellicano, E. (2021). 'I'm not just a guinea pig': Academic and community perceptions of participatory autism research. *Autism*, *25*(1), 148–163. https://doi.org/10.1177/1362361320951696

DeWeerdt, S. (2020, March 30th). *Autistic Burnout, Explained*. Spectrum News. www.spectrumnews.org/news/autistic-burnout-explained/

Digital Science. (2018-) Dimensions [Software] available from https://app.dimensions.ai. Accessed on November 23, 2021, under license agreement.

Dingfelder, H. E., & Mandell, D. S. (2011). Bridging the research-to-practice gap in autism intervention: An application of diffusion of innovation theory. *Journal of Autism and Developmental Disorders*, *41*(5), 597–609. https://doi.org/10.1007/s10803-010-1081-0

Fletcher-Watson, S., Adams, J., Brook, K., Charman, T., Crane, L., Cusack, J., Leekam, S., Milton, D., Parr, J. R., & Pellicano, E. (2019). Making the future together: Shaping autism research through meaningful participation. *Autism*, *23*(4), 943–953. https://doi.org/10.1177/1362361318786721

Frazier, T. W., Dawson, G., Murray, D., Shih, A., Sachs, J. S., & Geiger, A. (2018). Brief report: A survey of autism research priorities across a diverse community of stakeholders. *Journal of Autism and Developmental Disorders*, *48*(11), 3965–3971. https://doi.org/10.1007/s10803-018-3642-6

Ganuthula, V. R. R., & Sinha, S. (2019). The looking glass for intelligence quotient Tests: The interplay of motivation, cognitive functioning, and affect. *Frontiers in Psychology*, *10*. https://doi.org/10.3389/fpsyg.2019.02857

Garaigordobil, M. G., Larrain, E. L., Garaigordobil, M., & Larrain, E. (2020). Bullying and cyberbullying in LGBT adolescents: Prevalence and effects on mental health. *Comunicar. Media Education Research Journal*, 28(1).

Giri, A., Aylott, J., Giri, P., Ferguson-Wormley, S., & Evans, J. (2021). Lived experience and the social model of disability: conflicted and inter-dependent ambitions for employment of people with a learning disability and their family carers. *British Journal of Learning Disabilities*. https://doi.org/10.1111/bld.12378

Gomes, M. (2018). *A study of the effectiveness of people-first language*. Proceedings of the 4th Annual Linguistics Conference at UGA, The Linguistics Society at UGA: Athens, GA. 1–19.

Goodley, D. (2014). *Dis/ability Studies*. Taylor & Francis.

Happé, F., & Frith, U. (2020). Annual research review: Looking back to look forward – changes in the concept of autism and implications for future research. *Journal of Child Psychology and Psychiatry*, 61(3), 218–232. https://doi.org/10.1111/jcpp.13176

Harrop, C., Jones, D., Zheng, S., Nowell, S. W., Boyd, B. A., & Sasson, N. (2018a). Sex differences in social attention in autism spectrum disorder. *Autism Research*, 11(9), 1264–1275. https://doi.org/10.1002/aur.1997

Harrop, C., Jones, D., Zheng, S., Nowell, S., Boyd, B. A., & Sasson, N. (2018b). Circumscribed interests and attention in autism: The role of biological sex. *Journal of Autism and Developmental Disorders*, 48(10), 3449–3459. https://doi.org/10.1007/s10803-018-3612-z

Hedley, D., Uljarević, M., Foley, K.-R., Richdale, A., & Trollor, J. (2018). Risk and protective factors underlying depression and suicidal ideation in autism spectrum disorder. *Depression and Anxiety*, 35(7), 648–657. https://doi.org/10.1002/da.22759

Hedley, D., Uljarević, M., Wilmot, M., Richdale, A., & Dissanayake, C. (2017). Brief report: Social support, depression and suicidal ideation in adults with autism spectrum disorder. *Journal of Autism and Developmental Disorders*, 47(11), 3669–3677. https://doi.org/10.1007/s10803-017-3274-2

Hendricks, D. R., & Wehman, P. (2009). Transition from school to adulthood for youth with autism spectrum disorders: Review and recommendations. *Focus on Autism and Other Developmental Disabilities*, 24(2), 77–88. https://doi.org/10.1177/1088357608329827

Hens, K., Peeters, H., & Dierickx, K. (2016). The ethics of complexity. Genetics and autism, a literature review. *American Journal of Medical Genetics Part B: Neuropsychiatric Genetics*, 171(3), 305–316. https://doi.org/10.1002/ajmg.b.32432

Hillary, A. (2020). Neurodiversity and cross-cultural communication. In H.B. Rosqvist, N. Chown, & Stenning, A. (Eds.), *Neurodiversity Studies: A New Critical Paradigm* (Chapter 6). Routledge Advances in Sociology.

Hirvikoski, T., Mittendorfer-Rutz, E., Boman, M., Larsson, H., Lichtenstein, P., & Bolte, S. (2016). Premature mortality in autism spectrum disorder. *The British Journal of Psychiatry*, 208(3), 232–238. doi:10.1192/bjp.bp.114.160192.

Howard, K., Katsos, N., & Gibson, J. (2019). Using interpretative phenomenological analysis in autism research. *Autism*, 23(7), 1871–1876.

Hughes, J. M. F. (2016). *Nothing about us without us: Increasing neurodiversity in disability and social justice advocacy groups.* https://autisticadvocacy.org/wp-content/uploads/2016/06/whitepaper-Increasing-Neurodiversity-in-Disability-and-Social-Justice-Advocacy-Groups.pdf

Hull, L., Petrides, K. V., Allison, C., Smith, P., Baron-Cohen, S., Lai, M.-C., & Mandy, W. (2017). "Putting on my best normal": Social camouflaging in adults with autism spectrum conditions. *Journal of Autism and Developmental Disorders, 47*(8), 2519–2534. https://doi.org/10.1007/s10803-017-3166-5

Hume, K., Steinbrenner, J. R., Odom, S. L., Morin, K. L., Nowell, S. W., Tomaszewski, B., ... & Savage, M. N. (2021). Evidence-based practices for children, youth, and young adults with autism: Third generation review. *Journal of Autism and Developmental Disorders, 51,* 4013–4032. https://doi.org/10.1007/s10803-020-04844-2

Interagency Autism Coordinating Committee (IACC). (2011). *2011 strategic plan for autism spectrum disorder research.* https://iacc.hhs.gov/publications/strategic-plan/2011/strategic_plan_2011.pdf

Interagency Autism Coordinating Committee (IACC). (2020). *IACC Strategic Plan for Autism Spectrum Disorder (ASD) 2018-2019 Update.* www.iacc.hhs.gov/publications/strategic-plan/2019/strategic_plan_2019.pdf?version=3

Johnson, C. N., Ramphal, B., Koe, E., Raudales, A., Goldsmith, J., & Margolis, A. E. (2021). Cognitive correlates of autism spectrum disorder symptoms. *Autism Research, 14*(11), 2405–2411. https://doi.org/10.1002/aur.2577

Kanner, L. (1943). Autistic disturbances of affective contact. *Nervous Child, 2,* 217–250.

Kapp, S. K. (2020). Autistic community and the neurodiversity movement: Stories from the frontline. *Springer Nature.*

Kapp, S. K., Gillespie-Lynch, K., Sherman, L. E., & Hutman, T. (2013). Deficit, difference, or both? Autism and neurodiversity. *Developmental Psychology, 49*(1), 59–71. https://doi.org/10.1037/a0028353

Kasari, C., Gulsrud, A. C., Shire, S. Y., & Strawbridge, C. (2021). *The JASPER model for children with autism: Promoting joint attention, symbolic play, engagement, and regulation.* Guilford Publications.

Kirby, A. V., Diener, M. L., Dean, E. E., Darlington, A. N., Myers, A., & Henderson, J. (2021). Autistic adolescents' and their parents' visions for the future: How aligned are they? *Autism in Adulthood.* https://doi.org/10.1089/aut.2020.0061

Knutsen, J., Crossman, M., Perrin, J., Shui, A., & Kuhlthau, K. (2019). Sex differences in restricted repetitive behaviors and interests in children with autism spectrum disorder: An Autism Treatment Network study. *Autism, 23*(4), 858–868.

Lawson, A., & Beckett, A. E. (2020). The social and human rights models of disability: towards a complementarity thesis. *The International Journal of Human Rights, 25*(2), 348–379. https://doi.org/10.1080/13642987.2020.1783533

Leadbitter, K., Buckle, K. L., Ellis, C., & Dekker, M. (2021). Autistic self-advocacy and the neurodiversity movement: Implications for autism early intervention research and practice. *Frontiers in Psychology, 12,* 635–690. https://doi.org/10.3389/fpsyg.2021.635690

Lewis C. (2015). What is improvement science? Do we need it in education? *Educational Researcher, 44(1):54–61.*

Llewellyn, A., & Hogan, K. (2000). The use and abuse of models of disability. *Disability & Society*, *15*(1), 157–165. https://doi.org/10.1080/0968759 0025829

Lockwood, I., Walker, R. M., Latimer, S., Chaboyer, W., Cooke, M., & Gillespie, B. M. (2022). Process evaluations undertaken alongside randomised controlled trials in the hospital setting: A scoping review. *Contemporary Clinical Trials Communications*, 100894. https://doi.org/10.1016/j.conctc.2022.100894

Lovelace, T. S., Comis, M. P., Tabb, J. M., & Oshokoya, O. E. (2021). Missing from the narrative: A seven-decade scoping review of the inclusion of black autistic women and girls in autism research. *Behavior Analysis in Practice.* https://doi.org/10.1007/s40617-021-00654-9

McWade, B., Milton, D., & Beresford, P. (2015). Mad studies and neurodiversity: a dialogue. *Disability & Society*, 30(2), 305–309. https://doi.org/10.1080/09687 599.2014.1000512

Maenner, M. J., Shaw K.A., Bakian, A.V., Bilder, D.A., Durkin, M.S., Esler, A., Furnier, S.M., Hallas, L., Hall-Lande, J., Hudson, A., Hughes, M.M., Patrick, M., Pierce, K., Poynter, J.N., Salinas, A., Shenouda, J., Vehorn, A., Warren, Z., Constantino, J.N., ... Cogswell, M.E. (2021). Prevalence and characteristics of autism spectrum disorder among children aged 8 years—Autism and Developmental Disabilities Monitoring Network, 11 sites, United States, 2018. *MMWR. Surveillance Summaries, 70.* https://doi.org/10.15585/mmwr. ss7011a1

Maiano, C., Normand, C. L., Salvas, M. C., Moullec, G., & Aimé, A. (2016). Prevalence of school bullying among youth with autism spectrum disorders: A systematic review and meta-analysis. *Autism research, 9*(6), 601–615.

Mallipeddi, N. V., & VanDaalen, R. A. (2021). Intersectionality within critical autism studies: A narrative review. *Autism in Adulthood.* https://doi.org/ 10.1089/aut.2021.0014

Malone, K. M., Pearson, J. N., Manns, L., Palazzo, K., Riveria, A., & Martin, D. (under review). The scholarly neglect of black autistic adults in autism research. *Autism in Adulthood.*

Mandell, D. (2018). Dying before their time: Addressing premature mortality among autistic people. *Autism,* 22(3), 234–235. https://doi.org/10.1177/ 1362361318764742

Mandy, W. (2019). Social camouflaging in autism: Is it time to lose the mask? *Autism*, 23(8), 1879–1881. https://doi.org/10.1177/1362361319878559

Marsh, A., Spagnol, V., Grove, R., & Eapen, V. (2017). Transition to school for children with autism spectrum disorder: A systematic review. *World Journal of Psychiatry*, 7(3), 184–196. https://doi.org/10.5498/wjp.v7.i3.184

Mazzotti, V. L., Rowe, D. A., Kwiatek, S., Voggt, A., Chang, W.-H., Fowler, C. H., Poppen, M., Sinclair, J., & Test, D. W. (2021). Secondary transition predictors of postschool success: An update to the research base. *Career Development and Transition for Exceptional Individuals, 44*(1), 47–64. https://doi.org/ 10.1177/2165143420959793

Milton, D. E. M., Ridout, S., Kourti, M., Loomes, G., & Martin, N. (2019). A critical reflection on the development of the Participatory Autism Research

Collective (PARC). *Tizard Learning Disability Review, 24*(2), 82–89. https:// doi.org/10.1108/TLDR-09-2018-0029

Modini, M., Joyce, S., Mykletun, A., Christensen, H., Bryant, R. A., Mitchell, P. B., & Harvey, S. B. (2016). The mental health benefits of employment: Results of a systematic meta-review. *Australasian Psychiatry, 24*(4), 331–336. https:// doi.org/10.1177/1039856215618523

Morán, M. L., Hagiwara, M., Raley, S. K., Alsaeed, A. H., Shogren, K. A., Qian, X., Gómez, L. E., & Alcedo, M. Á. (2020). Self-determination of students with autism spectrum disorder: A systematic review. *Journal of Developmental and Physical Disabilities.* https://doi.org/10.1007/s10882-020-09779-1

Moses, T. (2018). Suicide attempts among adolescents with self-reported disabilities. *Child Psychiatry & Human Development, 49*(3), 420–433.

Mundy, P., Delgado, C., Block, J., Venezia, M., Hogan, A., & Seibert, J. (2003). *Early social communication scales (ESCS).* Coral Gables, FL: University of Miami.

Mundy, P., & Newell, L. (2007). Attention, joint attention, and social cognition. *Current Directions in Psychological Science, 16*(5), 269–274. https://doi.org/ 10.1111/j.1467-8721.2007.00518.x

Nabbijohn, A. N., van der Miesen, A. I. R., Santarossa, A., Peragine, D., de Vries, A. L. C., Popma, A., . . . VanderLaan, D. P. (2019). Gender variance and the autism spectrum: An examination of children ages 6–12 years. *Journal of Autism and Developmental Disorders, 49*(4), 1570–1585. https://doi.org/ 10.1007/s10803-018-3843-z

Nasamran, A., Witmer, S. E., & Los, J. E. (2017). Exploring predictors of postsecondary outcomes for students with autism spectrum disorder. *Education and Training in Autism and Developmental Disabilities, 52*(4), 343–35

National Academies of Sciences, Engineering, and Medicine (2015). *Mental disorders and disabilities among low-income children.* The National Academies Press. https://doi.org/10.17226/21780

National Autism Center. (2015). Findings and conclusions: National standards project, phase 2. www.nationalautismcenter.org/national-standards-project/resu lts-reports

Nicolaidis, C., Raymaker, D. (2015). Community-based participatory research with communities defined by race, ethnicity, and disability: Translating theory to practice. *In* Bradbury, H (Ed.), *The SAGE Handbook of Action Research.* (pp. 167–178). SAGE Publications Ltd. www.doi.org/10.4135/9781473921290

Nicolaidis, C., Raymaker, D., Kapp, S. K., Baggs, A., Ashkenazy, E., McDonald, K., Weiner, M., Maslak, J., Hunter, M., & Joyce, A. (2019). The AASPIRE practice-based guidelines for the inclusion of autistic adults in research as co-researchers and study participants. *Autism, 23*(8), 2007–2019. https://doi.org/ 10.1177/1362361319830523

Nicolaidis, C., Raymaker, D., McDonald, K., Dern, S., Ashkenazy, E., Boisclair, C., Robertson, S., & Baggs, A. (2011). Collaboration strategies in non-traditional community-based participatory research partnerships: Lessons from an academic–community partnership with autistic self-advocates. *Progress in Community Health Partnerships, 5*(2), 143–150. https://doi.org/10.1353/ cpr.2011.0022

Nicholas, D. B., Hodgetts, S., Zwaigenbaum, L., Smith, L. E., Shattuck, P., Parr, J. R., Conlon, O., Germani, T., Mitchell, W., Sacrey, L., & Stothers, M. E. (2017). Research needs and priorities for transition and employment in autism: Considerations reflected in a "Special Interest Group" at the International Meeting for Autism Research. *Autism Research*, 10(1), 15–24. https://doi.org/10.1002/aur.1683

Nicholas, D. B., & Klag, M. (2020). Critical reflections on employment among autistic adults. *Autism in Adulthood*, 2(4), 289–295. https://doi.org/10.1089/aut.2020.0006

Odom, S. L. (2021). Education of students with disabilities, science, and randomized controlled trials. *Research and Practice for Persons with Severe Disabilities*, 46(3), 132–145. https://doi.org/10.1177/15407969211032341

Office of Autism Research Coordination, on behalf of the Interagency Autism Coordinating Committee. (2021). *2017-2018 autism spectrum disorder research: Portfolio analysis report*.www.iacc.hhs.gov/publications/portfolio-analysis/2018/portfolio_analysis_2018.pdf?ver=2

Office of Autism Research Coordination (OARC), National Institute of Mental Health and Thomson Reuters, Inc. on behalf of the Interagency Autism Coordinating Committee (IACC). (2012). *IACC/OARC autism spectrum disorder research publications analysis report: The global landscape of autism research*. https://iacc.hhs.gov/publications/publications-analysis/2012/publications_analysis_2012.pdf

Office of Autism Research Coordination, National Institute of Mental Health, Autistica, Canadian Institutes of Health Research, and Macquarie University. (2019). *2016 international autism spectrum disorder research portfolio analysis report*. www.iacc.hhs.gov/publications/international-portfolio-analysis/2016/portfolio_analysis_2016.pdf

Pearson, J. N., Malone, K. M., & Stewart-Ginsburg, J. (under review). "We should all be welcome:" A discourse analysis of religious coping for black parents raising autistic children. *Journal of Disability & Religion*.

Pearson, J. N., Stewart-Ginsburg, J. H., Malone, K.M, & Avent Harris, J. R. (2021). Faith and FACES: Black parents' perceptions of autism, faith, and coping. *Exceptional Children*. https://doi.org/10.1177/00144029211034152

Pellicano, E., & Houting, J. (2021). Annual research review: Shifting from 'normal science' to neurodiversity in autism science. *Journal of Child Psychology and Psychiatry*. https://doi.org/10.1111/jcpp.13534

Pellicano, E., Dinsmore, A., & Charman, T. (2014). What should autism research focus upon? Community views and priorities from the United Kingdom. *Autism*, 18(7), 756–770. https://doi.org/10.1177/1362361314529627

Pellicano, L., Mandy, W., Bölte, S., Stahmer, A., Lounds Taylor, J., & Mandell, D. S. (2018). A new era for autism research, and for our journal. *Autism*, 22(2), 82–83. https://doi.org/10.1177/1362361317748556

Phung, J., Penner, M., Pirlot, C., & Welch, C. (2021). What I wish you knew: Insights on burnout, inertia, meltdown, and shutdown from autistic youth. *Frontiers in Psychology*, 4981.

Raymaker, D. M. (2020). Shifting the System: AASPIRE and the loom of science and activism. In S. K. Kapp (Ed.), *Autistic community and the neurodiversity movement: Stories from the frontline* (pp. 133–145). Springer. https://doi.org/10.1007/978-981-13-8437-0_10

Raymaker, D. M., Teo, A. R., Steckler, N. A., Lentz, B., Scharer, M., Delos Santos, A., Kapp, S. K., Hunter, M., Joyce, A., & Nicolaidis, C. (2020). "Having all of your internal resources exhausted beyond measure and being left with no clean-up crew": Defining autistic burnout. *Autism in Adulthood, 2*(2), 132–143. https://doi.org/10.1089/aut.2019.0079

Richter, M., Popa-Roch, M., & Clément, C. (2019). Successful transition from primary to secondary school for students with autism spectrum disorder: A systematic literature review. *Journal of Research in Childhood Education, 33*(3), 382–398. https://doi.org/10.1080/02568543.2019.1630870

Rifai, O. M., Fletcher-Watson, S., Jiménez-Sánchez, L., & Crompton, C. J. (2021). Investigating markers of rapport in autistic and nonautistic interactions. *Autism in Adulthood.* https://doi.org/10.1089/aut.2021.0017

Robison, J. E. (2019). Talking about autism—Thoughts for researchers. *Autism Research, 12*(7), 1004–1006. https://doi.org/10.1002/aur.2119

Roche, L., Adams, D., & Clark, M. (2021). Research priorities of the autism community: A systematic review of key stakeholder perspectives. *Autism, 25*(2), 336–348. https://doi.org/10.1177/1362361320967790

Rogers, S. J., & Dawson, G. (2020). *Early Start Denver Model for young children with autism: Promoting language, learning, and engagement.* Guilford Publications.

Roux, A. M., Shattuck, P. T., Cooper, B. P., Anderson, K. A., Wagner, M., & Narendorf, S. C. (2013). Postsecondary employment experiences among young adults with an autism spectrum disorder. *Journal of the American Academy of Child and Adolescent Psychiatry, 52*(9), 931–939. https://doi.org/10.1016/j.jaac.2013.05.019

Sandbank, M., Bottema-Beutel, K., Crowley, S., Cassidy, M., Dunham, K., Feldman, J. I., Crank, J., Albarran, S. A., Raj, S., Mahbub, P., & Woynaroski, T. G. (2020). Project AIM: Autism intervention meta-analysis for studies of young children. *Psychological Bulletin, 146*(1), 1–29. https://doi.org/10.1037/bul0000215

Sanderson, K. (2021). High-profile autism genetics project paused amid backlash. *Nature, 598*(7879), 17–18. https://doi.org/10.1038/d41586-021-02602-7

Shah, P., & Mountain, D. (2007). The medical model is dead – long live the medical model. *British Journal of Psychiatry, 191*(5), 375–377. https://doi.org/10.1192/bjp.bp.107.037242

Siddiqui, N., Gorard, S., & See, B. H. (2018). The importance of process evaluation for randomised control trials in education. *Educational Research, 60(3)*, 357–370.

Simonoff, E., Kent, R., Stringer, D., Lord, C., Briskman, J., Lukito, S., Pickles, A., Charman, T., & Baird, G. (2020). Trajectories in symptoms of autism and cognitive ability in autism from childhood to adult life: Findings from a longitudinal epidemiological cohort. *Journal of the American Academy of Child & Adolescent Psychiatry, 59*(12), 1342–1352. https://doi.org/10.1016/j.jaac.2019.11.020

Singer, J. (1999). Why can't you be normal for once in your life?: from a "Problem with No Name" to a new category of disability. In Corker, M and French, S (Eds.) *Disability Discourse* (pp. 59–67). Open University Press UK.

Singh, J., Illes, J., Lazzeroni, L., & Hallmayer, J. (2009). Trends in US autism research funding. *Journal of Autism and Developmental Disorders, 39*(5), 788–795. https://doi.org/10.1007/s10803-008-0685-0

Slocum, V., Eyres, R. M., Wolfe, P. S. (2021). Comprehensive sexuality and relationship education curriculum and teaching strategies. In Gibbon, T.C., Harkins Monaco, E. A., Bateman, D. F. (Eds.), *Sexuality education for students with disabilities* (pp. 125–142). Rowman & Littlefield.

Spectrum 10k. (nd). *Frequently asked questions.* https://spectrum10k.org/faqs/what-is-spectrum-10k/

Steinbrenner, J. R., Hume, K., Odom, S. L., Morin, K. L., Nowell, S. W., Tomaszewski, B., Szendrey, S., McIntyre, N. S., Yücesoy-Özkan, S., & Savage, M. N. (2020). *Evidence-based practices for children, youth, and young adults with autism.* The University of North Carolina at Chapel Hill, Frank Porter Graham Child Development Institute, National Clearinghouse on Autism Evidence and Practice Review Team. https://ncaep.fpg.unc.edu/sites/ncaep.fpg. unc.edu/files/imce/documents/EBP%20Report%202020.pdf

Steinbrenner, J. R., McIntyre, N., Rentschler, L. F., Pearson, J. N., Luelmo, P., Jaramillo, M. E., Boyd, B. A., Wong, C., Nowell, S. W., Odom, S. L., & Hume, K. A. (2022). Patterns in reporting and participant inclusion related to race and ethnicity in autism intervention literature: Data from a large-scale systematic review of evidence-based practices. *Autism.* https://doi.org/10.1177/136236 13211072593

Strang, J. F., van der Miesen, A. I., Caplan, R., Hughes, C., daVanport, S., & Lai, M.-C. (2020). Both sex- and gender-related factors should be considered in autism research and clinical practice. *Autism, 24*(3), 539–543. https://doi.org/10.1177/1362361320913192

Tan, G. T. H., Shahwan, S., Goh, C. M. J., Ong, W. J., Wei, K. C., Verma, S. K., Chong, S. A., & Subramaniam, M. (2020). Mental illness stigma's reasons and determinants (MISReaD) among Singapore's lay public – a qualitative inquiry. *BMC Psychiatry, 20*(1). https://doi.org/10.1186/s12888-020-02823-6

Test, D. W., Smith, L. E., & Carter, E. W. (2014). Equipping youth with autism spectrum disorders for adulthood: Promoting rigor, relevance, and relationships. *Remedial and Special Education, 35*(2), 80–90. https://doi.org/10.1177/0741932513514857

Tierney, S., Burns, J., & Kilbey, E. (2016). Looking behind the mask: Social coping strategies of girls on the autistic spectrum. *Research in Autism Spectrum Disorders, 23*, 73–83. https://doi.org/10.1016/j.rasd.2015.11.013

The White House. (2006). Combatting Autism Act of 2006 [Fact Sheet]. https://georgewbush-whitehouse.archives.goTv/news/releases/2006/12/20061 219-3.html

Tomasello, M. (1995). Joint attention as social cognition. In C. Moore, & P. J. Dunham (Eds.), *Joint attention: Its origins and role in development* (pp. 103–130). Hillsdale, NJ: Lawrence Erlbaum Associates Inc.

Tomasello, M., & Farrar, M. J. (1986). Joint attention and early language. *Child Development, 57*(6), 1454–1463. https://doi.org/10.2307/1130423

Tomaszewski, B., Kraemer, B., Steinbrenner, J. R., Smith DaWalt, L., Hall, L. J., Hume, K., & Odom, S. (2020). Student, educator, and parent perspectives of self-determination in high school students with autism spectrum disorder. *Autism Research, 13*(12), 2164–2176. https://doi.org/10.1002/aur.2337

U.S. Department of Health and Human Services. (2017 October). *Report to Congress: Young adults and transitioning youth with autism spectrum disorder.* www.hhs.gov/sites/default/files/2017AutismReport.pdf

Verhoeff, B. (2015). Fundamental challenges for autism research: the science–practice gap, demarcating autism and the unsuccessful search for the neurobiological basis of autism. *Medicine, Health Care and Philosophy, 18*(3), 443–447. https://doi.org/10.1007/s11019-015-9636-7

Warrier, V., Greenberg, D. M., Weir, E., Buckingham, C., Smith, P., Lai, M.-C., Allison, C., & Baron-Cohen, S. (2020). Elevated rates of autism, other neurodevelopmental and psychiatric diagnoses, and autistic traits in transgender and gender-diverse individuals. *Nature Communications, 11*(1), 3959. https://doi.org/10.1038/s41467-020-17794-1

Wehmeyer, M. L. (2020). Self-determination in adolescents and adults with intellectual and developmental disabilities. *Current Opinion in Psychiatry, 33*(2), 81–85. https://doi.org/10.1097/YCO.0000000000000576

West, E. A., Travers, J. C., Kemper, T. D., Liberty, L. M., Cote, D. L., McCollow, M. M., & Stansberry Brusnahan, L. L. (2016). Racial and ethnic diversity of participants in research supporting evidence-based practices for learners with autism spectrum disorder. *The Journal of Special Education, 50*(3), 151–163.

Chapter 19

Aging and Autism Spectrum Disorder

Danielle A. Waldron, [1,2] *Jacquelin A. Sauer,* [1] *and*
Megan M. Anderson [1]

[1] Stonehill College, Department of Healthcare Administration
[2] University of Massachusetts Boston, Department of Gerontology

Today, almost all of us know a child with autism spectrum disorder (ASD). These children, however, are growing up and eventually, will grow old too. As adult children with ASD begin to outlive their aging parents for the first time, existing healthcare, social services, and aging infrastructures are ill-equipped to support them in older adulthood (Wright, Wright, D'Astous, & Wadsworth, 2019). Before looking ahead, however, we must look back in time to understand the gravity of this situation. Chapters 1 through 3 provide a more comprehensive historical perspective on the diagnosis of ASD, but the year 1980 is the most relevant in the context of aging. In 1980, the DSM-III recognized ASD as its own diagnosis with specific diagnostic criteria under a form of pervasive developmental disorder for the first time (American Psychological Association (APA), 1980; Rosen, Lord, and Volkmar, 2021). This means that the first, large cohort of children diagnosed with ASD in 1980 are only approximately 41-years-old today. Adults with ASD older than 41-years-old may have received an alternate or misdiagnosis prior to 1980, sought a late-life diagnosis, or self-diagnosed themselves with ASD.

An estimated 1 in 54 children live with ASD today, a drastic increase from 1 in 150 children diagnosed with ASD in 2000 (CDC, 2020). Estimates suggest between 707,000 and roughly 1.1 million adolescents with ASD will transition to adulthood over the next 100 years (Shattuck, 2019). They will join the estimated nearly 5.5 million adults (~2.2% of U.S. adults) aged 18+ years living with ASD today (Dietz et al., 2020). ASD diagnoses will likely continue to climb through 2060 unless researchers identify risks for ASD and begin preventing the condition (Blaxill, Rogers, & Nevison, 2021), which would undoubtedly pose troubling ethical concerns for the ASD community.

Adults with ASD have a shortened life expectancy compared to the general population, but it is unclear how much shorter. Some researchers suggest that life expectancy ranges between 36 years to 54 years on average, a staggering divergence from the life expectancy of 79 years in the general population (CDC, 2017; Guan & Li, 2017; Hirvikoski et al., 2016). These

DOI: 10.4324/9781003255147-23

estimates are conservative; they exclude adults and older adults who may live long, fulfilling lives with few supports, yet have never sought a formal ASD diagnosis and slide under the radar of tracking systems. Barnard-Brak and colleagues (2019) who used the same National Vital Statistics System data as Guan and Li (2017) found a life expectancy of 68 years in the ASD population compared to the general population's 72-year life expectancy between 1999 and 2015 after adjusting for changes in ASD prevalence rates. Despite some mixed findings on life expectancy, adults with ASD experience a multitude of physical and mental health comorbidities at younger ages than the general population, and there are few specialized infrastructures to support them after they outgrow child services at 18-22 years of age (Croen et al., 2015; Weir et al., 2021). Some say that ASD has more of an influence on poor health status than aging; women with ASD being even worse off than younger adults and men with ASD (Rydzewska et al., 2019). Increasing wellness and longevity in those aging with ASD are top priorities for the current and future aging cohorts of individuals with ASD and their families.

This chapter uses the "Global Age-Friendly Cities" Framework (2007), created by the World Health Organization (WHO), here forth called the "Age-Friendly Community" framework (AARP, 2021; Central Oregon COA, 2022) (see Figure 19.1).

There are eight Age-Friendly Community domains, including respect and social inclusion, community support and health services, social participation, transportation, housing, outdoor spaces and buildings, civic participation and employment, and communication and information. Today, 1,114 age-friendly cities and communities across 44 nations serve approximately 262 million people, making this framework widely respected and recognized in aging research, policy, and practice (WHO, 2021). This chapter explores each of the eight domain's challenges and supportive policies and programs in the context of aging with ASD. Given the shortened life expectancies, accelerated aging, and a lack of data on this population, the construct of aging is more fluid here than aging research in the general population, which typically only includes those 65 years or older. Case studies of adults and older adults with ASD presented at the end of the chapter offer an opportunity for readers to engage deeply with the interconnectedness of these topic areas.

Respect and Social Inclusion

Challenges

Approximately 60% of adults with ASD reportedly experience bad or very bad social outcomes (e.g., employment, friendship, relationships, and independent living), and this is perhaps amplified by ageism (i.e.,

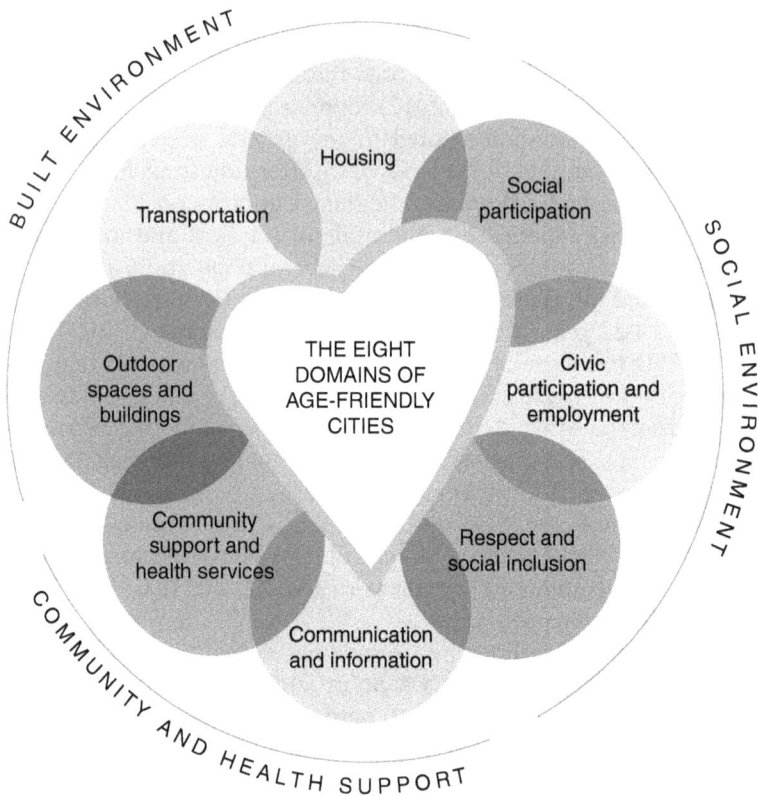

Figure 19.1 Age Friendly Communities.

Notes: From "Age Friendly Communities: A Step Forward for Older Adults." Image Courtesy of the Council on Aging of Central Oregon, Copyright 2022.

discrimination based on age) in later life (Howlin et al., 2013). Many adults with ASD report having no friends, no romantic partners, and few have children, and it is concerning that these social networks will continue to narrow as these individuals age (Howlin et al., 2013; Waldron, Coyle, Kramer, & Jeckel, 2018). Society can neither identify their disability nor understand them, believing that those with ASD must be genius savants with a specialized skill or have an ID (Singer, 1999).

Additionally, many adults with ASD experience the impact of intersectionality, or the ways in which being a member of multiple minorities or marginalized groups across race/ethnicity, gender, LGBTQ+, age, and disability amplifies discrimination in additive or multiplicative ways (Crenshaw, 1989; Martino and Schormans, 2018; Hillier et al., 2019). A tendency to focus exclusively on a person's ASD diagnosis can limit and/or oppress other essential aspects of their being (Cascio et al., 2021). Cascio and colleagues (2021) call into question the ethics of ASD research, which often lacks women, non-verbal persons, those in racial/ ethnic minorities, older adults, and other marginalized communities. This may lead to an inequitable understanding of diverse experiences and support needs in such groups.

Social resources are unequally distributed in the adult population with ASD across racial/ethnic groups. Here, "Hispanic" is used rather than "Latinx" because of the terminology used by California Department of Developmental Services. An analysis of non-medical expenditures (e.g., supplemental employment and work programs, community care, day-care, transportation, respite) of adults with ASD served by the California Department of Developmental Services from FY 2012–2013 indicated disparities in spending for adults (18+ years) across race/ethnicity: non-Hispanic white individuals ($31,008), non-Hispanic African Americans ($26,831), non-Hispanic Other Race ($25,395), non-Hispanic Asians ($22,993), and Hispanics ($18,083) (Leigh et al., 2016). Disparities in spending within the ASD and ID community persisted across race/ethnicity; non-Hispanic white persons accumulated the highest expenditure total, which was approximately 38% higher than their non-Hispanic African American, 41% higher than non-Hispanic Other Race, 56% higher than non-Hispanic Asian, and 89% higher than their Hispanic counterparts (Leigh et al., 2016). As our aging nation and world become increasingly diverse, equitable distribution of funding across race/ethnicity is critical in supporting older adults with ASD with particular focus on older adults with both ASD and ID.

There are also inequities across gender in ASD assessment, treatment, and research over the lifespan (Lai & Baron-Cohen, 2015). Diagnostic tools, originally developed and normed for men, are not inclusive of the female ASD profile and, in turn, underdiagnose and/or misdiagnose females with ASD (Lai et al., 2011). The diagnostic rate, believed to be 4:1 male to female, varies with age and ID (Nicholas et al., 2008; Fombonne, 2009). For example, females with stronger verbal skills and higher IQs who meet the criteria for ASD are less likely to be diagnosed or are diagnosed much later in life than their male counterparts (Loomes, Hull & Mandy, 2017). Researchers suggest that numerous factors, such as greater social motivation, a tendency to study the social behavior of others, and the frequent masking of ASD symptoms, contribute to lower rates of ASD diagnosis in females (Gould & Ashton-Smith, 2011). Females with ASD who have an ID often have their needs either overlooked or identified much later in life, depriving them of crucial support that follows a diagnosis, as well as the opportunity to understand themselves, physically, emotionally, and intellectually, and adapt successfully in a world that was not designed to accommodate their needs (Zener, 2019).

Recent research suggests there is an increase in adults with ASD who identify as part of the LGBTQ+ community (George & Stokes, 2018; Dewinter, De Graaf & Beeger, 2017; van der Meisen et al., 2018; Rudolph et al., 2017). However, adults with ASD are more likely to struggle with expressing their gender and sexuality due to ongoing ASD stereotyping and victimization. The chapter of this book on sexuality provides a more comprehensive look at sexuality and ASD, but this section focuses on impact on well-being. Compared to heteronormative populations, individuals who belong to sexual and gender minority groups experience poorer mental health, such as the increased risk of depressive and anxiety disorders, reported lower life satisfaction and higher rates of suicide, which are already four times higher for the ASD population (George & Stokes, 2018; Croen et al., 2015). Research shows that an individual's mental health worsens as their minority group membership increases, especially in adults with ASD; for example, an individual with ASD and gender dysmorphia had worse mental health than those who only had ASD (George & Stokes, 2018). These increased rates of mental health issues among LGBTQ+ individuals and individuals with ASD result from stigma and marginalization connected to living outside of mainstream socio-cultural norms and stress associated with various forms of victimization, including verbal abuse, physical acts of violence, sexual assault, employment discrimination, reduced medical care, and harassment from authority (Sandfort, Melendez, & Diaz, 2007; Meyer, 2003).

Supportive Policies and Programs

The transition from youth to adulthood is a critical period to set people up for successful social inclusion over the lifespan. Findings from Eilenberg and colleagues' study (2019) indicate that transition-age youth who identified as either low income or part of a racial minority group were less likely to live independently, engage in social events, be employed, seek higher education or partake in transitional preparatory meetings later on in life. These disadvantages in transition put them behind their non-Hispanic white and higher-income peers from the start of adulthood, making it increasingly difficult for them to "catch up" to these educational, occupational, and social gains over time (Eilenberg et al., 2019).

La Roche and colleagues (2018) identified a series of action steps to generate culturally sensitive options for those with ASD seeking support or services. Though aimed at clinicians, these suggestions extend to culturally appropriate social service delineation. La Roche and colleagues (2018) challenge providers to 1) become more aware of one's own cultural beliefs, traditions, values, bias, and privilege and 2) use instruments such as the Cultural Formulation Interview (CFI), which asks questions such as "What do others in your family, your friends, or others in your community think is causing your problem?" or people "...come from different backgrounds or have different expectations. Have you been concerned about this and is there anything that we can do to provide you with the care you need?" to assess how individuals with ASD and their families see their challenges and what they perceive as solutions (La Roche et al., 2018, p. 109).

McCarthy, Chaplain, and Underwood (2015) describe a national strategy to improve social inclusion for adults with ASD in the UK, which set forth 15 priority items presented in *Think Autism: An Update* (Department of Health, 2014). The National Autistic Society also offers a framework, "SPELL," that encourages a more ASD-friendly culture; the major tenets include structure, positive approach, empathy, low arousal in settings, and links to the community (Roberts et al., 2011; Beadle-Brown et al., 2009; Beadle-Brown & Mills, 2010). Otero and Copeland (2020) propose the inclusion of individual's hopes for social interaction, with whom they wish to interact, and the skills needed to accomplish these goals in assessments of adults with ASD. Siblings Focusing on Relationships, Well-being, and Responsibility Ahead (FORWARD), a pilot study at Boston University helps siblings of adults with ASD plan for their futures (Family-Based Planning for Autism in Adulthood, n.d.). Perhaps best practices for supporting the futures of individuals aging with ASD should incorporate both person-centered and family-centered planning.

Community Support and Health Services

Challenges

At ages 65 years and older, 66.2% of adults with ASD report poor health compared to 45.6% in the population without ASD (Rydzeska et al., 2019). Compared to the general population, adults with ASD present with a significantly higher prevalence of psychiatric conditions, such as anxiety disorder, attention deficit disorder, dementia, depression, obsessive-compulsive disorder, suicide attempts, and others (Croen et al., 2015; Weir et al., 2021). Barnard-Brak and colleagues (2019), however, contest that adults with ASD die of dementia less often than people without ASD. Women with ASD present more often with anxiety, depression, bipolar disorder, suicide attempts, and schizophrenia, while men with ASD present more often with obsessive-compulsive disorder, attention deficit disorder, alcohol, and drug problems (Croen et al., 2015). Croen and colleagues (2015) report that women with ASD are more likely to experience dementia than men with ASD, while Barnard-Brak and colleagues (2019) report the opposite. Adults with ASD are significantly more likely than the general population to experience an extensive array of physical comorbidities, such as diabetes, obesity, gastrointestinal disorders, genetic disorders, and more (Croen et al., 2015; Weir et al., 2021). Women with ASD experience many of these physical health comorbidities more often than men with ASD (Croen et al., 2015; Weir et al., 2021). Individuals with ASD experience these comorbidities, which are expected in a much older population, beginning in their late 20s to early 40s, evidence of accelerated aging in this group.

Compared to adults without ASD, adults with ASD reported poorer communication with clinicians, lower healthcare self-efficacy, poorer chronic condition management, fewer tetanus vaccines, and fewer pap smears (Nicolaidis et al., 2013). Adults with ASD reported more significant unmet needs across physical health, mental health, and prescription medications, and greater emergency room usage compared to their peers in the general population (Nicolaidis et al., 2013). The most recent Medicaid data available for adult enrollees with ASD (2008) indicate that approximately 56% of adult Medicaid enrollees (i.e., age 18–64 years) with ASD were white, followed by 22% black, 7% Hispanic or Latinx, and 15% other races, which included American Indian or Alaska Native, Asian, Native Hawaiian or Other Pacific Islander (Jariwala-Parikh et al., 2019). During this time, the general population's racial distribution of Medicaid enrollees (age 18–64 years) painted a slightly different picture: 43% white, 23% black, 27% Hispanic or Latinx, and 7% "Other" (Kaiser Family Foundation, 2020). These demographics offer a new perspective on a notion recognized in the childhood ASD literature; non-Hispanic white persons are diagnosed with ASD earlier in life and more often than in minority groups, particularly for Latinx populations. Medicaid medical expenditure data suggest that white adults with ASD (i.e., age 18–64 years) were significantly less likely to visit the Emergency Room (ER) than black adults and adults of other races with ASD and also used outpatient services less often than black adults with ASD from 2006–2008 (Jariwala-Parikh et al., 2019). It is unlikely that non-Hispanic white individuals with ASD have less access to healthcare services because of their higher social privilege and access to resources. Therefore, this finding might indicate that non-Hispanic white adults with ASD are either healthier than their peers in racial minority groups, or perhaps they received earlier diagnoses and support in childhood. Thus, they use ER and outpatient services less frequently in adulthood.

There are other issues surrounding healthcare such as long waitlists, cost, and availability of specialty care. Pediatric providers cut off services at a certain age, and finding adult providers is extremely difficult. In the US, there are not enough developmental disability and mental health specialists, so many individuals go without healthcare services or insurance, and lower-income countries are likely even worse off (King et al., 2020). Very little is known about ASD and the use of long-term services and supports (LTSS). Older adults in skilled nursing facilities (SNFs) may experience triggering sensory input (e.g., touch), challenges with socialization (e.g., shared mealtimes), and changes in routine (e.g., alternating staff) (Smith, 2018). Managers in long term care settings in England largely report a lack of communication and "sensory-friendly" training on dementia units (Leroi et al., 2021, p. 1522).

Approximately 77% of 922 physician respondents from Kaiser Permanente Northern California rated their ability to care for adults with ASD as fair/poor (Zerbo et al., 2015). Many did not know how many adult patients they had with ASD; some did not know adults could even have ASD, believing it was a childhood condition, and nearly half of respondents lacked confidence in identifying female patients with ASD in patients with ID (Zerbo et al., 2015; Tromans et al., 2019). Surveyed physicians also largely lacked confidence in caring for adults with ASD, and reported inconsistencies in training amongst healthcare professionals only reinforce the need for universal ASD training for clinicians (Tromans et al., 2019; Smith, 2018; Nicolaidis et al., 2021). This is all, of course, highly problematic. A telling quote reported by a practitioner of 25 years in Zerbo and colleagues' study states, "I think that ...we need education. I mean, autism was like "Rain Man"[reference to the 1988 film] when I was in medical school. There wasn't anything else besides that: it was Rain Man or nothing" (Zerbo et al., 2015 p. 4008). Highly experienced medical professionals should not look to the big screen to learn about a condition affecting nearly 5.5 million adults aging in the U.S. today and many more globally.

In 2016 and 2017, a special interest group with members from the US, UK, Netherlands, Italy, Norway, Denmark, Canada, Taiwan, and Australia at the International Society of Autism expressed the following concerns for the future of adults aging with ASD: lack of information about ASD and dementia, validity and reliability of diagnostic testing in later life, especially when a person cannot recall their own medical and life histories, medication overuse, and what treatments are the best options for comorbid physical and mental health conditions (Roestorf et al., 2019).

Supportive Policies and Programs

Providers are, however, willing to train and learn more about this population, and some have already begun (Zerbo et al., 2015). Nurses at Loudon Hospital in Virginia spearheaded a project to make their children's hospital more sensory-friendly on behalf of patients with ASD (Wood et al., 2019), and these sensory modifications may help people with ASD over the life course. Emergency rooms tend to be bright, noisy, foul-smelling, and patient exams, themselves, elicited sensory overload with insufficient communication between patients with ASD and staff (Wood et al., 2019). Their team implemented the following solutions: specialized kits with headphones, fidget toys, and a storyboard about what to expect in the emergency room, a rolling cart with similar items, dimmed lights in exam rooms, signs on patients' doors requesting permission before entry, private rooms, white noise machines, expedited wait times, and education for staff on communicating with patients with ASD (Wood et al., 2019). Owen and colleagues (2020) suggest tailored communication techniques in clinical settings, such as information cards with an individual's unique preferences, use of basic sign language, visual pain indicators, and an option to pretend to do a procedure before doing it to make the patient more familiar. The model (Figure 19.2) illustrates other patient, provider, and systemic-level factors that may help guide healthcare interactions for people with ASD (Nicolaidis et al., 2015).

Other supports, such as the Hospital and Depression Assessment Tool (HADS), can help inform family and the care team about specific issues and unmet needs in mental health (Zigmond & Snaith, 1983). The Caregiver Skill Training, a WHO pilot program, teaches caregivers about ASD in thirty countries across the globe (Salmone et al., 2018). The Autism Accommodations Tool and the Adult Autism Healthcare

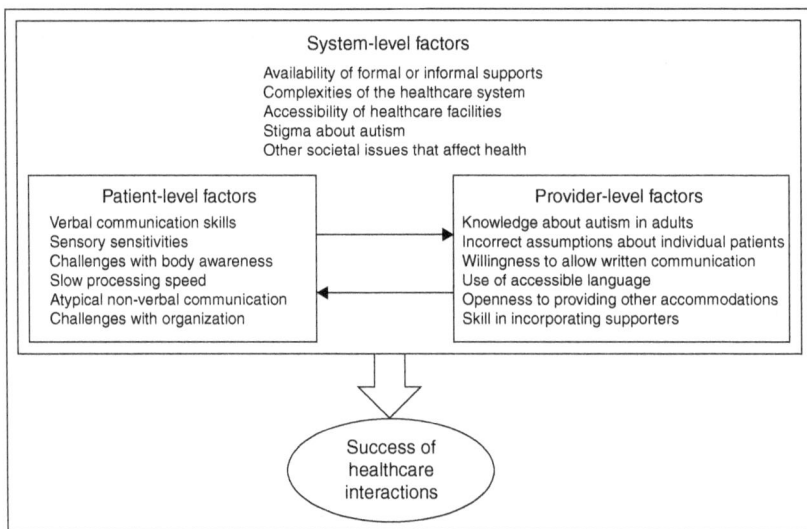

Figure 19.2 Patient-, Provider-, and System-level Factors Affecting the Participants Experiences with Healthcare.

Notes: From "Respect the way I need to communicate with you": Healthcare experiences of adults on the autism spectrum" by Nicolaidis, C., Raymaker, D. M., Ashkenazy, E., McDonald, K. E., Dern, S., Baggs, A. E., Kapp, S. K., Weiner, M., & Boisclair, W. C., 2015, *Autism, 19*(7), 824–831, Copyright 2021 by The Authors.

Provider Self-Efficacy Scale (ASPIRE) might also help providers target and improve their insufficiencies in treating patients with ASD once it is further tested (Nicolaidis et al., 2021; Nicolaidis et al., 2016). Roestorf and colleagues (2019) propose an international database to share information amongst researchers, providers, and relevant stakeholders. A centralized source that expedites sharing of tools such as these and critical information about ASD across countries would support global aging with ASD.

To help improve the competency of providers, Smith (2018) suggests that SNFs share case study data on their experiences with older adults with ASD, as well as look to identification tools such as Autism Spectrum Quotient, which does not diagnose ASD officially but identifies those who likely have ASD (Baron-Cohen et al., 2001). This is practical for SNFs given scarce resources to bring in clinicians to formally diagnose individuals.

Outdoor Spaces and Buildings

Challenges

Kinnaer and colleagues (2016) found four common challenges faced by adults with ASD in the material world: sensory challenges, unpredictability, self-growth and development, and physical safety and well-being in robust environments. The unique sensory experiences of adults with ASD play an essential role in their perception and utilization of the environment. Outdoor and indoor spaces can either exacerbate or decrease the sensory experiences of adults with ASD. Numerous public spaces, such as educational and healthcare settings, human resource offices, legal offices, modes of public transportation, and grocery stores, are oversaturated with sensory stimuli that can cause anxiety in adults with autism, preventing them from utilizing these spaces (Morgan, 2019). An environment cautious of external and internal stimuli can create a safe and accessible space that encourages self-development and personal growth in adults with ASD. Unplanned social situations, uncontrollable sensory stimuli, and unpredictable activities can discourage adults with ASD from participating in their environment. This lack of participation in the physical environment can inhibit personal growth and development for adults with ASD.

Supportive Policies and Programs

Researchers suggest consultants meet with individuals with ASD and their families before creating new buildings and spaces (Roberts et al., 2011). Providing a range of spaces for different social situations and experiences and areas with numerous visible exits allow adults with ASD to have control over their environment, reducing stress and anxiety during unpredictable situations (Kinnaer et al., 2016). The Helen Hamlyn Center for Design and Kingwood Trust organization designed and evaluated accessible and inclusive gardens for adults with ASD in London at Kingwood College (Gaudion & McGinley, 2012). The design team used data collected from existing activity timetables, interviews with adults with autism and their caregivers, shadowing a horticulturist, and various workshops to create seven outdoor spaces. The combination of these seven spaces (escape, exercise, occupation, sensory, social, transition, and wilderness spaces) offers an inclusive and beautiful garden for adults with autism to advance their social development, physical activity, and independence while decreasing anxiety-inducing triggers, such as unpredictability. These recommendations for outdoor spaces may translate to nearly any outdoor venue looking to increase sensory accommodations for adults with ASD.

Escape

The first green space provided a 'hidden' area in the garden where adults with ASD could sit under natural canopies formed by trees. These spaces allow adults with ASD to 'hide' in a semi-transparent yet hidden area where they continue to observe their surroundings while escaping uncomfortable situations or experiences and overwhelming stimuli.

Exercise

Kingwood College incorporated age-appropriate exercise equipment in their garden (e.g., sunken trampoline to encourage jumping) to foster physical activities. In addition, Kingwood College designed a specific space with subtly curved fencing and rubber mulch flooring to safely guide a person to gardening and exercise equipment.

Occupation

The occupational green space was designed to incorporate people's natural interests and abilities, such as repetition, routine, pattern, and attention to detail. Kingwood College achieved this through providing clear visual instructions, organizational materials (e.g., activity charts), solitary garden activities that require little movement (e.g., picking up sticks or planting seeds), plants that grow quickly for adults with short attention spans, plants of interest or preference, and crafting activities (e.g., building bird feeders).

Sensory

To create a welcoming environment for adults with ASD to explore new stimuli, Kingwood College designed a series of sensory 'rooms' that grouped senses by visual (i.e., plant color), texture, noise, smell, and temperature. Furthermore, Kingwood College provided clear signs and orientation toward each sensory 'room,' allowing adults with autism to explore specific sensory experiences of interest while avoiding others.

Social

It is important to include visible and accessible opportunities for adults with autism to engage in social interactions and group activities in outdoor spaces. To foster social development, Kingwood College designed an open area connected to a summer house that could be used for group activities such as barbecues, crafts, and games.

Transition

Transitioning from space to space can overwhelm adults with ASD since each space offers different stimuli and experiences. Kingwood College suggests that the best way to ease transitions between spaces is to provide indicators between each space, such as signs or structural markers.

Wilderness

Kingwood College designed this green space to engage adults with ASD in a more natural environment while encouraging social development, special interests, and physical exercise. To create an inclusive and enjoyable space for adults with autism, many theaters, sporting arenas, and stadiums now offer sensory-friendly rooms. Generally, these sensory-friendly rooms are sound-proofed and contain small toys or objects adults with autism can use to relieve stress. Furthermore, several stadiums offer sensory-friendly bags to children and adults with ASD at the beginning of the sporting event and contain fidget toys, noise-canceling headphones, sunglasses, etc.

Social Participation

Challenges

All of the above domains of age-friendly livability may negatively influence social participation in adults with ASD. It is difficult to participate in social events when outcasted, ill, or overwhelmed by a space. Adults with ASD reported the following number of days a year taking part in these activities, on average: walking/exercising (117 days), hobbies (54 days), time with relatives (48 days), recreational activities (33 days), time with coworkers (30 days), time with friends/neighbors (24 days), religious services (19 days), traveling (5 days), and social event-religious group (3 days) (DaWalt et al., 2019). This level of social participation is less than the general population, and adults with ASD living with their families experienced further negative social impact and higher levels of family social isolation (DaWalt et al., 2019). Social anxiety also often complicates the social experiences of adults with ASD, particularly those who want to engage with others but worry about failing in social situations (Maddox & White, 2015). Individuals with more severe ASD and high social anxiety are more likely to want to spend time alone (Chen et al., 2015).

A study assessing friendships of adults with ASD (age 18-81 years) found that people with ASD rated their friendships poorer than those without ASD (Sedgewick, Leppanen, & Tchanturia, 2019; Baron-Cohen & Wheelwright, 2003). Adults and older adults with ASD report a longing for friendship, social connectivity, and closeness, but they have difficulty communicating or initiating such companionship (Muller, Schuler, and Yates, 2008; Waldron et al., 2021). Sedgewick and colleagues (2019) went on to report that adults with ASD's relationships with best friends and romantic partners did not vary from the comparison group. Perhaps, for some adults with ASD, friendship is more about quality than quantity. This was true for those who had such relationships, but many do not have such relationships. One participant in Muller and colleagues' study (2008) expressed this articulately, craving "a little bit more closeness and friendship without getting too close, because I myself have a very limited tolerance of closeness in relationships" (p. 180). The goal of getting close, but not too close, further complicates social participation and friendship in this group.

Supportive Policies and Programs

Muller and colleagues (2008) suggested the following social supports to help increase social participation for adults with ASD: external support, communication supports, self-care, and open-mindedness or supportive attitudes (e.g., understanding companions). Evidence suggests that social skills training intervention decreases social isolation and improves social skills in adults with ASD (Gantman et al., 2012). Community groups, such as music therapy, are an innovative social activity that anyone can participate in (Shiloh & Blythe, 2014). At their musical performances, "The Musical Autist," a non-profit developed by C.J. Shiloh, show-goers proudly tout their motto "hand flapping allowed," which welcomes self-stimulation that our culture sometimes tries to shut down (Shiloh & Blythe, 2014). "The Musical Autist," advocates for acceptance and access to the community for people with ASD and everyone through a shared love of music (Shiloh & Blythe, 2014, p. 114). Community gardens, such as the Kingwood College in London, also offer physically and socially engaging activities for adults with autism. Older adults with ASD may also engage in Medicare's SilverSneakers Program or partake in Special Olympics to increase both their physical activity and social engagement (Stancliffe et al., 2017; Waldron et al., 2021).

Transportation

Challenges

"Transportation can be the biggest barrier to adults living productive and joyful lives and is the key to success in the workplace, in the community and in gaining personal independence" (Advancing the Futures for Adults with Autism, 2009, p. 8). In addition, transportation is costly for families if an individual is unable to navigate public transit; one mother reported spending $700 a month on her adult daughter's transportation (Lubin & Feely, 2016). Other parents report having to drive their adult children with ASD themselves because of safety concerns or no other available options (Lubin & Feely, 2016). This worsened during the COVID-19 pandemic when day habilitation and community programs sold their fleets of vehicles to stay financially afloat and/or could not find contracted drivers to transport adults with ASD. Some adults with ASD also report difficulty with public transit systems. They report challenges getting to the bus/train stop, paying fares, engaging with drivers, coping with fear and anxiety of unpredictability of stimuli, finding a seat, and they and their guardians fear their vulnerability to crime (Deka et al., 2016; Kinnaer et al., 2016). In Canada, when it comes to transportation for people with ASD, "currently [experience] a patchwork of services, availability, quality and access" (Dudley & Zwicker, 2016, p. 2). Such inconsistency in routes and fragmented services make accessing public transit extremely challenging and unpredictable for people with ASD who often thrive in routines.

So, how do these individuals get around? In a recent study by Deka and colleagues (2016), primary modes of transit for adults with ASD over the previous three months suggested the following; only approximately 1.6% of respondents drove themselves, while 35.8% were passengers in a car with family, 7.3% rode in a car with friends, 6.3% rode in a car with a volunteer, 15% reported walking, 6.6% used a complimentary disability transit made possible by the Americans with Disability Act, 11.6% rode a public bus or van, 3.9% used a taxi or hired car, and small percentages of respondents reported other transit usage, such as that provided by schools, day habilitation programs, group homes, and other services. Nearly half of respondents reported needing transportation to get to work, and 58% needed support getting to educational, vocational, or job training (Deka et al., 2016). People also needed transportation for errands, religious services, appointments, and visits to see friends and family (Deka et al., 2016).

Of course, when people cannot get to the places they want or need to go, this has negative consequences on their lives. Some people lose their jobs, experience social isolation or depression, and cannot make it to doctor appointments, a grave concern for individuals with medical complexities (Lubin & Feely, 2016). Zalewska and colleagues (2016) found that young adults with ASD who could drive themselves or had another mode of independent transportation, such as biking or walking, were significantly more likely to have a job. Still, older adults with ASD may be less likely to sustain such physical activity as a mode of transit.

Though older adult drivers rank behind teenagers and young adults when it comes to crash rates, they suffer from the highest rates of fatality in car crashes because of their often-declining overall health status (Tefft, 2017). Not much is yet known about older drivers with ASD. However, limited research available on driving proficiency in adults with ASD suggests mixed findings. About a third of adolescents with ASD attain their license compared to nearly 84% of adolescents in the general population, and they do so approximately nine months later than their peers without ASD (Curry et al., 2018). Bishop and colleagues (2017) found that drivers (age 16–30 years) without ASD responded significantly faster to social hazards (e.g., child pedestrian, a cyclist in the road) than non-social hazards (e.g., a head-on crash) using a driving simulation, while adults with ASD did not differentiate between which types of hazards needed a fast-acting response (Bishop et al., 2017). Cox and colleagues (2015) found that adults with ASD (age 15–23 years) demonstrated slower steering response times and showed worse tactical driving (e.g., hitting the car ahead, swerving, lane changes) than drivers without ASD. Some of these challenges are working memory issues or difficulty processing information from driving inputs (e.g., road signs, pedestrians) while performing a task (e.g., braking, steering).

Supportive Programs and Policies

A range of solutions may help support adults and older adults with ASD as they navigate transportation. Some of these suggestions may also benefit the general population, such as improving the reliability of public transit altogether; though costly, reconstructing public transit is perhaps the most effective strategy (Dudley & Zwicker, 2016). Dudley and Zwicker (2016) suggest training adults with disabilities on how to use public transportation, as done in Ontario as part of "The Passport Program." Additionally, Europe bolster their transit with staff at transfers, audio support, technology, and clear signage to help people navigate public transit (International Transport Forum, 2009). Given that adults with ASD experience accelerated aging and have shortened life expectancies, perhaps transportation companies could widen their age range or remove age restrictions altogether to better accommodate adults with disabilities who may not meet their age qualifications.

Increasing the number of capable drivers with ASD would also help relieve transportation-related stressors. After reviewing the literature of 22 studies on vehicle transportation challenges for individuals with ASD (ages 2 years–35 years) across six countries, Lindsay (2016) declared "an urgent need for further transportation-related training and support for people with ASD" encouraging training and driving lessons for people with ASD, advocacy from clinicians and educators for more programming, options, and training to support these drivers, and more research (p. 837).

Housing

Challenges

As parents age and are unable to care for their adult children with ASD at older ages, housing is a critical concern for this population and their loved ones. In a recent study, 22 participants with ASD were surveyed; approximately 14% of participants were living alone, 73% were living with parents, and 14% did not answer (Lubin & Feeley, 2016). While not all individuals with ASD are capable or ready to live entirely independently, there are several options for housing based on individuals' needs. This does not, however, come without concerns. There have been many cases of abuse within these types of living options. In the State of Massachusetts, according to the Disabled Persons Protection Commissioner annual report, 2,214 cases of alleged abuse of people with disabilities were sent to the district attorney's office in FY 2019 (Commonwealth of MA, 2019).

As adults with ASD age, however, they may want to relocate to finally exert their independence and gain a sense of freedom. However, finding accessible and affordable housing can be complicated for this group. Owning a home, the ultimate sign of self-independence, can be mentally and physically discouraging for adults with ASD (Kinnaer et al., 2016). For an adult with ASD, maintaining a home and doing daily tasks (e.g., cleaning, doing laundry, cooking) can be discouraging, uninteresting, and unimportant (Kinnaer et al., 2016). Finding and financing caregiver support are often two key challenges. If adults with ASD fail to maintain their homes, they could be at risk for physical health complications. In addition, forgetfulness, lack of depth perception, and difficulty with temperature regulation may make living alone dangerous for adults with ASD (Kinnaer et al., 2016).

Supportive Programs and Policies

There are a few options for housing available to adults with ASD made possible by the U.S Supreme Courts 1999 landmark decision in the Olmstead v. L.C, which found the unjustified segregation of people with disabilities is a form of unlawful discrimination under the Americans with Disabilities Act. Today, the Olmstead Act of 1999 defends the civil rights of individuals with ASD to live in the community when "community placement is appropriate, the transfer from institutional care to a less restrictive setting is not opposed by the affected individual, and the placement can be reasonably accommodated, taking into account the resources available to the State and the needs of others with mental disabilities." (Olmstead v. L.C., 1999, p. 587). Adults with ASD may live independently, with family or friends, group homes, adult foster care, or institutional care facilities. In Mission, Kansas, "The Mission Project" provides a safe and supportive community for adults with disabilities, such as ASD, that offers jobs, services, retail, entertainment, parks, and community centers, all within walking distance (2021). Institutions are a last resort for adults with ASD, given the trauma, abuse, and neglect associated with institutional care for individuals with disabilities prior to the Olmstead Act of 1999. Therefore, smaller group homes may be a better option than nursing homes, especially for those who experience social and sensory overwhelm as part of their ASD.

Civic Participation and Employment

Challenges

As described in Chapter 16, civic participation and employment are often difficult for people with ASD. An inconsistent work history over the adult lifespan sets people up for financial instability in late life. In Canada, approximately 74% of adults are employed, compared to 22% of adults with ASD (Bizier et al., 2015). In the U.S., Howlin and colleagues (2013) reported that 55% of adults with ASD had either never worked or reported sustained unemployment, and an additional 15% worked either in a sheltered workshop or volunteered, suggesting that a total of 70% of the 60 participants with ASD received little or no employment income. Approximately 20% worked in skilled labor jobs (Howlin et al., 2013).

There are several barriers to employment for this group. Stigma surrounding ASD can impede employment of adults with ASD (Scott et al., 2017; Johnson & Joshi, 2016). Communication challenges also impede employment for people with ASD, and some people with ASD believed that disclosing their ASD diagnosis led to a lack of hire (Nicholas, Zwaigenbaum, et al., 2018; Walsh et al., 2017). Adults with ASD may feel "demoralized and more reluctant to pursue future employment" after being under-supported at or let go from a job (Nicholas, Zwaigenbaum, et al., 2018, p. 699). Continued failures and disappointment in employment may accumulate over the lifetime, making aging with ASD all the more difficult

Supportive Policies and Programs

A model adapted from Bronfenbrenner's ecological systems theory (1977) uses nested levels to explain how barriers and supports to the employment of persons with ASD manifest at the individual, family, agency, workplace/employer, community support, and public policy levels (Nicholas, Mitchell, et al., 2018).

Another integrated model presented in Figure 19.3 incorporates structural/programmatic issues, family navigation and support, community/workplace capacity, and tailored individual supports as the four pillars of access, engagement, and retention invocations (Nicholas, Zwaigenbaum et al., 2018). These two models may offer guidance as communities and employers increasingly integrate adults with ASD into the workforce.

Walsh and colleagues (2017) launched a pilot training program, "ACCESS," to increase social skills in adults with ASD in an attempt to increase employment. Participants with ASD and ID showed statistically significant increases in the following social skills: peer (e.g., listening, greeting, negotiating, expressing negative emotion), adult-related (e.g., doing quality work, working independently, responding), and self-related (e.g., organizing, self-control, self-esteem). Social skills are often complex for people with ASD, which impedes their employability. The Massachusetts Inclusive Concurrent Enrollment Initiative (MAICEI) is a program available at several community colleges and state universities in MA that offers job skills training, course offerings, professional etiquette seminars, and coaching to 18–22-year-olds with ASD (Massachusetts Department of Education, 2022). Options such as this for older adults with ASD would support professional development over the lifespan. Employers of adults with ASD generally report positive experiences in hiring adults with ASD included improvements in workplace inclusion, strong work ethic, and good quality of work with great attention to detail by employees with ASD (Scott et al., 2017). Only 19% reported struggles in relations between employees with and without ASD. People

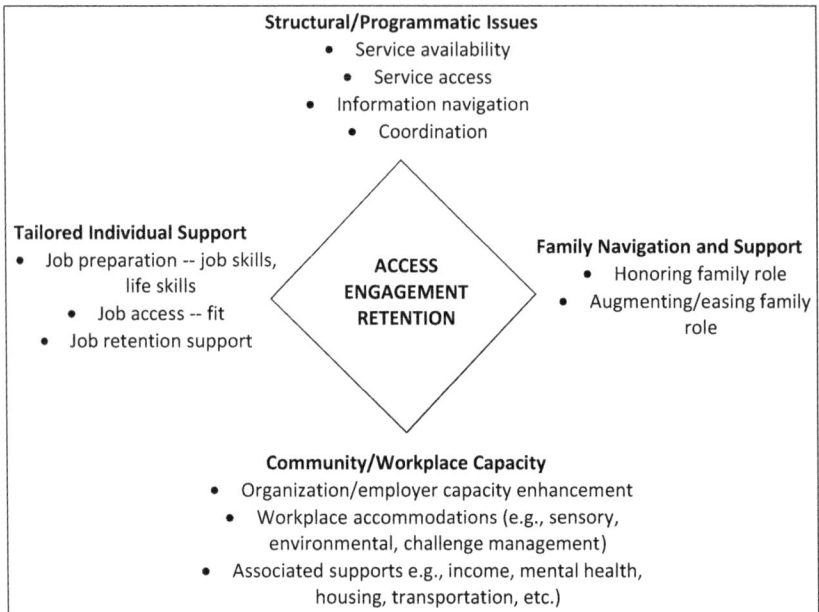

Figure 19.3 Integrated Resources for Vocational Opportunity Advancement in ASD.

Notes: From "Evaluation of employment-support services for adults with autism spectrum disorder" by Nicholas, D. B., Zwaigenbaum, L., Zwicker, J., Clarke, M. E., Lamsal, R., Stoddart, K. P., Carroll, C., Muskat, B., Spoelstra, M., & Lowe, K. 2018, *Autism*, 22(6), 693–702, Copyright 2021 by The Authors.

with ASD were more likely to work part-time and earned $1.65 less an hour than their neurotypical peers. Employers incurred no additional costs for the training and supervision of adults with ASD compared to those without ASD.

Communication and Information

Challenges

Communication has implications for how one attains and processes information and engages in all aspects of life. Communication problems and corresponding social isolation are likely to have health-related consequences in older adulthood for individuals with autism (American Psychiatric Association (APA, 2013). Communication skills and language abilities of individuals with autism vary, as outlined in chapter eight. Communication impairments of individuals with ASD tend to persist throughout life and lead to poorer social and health outcomes, such as lower employment rates, worsened mental health, poor academic outcomes, and fewer social relationships later in life (Cimera & Cowan, 2009; Whitehouse et al., 2009; Howlin et al., 2013). Some adults with ASD and their families underutilize available occupational therapy, physiotherapy, speech and language therapy, and counseling (Howlin et al., 2013), while others simply cannot afford services. Poor communication skills may significantly impact individuals with ASD as they grow older, but more research is needed in this realm.

Supportive Policies and Programs

Augmentative and alternative communication (AAC) systems (i.e., writing, drawing, and pointing to objects or images) are effective communication tools for individuals with ASD (Ganz et al., 2013; Gordon et al., 2011; Hidecker, 2010). However, there are very few studies that involve adults with ASD who have complex communication needs. A case study by Hong et al. (2014) found significant associations between the caregiver support and the user's appropriate use of an Apple iPad equipped with the app Tap to Talk™. This app displays pictures and outputs a word, developed for all age groups who rely on AAC systems to communicate.

Difficulties with social-emotional reciprocity, social approach, conversation, reduced sharing of interests or emotions, and difficulty initiating or responding to social interactions can interfere with social conversation and social relationships for individuals with ASD (Koegel et al., 2016). In a 2016 study, three adults ages 19–26 with ASD who experienced social difficulties in empathetic communication skills underwent weekly intervention sessions (about 40 minutes long) using video feedback (Koegel et al., 2016). All three participants showed significant improvement in targeted communication skills and empathy expression, increased use of empathetic verbal questions throughout their conversations, and felt more confident in their ability to communicate with others after the intervention (Koegel et al., 2016). Of the three participants, two showed long-term improvement in empathetic communication skills (Koegel et al., 2016). The two studies suggest that intervention effectively increases communication skills for adults with ASD. In addition, these studies lay a foundation for future research in social communication with larger sample sizes and in older adults with ASD.

Conclusion

Our society is ill-prepared to support the aging population with ASD across the eight domains of livability: respect and social inclusion, community support and health services, social participation, transportation, housing, outdoor spaces and buildings, civic participation, and employment, and communication and information, as defined by the Age-Friendly Communities Framework. Raymaker and colleagues (2020) put aging with ASD in perspective with their definition of "autistic burnout: a syndrome conceptualized as resulting from chronic life stress and a mismatch of expectations and abilities without adequate support. It is characterized by pervasive, long-term (typically 3+ months) exhaustion, loss of function, and reduced tolerance to stimulus" (p. 133). The implications are greater for the "autistic burnout" of older adults having spent an entire life course dealing with great stress and little support.

Communities, healthcare systems, social systems, public works, and many other stakeholders must take responsibility and concrete action to reform systems to best accommodate aging persons with ASD and future cohorts. As Age-Friendly Communities gain momentum across the globe, communities behind these initiatives must consider those aging with ASD. As the prospect of long term "autistic burnout" looms for the soon to be millions of people aging with ASD, research on aging and ASD is *just* now emerging. The following case studies provide the stories of adults with ASD at varied stages in their aging journeys and provide context as to how these individuals navigate challenges across the eight domains of livability.

Case Studies

Case Study 1

Warren, a 29-year-old man with ASD, participated in the interview using his communication device along with his mother/guardian, Rosalie. He received his diagnosis at the age of two and a half years old after some regression in his speech. Shortly after his diagnosis, his family moved to Australia for about five years. They were told that a family with a special needs child should not leave the states but do not think the care they received abroad impacted Warren's health or quality of life today. Warren has diabetes, epilepsy, and Celiac disease, and no mental health conditions. He enjoys swimming, walking, and working out with his personal trainer and has a broad palate when it comes to food! His mother serves as his care coordinator. Warren lives with his mother, father, and one brother in a town in Massachusetts. He attends a day program for adults with disabilities but cannot go out into the community to volunteer as he used to because of COVID-19. Though fully vaccinated, the risk of illness remains too high. His mother drives him to and from his program because the driver assigned to him has no training in responding to seizures, and this is also a risk not worth taking.

The family's concerns regarding aging include housing, navigating systems such as Medicaid, Warren's future finances, his accelerated aging, and his parents' own aging. Rosalie envisions Warren living with a live-in staff person in an apartment across the hall from herself and her husband within a community of families with similar dynamics. Still, Warren's brothers want him to stay at home with them in the future. Their parents do not want to leave them with this responsibility. Rosalie also does not know how much a live-in staff person will cost in the long run, so Warren's father plans to work "until he dies" to save as much money as possible for Warren. Warren receives support from Social Security, has MassHealth, and will be a lifelong beneficiary of his father's employer's private health insurance plan. Keeping track of the paperwork for these programs is a bit of a nightmare. Each year, someone needs to reapply for Warren's private health insurance in order for him to maintain this benefit. Quite frankly–it is all too much. Rosalie worries about passing this burden on to Warren's brothers, his future guardians. Rosalie is also concerned about how adults with ASD accumulate health comorbidities earlier in life than most. She and her husband are aging, too, making the future full of uncertainty. Though she is grateful for their health at the moment, she fears the future.

Case Study 2

Cameron, a 57-year-old non-binary autistic person living in the midwestern region of the U.S, raised their/her four children as a single mother after a divorce. They/she remains close with their/her childhood best friend, and they are both happily grandmothers! They/she describes their/her health as fragile; Cameron has Ehlers-Danlos syndrome, a rare connective tissue disorder that makes their/her joints hyperextend, mast cell activation syndrome that can trigger allergic reaction-like symptoms, and post-traumatic stress disorder (PTSD). Cameron received an ASD diagnosis at age 41 after one of their/her children received a diagnosis, and the child's psychologist suggested they/she, too, get an assessment.

Growing up, they/she had a difficult time with sensory input in school. Their/her teachers believed that they/she had hearing loss, but Cameron could hear *everything*, and this was too much, so they/she zoned out in class sometimes. Though Cameron excelled in the classroom, their/her parents brought them/her to several specialists to address social concerns. At the time, physicians believed only boys, not girls could have ASD. Upon reflecting on their/her childhood, Cameron felt pressured by culture to act in a certain way, taught to "mask" to fit into a social setting, and misgendered as female (e.g., given a baby doll to play with and reprimanded when they/she was disappointed), despite feeling like they/her were a person, not a gender.

Today, Cameron lives in a society that oppresses both LGBTQ+ persons and autistic individuals. People are disrespectful and sometimes downright cruel, especially online. To the point where they/she does not believe they/she would have come out as autistic if they/she knew what backlash lay ahead. Cameron only mentions their/her ASD in conversation when absolutely necessary even in a medical setting to avoid negative consequences, such as not getting a ventilator during the COVID-19 pandemic based on rationing of care by disability status. Cameron directs an autistic advocacy organization and previously had a long, fruitful career as a social worker for children at risk of entering the foster care system. She gets around in their/her own car but waited until their/her mid-twenties to attain a driver's license because of a fear of driving and the overwhelm of too many moving parts to keep track of while behind the wheel. While Cameron doesn't often think about the future or aging, their/her established patterns of routine and behavior suggest they/she will put their/her best foot forward. They/she have already built their/her life in a way that minimizes the challenges associated with ASD. Their/her home has lighting and noise levels that do not trigger their/her sensory sensitivities, and they/she even plans their/her afternoon walk to face away from the bright setting sun. Cameron's suggestion for children soon to be aging with ASD is to be yourself and do not waste time trying to befriend anyone who doesn't easily accept you.

Case Study 3

Cheryl is a 60-year-old woman living with ASD in Essex in the UK. She has three children with ASD and several other neurotypical children. Cheryl received her ASD diagnosis at age 55 after her manager at the autism advocacy center she worked at suggested that she get assessed. Due to wait times up to five years in the UK's National Health Service, she opted for an assessment through a private practice, which cost £1500, the equivalent of nearly $2,000 in U.S. currency. At first, Cheryl told almost no one about her diagnosis, but now she feels comfortable sharing. She is of relatively good health but has asthma, and right now, a fractured shoulder. Cheryl also has depression and anxiety that are at times crippling but right now managed with medications prescribed by two General Practitioners (GP). Cheryl walks 12,500 steps every day and abides by a healthy vegetarian diet. She neither drinks nor smokes. Cheryl reports having very consistent employment as a welfare advisor in the courts, and in fact, hasn't taken one day off in twelve years, aside from holidays. She owns her own home and saves most of her money, a lasting repercussion of an impoverished childhood.

She had one or two childhood friends but did not like to go out and do things with them. Cheryl's mother sold her into a pedophile ring in childhood, where Cheryl sadly experienced horrible sexual abuse, but does not believe she experiences life-altering trauma from this abuse. She doesn't dwell on the sadness; it is something that happened, but she has moved on and says that in this regard, "autism is my saving grace." Estranged from most of her family, she looks to her four or five friends for companionship. She is pleased with her friendships, except for when they do things like take her to the theater, which she hates because you must sit near people. She has had "a load of [romantic] relationships," most notably two husbands. expressing that her own emotions felt like too much to handle in each relationship, never mind that of her partners'.

Cheryl fears aging because she may need to go into a hospital; she is "petrified" of hospitals" because of the forced socialization, yet also fears social isolation when her adult children move out. She also wonders, "What if I get dementia?" and dreads the thought of nursing homes, again because of socialization, but also because of sensory overwhelm, such as loud TVs and even the sound of other residents turning newspapers.

Case Study 4

At 88 years old, Matthew sits in his kitchen reflecting on a life of isolation; 'I didn't slip through the cracks [of the system]...I was free falling.' Though diagnosed in childhood with ADHD, depression, and a learning disability, Matthew didn't receive his Asperger's and ASD diagnoses until he was 70 years old. This late-life diagnosis, however, meant everything to him. So many things made sense in hindsight. He reports having no friends and no close relationships over his life course. He has never had sex or an intimate partner but identifies as bisexual with a gay leaning. Matthew battled cancer in his sixties, and when asked who supported him through that, he said: "mostly myself." He provided care to his aging mother in failing health years later. As a child, Matthew struggled in school and then joined the military in WWII, which he described as a "disaster." No one understood or accepted Matthew for who he was, and he did not get along with other people, something that negatively impacted nearly every aspect of his life. He went on to get a Masters in English but never attained stable employment, jumping from job to job and state to state more often than most.

Today, Matthew lives alone in assisted housing. He attends a support group with others on the spectrum once a week and has an in-home aid who helps him with groceries and other day-to-day tasks, weekly. Matthew calls his brother on Thursdays at 7 pm, and though they now have aging in common, he wouldn't describe their relationship as close. Matthew's health is deteriorating; he has high cholesterol, high blood pressure, prostatic hyperplasia, anemia, an overactive thyroid, kidney stones, depression, and anxiety. He has Medicare, as well as private health coverage to offset the cost of prescription drugs not covered by Medicare Part D. He manages his own medications, walks 7-8,000 steps daily, eats a primarily healthy vegetarian diet, and manages his own finances. Matthew walks everywhere because he fears driving and can recite statistics of fatalities in motor vehicle crashes each year off the top of his head. He receives financial support through Social Security, but not as much he would if he had stable employment in his younger years. His greatest fear is that he will outlive his financial means, and his greatest coping mechanism for life's challenges is sleeping.

Case Study Discussion Questions

1. How does Warren's transportation compare to the other case studies?
2. What are some of the concerns the family has due to Warren's aging?

3. What signs did Cameron show in their/her earlier years that made sense to them/her after being diagnosed with ASD so late in his adulthood?
4. What are some reasons why Cameron may be hesitant to open up about their/her diagnosis?
5. How has Cheryl shown that she is capable of taking care of herself being an adult with ASD?
6. Describe her adult communication and relationship skills.
7. What are some of Cheryl's fears of aging that could be related to her ASD diagnosis?
8. What signs did Matthew show in his earlier years that made sense to him after being diagnosed with ASD so late in his adulthood?
9. Should Matthew be concerned about outliving his financial means? Why?
10. Describe Matthew's housing situation in comparison to the other case study participants.

References

AARP. (2021). AARP Network of Age-Friendly States and Communities. www. aarp.org/livable-communities/network-age-friendly-communities/

Advancing futures for adults with autism (AFAA). (2009). Retrieved March 27, 2022, from www.afaa-us.org/storage/documents/AFAA_2009_Think_Tank_R eport__Addendum.pdf

Age friendly communities. Council on Aging of Central Oregon.(COA) (2020). Retrieved March 28, 2022, from www.councilonaging.org/blog/age-friendly-communities/

American Psychiatric Association. (1980). Diagnostic and statistical manual of mental disorders (3rd ed., text rev.). Washington, DC: Author.

American Psychiatric Association. (2013). Diagnostic and statistical manual of mental disorders (5th ed., text rev.). Washington, DC: Author.

Baron-Cohen, S., Wheelwright, S., Skinner, R., Martin, J., & Clubley, E. (2001). The autism-spectrum quotient (AQ): Evidence from Asperger syndrome/high-functioning autism, males and females, scientists and mathematicians. Journal of Autism and Developmental Disorders, 31(1), 5–17. https://doi.org/10.1023/a:1005653411471

Baron-Cohen, S., & Wheelwright, S. (2003). The Friendship Questionnaire: An investigation of adults with Asperger syndrome or high-functioning autism, and normal sex differences. Journal of Autism and Developmental Disorders, 33(5), 509–517. https://doi.org/10.1023/a:1025879411971

Beadle-Brown, J., Roberts, R. and Mills, R. (2009). "Person-centred approaches to supporting children and adults with autism spectrum disorders." Tizard Learning Disability Review, 14(3), 18–26. https://doi.org/10.1108/135954 74200900024

Beadle-Brown, J. and Mills, R. (2010). Understanding and Supporting Children and Adults on the Autism Spectrum, Pavilion Publishing, Brighton.

Bishop, H. J., Biasini, F. J., & Stavrinos, D. (2017). Social and Non-social Hazard Response in Drivers with Autism Spectrum Disorder. *Journal of Autism and Developmental Disorders,* 47(4), 905–917. https://doi.org/10.1007/s10 803-016-2992-1

Bizier, C., Fawcett, G., Gilbert, S., & Marshall, C. (2015). Develop- mental disabilities among Canadians aged 15 years and older, 2012. Statistics Canada Catalogue no. 89-654-X2015003. Retrieved from www150.statcan.gc.ca/n1/pub/89-654-x/89-654-x2015003-eng.pdf

Blaxill, M., Rogers, T., & Nevison, C. (2021). Autism Tsunami: the Impact of Rising Prevalence on the Societal Cost of Autism in the United States. *Journal of Autism and Developmental Disorders,* 1–17. https://link.springer.com/arti cle/10.1007/s10803-021-05120-7

Bronfenbrenner, U. (1977). Toward an experimental ecology of human development. *American psychologist, 32*(7), 513. https://psycnet.apa.org/doi/10.1037/0003-066X.32.7.513

Cascio, M. A., Weiss, J. A., & Racine, E. (2021). Making autism research inclusive by attending to intersectionality: a review of the research ethics literature. *Review Journal of Autism and Developmental Disorders, 8*(1), 22–36. https://doi.org/10.1007/s40489-020-00204-z

CDC. (2017). Life expectancy. Retrieved January 25, 2018 from www.cdc.gov/nchs/fastats/life-expectancy.htm

CDC. (2020). Data & Statistics on Autism Spectrum Disorder. Retrieved from www.cdc.gov/ncbddd/autism/data.html

Chen, Y. W., Bundy, A., Cordier, R., Chien, Y. L., & Einfeld, S. (2016). The experience of social participation in everyday contexts among individuals with autism spectrum disorders: An experience sampling study. *Journal of Autism and Developmental Disorders, 46*(4), 1403–1414. https://doi.org/10.1007/s10 803-015-2682-4

Cimera, R. E., & Cowan, R. J. (2009). The costs of services and employment outcomes achieved by adults with autism in the US. *Autism, 13*(3), 285-302.

Commonwealth of Massachusetts. (2019). *DPPC annual report (FY2019).* DSpace Home. Retrieved March 27, 2022, from https://archives.lib.state.ma.us/handle/2452/808658

Cox, S. M., Cox, D. J., Kofler, M. J., Moncrief, M. A., Johnson, R. J., Lambert, A. E., Cain, S. A., & Reeve, R. E. (2016). Driving Simulator Performance in Novice Drivers with Autism Spectrum Disorder: The Role of Executive Functions and Basic Motor Skills. *Journal of Autism and Developmental Disorders, 46*(4), 1379–1391. https://doi.org/10.1007/s10803-015-2677-1

Crenshaw, K. (1989). Demarginalizing the intersection of race and sex: ablack feminist critique of antidiscrimination doctrine, feminist theory and antiracist politics. University of Chicago Legal Forum, 139–167.

Croen, L. A., Zerbo, O., Qian, Y., Massolo, M. L., Rich, S., Sidney, S., & Kripke, C. (2015). The health status of adults on the autism spectrum. *Autism, 19*(7), 814–823. https://doi.org/10.1177/1362361315577517

Curry, A. E., Yerys, B. E., Huang, P., & Metzger, K. B. (2018). Longitudinal study of driver licensing rates among adolescents and young adults with autism spectrum disorder. *Autism: The International Journal of Research and Practice,* 22(4), 479–488. https://doi.org/10.1177/1362361317699586

DaWalt, L. S., Usher, L. V., Greenberg, J. S., & Mailick, M. R. (2019). Friendships and social participation as markers of quality of life of adolescents and adults with fragile X syndrome and autism. *Autism,* 23(2), 383–393. https://doi.org/10.1177/1362361317709202

Deka, D., Feeley, C., & Lubin, A. (2016). Travel Patterns, Needs, and Barriers of Adults with Autism Spectrum Disorder. *Transportation Research Record,* 2542(1), 9–16. https://doi.org/10.3141/2542-02

Dewinter J, De Graaf H, Begeer S. (2017). Sexual Orientation, Gender Identity, and Romantic Relationships in Adolescents and Adults with Autism Spectrum Disorder. *J Autism Dev Disord,* 47(9):2927–2934. https://doi.org/10.1007/s10803-017-3199-9

Department of Health. (2014). Think Autism. Fulfilling and Rewarding Lives, the strategy for Adults With Autism in England: An Update. Department of Health, London.

Dietz, P. M., Rose, C. E., McArthur, D., & Maenner, M. (2020). National and state estimates of adults with autism spectrum disorder. *Journal of Autism and Developmental Disorders,* 50(12), 4258–4266. https://doi.org/10.1007/s10803-020-04494-4

Dudley, C., & Zwicker, J. D. (2016). Mind the gap: Transportation challenges for individuals living with autism spectrum disorder. *The School of Public Policy Publications,* 9, 1–5. https://doi.org/10.11575/sppp.v9i0.42559

Eilenberg, J. S., Paff, M., Harrison, A. J., & Long, K. A. (2019). Disparities based on race, ethnicity, and socioeconomic status over the transition to adulthood among adolescents and young adults on the autism spectrum: a systematic review. *Current Psychiatry Reports,* 21(5), 1–16. https://doi.org/10.1007/s11920-019-1016-1

Family-Based Future Planning For Autism In Adulthood. Family-based future planning for autism in adulthood. (n.d.). Retrieved March 27, 2022, from https://sites.bu.edu/familyfuture/

Fombonne, E. (2009). Epidemiology of pervasive developmental disorders. *Pediatric Research,* 65(6), 591–8. https://doi.org/10.1203/pdr.0b013e31819e7203

Gantman, A., Kapp, S. K., Orenski, K., & Laugeson, E. A. (2012). Social skills training for young adults with high-functioning autism spectrum disorders: A randomized controlled pilot study. *Journal of Autism and Developmental Disorders,* 42(6), 1094–1103. https://doi.org/10.1007/s10803-011-1350-6

Ganz, J. B., Hong, E. R., & Goodwyn, F. D. (2013). Effectiveness of the PECS Phase III app and choice between the app and traditional PECS among pre-schoolers with ASD. *Research in Autism Spectrum Disorders,* 7, 973–983 http://dx.doi.org/10.1016/j.rasd.2013.04.003

Gaudion, K., and McGinley, C. (2012). Outdoor Environments for Adults with Autism. *Helen Hamlyn Center for Design, Royal College of Art.* ISBN: 978-1-907342-64-6

George, R., Stokes, M. A. (2018). "A Quantitative Analysis of Mental Health Among Sexual and Gender Minority Groups in ASD", *J Autism Dev Disord.* Jun;48(6):2052–2063. https://doi.org/10.1007/s10803-018-3469-1

Gordon, K., Pasco, G., McElduff, F., Wade, A., Howlin, P., & Charman, T. (2011). A communication-based intervention for nonverbal children with autism: What changes? Who Benefits? *Journal of Consulting and Clinical Psychology, 79,* 447-457. doi:10.1037/a0024379

Gould, J. and Ashton-Smith, J. (2011), Missed diagnosis or misdiagnosis? Girls and women on the autism spectrum. *Good Autism Practice, 12*(21), 34–41.

Hidecker, M. J. C. (2010). Early AAC Intervention: Some International Perspectives. *Perspectives on Augmentative and Alternative Communication, 19*(1), 3-4.

Hillier, A., Gallop, N., Mendes, E., Tellez, D., Buckingham, A., Nizami, A., & O'Toole, D. (2019). LGBTQ + and autism spectrum disorder: Experiences and challenges. *International Journal of Transgender Health, 21*(1), 98–110. https://doi.org/10.1080/15532739.2019.1594484

Hirvikoski, T., Mittendorfer-Rutz, E., Boman, M., Larsson, H., Lichtenstein, P., & Bölte, S. (2016). Premature mortality in autism spectrum disorder. *The British Journal of Psychiatry, 208*(3), 232–238. https://doi.org/10.1192/bjp.bp.114.160192

Hong, E. R., Ganz, J. B., Gilliland, W., & Ninci, J. (2014). Teaching caregivers to implement an augmentative and alternative communication intervention to an adult with ASD. *Research in Autism Spectrum Disorders, 8,* 570–580. https://do/10.1016/j.rasd. 2014.01.012

Howlin, P., Moss, P., Savage, S., & Rutter, M. (2013). Social outcomes in mid-to later adulthood among individuals diagnosed with autism and average nonverbal IQ as children. *Journal of the American Academy of Child & Adolescent Psychiatry, 52*(6), 572–581. https://doi.org/10.1016/j.jaac.2013.02.017

International Transport Forum. (2009). *Cognitive Impairment, Mental Health and Transport Design with Everyone in Mind.* Retrieved March 27, 2022, from www.itf-oecd.org/sites/default/files/docs/09cognitive.pdf

Jariwala-Parikh, K., Barnard, M., Holmes, E. R., West-Strum, D., Bentley, J. P., Banahan, B., & Khanna, R. (2019). Autism prevalence in the medicaid program and healthcare utilization and costs among adult enrollees diagnosed with autism. *Administration and Policy in Mental Health and Mental Health Services Research, 46*(6), 768–776. https://doi.org/10.1007/s10 488-019-00960-z

Kaiser Family Foundation. (2020). Distribution of the nonelderly with Medicaid by Race/Ethnicity. Retrieved November 29, 2021, from www.kff.org/medicaid/state-indicator/medicaid-distribution-nonelderly-by-raceethnic ity/?currentTimeframe=11&sortModel=%7B%22colId%22%3A%22Locat ion%22%2C%22sort%22%3A%22asc%22%7D

King, C., Merrick, H., & Le Couteur, A. (2020). How should we support young people with ASD and mental health problems as they navigate the transition to adult life including access to adult healthcare services. *Epidemiology and Psychiatric Sciences, 29,* e90. https://dx.doi.org/10.1017%2FS204579601 9000830

Kinnaer, M., Baumers, S., & Heylighen, A. (2016). Autism-friendly architecture from the outside in and the inside out: an explorative study based on autobiographies of autistic people. *Journal of Housing and the Built Environment, 31*(2), 179–195. www.jstor.org/stable/43907378

Koegel, L. K., Ashbaugh, K., Navab, A. et al. (2016). Improving Empathic Communication Skills in Adults with Autism Spectrum Disorder. J Autism Dev Disord 46, 921–933 https://doi.org/10.1007/s10803-015-2633-0

La Roche, M. J., Bush, H. H., & D'Angelo, E. (2018). The assessment and treatment of autism spectrum disorder: A cultural examination. *Practice Innovations, 3*(2), 107. https://psycnet.apa.org/doi/10.1037/pri0000067

Lai, M. & Baron-Cohen, S. (2015). Identifying the lost generation of adults with autism spectrum conditions. *Lancet Psychiatry, 2*(11), 1013–27 https://doi.org/10.1016/s2215-0366(15)00277-1

Lai, M. C., Lombardo, M. V., Pasco, G., Ruigrok, A. N., Wheelwright, S. J., Sadek, S. A., ... & Baron-Cohen, S. (2011). A behavioral comparison of male and female adults with high functioning autism spectrum conditions. *PloS one, 6*(6), e20835. https://doi.org/10.1371/journal.pone.0020835

Leigh, J. P., Grosse, S. D., Cassady, D., Melnikow, J., & Hertz-Picciotto, I. (2016). Spending by California's Department of Developmental Services for persons with autism across demographic and expenditure categories. *PLoS One, 11*(3),) e0151970. https://doi.org/10.1371/journal.pone.0151970

Leroi, I., Chauhan, N., Hann, M., Jones, L., Prew, S., Russell, G., Sturrock, R., Taylor, J., Worthington, M., & Dawes, P. (2021). Sensory Health for Residents with Dementia in Care Homes in England: A Knowledge, Attitudes, and Practice Survey. *Journal of the American Medical Directors Association, 22*(7), 1518–1524. https://doi.org/10.1016/j.jamda.2021.03.020

Lindsay, S. (2016). Systematic review of factors affecting driving and motor vehicle transportation among people with autism spectrum disorder. *Disability Rehabilitation 39*(9), 837–846, https://doi.org/10.6084/m9.figshare.3153829

Loomes, R., Hull, L. and Mandy, W. (2017), What is the male-to-female ratio in autism spectrum disorder? A systematic review and meta-analysis, *Journal of the American Academy of Child and Adolescent Psychiatry, 56*(6), pp. 466–74. https://doi.org/10.1016/j.jaac.2017.03.013

Lubin, A., & Feeley, C. (2016). Transportation Issues of Adults on the Autism Spectrum. *Transportation Research Record, 2542*(1), 1–8. https://doi.org/10.3141/2542-01

Maddox, B. B., & White, S. W. (2015). Comorbid social anxiety disorder in adults with autism spectrum disorder. *Journal of Autism and Developmental Disorders, 45*(12), 3949–3960. https://doi.org/10.1007/s10803-015-2531-5

Martino, A. S., & Schormans, A. F. (2018). When good intentions back-fire: university research ethics review and the intimate lives of people labeled with intellectual disabilities. *Forum: Qualitative Social Research, 19*(3), 1–18. https://doi.org/10.17169/fqs-19.3.3090

Massachusetts Department of Education. (2022). *Massachusetts Inclusive Concurrent Enrollment Initiative (MAICEI)*. Inclusive Concurrent Enrollment (MAICEI) / Strategic Initiatives / Massachusetts Department of Higher Education. Retrieved March 28, 2022, from www.mass.edu/strategic/maicei.asp

McCarthy, J., Chaplin, E., & Underwood, L. (2015). An English perspective on policy for adults with autism. *Advances in Autism*, 1–8.

Meyer, I. H. (2003). Prejudice, social stress, and mental health in lesbian, gay, and bisexual populations: Conceptual issues and research evidence. *Psychological Bulletin, 129*(5), 674–697. https://doi.org/10.1037/0033-2909.129.5.674

Mission Project, Inc. (2022). Retrieved from www.themissionproject.org/

Morgan, H. (2019). Connections Between Sensory Sensitivities in Autism; the Importance of Sensory Friendly Environments for Accessibility and Increased Quality of Life for the Neurodivergent Autistic Minority. *PSU McNair Scholars Online Journal, 13*(1), 11.

Müller, E., Schuler, A., & Yates, G. B. (2008). Social challenges and supports from the perspective of individuals with Asperger syndrome and other autism spectrum disabilities. *Autism, 12*(2), 173–190. https://doi.org/10.1177/13623 61307086664

Nicholas, D. B., Mitchell, W., Dudley, C., Clarke, M., & Zulla, R. (2018). An Ecosystem Approach to Employment and Autism Spectrum Disorder. *Journal of Autism and Developmental Disorders, 48*(1), 264–275. https://doi.org/ 10.1007/s10803-017-3351-6

Nicholas, D. B., Zwaigenbaum, L., Zwicker, J., Clarke, M. E., Lamsal, R., Stoddart, K. P., Carroll, C., Muskat, B., Spoelstra, M., & Lowe, K. (2018). Evaluation of employment-support services for adults with autism spectrum disorder. *Autism, 22*(6), 693–702. https://doi.org/10.1177/136236131 7702507

Nicholas, J., Charles, J., Carpenter, L., King, L., Jenner, W. and Spratt, E. (2008), Prevalence and characteristics of children with autism-spectrum disorders. *Annals of Epidemiology, 18*(2), 130–6. https://doi.org/10.1016/j.annepi dem.2007.10.013

Nicolaidis, C., Raymaker, D., McDonald, K., Dern, S., Boisclair, W. C., Ashkenazy, E., & Baggs, A. (2013). Comparison of healthcare experiences in autistic and non-autistic adults: a cross-sectional online survey facilitated by an academic-community partnership. *Journal of General Internal Medicine, 28*(6), 761–769. https://doi.org/10.1007/s11606-012-2262-7

Nicolaidis, C., Raymaker, D. M., Ashkenazy, E., McDonald, K. E., Dern, S., Baggs, A. E., Kapp, S. K., Weiner, M., & Boisclair, W. C. (2015). Respect the way I need to communicate with you": Healthcare experiences of adults on the autism spectrum. *Autism, 19*(7), 824–831. https://dx.doi.org/10.1177%2F1 362361315576221

Nicolaidis, C., Schnider, G., Lee, J., Raymaker, D. M., Kapp, S. K., Croen, L. A., Urbanowicz, A., & Maslak, J. (2021). Development and psychometric testing of the AASPIRE adult autism healthcare provider self-efficacy scale. *Autism, 25*(3), 767–773. https://doi.org/10.1177/1362361320949734

Nicolaidis, C., Raymaker, D., McDonald, K., Kapp, S., Weiner, M., Ashkenazy, E., ... & Baggs, A. (2016). The development and evaluation of an online healthcare toolkit for autistic adults and their primary care providers. *Journal of General Internal Medicine, 31*(10), 1180–1189. https://doi.org/10.1007/s11 606-016-3763-6

Olmstead v. L.C., 527 U.S. 581 (1999).

Otero, T., & Copeland, S. (2020). Facilitating Social Inclusion of Individuals with Autism Spectrum Disorder. *Interprofessional Care Coordination for Pediatric Autism Spectrum Disorder.* 341–355.

Owen, A. M., Gary, A., & Schnetter, V. (2020). Nursing care of patients with autism spectrum disorder. *Nursing made Incredibly Easy, 18*(2), 28–36. https://doi.org/10.1097/01.NME.0000653180.86134.05

Raymaker, D. M., Teo, A. R., Steckler, N. A., Lentz, B., Scharer, M., Delos Santos, A., Kapp, S. K., Hunter, M., Joyce, A., & Nicolaidis, C. (2020). "Having All of Your Internal Resources Exhausted Beyond Measure and Being Left with No Clean-Up Crew": Defining Autistic Burnout. *Autism in Adulthood, 2*(2), 132–143. https://doi.org/10.1089/aut.2019.0079

Roberts, R., Beadle-Brown, J., & Youell, D. (2011). Promoting social inclusion for children and adults on the autism spectrum–reflections on policy and practice. *Tizard Learning Disability Review, 16*(4), 45–52. https://doi.org/10.1108/13595471111172840

Roestorf, A., Bowler, D. M., Deserno, M. K., Howlin, P., Klinger, L., McConachie, H., ... & Geurts, H. M. (2019). Older Adults with ASD: The Consequences of Aging. Insights from a series of special interest group meetings held at the International Society for Autism Research 2016–2017. *Research in Autism Spectrum Disorders, 63*, 3–12. https://doi.org/10.1016/j.rasd.2018.08.007

Rosen, N. E., Lord, C., & Volkmar, F. R. (2021). The Diagnosis of Autism: From Kanner to DSM-III to DSM-5 and Beyond. *Journal of Autism and Developmental Disorders*, 1–18. https://doi.org/10.1007/s10803-021-04904-1

Rudolph, C.E.S., Lundin, A., Åhs, J.W. *et al.* Brief Report: Sexual Orientation in Individuals with Autistic Traits: Population Based Study of 47,000 Adults in Stockholm County. *J Autism Dev Disord* 48, 619–624 (2018). https://doi.org/10.1007/s10803-017-3369-9

Rydzewska, E., Hughes-McCormack, L. A., Gillberg, C., Henderson, A., MacIntyre, C., Rintoul, J., & Cooper, S. (2019). General health of adults with autism spectrum disorders–A whole country population cross-sectional study. *Research in Autism Spectrum Disorders, 60*, 59–66. https://doi.org/10.1016/j.rasd.2019.01.004

Salomone, E., Pacione, L., Shire, S., Brown, F. L., Reichow, B., & Servili, C. (2019). Development of the WHO caregiver skills training program for developmental disorders or delays. *Frontiers in Psychiatry, 10*, 769. https://dx.doi.org/10.3389%2Ffpsyt.2019.00769

Sandfort, T. G., Melendez, R. M., & Diaz, R. M. (2007). Gender non-conformity, homophobia, and mental distress in Latino gay and bisexual men. *Journal of Sex Research, 44*(2), 181–189. https://doi.org/10.1080/00224490701263819

Scott, M., Jacob, A., Hendrie, D., Parsons, R., Girdler, S., Falkmer, T., & Falkmer, M. (2017). Employers' perception of the costs and the benefits of hiring individuals with autism spectrum disorder in open employment in Australia. *PloS one, 12*(5), e0177607. https://doi.org/10.1371/journal.pone.0177607

Sedgewick, F., Leppanen, J., & Tchanturia, K. (2019). The Friendship Questionnaire, autism, and gender differences: a study revisited. Springer Science and Business Media LLC. https://doi.org/10.1186/s13229-019-0295-z

Shattuck, P. (2019). Growing numbers of young adults on the autism spectrum. Retrieved November 29, 2021, from https://drexel.edu/autismoutcomes/blog/overview/2019/June/Growing-numbers-of-young-adults-on-the-autism-spectrum/

Shiloh & Blythe, A. (2014). Keywords autism community music therapy (CoMT) disability rights music therapy Neurodiversity self-advocacy. https://doi.org/ 10.1386/ijcm.7.113_1

Singer, J. (1999). Why can't you be normal for once in your life? From a problem with no name to the emergence of a new category of difference. *Disability Discourse*, 59–70.

Smith, P. A. (2018). On the Horizon: Older Adults With Autism in a Changing Health Care Environment. *Perspectives of the ASHA Special Interest Groups, 3*(15), 4–14. https://doi.org/10.1044/persp3.SIG15.4

Stancliffe, R. J., & Anderson, L. L. (2017). Factors associated with meeting physical activity guidelines by adults with intellectual and developmental disabilities. *Research in Developmental Disabilities, 62*, 1–14. https://doi.org/ 10.1016/j.ridd.2017.01.009

Tefft, B.C. (2017). *Rates of Motor Vehicle Crashes, Injuries and Deaths in Relation to Driver Age, United States, 2014–2015* (Research Brief). Washington, D.C.: AAA Foundation for Traffic Safety.

Tromans, S., Chester, V., Kapugama, C., Elliott, A., Robertson, S., & Barrett, M. (2019). The PAAFID project: exploring the perspectives of autism in adult females among intellectual disability healthcare professionals. *Advances in Autism, 5(3)* 157–170. https://doi.org/10.1108/AIA-09-2018-0033

van der Miesen AIR, Hurley H, Bal AM, de Vries ALC. Prevalence of the Wish to be of the Opposite Gender in Adolescents and Adults with Autism Spectrum Disorder. *Arch Sex Behav.* 2018 Nov;47(8):2307–2317. https://doi.org/ 10.1007/s10508-018-1218-3

Waldron, D. A., Coyle, C. E., Kramer, J., & Jeckel, D. (2018). Supporting pioneers: Building better networks for adults aging with Autism. *Innovation in Aging, 2*(Suppl 1), 804. https://dx.doi.org/10.1093%2Fgeroni%2Figy 023.2988

Waldron, D.A., Coyle, C., & Kramer, J. (2021). Aging on the Autism Spectrum: Self-care Practices and Reported Impact on Well-Being. *Journal of Autism and Developmental Disorders,* https://doi.org/10.1007/s10803-021-05229-9

Walsh, E., Holloway, J., & Lydon, H. (2017). An evaluation of a social skills intervention for adults with autism spectrum disorder and intellectual disabilities preparing for employment in Ireland: A pilot study. *Journal of Autism and Developmental Disorders, 48*(5), 1727–1741. https://doi.org/10.1007/s10 803-017-3441-5

Weir, E., Allison, C., Warrier, V., & Baron-Cohen, S. (2021). Increased prevalence of non-communicable physical health conditions among autistic adults. *Autism, 25*(3), 681–694. https://doi.org/10.1177%2F1362361320953652

WHO. (2021). About the global network for age-friendly cities and communities – age-friendly world. Retrieved November 29, 2021, from https://extranet. who.int/agefriendlyworld/who-network/

Whitehouse, A. J., Watt, H. J., Line, E. A., & Bishop, D. V. (2009). Adult psychosocial outcomes of children with specific language impairment, pragmatic language impairment and autism. *International Journal of Language & Communication Disorders, 44*(4), 511-528.

Wood, E. B., Halverson, A., Harrison, G., & Rosenkranz, A. (2019). Creating a sensory-friendly pediatric emergency department. *Journal of Emergency Nursing, 45*(4), 415–424. https://doi.org/10.1016/j.jen.2018.12.002

Wright, S. D., Wright, C. A., D'Astous, V., & Wadsworth, A. M. (2019). Autism aging. *Gerontology & Geriatrics Education*, 40(3), 322–338. https://doi.org/10.1080/02701960.2016.1247073

Zalewska, A., Migliore, A., & Butterworth, J. (2016). Self-determination, social skills, job search, and transportation: Is there a relationship with employment of young adults with autism? *Journal of Vocational Rehabilitation, 45*(3), 225–239. https://doi.org/10.3233/JVR-160825

Zener, D. (2019). Journey to diagnosis for women with autism. *Advances in Autism. 5*(1), 2–13. https://doi.org/10.1108/aia-10-2018-0041

Zerbo, O., Massolo, M. L., Qian, Y., & Croen, L. A. (2015). A study of physician knowledge and experience with autism in adults in a large integrated healthcare system. *Journal of Autism and Developmental Disorders, 45*(12), 4002–4014. https://doi.org/10.1007/s10803-015-2579-2

Zigmond A.S. & Snaith R.P. (1983). The hospital anxiety and depression scale. *Acta Psychiatrica Scandinavica 67*, 361–370.

Chapter 20

Social Media, Digital Inclusion, and Internet Safety

Mary Jo Krile[1] and David F. Cihak[2]
[1]Department of Teaching, Learning, and Educational Leadership, Eastern Kentucky University
[2]Department of Theory and Practice in Teacher Education, University of Tennessee, Knoxville

A Digital Inclusion Case Study

Ella is a 17-year-old with autism spectrum disorder (ASD) who lives in a small rural town. Every summer, Ella attends an autism summer camp where she has developed strong friendships with other campers. However, these friends live long distances away from Ella. During the school year, Ella can only keep in contact with her camp friends through calling them on her mother's mobile phone. When Ella turned 16-years-old, her older brother, Steve, noticed that Ella was lonely and had few local friends she felt understood her. He wanted Ella to be able to communicate with her camp friends more frequently. This prompted Steve to ask their parents to consider letting Ella use social media (SM). While Ella's parents had concerns about Ella's online safety, they agreed that Ella needed to maintain her relationships with her camp friends and others who understood ASD. Ella's parents gave Steve permission to help Ella learn how to safely navigate and use SM. Steve helped Ella set up Facebook and Instagram accounts. He helped her complete her profiles, set safe privacy settings, learn how to message her friends, post updates, share content, and maintain her online safety. He also taught her about the dangers of SM, including predators, scams, and cyberbullying. Once Ella's profiles were complete, she began engaging with her friends through messages and posts. A few months later, Ella noticed that one of her friends started using hashtags about ASD, such as #autismisawesome, #asdrocks, #autismawareness, and #autismacceptance. Out of curiosity, Ella clicked on these hashtags. She found that this took her to all posts that used these hashtags. Ella was excited that she found a whole community of people using autism hashtags. She began reading posts of others who advocated for the autism community through SM or posted about their own experience having autism. Ella enjoyed seeing a whole community of others who shared similar experiences and excitedly showed her parents and brother what she had found. Steve was proud that his sister was finding a larger autism community. He decided to help Ella find SM groups and pages

DOI: 10.4324/9781003255147-24

that supported the autism community. He also helped her find pages and groups that fit her interests. This allowed Ella to begin engaging with others on these groups and pages. She began sharing her own experience with autism with others in these SM groups, as well as giving support to others having difficult times. Ella's parents were ecstatic that Ella was meeting others she felt were like her, as well as reading posts from others that demonstrated self-advocacy and self-determination. They were excited that Ella was seeing this modeling from others with autism and learning from it. However, they still had concerns with Ella's safety. It was not long before Ella began receiving friend and follower requests, as well as messages, from strangers claiming to be in these groups. She began friending and following these strangers. She also was interested in responding to the strangers who messaged her. Steve began to become concerned when Ella shared with him that a stranger was asking for her address and phone number. He discussed these concerns with their parents. Steve and his parents decided that they needed to find a class for Ella to take so she could learn more about digital citizenship and how to address online dangers. Ella's parents started advocating for Ella to learn about SM and internet safety at school, as well as the summer camp she attends. They also began to search for resources and strategies that educators and camp counselors could use when teaching this topic. Their hopes were for Ella to continue using SM and the internet to be part of the larger autism community and learn about self-determination and advocacy from others online. Ella's parents also hope for Ella to master mitigating the dangers that arise when using SM so that she can continue to engage with others online without putting herself in danger.

Introduction

In the above case study, Ella experienced both benefits and risks to digital inclusion. She was able to use online platforms, such as social media (SM) and the internet, to maintain long-distance friendships, engage with a larger autism community, observe self-advocacy done by others, and feel connected to others she felt understood her. While these benefits were experienced by Ella, she also faced dangers. These dangers came in the form of strangers messaging and sending friend or follow requests to her. Online strangers can be beneficial in forming relationships with others, especially when it comes to online dating. However, strangers can also be predators who seek to harm others. Other risks that Ella could experience include cyberbullying, scams, identity theft, and being sent illicit content without being asked permission. In this chapter, digital inclusion will be defined, benefits and risks individuals with autism spectrum disorder (ASD) experience from

digital inclusion will be discussed, and instructional strategies and resources to promote cyber safety and digital inclusion for individuals
with ASD will be included.

Defining Digital Inclusion

Prior to examining digital inclusion for individuals with ASD, one must
have an understanding of the digital inclusion concept. According to the
Institute of Museum and Library Sciences et al. (2012), digital inclusion occurs when individuals are able to access and use technology.
Furthermore, the three digital inclusion principles of access, adoption,
and application must be present (Becker et al., 2012). The first principle
of digital inclusion, access, addresses the necessities required for individuals and communities to be able to access technology and connect to
the internet. Among these infrastructure necessities are technology and
internet availability, affordability, and accessibility. The second digital
inclusion principle, adoption, focuses on providing individuals and communities with the knowledge, resources, and strategies needed to overcome any barrier that may be faced when accessing and using technology.
Technology relevance (the benefits of using technology to achieve desirable outcomes), digital literacy skills (ability to find, evaluate, and use
digitally presented information), and consumer safety (safely navigating
the digital world) are the areas in which information must be given for
the adoption principle to occur. It is also important to note that the principle of adoption covers all areas of technology. This ranges from basic
technology use, such as hardware, software, and application use, to use
of the internet and SM platforms.

Lastly, the principle of application addresses the use of technology to
benefit and enhance the lives of individuals (Becker et al., 2014; Institute
of Museum and Library Services et al., 2012).

The focus of this book chapter will be on the second principle of
digital inclusion, adoption, and how it pertains to individuals with
ASD. Additionally, since the principle of adoption covers all areas of
technology use, the emphasis for this chapter will be on the adoption
of online platforms by individuals with ASD. For the purposes of this
chapter, online platforms will be defined as the use of the internet and
SM platforms. Furthermore, SM will be defined as any online platform
in which users can create and share a variety of content (Bolton et al.,
2013). This includes everything from specific apps, such as Facebook,
YouTube, Instagram, Snapchat, and Twitter, to dating apps, chatrooms,
and blogs. In the following section, the impact and experiences of individuals with ASD adopting the use of these online platforms will be
reviewed.

Digital Inclusion for Individuals with Autism

In Ella's case study, she was an adolescent with ASD who went from not using any SM to having only an Instagram and Facebook account. Research has indicated that online platform use by individuals with ASD has consistently been significantly less than those without ASD (Begara Iglesias et al., 2019; Mazurek et al., 2012; Mazurek, 2013; Mazurek & Wenstrup, 2013). Despite this limited use of online platforms, individuals with ASD who do use online platforms have experienced benefits from this use. These benefits have included increased and improved social interactions (Gillespie-Smith et al., 2021; Kuo et al., 2014; Mazurek, 2013; Van Schalkwyk et al., 2017), building and maintaining relationships/community (Gillespie-Smith et al., 2021; Suzuki et al., 2020; Wang et al., 2020), increased skills (Molin et al., 2015; Raghavendra et al., 2015; Raghavendra et al., 2018), and increased happiness/self-esteem (Brosnan & Gavin, 2021; Molin et al., 2015; Ward et al., 2018).

Online Platform Use by Individuals with ASD

While research analyzing the online platform use of individuals with ASD is scarce, all results of these studies have indicated that individuals with ASD use online platforms significantly less than those without disabilities (Alhujaili et al., 2022; Begara Iglesias et al., 2019; Kuo et al., 2013; Mazurek et al., 2012; Mazurek, 2013; Mazurek & Wenstrup, 2013; MacMullin et al., 2016). Additionally, this research has shown that individuals with ASD not only favor different online platforms than those without disabilities (Alhujaili et al., 2022), but also use these platforms for different reasons (Alhujaili et al., 2022, Mazurek et al., 2012; Mazurek, 2013; Mazurek & Wenstrup, 2013). Among all SM platforms, YouTube (Alhujaili et al., 2022) and Facebook (Alhujaili et al., 2022; Ward et al., 2018) were most favored for individuals with ASD. In contrast, individuals without ASD most favored Snapchat and Instagram. When asked the reason for using SM, the most cited among individuals with ASD was that of entertainment purposes. The least cited reasons for SM use were social interaction and academic purposes. However, the main reason for SM use among individuals without ASD was that of social interaction (Alhujaili et al.). Research analyzing the time spent on SM has also shown a difference between individuals with ASD and those without. Mazurek & Wenstrup surveyed parents of adolescents with ASD and asked them to compare the SM use of their child with ASD to that of their child without ASD. Results of this study demonstrated that adolescents with ASD spent a total average of 0.2 hours per day using SM (including email, SM, and sending text messages). This was significantly less than the 1.0 hours per day that their typically developing siblings spent using SM.

Similar to SM use, entertainment purposes (such as viewing online videos and playing online games) has been cited as the main reason individuals with ASD use the internet. In a 2013 study, Kuo et al., surveyed 91 adolescents with ASD. Results of this survey indicated that the 84% of respondents visit websites for entertainment purposes and finding information, 78% for playing video games, 30% for email, 23% for social networking programs, 22% for instant messaging programs, and 13% for chat rooms. Additionally, the screen time of adolescents with ASD has also been examined. Mazurek and Wenstrup (2013) found that adolescents with ASD spent more time (an average of 4.5 hours per day) engaged with screen-based media (television and online games). Additionally, it was found that the majority of online games played by adolescents with ASD were single player. This internet use research demonstrates that individuals with ASD use the internet, but favor using it in ways that are more solitary. Overall, social interaction has not been found to be a significant reason individuals with ASD use the internet.

While the amount of research that analyzes actual use of online platforms is limited, these use statistics demonstrate consistent trends. First, it is evident that while individuals with ASD use online platforms, their use is significantly lower than individuals without ASD. There are many reasons as to why this may be the case. One of these reasons can be contributed to individuals with ASD being vulnerable to cyber victimization (Gillespie-Smith et al., 2021; Iglesias et al., 2019; Sallafranque-St-Louis & Normand, 2017) and not having the strategies to mitigate these online dangers. The second consistent trend is that individuals with ASD tend to use online platforms less for social interactions, but more for solitary entertainment purposes. While online platforms offer less anxiety inducing and more visual means of communication (ex. use of emojis, pictures, memes, gifs, etc.), digital literacy skills and learning the social rules of the internet (i.e. netiquette) are still needed in order to engage in online social interactions. Without these skills, communicating with others in online settings can be difficult. Digital literacy and netiquette skills must be taught to individuals with ASD in ways similar to that of face-to-face social skills. With this knowledge, online social interactions for individuals with ASD may increase and become easier.

Benefits of Online Platform Use for Individuals with ASD

As seen in Ella's case study, digital inclusion for individuals with ASD can offer many benefits. Ella experienced the benefits of seeing others model self-advocacy, connecting with others within the ASD community, and maintaining long-distance relationships with her friends. These benefits are among several that individuals with ASD experience from online platform use. In the following paragraphs, the benefits individuals with ASD experience from using online platforms will be examined.

Increased and Improved Social Interactions

Improved and increased social interaction have been found to be one of the major benefits individuals with ASD experience from using online platforms (Gillespie-Smith et al., 2021; Kuo et al., 2014; Mazurek, 2013; Van Schalkwyk et al., 2017). It has been noted that individuals with ASD who interact with others using online platforms have reported a greater quality of friendships with others (Kuo et al., 2014; Mazurek, 2013; Van Schalkwyk et al., 2017), greater security in friendships, and more positive overall friendships (Kuo et al., 2014). Furthermore, individuals with ASD have expressed that SM offers a more comfortable way to communicate and engage with others (Gillespie-Smith et al., 2021; Mazurek, 2013). For example, when interviewed about online social interactions, parents and adolescents with ASD reported that adolescents with ASD experienced more ease when making new friends and talking with others online, due to not have deal with the social anxiety that occurs in face-to-face interactions (Gillespie-Smith et al., 2021). Other reasons online interactions have been cited as easier and/or a better experience than face-to-face interactions include online platforms offering a more relaxed mean of social interaction (Gillespie-Smith et al., 2021) and universally accepted visual mode of communication (Krile, 2020; Raghavendra et al., 2015). For example, in online interactions, the use of body language, facial expressions, and other social rules necessary for face-to-face interactions are not required as often (Burke et al., 2010; Van Schalkwyk et al., 2017). Additionally, online platforms have a built-in visual mean of communication that is age appropriate (i.e., emojis, memes, stickers, reactions, and gifs) (Krile, 2020; Raghavendra et al., 2015). Each of these components of online interactions allow interacting with others to be easier and less anxiety inducing for individuals who already struggle with social interactions due to social skill needs.

Building and Maintaining Relationships/Community. Other benefits individuals with ASD can experience from using online platforms is that of becoming involved with a larger autism community (Antunes & Dhoest, 2018), as well as building and maintaining relationships with others (Antunes & Dhoest, 2018; Gillespie-Smith et al., 2021; Suzuki et al., 2020; Wang et al., 2020). In Ella's case study, her use of SM led to finding a place in a larger autism community. Through the use of hashtags, Ella was able to find a whole community of others who share experiences with ASD. This community can range from individuals with ASD to advocates, relatives, educators, and service providers of individuals with ASD. In a 2018 study, Antunes and Dhoest examined the online autism community in Brazil. Findings of this study indicated two forms of online autism communities. The first of these types, *autistic communities*, were formed by, and comprised of, primarily individuals with ASD. It is important to note that the researchers found this community to not be exclusive to only individuals with ASD. Instead, it was found that this community, "makes it clear that their group is made by and for people with autism" (Antunes & Dhoest, 2018, p. 5). These *autistic communities* where where individuals with ASD went to find information and receive social support. For example, one of Brazil's Facebook *autistic community* groups consisted of individuals with ASD. In this group, members would have discussions about how ASD impacts their lives and personality. Discussions wer often had between community members on what characteristics of ASD they have and how they cope with them, as well as the challenges they experience with social interactions, finding romantic relationships, and mental health. The other type online ASD communities, *autism communities*, were comprised of individuals with ASD and those without ASD. It is in these communities where more controversial topics pertaining to ASD were more frequently discussed.

Individuals with ASD have used online platforms to make new relationships, including that of long-distance friendships with others from other countries (Gillespie-Smith et al., 2021) and romantic relationships (Brosnan & Gavin, 2021; Gillespie-Smith et al., 2021; Roth & Gillis 2015; Sallafranque-St-Louis & Normand, 2017; Wang et al., 2020). In a 2020 study, Wang et al., interviewed eight adults with autism. Findings of this study indicated that adults with autism found SM to be beneficial for staying in contact with friends and family who have moved away. It was also noted that interviewees used SM to engage more frequently with local friends, as it did not require the transportation needs of face-to-face meetings.

While some individuals with ASD mainly use online platforms to build mutual friendships, many have begun to turn to online platforms for dating purposes (Brosnan & Gavin, 2021; Roth & Gillis, 2015; Sallafranque-St-Louis & Normand, 2017; Wang et al., 2020). Roth & Gillis (2015) surveyed 17 individuals with ASD regarding online dating. Fifty-three percent of survey respondents reported having tried online dating. Results of this survey indicated that the respondents perceived online dating as easier than face-to-face dating. Additionally, respondents experienced success with online dating. Both long-term and long-distance relationships with others were achieved through the use of dating websites. The average length of relationships experienced among respondents was 2.65 years. Benefits that respondents experienced from online dating included making their own profile for others to see prior to the dating process, having information about others before starting the dating process, meeting people without having to experience anxiety inducing face-to-face situations, and having more people to choose from. When asked about drawbacks of online dating, respondents cited safety concerns, not knowing the history of potential dates, being victimized, transitioning from all online communication to meeting face-to-face, dealing with rejection from potential dates, and having too many dating profiles to browse.

As the above online relationships research has indicated, individuals with ASD can experience success when making and maintaining relationships online. Additionally, individuals with ASD can be successful in using online dating as a means of forming romantic relationships with others. In order to promote this success, it is important to teach online safety skills and the benefits/dangers of online relationships. Lastly, it is also essential to teach individuals with ASD how to set and follow through with boundaries when interacting with others online, especially in online dating situations.

Increased Skills

Using online platforms can result in increased academic, self-advocacy, self-determination, and social skills. All online platforms require the use of reading, written expression, social, technology/digital literacy, and communication skills. As one continues to access online platforms, the requirement for these skills are increased. When skills are used more frequently, this can result in improvement of skills. Research has found that use of online platforms has resulted in the use of clearer and more meaningful communication (Raghavendra et al., 2015), improved word recognition (Raghavendra et al., 2018), and increased confidence in written and spoken communication (Raghavendra et al., 2015). Additionally, research has shown that online platform use offers opportunities for one to gain more awareness of their disability (Molin et al., 2015). In Ella's case study, she was able to see others with ASD model self-advocacy skills and learn more about ASD. This resulted in her parents seeing Ella begin to share her experiences with ASD with others, as well as talk about ASD more. As Ella engaged more with the online ASD community, she was able to gain more awareness about ASD. She was also offered a place to share her own experiences with others who would understand these experiences. Through the use of online groups and pages for ASD, Ella can have a safe place to learn more about ASD and increase her use of reading, written expression, communication, social, and technology/digital literacy skills.

Increased Happiness/Self-Esteem

The last benefits of online platform use individuals with ASD can experience, include that of increased happiness and self-esteem. In a 2018 study, Ward et al. analyzed the relationship between SM use and happiness in adults with ASD. Results of this study indicated that SM use (specifically that of Facebook) in moderation led to increased happiness. However, it was noted that too much SM use led to lowered rates of happiness. Therefore, online platform use with moderation is key. Research has also shown that online platform use can help individuals with ASD combat boredom, pursue special interests (Ward et al., 2018), and create a self-presentation they favor (Brosnan & Gavin, 2021; Molin et al., 2015). When creating online profiles and sharing content online, an individual can choose what is shared. In other words, how one presents themselves online can be self-selected and reflect an identity they want others to see. Individuals with ASD who do not want to share that they have ASD do not have to include this on their profile. Whereas, those who want to self-disclose that they have ASD can share this on their profile and have it be a part of their online identity. In face-to-face social situations, this opportunity to choose the identity that others see is often not available. Being able to self-select and personally build your own online identity can increase self-esteem and happiness. Furthermore, online platforms offer communities through pages, websites, blogs, and groups. These communities offer opportunities for individuals to give and gain support from others. Through gaining support from others in the ASD community, individuals with ASD may be able to increase their confidence, happiness, and self-esteem. As with Ella's case study, she found a larger ASD community in which she could engage. This community offered her a safe place to learn more about ASD, find resources, gain support, and give support. Each of these aspects of online communities can afford individuals with ASD a place to gain further acceptance and increase their self-esteem and happiness.

Risks of Using Online Platforms

In Ella's case study, Ella received messages and friend requests from strangers. Furthermore, some of these strangers began asking for her address and phone number. While some of these strangers may be potential friends with good intentions, there is also the risk of them being individuals who have the intention of causing harm. These harmful intents can range from hacking accounts, stealing personal information, cyberbullying, and/or being predators who have intentions of committing crimes. All individuals who use online platforms have the potential to be the victim and/or perpetrator of online dangers. In the following paragraphs, the dangers individuals with ASD experience with online platform use will be examined.

Victims

Research has indicated that individuals with ASD have been victims of online dangers. These online dangers have ranged from impersonation, sexual advances without consent (Iglesias et al., 2019; Sallafranque-St-Louis & Normand, 2017), being mocked, being verbally bullied online, facing online exclusion (Iglesias et al., 2019), receiving abusive interactions, and talking to a stranger posing as someone else (Gillespie-Smith et al., 2021). Of these dangers, research has indicated that individuals with ASD experienced being a victim of all these online platform dangers. In a 2019 study, Inglesias et al. found that individuals with ASD most often experienced being picked on, insulted, or made fun of on SM. A 2020 study by Gillespie-Smith at al. mirrored this result, as participants commented on being abused, receiving hate comments, being judged, and getting much criticism when using online platforms. The second highest area of online victimization experienced by individuals with ASD was online exclusion, specifically in the area of being removed from, or not accepted on, an online platform. The areas found to be where the least victimization occurred for individuals with ASD included: being forced to do something humiliating, someone recording it, and others posting it online; being pressured to do sexual acts and having others threatening to post the intimate pictures or videos online; and someone posting compromising pictures or videos of the individual without their consent (Iglesias et al., 2019).

Perpetrators

Individuals with ASD have also been found to engage in perpetrating online dangers. Impersonation and verbal cyberbullying have been cited as the online dangers in which individuals with ASD most frequently commit. The area found to be the most frequently perpetrated by individuals with ASD was that of mocking someone on SM with offensive or insulting comments (Iglesias et al., 2019). While the statistics of individuals with ASD committing these online dangers are significantly lower than the online victimization of individuals with ASD statistics, it is important to take measures in teaching the repercussions of perpetrating online dangers. These repercussions can range from being banned from using online platforms to building a negative digital footprint (which can negatively impact future opportunities, such as employment, postsecondary education, and any other opportunity in which one completes an application).

Online platform use offers many benefits for individuals with ASD. Among these benefits are that of finding and engaging with a community that is likeminded and offers support. There are also dangers that may be experienced by individuals with ASD when they use online platforms. To be able to afford individuals with ASD the most beneficial experience when using online platforms, it is essential to provide them with the knowledge and skills needed to mitigate any victim or preparator dangers that may occur.

This can be done through the formation of online safety strategies specifically for individuals with ASD, having the hard conversations about online dangers (i.e., predators, scams, etc.), and offering many safe opportunities for practice. These are some of the instructional strategies that are discussed and provided within the instructional strategies portion of this chapter.

Areas for Future Research

Existing literature, while minimal, has explored the online platform use of individuals with ASD, benefits and risks associated with this online platform use, and perspectives regarding using online platforms. As this research is minimal, there is a need for further research in these areas to contribute to the existing literature. It is also noted that the perspectives the educators, caretakers, and support staff of individuals with ASD have not been explored. There is a need for this research, as many of these individuals may indicate specific needs for resources and support in the area of digital inclusion for individuals with ASD. Additionally, there is a need for research in the areas of netiquette, digital footprints/online reputations, technology addiction, and coping of emotions that occur with online interactions as it pertains to individuals with ASD. Lastly, there is a lack of research that analyzes the use of instructional strategies to promote safe digital citizenship practices for individuals with ASD. Future research done in this area must focus on the development of these strategies and use of sound research methods to examine the effectiveness of developed strategies.

Instructional Strategies for Internet Safety and Online Platform Use

Instructional strategies for promoting internet safety and online platform use for individuals with ASD are limited. As a digital literacy instructor for young adults with intellectual and/or developmental disabilities, Krile (2021) has developed and implemented strategies specifically for teaching these skills to individuals with ASD. These strategies incorporate the use of evidence-based teaching practices. Among these strategies is that of using visual checklists, developing rules for netiquette, and creating safe opportunities for practice. In the following section, these strategies are described. Additionally, online resources that provide lesson plans, discussion guides for parents, and other resources regarding online platform safety are included.

Visual Checklists

Krile (2020) created a visual checklist that can be used by individuals with intellectual and/or developmental disabilities to ensure online safety. This resource (provided in Figure 20.1) uses a checklist to help individuals

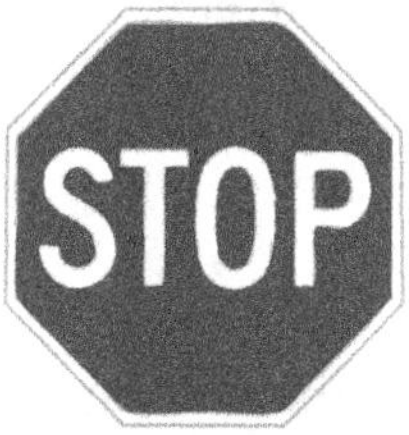

Figure 20.1 Online Safety Visual Checklist.
Source: *Taken from (Krile, 2020).

identify the safety level (safe vs. dangerous) of an electronic message and determine what actions (reply to the message or do not reply and tell a trusted adult immediately) to take as a result of the safety level.

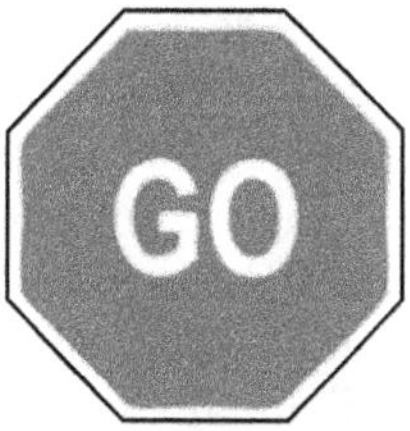

To use this checklist, individuals begin with the first checkbox on the Stop portion of the checklist. If the individual does not know the person who sent the message, they would check the box. If they do know the sender, they would leave the box unchecked. Using the same system for checking the box (yes results in box being checked and no results in box being left unchecked) the individual then progresses through the remaining three checkboxes on the Stop portion. If at the end of the Stop checklist, one or more of the boxes are checked, the individual would stop, identify the message as dangerous, and talk to a trusted adult (an adult the individual identifies as someone they trust and feel comfortable talking about online dangers with). If none of the boxes in the Stop portion are checked, the individual would progress to the Go portion of the checklist and repeat the process. If all boxes remain unchecked, the message can be identified as safe and can be replied to. Prior to using this checklist, Krile stated that it is important to define each of the checklist statements with the individual using the checklist. This clears any ambiguity and allows the individual using the checklist to understand the criteria for a safe or dangerous message. The definitions Krile formed for each checklist statement are provided in the following table. (See Table 20.1.)

Developing Rules for Netiquette

Netiquette refers to the social rules and behaviors used in online settings (Sorbring et al., 2017). In other words, it is the etiquette of the internet. As with many online situations, one does not see the reactions (including facial expressions and body language) of the person receiving sent messages. Due to this, it is much easier for one to exhibit online behaviors that may be offensive to others. It is also easy for one to forget when a camera or microphone is on. This can result in a person exhibiting embarrassing behaviors or saying inappropriate, offensive, or confidential information. All of these situations are reasons why it is important to develop and teach netiquette rules. Refer to Table 20.2 for some netiquette rules that Krile (2021) developed specifically for individuals with ASD. These rules can be taught and modeled to individuals with ASD. Included in the table are definitions of each netiquette rule and information about when to use the specific rules. When netiquette rules are not followed, corrective feedback about the netiquette rule should be given. This feedback should include reminders of the specific netiquette rule and how to correct a post or message so that it follows the netiquette rule.

Creating Safe Opportunities for Practice

Due to online risks having the ability to create immediate harmful effects, it is important to create safe opportunities in which individuals with

Table 20.1 Visual Checklist Criteria Definitions

Checklist Statement	Definition
I do not know the person who sent the message.	A person we do not know in real life, including celebrities.
The message is inappropriate.	Message that uses curse words; says mean things; tells one to do actions that are harmful or do not want to be done; and/or say, do, or ask for things that are sexual in nature.
The message bothers me.	Reading the message results in feeling upset, irritated, angry, or sad.
The person asked for personal information.	The message asks for personal information such as date of birth, phone number, address, social security number, debit/credit card information, and banking information.

Table 20.2 Netiquette Rules

Netiquette Rule	What it Means	When to Use
Twitter Rule	Messages should be kept under the 240-character limit that Twitter uses for Tweets	When users frequently send extremely lengthy messages to others
1:1:1 OR 1:24:1 Rule	Send 1 message. Wait a minimum of 1 day for a reply, then send 1 more message. Repeat process as necessary. Also teach that it is okay if someone does not reply. Note: This rule does not apply in emergency situations!	When users do not wait for replies from others and/or frequently message others to the point where it could be considered harassment
Grandma Rule: "If you don't want your Grandma to see it, don't post it!" *Note: Use the name/role of any individual important to the user in place of "Grandma." This can include family members, teachers, employers, coaches, etc.	If you don't want someone who is a role model to you to see something, you should not post it. Think twice before you post because others see what you post and can find it, even if it gets deleted.	When teaching the concepts of oversharing, digital footprints, and online reputations.
Golden Rule: "Treat others online how you want to be treated online."	Be kind to others in online settings and treat them the way you want to be treated.	When teaching what to share/post online
Keep it Positive	Keep posts and comments positive. You have the power to make someone smile and make a difference to at least one person with your post. By keeping it positive, you are making the world a happier place! Negative posts make others feel bad and can build a negative online reputation.	What teaching what to share/post online

Source: *Taken from Krile (2021).

ASD can make mistakes, ask questions, and learn from mistakes without harmful effects. Safe opportunities for practice can be done through online learning modules/quizzes or printed messages. In Figures 20.2 and 20.3, there are two examples of game cards and online quizzes that Krile (2021) created to provide digital literacy students with ASD safe opportunities for practicing how to identify and address predators, scams, and cyberbullies.

Figure 20.2 has an example of game cards created on Microsoft PowerPoint slides. Each card contains a message for an individual to read. After reading a message, a discussion can be had on if the message is: (a) safe or dangerous; (b) from a predator, cyberbully, scammer, or real friend; and (c) how the message should be addressed (replied to, or blocked and reported). These cards can be used in a drill and practice style, in which individuals continually review and practice with them. Games such as I Have, Who Has; Go Fish; Memory; etc. can also be played with them. Another example of providing a safe opportunity for practice can be seen in Figure 20.3.

This image has an example of an online quiz question created within an online learning management system. Each quiz question contains a premade message to be read. After reading the message, the individual will choose if the message is safe or dangerous and if they would reply to the message. All dangerous messages should not be replied to. Additionally, these opportunities for practice can be used in conjunction with the visual checklist discussed in the above paragraphs (and provided in Figure 20.1). Individuals can have a laminated printed out version of this checklist and check off the boxes that apply with a dry erase marker. This checklist can then be erased and reused throughout all practice opportunities.

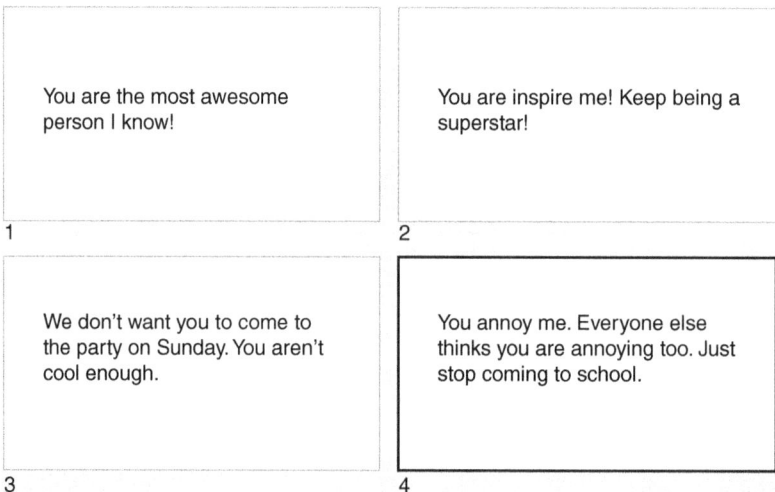

You are the most awesome person I know!	You are inspire me! Keep being a superstar!
1	2
We don't want you to come to the party on Sunday. You aren't cool enough.	You annoy me. Everyone else thinks you are annoying too. Just stop coming to school.
3	4

Figure 20.2 Identify the Cyberbully and Predator Game Cards.
*Taken from Krile (2021).

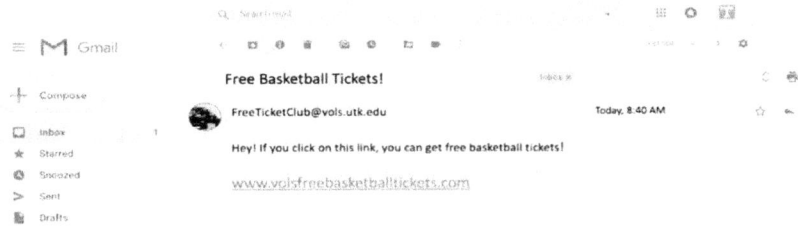

Question 1 — 0 pts

Is this email safe or dangerous?

○ Safe

○ Dangerous

Question 2 — 0 pts

Would you reply to this email?

○ Yes

○ No

Figure 20.3 Identifying and Addressing Dangerous Messages Quizzes.
*Taken from Krile (2020).

While progressing through these opportunities for practice, it is important to provide corrective feedback. For example, when an individual identifies a message from a scammer as safe to reply to, corrective feedback should be given. This feedback should include information about how scams steal personal information and are often too good to be true. As a result of a scam, your information is stolen and the item you wanted does not arrive. In *Post, update, tweet, or snap? Promoting safe social media use for young adults with intellectual disability,* Krile (2020) discussed an incident in which a participant indicated knowledge that a message was a scam. However, the participant still marked the message as safe and okay to reply to because of a great desire to win the free cruise offered in the message. Corrective feedback in this situation should include information about the free cruise ticket being fake and resulting in the individual having their sent information stolen and used for identity theft purposes.

It is also important to have a crisis plan ready if any message creates emotional harm to an individual or an individual reports a cybercrime. For example, an individual who may have been cyberbullied in real life may get upset when reading messages from cyberbullies. When this occurs, it is essential to discuss the emotions that occur from these messages and how to cope with them (i.e., talking to a trusted adult or friend). Lastly, it is essential to be aware of cybercrimes. If during these opportunities for practice an individual reports having had a cybercrime committed against them (ex. being asked for nude pictures or sent pornographic images when the individual is under the age of 18) or having committed a cybercrime themselves, it is critical that the report is taken seriously and investigated. Having a crisis plan ready for addressing emotional distress or cybercrimes will keep one prepared for situations in which this occurs.

Online Resources

There are several online websites that have been developed to provide educators, families, and service providers with resources specific to teaching and promoting online safety and digital citizenship. Among these websites, only two are formed specifically to give resources for teaching these concepts to individuals with ASD. These two websites (Digital Citizenship 4 All and Digitability) are given in the following table (see Table 20.3). Also included on this table are other websites that can be used. However, many of these resources may have to be adapted for individuals with ASD.

Conclusion

In Ella's case study, she was experiencing benefits and dangers from using SM. The online dangers Ella experienced (receiving messages and friend requests from strangers, as well as being asked for her address and phone number) are among several that individuals with ASD can experience. Much like Ella's parents and older brother, many practitioners and service providers working with individual with ASD are concerned about dangers such as these. The strategies and resources given in this chapter can assist with teaching internet safety and promoting digital inclusion for individuals with ASD. For example, Ella's parents and older brother were searching for online resources to assist Ella's teachers and camp counselors in teaching internet safety and use to Ella. The online resources given in Table 20.3 consist of resources that can be used for this purpose. However, Ella's parents may want to recommend starting with the two websites (Digital Citizenship 4 All and Digitability) formed specifically for individuals with ASD and/or intellectual disability.

Table 20.3 Websites for Teaching Online Safety and Digital Citizenship

Online Resource	Website	Resources Provided
Common Sense Media	https://www.commonsense.org/education/	Digital citizenship lesson plans for teachers, games for students, and free resources for families. Topics covered include addressing online safety risks, digital footprint, and netiquette.
Digital Citizenship 4 All	https://dc4all.com *To be published for the public in summer 2022.	Lessons and resources for teachers, parents/guardians/caretakers, and individuals with ASD and/or ID. Contains pages for individuals with ASD and/or ID to interact with learning materials and learn skills for digital citizenship and internet safety.
Digitability	https://digitability.com/	Subscription based transition curriculum. Contains curriculum for digital citizenship formed specifically for individuals with ASD and/or ID.
Digital Learn	https://training.digitallearn.org/	Courses on learning computer basics, social media (only Facebook and Pinterest), Microsoft tools, and Linkedin.
Digital Futures Initiative	https://www.dfinow.org/all-courses/	Digital citizenship lessons for students in 6th, 7th, 8th, and 9th grade.
Northstar Digital Literacy	https://www.digitalliteracyassessment.org/	Online assessments and learning modules for learning essential computer skills, software skills, and using technology in daily life. Topics covered include social media, information literacy, and digital footprint.
Thorn	https://parents.thorn.org/	Resource for parents on that contain guides for discussing online platform risks with their child. Topics include sexting and nudes, device access and monitoring, using balanced approaches, online platforms (all platforms are discussed) and stranger danger 2.0.
NetSmartz	https://www.missingkids.org/netsmartz/home	Online safety education program for children. Lessons and resources cover the topics of social media, sexting and sextortion, livestreaming, Smartphones, online enticement, and cyberbullying.

To further address the online dangers that Ella was experiencing, as well as mitigate any other dangers that could arise, the various instructional strategies mentioned in the chapter can be used. When addressing the messages Ella receives from strangers, Ella's parents, brother, teachers, or camp counselors can use the visual checklist provided in this chapter. They can also create safe opportunities for her to practice using the checklist. Once Ella has mastered identifying the safety level of electronic messages, she can independently use the checklist to determine the steps she should take to address received messages. When teaching Ella to address other online dangers, more opportunities for practice can be created to reflect the danger topic being taught (e.g., cyberbullying, scams, etc.). In these opportunities for practice, messages can be created to simulate messages that would be sent in these online danger situations. For example, a created message for a scam would ask for personal information, be from an unknown sender, contain a lengthy link to an unknown website, and/or contain misspelled words. Lastly, Ella can be taught netiquette rules, such as those provided in this chapter, to learn the social rules of the internet. These netiquette rules can assist Ella with creating an online reputation that will be beneficial for achieving future goals (such as employment), as well as success when virtually connecting with others. Similar to Ella, all individuals with ASD need to be equipped with the knowledge and skills needed to safely, and independently, navigate the online world. With these skills, individuals with ASD can be truly digitally included, experience a broader and more open world, and be further empowered.

References

Alhujaili, N., Platt, E., Khalid-Khan, S., & Groll, D. (2022). Comparison of social media use among adolescents with autism spectrum disorder and non-ASD adolescents. *Adolescent Health, Medicine, and Therapeutics, 13,* 15–21. https://doi.org/10.2147/AHMT.S344591

Antunes, D. & Dhoest, A. (2018). Autism and social media: The case of Brazil. *Observatorio Journal, 12*(4), 1–12. https://doi.org/10.15847/obsOBS1242 0181298

Becker, S., Coward, C., Crandall, M., Sears, R., Carlee, R., Hasbargen, K., & Ball, M. A. (2012). Building digital communities. A framework for action. Institute of Museum and Library Services. https://www.imls.gov/publications/building-digital-communities-frameworkaction

Begara Iglesias, O., Gómez Sánchez, L. E., & Alcedo Rodríguez, M. D. L. Á. (2019). Do young people with Asperger syndrome or intellectual disability use social media and are they cyberbullied or cyberbullies in the same way as their peers?. *Psicothema.*

Bolton, R. N., Parasuraman, A., Hoefnagels, A., Migchels, N., Kabadayi, S., Gruber, T., Loureiro, Y. K., & Solnet, D. (2013). Understanding Generation Y and their use of social media: A review and research agenda. *Journal of Service Management, 24*(3), 245–267. https://doi.org/10.1108/09564231311326987

Brosnan, M. & Gavin, J. (2021). The impact of stigma, autism label, and wording on the perceived desirability of the online dating profiles of men on the autism spectrum. *Journal of Autism and Developmental Disorders, 51*, 4077–4085. https://doi.org/10.1007/s10803-020-04830-8

Burke, M., Kraut, R., & Williams, D. (2010). Social use of computer mediated communication by adults on the autism spectrum. *Computer Supportive Cooperative*, 425–434. https://doi.org/10.1145/1718918.1718991

Digitability. (n.d.). Digitability: Be work ready. https://digitability.com/

Digital Futures Initiative. (n.d.). All courses. www.dfinow.org/all-courses/

Gillespie-Smith, K., Hendry, G., Anduuru, N., Laird, T., & Ballantyne, C. (2021). Using social media to be 'social': Perceptions of social media benefits and risk by autistic young people and parents. *Research in Developmental Disabilities, 118*, 1–11. https://doi.org/10.1016/j.ridd.2021.104081

Institute of Museum and Library Services, University of Washington Technology & Social Change Group, & International City/County Management Association. (2012). Building digital communities: Getting started. Washington, DC: Institute of Museum and Library Services.

Krile, M. J. (2020). *Post, update, tweet, or snap? Promoting safe social media use for young adults with intellectual disability.* (Publication No: 5850) [Doctoral Dissertation, University of Tennessee]. Tennessee Research and Creative Exchange. https://trace.tennessee.edu/utk_graddiss/5850/

Krile, M. J. (2021, June 3). *Online social networks and learning for individuals with intellectual and developmental disabilities: Risk and strategies* [Live interactive webinar]. Summer Learning Series, Maryland Center for Developmental Disabilities at Kennedy Krieger Institute, Baltimore, MD.

Kuo, M. H., Orsmond, G. I, Coster, W. J., & Cohn, E. S. (2014). Media use among adolescents with autism spectrum disorder. *Autism: The International Journal of Research and Practice, 18*(8), 914–923. https://doi.org/10.1177/1362361313497832

MacMullin, J. A., Lunsky, Y., & Weiss, J. A. (2016). Plugged in: Electronics use in young and young adults with autism spectrum disorder. *Autism, 20*(1), 45–54. https://doi.org/10.1177/1362361314566047

Mazurek, M. O. (2013). Social media use among adults with autism spectrum disorders. *Computers in Human Behavior, 29*(4) 1709–1714. https://doi.org/10.1016/j.chb.2013.02.004

Mazurek, M. O., Shattuck, P. T., Wagner, M., & Cooper, B. P. (2012). Prevalence and correlates of screen-based media use among youths with autism spectrum disorders. *Journal of Autism and Developmental Disorders, 42*(8), 1757–1767. https://doi.org/10.1007/s10803-011-1413-8

Mazurek, M. O. & Wenstrup, C. (2013). Television, video game, and social media use among children with ASD and typically developing siblings. *Journal of Autism and Developmental Disorders, 43*(6), 1258–1271. https://doi.org/10.1007/s10803-012-1659-9

Molin, M., Sorbring, E., & Löfgren-Mårtenson, L. (2015). Teachers' and parents' views on the internet and social media usage by pupils with intellectual

disabilities. *Journal of Intellectual Disabilities, 19*(1), 22–33. https://doi.org/
10.1177/1744629514563558

National Center for Missing & Exploited Children. (n.d.). NetSmartz. www.miss
ingkids.org/netsmartz/home

Northstar. (n.d.). Learn it, know it, show it. www.digitalliteracyassessment.org/

Public Library Association. (n.d.). Tools and resources for trainers. Digital Learn.
https://training.digitallearn.org/

Raghavendra, P., Newman, L., Grace, E., & Wood, D. (2015). Enhancing social
participation in young people with communication disabilities living in rural
Australia: Outcomes of a home-based intervention for using social media.
Disability and Rehabilitation, 37(17), 1576–1590. https://doi.org/10.3109/
09638288.2015.1052578

Raghavendra, P., Hutchinson, C., Grace, E., Wood, D., & Newman, L. (2018).
"I like talking to people on the computer": Outcomes of a home-based intervention to develop social media skills in youth with disabilities living in rural
communities. *Research in Developmental Disabilities, 76,* 110–123. https://
doi.org/10.1016/j.ridd.2018.02.012

Roth, M. E. & Gillis, J. M. (2015). "Convenience with the click of a mouse": A
survey of adults with autism spectrum disorder on online dating. *Sexuality and
Disability, 33,* 133–150. https://doi.org/10.1007/s11195-014-9392-2

Sallafranque-St-Louis, F., & Normand, C. L. (2017). From solitude to solicitation: How people with intellectual disability or autism spectrum disorder
use the internet. *Cyberpsychology: Journal of Psychosocial Research on
Cyberspace, 11*(1). https://doi.org/10.5817/CP2017-1-7

Sorbring, E., Molin, M., & Löfgren-Mårtenson, L. (2017). "I'm a mother, but
I'm also a facilitator in her every-day life": Parents' voices about barriers and
support for internet participation among young people with intellectual disabilities. *Cyberpsychology: Journal of Psychosocial Research on Cyberspace,
11*(1). https://doi.org/10.5817/CP2017-1-3

Suzuki, K., Oi, Y., & Inagaki, M. (2020). The relationships among autism spectrum disorder traits, loneliness, and social networking service use in college
students. *Journal of Autism and Developmental Disabilities, 51,* 2047–2056.
https://doi.org/10.1007/s10803-020-04701-2

Thorn. (n.d.). Be your kid's safety net. Thorn for Parents. https://parents.
thorn.org/

Van Schalkwyk, G. I., Marin, C. E., Ortiz, M., Rolison, M., Qayyum, Z.,
McPartland, J. C., Lebowitz, E. R., Volkmar, F. R., & Silverman, W. K. (2017).
Social media use, friendship quality, and the moderating role of anxiety in ado-
lescents with autism spectrum disorder. *Journal of Autism and Developmental
Disorders, 49*(9), 2805–2813. https://doi.org/10.1007/s10803-017-3201-6

Wang, T., Garfield, M. J., Wisniewski, P., & Page, X. (2020). Benefits and challenges for social media users on the autism spectrum. *Computer Supported
Cooperative Work 2020 Conference Companion.* https://doi.org/10.1145/
3406865.3418322

Ward, D. M., Dill-Shackleford, K. E., & Mazurek, M. O. (2018). Social media
use and happiness in adults with autism spectrum disorder. *Cyberpsychology,
Behavior, and Social Network, 21*(3). https://doi.org/10.1089/cyber.2017.0331

Chapter 21

Interactions with First Responders and Medical Providers

Lindsay L. Diamond,[1] Lindsey B. Hogue,[1] Jamie Prosser,[2] and Kochy Tang[3]
[1]University of Nevada, Reno
[2]Las Vegas Metropolitan Police Department, Las Vegas
[3]M Family Care, Henderson, Nevada

Interactions with First Responders and Medical Providers

First responders and medical professionals play a critical role in the care of individuals with ASD spectrum disorder (ASD). From routine dental or doctor's appointments to emergency situations such as car accidents, fires, and even non-emergency situations, first responders and medical professionals should be prepared to assist and treat individuals across a variety of environments. Furthermore, with the continuous rise in the prevalence of ASD (1 in 44; CDC, 2022) it is likely that first responders and medical providers will have more contact with individuals with ASD supporting the need to be aware of the characteristics of ASD and how to provide the best care to individuals with ASD. Unlike a routine visit to a doctor or a dentist, interactions with first responders are often not planned and it is very likely the first responder will not be aware if an individual has ASD. Thus, having a general understanding of ASD and strategies of how to approach an individual with communication and social differences will allow first responders to better handle emergency and non-emergency situations.

First Responders

First responders are the initial individuals who arrive to the scene of an emergency and are comprised of emergency medical technicians (EMTs), firefighters, and law enforcement officers (LEOs). During emergency and non-emergency situations the responsibility of a first responder is to ensure the protection, safety, and emergency treatment of all individuals who require assistance during various situations. When first responders arrive to a call for service, LEOs are often the first to enter and clear a scene. By securing the scene, the LEO is doing their best to allow safe entry for EMTs and firefighters who may need to render aid. During this

DOI: 10.4324/9781003255147-25

time, LEOs must be direct, assertive, and take charge of the people and events that are occurring. This type of authority may be perceived as aggressive or intrusive by victims, offenders, and bystanders. Emergency situations can be stressful for individuals with ASD and may cause an individual to demonstrate inappropriate responses such as engaging in self-stimulatory behavior, looking away, not responding, running, or yelling when a first responder provides a verbal request or directive (Diamond & Hogue, 2021a). The demonstration of these types of behaviors may result in unplanned interactions with LEOs (Diamond & Hogue, 2021a; Perry & Carter-Long, 2016), and may even result in a more aggressive response from a first responder due to the lack of awareness of a disability (McGonigle et al., 2014).

Emergency Scenario

One evening, the Gutierrez family was spending a typical evening at home when they experienced an unfortunate encounter with first responders, specifically LEOs. Claudia and George were preparing dinner when they called Andrew downstairs to help. Upon entry to the kitchen, Andrew became very upset because he did not want pasta for dinner, he wanted pizza. Claudia explained to Andrew that pizza was not an option that evening which sent Andrew into a meltdown. He began yelling at Claudia and throwing dishes across the kitchen. As plates were shattering, George tried to calm Andrew down but instead he started pushing and punching his dad. After approximately 30 minutes of trying to calm Andrew down, George instructed Claudia to call 911 for help. As LEOs arrived at their house they were informed that Andrew has ASD and that George needed help holding him down. As the LEOs assessed the scene they removed George to ensure his safety and attempted to help Andrew by talking to him. However, this talking seemed to escalate the situation and Andrew became more upset. When he gets upset, he "turns into superman" and has this strength that comes out of nowhere. As he was spoken to, he charged toward the LEO and started throwing punches. The LEO made many attempts to calm Andrew down, but he continued yelling and began kicking, and flailing his limbs. This outburst resulted in Andrew kicking one of the LEOs. This immediately changed the direction of this call for service as Andrew would now be detained for hitting the officer. Andrew was placed on a 72-hour hold and the EMTs on scene transported him to the emergency room. While in the emergency room he was handcuffed and sedated to protect the professionals trying to render aid. This obviously upset Claudia and George as they only wanted help and now, they are in a completely different situation. Thankfully after the 72-hour hold,

Andrew was released to his parents, and no charges were pressed against Andrew but this left lasting concerns for his parents.

Situations similar to this one with the Gutierrez family occur frequently and include individuals with ASD of all ages. Just as Claudia and George have done many times, parents, and guardians call 911 for assistance with situations they cannot gain control over. However, as individuals with ASD grow in strength and size, reliance on first responders pose a problem as seen with the Gutierrez family. Concerns of seeking help from first responders are evident as these situations often end up escalating due to unforeseen circumstances. Specifically, parents of individuals with ASD report feeling nervous that their child may not be able to communicate with first responders and fear that unplanned interactions with LEOs may lead to arrest (Diamond & Hogue, 2021b). Therefore, it is imperative that parents, individuals with ASD, and first responders are prepared to interact with each other across a variety of emergency and non-emergency situations.

Interactions with First Responders

Over the past twenty-five years researchers have sought to provide more accurate data regarding the actual number of individuals with disabilities including those with ASD who encounter first responders, specifically LEOs. In 1998, The Crime Victims with Disabilities Awareness Act (P.L. 105-301) mandated the collection of crime statistics to shed light on the rate and type of crimes against people with disabilities in the United States (Bureau of Statistics, 2021). The National Crime Victimization Survey (NCVS) is collected to estimate the number of crimes against people with disabilities by number and type. Although this survey is used across multiple disciplines to report crime statistics the survey is limited in accuracy due to the types of disability categories. Specifically, the survey collects data on six broadly defined categories of disabilities: a) hearing, b) vision, c) cognitive, d) ambulatory, e) self-care, and f) independent living. The most recent report summarizes data from 2017 to 2019, which indicates individuals with disabilities were victims of 26% of all nonfatal violent crimes, with the highest rate of victimization against individuals with cognitive disabilities (Bureau of Statistics, 2021). Additionally, individuals with disabilities over the age of 12 are more likely to be victims of violent crimes than their non-disabled peers. While this information from this report is helpful to generally shed light on crimes against individuals with a disability, the data is fragmented at best and does not provide a true estimate for the crimes specific to individuals with ASD.

Due to the lack of a well-defined universal data collection system, some researchers have sought to determine the amount and type of interactions between individuals with ASD and first responders (Gibbs & Haas, 2020; Rava et al., 2017; Tint et al., 2017; Tint et al., 2019;). Using the National Longitudinal Transition Study-2 (NLTS2) data set representing 920 individuals with ASD, Rava et al. (2017) sought to determine the percentage of transition-aged youth with ASD who have been stopped or questioned by LEOs. Results of this analysis indicate that approximately 8% of individuals with ASD who were 14 to 15 years old were stopped and questioned by LEOs with less than 1% of these interactions resulting in arrest. However, by the age of 21 the percentage of individuals with ASD being stopped and questioned increased to 20% with almost 5% resulting in arrest (Rava et al., 2017). Furthermore, the results of this analysis indicate that females with ASD are less likely to have interactions with LEOs than males and individuals with ASD who display external behaviors are more likely to be stopped and questioned by LEOs (Rava et al.). Overall, these results suggests that although there are a high number of interactions between LEOs and youth with ASD, the rate of arrests remains low.

Using parent report data, researchers further explored the contextual correlates between individuals with ASD and LEOs (Tint et al., 2017). A total of 284 parents completed approximately four surveys over a 14-month period to report various types of involvement with LEOs. Results of the surveys indicate that one in six individuals with ASD encountered LEOs across a variety of situations (e.g., elopement, physical/verbal aggression with others, victim of aggression) during the study period and were more likely to occur among older individuals with ASD who were living outside the home. Specifically, parents reported the most common contact with LEOs was due to concerns surrounding the display of aggressive verbal or physical behavior and caregiver strain. These situations were often resolved with crisis resolution, physical restraint, or transportation to the emergency room but not arrest and in some cases, parents perceived the LEOs as having a calming effect on the situation (Tint et al.).

Perceptions of First Responders

A study conducted by Diamond and Hogue (2021b) sought to determine the perceptions and needs of individuals with ASD based on caregiver report. Results of this focus group indicated caregivers of individuals with ASD have many concerns regarding potential interactions with first responders, specifically LEOs. Caregivers report when they see a EMT or firefighter they are relieved because these first responders are on scene to provide help to those in need. Whereas when they see a LEO, they immediately panic and think about what could go wrong in the situation or think about what might happen to their child if they display the wrong behaviors. Because of these concerns, caregivers suggest that more opportunities are needed for individuals with ASD interact with all first responders outside of emergency situations.

In addition to the perceptions of caregivers, it is important to understand the perceptions and experiences of individuals with ASD. Tint et al. (2019) conducted a study to gain an understanding of the satisfaction of care during interactions with LEOs and other professionals in the emergency department. A total of 40 adults with ASD between the ages of 18 and 61 years old participated in the survey. Participants reported having at least one engagement with a LEO or emergency department over a 15-month period. Emergency services resulting in interactions with LEOs were based on a variety of needs (e.g., care of others, violation of court order, victim of aggression, psychiatric crisis; Tint et al.). Some participants reported feeling increased agitation during their interactions with LEOs. However, others reported the LEO having a calming effective and expressed an overall level of satisfaction with interactions. Conversely, participants with who reported receiving emergency services in the emergency department expressed lower levels of satisfaction with emergency personnel. These interactions were most commonly due to the participant posing harm to themselves or others and medical needs (e.g., allergic reaction, refill of prescription; Tint et al.).

Gibbs & Haas (2020) further explored the experiences and perspectives of interactions between LEOs and adults with ASD during a five-year period. A total of 50 adults with ASD and 61 caregivers participated in this survey and some participants completed interviews. Twelve participants with ASD reported interactions due to traffic violations, 27 of the participants were victims of crimes (e.g., sexual assault, physical assault, harassment), while five were suspects of crimes (e.g., sexual offences, physical assault, drug offences; Gibbs & Haas, 2020). Caregivers reported individuals with ASD commonly interacted with LEOs to seek help or assistance. In addition to seeking help, 38 caregivers indicated that individuals with ASD were often suspects of crimes or sexual offenses, victims of violent crimes or harassment. Across participants, a total of 183 interactions with LEOs were reported. During 109 of these interactions, caregivers were satisfied with the interactions while adults with ASD were unsatisfied during 74 of these situations (Gibbs & Haas). In addition to gaining an understanding of the type of interactions and levels of satisfaction, Gibbs and Haas also sought to determine if individuals with ASD or their caregivers choose to disclose their diagnosis to LEOs. Adults with ASD reported lower rates of disclosure compared to caregivers. However, disclosures were most often made to explain communication difficulties, anxiety, and violent or other externalizing behaviors. Results of these studies (Diamond & Hogue, 2022; Tint et al., 2019; Gibbs & Haas, 2020) provide valuable insight to the experiences and perceptions of individuals with ASD and their caregivers when interacting with first responders. Furthermore, these results support the ongoing call to ascertain the knowledge and comfort levels of first responders during calls for service involving individuals with ASD.

Disability Awareness of First Responders

Although first responders receive ample amounts of training prior to beginning and during their career to be prepared for a variety of situations, training surrounding knowledge about disabilities, including ASD is lacking (Diamond & Hogue, 2021a; McGonigle et al., 2014). Because of this lack of training, people with disabilities, including those with ASD continue to experience non-lethal and deadly interactions with police, raising concerns regarding law enforcement officers' ability to differentiate between a mental illness and a disability (Perry & Carter-Long, 2014; 2016). To develop specific training for first responders, ongoing research has attempted to describe the perceptions and needs of first responders when responding to calls for service involving individuals with ASD. While most of the literature focuses on LEOs, little to no research had included firefighters while some studies have included EMTs.

McGonigle et al. (2014) conducted a study to determine the caregiver perceptions of the level of care of individuals with ASD when being treated by emergency service personnel (e.g., EMT, paramedics, and emergency room nurses). Data collected through this assessment indicated that caregivers reported that emergency personnel do not understand the communication and behavioral needs of individuals with ASD which often leads to the unnecessary arrest, sedation, or restraint. Results of a needs assessment conducted by McGonigle et al. (2014) were used to guide the development of a didactic training about ASD designed to develop knowledge of ASD, dispel myths, educate personnel on medical issues surrounding ASD, and apply knowledge learned through practical application (McGonigle et al., 2014). A total of 110 medical personnel engaged across three training session and completed pre- and post-assessments to measure their acquisition of knowledge of ASD and comfort levels in treating patients with ASD. Pre-and post-assessments demonstrate participants gained knowledge of ASD which increased their levels of comfort when treating patients with ASD (McGonigle et al).

Additional research conducted by Wachob and Pesci (2017) sought to determine the knowledge and comfort of EMTs and paramedics when treating individuals with ASD. A total of 73 EMTs and paramedics completed the survey. Results indicate that EMTs and paramedics who know someone with ASD (e.g., family member, acquaintance) or received prior training about ASD had higher levels of knowledge and comfort when treating individual with ASD (Wachob & Pesci, 2017).

Additionally, EMTs and paramedics with experience on over 10 calls for services to treat individuals with ASD had higher levels of comfort in providing appropriate care. Overall, levels of knowledge and comfort were higher among female EMTs and paramedics and both male and females between the ages of 26 and 45 years of age with fewer years of experience. However, while comfortable the EMTs and paramedics did not feel that they had enough training or access to resources to provide the best care to individuals with ASD (Wachob & Pesci). Ultimately, these results suggest that the younger first responders may have more knowledge of ASD increasing their understanding of how to communicate with and treat individuals with ASD, but they need more training and resources.

As well as the investigation of the knowledge and comfort levels of EMTs and paramedics when providing treatment to individuals with ASD, researcher have explored the perceptions and needs of LEOs when responding to calls for service including individuals with ASD. Crane et al. (2016) conducted a study to understand the perceptions and experiences of LEOs when providing support to individuals with ASD, and their training needs. A total of 394 LEOs of all ranks responded to the survey. LEOs reported that involvement with individuals diagnosed with ASD were typically due to the person being a victim, witness, or a suspect of violent crimes such as domestic violence, criminal damage, sex offenses, and harassment (Crane et al., 2016). LEOs also reported that individuals often disclosed their diagnosis of ASD during contact making it easier to adjust their tactics on scene and allows for a department assigned appropriate adult (AA) to be present on scene to provide support to the individual with ASD. However, LEOs reported a lack of satisfaction with the department assigned AA and indicated they prefer an AA who was a family member or other support individual who was familiar with the individual's needs (Crane et al., 2016). Of the LEOs who participated in the study, almost 50% were knowledgeable and felt comfortable handling calls for service that include individuals with ASD. Specifically, the LEOs who were trained felt comfortable applying the knowledge and skills learned to modify techniques on scene. However, LEOs felt the training received was too simplistic and did not focus enough on ASD. This information is informative for researchers to understand the urgency and importance of providing a specific and well-designed training to support he needs of LEOs when responding to calls for service that include individuals with ASD.

Railey et al. (2020) conducted semi-structured interviews to explore LEOs knowledge of ASD, the most common type of interactions experienced, and the specific training needs of the LEOs. Seventeen participants representing LEOs, caregivers, and adults with ASD were included in this study. Data analysis of the interviews indicate that LEOs (n=6) gain knowledge and understanding thought experiences with family members who have ASD, individuals with ASD, mothers who are teachers or social workers, and through work experience and trainings. LEOs reported experience handling calls for service that included individuals with ASD who were domestic situations, sexual assault, externalizing behaviors, aggression, and child elopement (Railey et al., 2020). Many LEOs reported being aware of behavioral characteristics of individuals with ASD when on scene (e.g., sensory needs, eye contact, repetitive behaviors) and describe positive interactions with individuals with ASD. LEOs noted that caregivers were sometimes helpful in providing information about the individuals interests and communication preferences. The LEOs who participated in this study provided helpful information regarding the need for mandatory training on ASD to learn about the characteristics and commonly seen behaviors of ASD, as well as the communication needs. The LEOs further highlighted the importance of understanding how the characteristics often seen among individuals with ASD might resemble behaviors of someone who is intoxicated (Railey et al., 2020). The adults with ASD and caregivers included in this study emphasized the need for LEOs to be trained on the characteristic and behaviors typically seen among individuals with ASD and the importance of community involvement to increase the number of positive interactions (Railey et al., 2020). These perceptions of LEOs and suggestions for training align with the results of research conducted to explore needs and perceptions of LEOs across multiple law enforcement agencies (Diamond & Hogue, 2022).

Diamond & Hogue (2022) conducted two semi-structured focus groups with 13 LEOs from a variety of agencies across a large Western State to determine the current perspectives of LEOs regarding people with disabilities, including ASD and their current training needs. Results of this study further support previous research indicating the LEOs, EMTs, and paramedics perceptions are shaped by personal connections (e.g., a family member with ASD, friends or coworkers), experiences providing support to individuals with disabilities when responding to calls for service (e.g., traffic stops, critical events) or during other community activities (e.g., classroom visits, community outreach activities; Diamond & Hogue, 2022; Railey et al., 2020; Wachob & Pesci, 2017), and training experiences (e.g., mandatory training, voluntary training; Diamond & Hogue). Results regarding the specific training needs and suggestions of LEOs also aligns with previous research suggesting the need for initial and ongoing training about ASD (Railey et al., 2020; Wachob & Pesci, 2017), other disabilities (Diamond & Hogue, 2022; Modell & Mak, 2008), and the differences between disabilities such as autism and mental illness (Diamond & Hogue, 2022; Gardner et al., 2019; Modell & Mak, 2008). Additionally, training should use a collaborative approach (e.g., LEO, education professional, adult with ASD; Diamond & Hogue, 2022; Kelley & Hassett-Walker, 2016; Viljoen et al., 2017) that provides an overview of common characteristics, strategies to promote successful interactions, and role-play (Diamond & Hogue).

Based on the consistent call for ASD awareness training, Love et al., (2020) conducted a study to determine the effectiveness of the Emergency Network Autism Community Training (ENACT). ENACT is an in-person training format consist of lecture, discussion, and short videos to teach LEOs to recognize ASD and strategies to support individuals with ASD. The two-hour training was implemented with 224 first responders (e.g., LEOs, paramedics, firefighters). First responders reported increased confidence in handling calls for service including individuals with ASD after attending the training (Love et al., 2020). The Results of this study support the implementation of training for first responders that may help improve interactions between individuals with ASD and first responders but recognizes the need for more rigorous research to determine the effectiveness of the trainings (Love et al., 2020).

Overall, the result of ongoing research supports the need for first responders to be better prepared to interact with individuals with ASD (Crane et al., 2016; Diamond & Hogue, 2022; Love et al., 2020; McGonigle et al., 2014; Railey et al., 2020; Wachob & Pesci, 2017). However, consistency in the design and implementation of first responder training is lacking (Diamond & Hogue, 2021a; Modell & Mak, 2008). Thus, it is important for developers of these trainings to follow guidelines based in research to ensure the needs of first responders are met.

First Responder Training

First responders training should encompass a multi-pronged approach that includes training first responders (Diamond & Hogue, 2022; Love et al., 2020; McGonigle et al., 2014), individuals with ASD (Diamond & Hogue, 2021a; Gardner et al., 2019; Modell & Mak, 2008), and caregivers (Diamond & Hogue, 2021b). This multi-pronged approach should be used to increase the likelihood of positive interactions between first responders and individuals with ASD. Furthermore, disability awareness training including, ASD specific training, should be implemented prior to and throughout the career of first responders (Diamond & Hogue 2021; Diamond & Hogue 2022; Railey et al., 2020; Wachob & Pesci, 2017). LEOs and firefighters should receive substantial training specific to ASD during initial academies and annual recertification or refresher trainings (Diamond & Hogue, 2022). Additionally, EMTs and other emergency medical staff should receive training during coursework and ongoing continuing education. By attending initial and yearly training, first responders will become knowledgeable about the characteristic and manifestation of ASD across the lifespan. Initial research indicates that first responders who attend training demonstrate higher levels of comfort, when providing care to individuals with ASD (Love et al., 2020; McGonigle et al., 2014).

The multi-pronged approach is designed to focus on training first responders and individuals with ASD to promote positive interactions. The first prong to this approach focuses on teaching the first responder to understand the characteristics of ASD and to develop strategies for handling calls for service involving individuals with ASD (Diamond & Hogue, 2021a). The format of training first responders aligns with the training designed for the individual with ASD. First, the first responder must gain knowledge and understating of ASD. Second, the first responder develops the skills and strategies to interact with individuals with ASD. Third, through application, the first responders review videos and case studies of first responders' interactions with individuals with ASD. Lastly, the training should provide ample times for reflection (Diamond & Hogue, 2021a).

The second and third prongs to this approach to provide caregivers and educators with the support and training needed to successfully teach the individual with ASD the skills needed to recognize, respond to, and comply with first responders (Diamond & Hogue 2021a; Diamond & Hogue 2021b). The second prong to this approach focuses on first training the individual with ASD to understand who a first responder is and what their roles is in society. Second, the individual with ASD should be taught how to communicate with first responders, especially LEOs. During this instruction, individuals are taught to stop, look, listen, and follow the direction of the first responder (Diamond & Hogue). This set of skills will ensure the individual is prepared when they encounter LEOs and other first responders during novel events. Third, the training should implement video modeling and role paly to allow for the application and practice of the new skills. Fourth, the training should provide multiple opportunities for reflection (Diamond & Hogue). This prong should be implemented by educators and practiced across a variety of environments to promote generalization of these skills for the individual with ASD.

Educators can implement embedded learning opportunities to teach individuals with ASD about first responders beginning in preschool (Diamond & Hogue, 2021a). For example, educators can invite first responders to the school to visit the classroom during career week, literacy week, or at other times during the school year. Educators can also schedule visits to local fire and police stations to tour the building and first responder's vehicles (e.g., police car, firetruck, ambulance; Diamond & Hogue, 2021a).

The third and final prong focuses on using the same embedded educational model with caregivers. This approach will provide opportunities for caregivers to implement discussions of first responders in the home, during public outings, and while watching television. Throughout these daily events, caregivers can promote positive conversations about first responders that describe who first responders are, what they wear, the cars they drive, and talk about what they do to help (Diamond & Hogue 2021b). When possible, caregivers can model positive interactions when by waving and saying hello to first responders.

This multi-pronged approach focuses on preparing first responders to understand ASD and incorporates training to support individuals with ASD to understand who first responders are and the role they hold in society and ideas for caregivers and educators to support positive interactions.

When designing content and training materials first responders it is important to include multiple stakeholders (e.g., first responders, educators, individuals with ASD; Diamond & Hogue, 2022; Kelley & Hassett-Walker, 2016; Viljoen et al., 2017) to ensure the needs of the first responders are met (Diamond & Hogue, 2021a). Content for the training should be developed using the individual expertise and experience of the targeted stakeholder group. This will increase the buy-in of participants and ensure the content is appropriate for the population being receiving training (Diamond & Hogue, 2021a). Providing strategies to promote successful interactions will be central to the success of the training.

Suggestions for Interactions

To engage in positive interactions with individuals with ASD, first responders should develop an understanding of the social behavioral, communication, and sensory needs commonly associated with ASD (Diamond & Hogue, 2022; McGonigle et al., 2014; Railey et al., 2020). Because ASD presents a unique set of behaviors that are different among everyone it is important to be aware of common externalizing behaviors that may

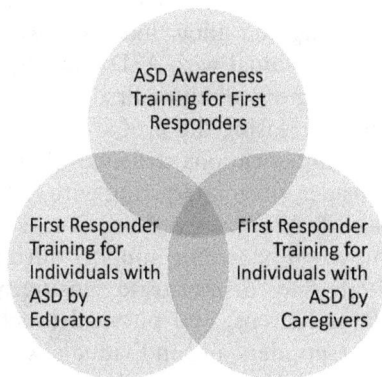

Figure 21.1 Multi-Pronged Approach to Training.

be observed as these behaviors may be misinterpreted as noncompliant and sometimes perceived as under the influence of a controlled substance (e.g., fidgeting, hand flapping, visual fixations, verbal outburst). Social behavioral interactions may too present challenges for an individual to interact with first responders. Behaviors such as a lack of eye contact or an inability to follow complex directions might be misinterpreted as noncompliant and could result in more aggressive tactics from first responders (Diamond & Hogue, 2021a). In addition to understanding behaviors, it is important for first responders to recognize the communication needs of individuals with ASD.

The ability to successfully communicate with individuals who have ASD and other communicative needs is imperative to ensuring the best outcome (Depew & Thistle, 2021; Diamond & Hogue, 2021a). During emergency and non-emergency situations, individuals with ASD may have difficulty responding appropriately to commands or directives given by first responders. A loud tone of voice, speaking too quickly, and providing complex directives may results in an inappropriate response from an individual with ASD (e.g., delayed verbal response, yelling, refusal to respond, walking or turning away). DePew & Thistle conducted interviews with a first responders representing each type of agency (EMTs, firefighters, and LEOs) to determine how first responders might respond to hypothetical circumstances with individuals who have communication difficulties and to understand prior training received. Results of this research indicate that two of the participants had some communication training one of which was a training about ASD, and the third first responder reported no training. Each of the participants in this study indicated a reliance on basic department procedures learned through training (DePew & Thistle, 2021). LEOs tend to demonstrate strong problem-solving skills which is helpful when dealing with individuals who demonstrate communication deficits (DePew & Thistle). When communicating all first responders should keep an open mind, slow down when speaking, and allow increased wait time when a call for service includes an individual with ASD. Having knowledge of general communication strategies will allow first responders to adapt to the needs of the individual increasing the probability of positive outcomes. Table 21.1 provides communications strategies that may be helpful for first responders to consider when interacting with individuals with ASD.

Many individuals with ASD present unique sensory needs that may require consideration when providing support during calls for service. Specifically, individuals may demonstrate sensitivity to lights on vehicles, the sound of loud sirens, and physical touch. It is in the best interest of both first responders and individuals with ASD for first responders to be aware of these sensitives (Diamond & Hogue, 2021a). When possible, first responders might consider turning off the lights and sirens on emergency vehicles, avoid shining flashlights directly at

Table 21.1 Communication Strategies for First Responders

Communication Type	Strategies to Adjust Communication	Reasoning for Communication Adjustment
Nonverbal Communication	Use a nonauthoritarian stance Avoid quick movements Do not touch unexpectedly	Individual may be intimidated by the perceived aggression of the stance, reactive to fast movements of the hands or body, and may have an aversion to touch.
Verbal Communication	Speak slowly Use a calm tone of voice Provide clear and short directives	Individual may have difficulty following directions that are provided quickly, have an aversion to loud voices, and may not be able to follow complex direction.

Note. Strategies were adapted from Diamond & Hogue (2021a).

the individual, and provide a quiet and calm space to provide care. In addition to understanding the social behavior, communication, and sensory needs of individuals with ASD, first responders should be conscious of how their behavior that might be misinterpreted. For example, the mere presence of an LEO often intimidates individuals and may cause an individual to shut down or have an inappropriate response (Diamond & Hogue, 2021a).

First responders have an immense amount of responsibility to ensure timely, effective, and safe treatment of individuals with ASD across non-emergency and emergency situations. Participating in ongoing training to develop a comprehensive understanding of ASD and the unique characteristics associated with ASD will prepare first responders for positive interactions. In addition to first responders, medical professionals should also understand the nuances of ASD in order to provide effective care across a variety of medical settings.

Medical Providers

Medical Scenario

Kong (2015), a pediatrician in Alabama, described a recent emergency room visit for a child with ASD. The child had been vomiting for about a week and had a persistent fever. He was non-verbal and generally good natured, although recently had exhibited crying and self-injurious behaviors such as head-hitting. The child's father described him as "wobbly." The emergency room physician examined the child through a basic workup and an X-ray of the child's kidney, ureter, and bladder, and found no cause for concern. The physician *noted tachycardia (e.g., a heart rate over 100 beats per minute) and agitation. The child was released from the emergency room with a diagnosis of viral gastroenteritis. His family was told to provide him with hydration and over-the-counter fever medication. Over the next twelve hours, the child's conditioned worsened, and the family returned to the emergency room. The child was intubated, admitted to the intensive care unit, and diagnosed with bacterial meningitis. He survived the bacterial meningitis but required a ventricular shunt and he now has paraplegia of his lower extremities due to an infection involving his spinal cord. Kong (2015) used this sad example to highlight the difficulties in caring for patients with ASD in emergency settings, particularly those who struggle with communication. Kong (2015) explained that further examination revealed the head-hitting to be a new behavior that had increased as the vomiting and fever increased. In hindsight, this new behavior was the clue that the child had the new symptom of a headache. Along with the other symptoms of vomiting and fever, the emergency room staff would have evaluated the child for bacterial meningitis sooner.*

(Kong, 2015)

Considerations for Providers

Medical providers include doctors, nurses, and dentists. There are several components for medical providers who work with children and adolescents with ASD to consider. Doctors may struggle with working with patients with ASD because of the complexity of the disorder as well as a lack of training and knowledge about ASD (Morris et al., 2019). Also, young people with ASD can have extensive comorbid health problems such as constipation, sleep issues, seizures, and psychiatric symptoms (Kalb et al., 2019; Mandell et al., 2019; Mazurek et al., 2017; Myers & Johnson, 2007; Richdale, 1999; Wang et al., 2011).

In addition to considerations regarding comorbid health issues, there are some characteristics of ASD that can provide challenges for medical providers. In the emergency room setting, young people with ASD might struggle due to sensory issues, communication issues, or cognitive deficits (McGonigle et al., 2014; Nicholas et al., 2016). The bright lights, beeping machines, and unfamiliar people in an emergency room may upset a person with ASD, and communication issues and cognitive deficits may make it difficult for people with ASD to express their health needs (Austriaco et al., 2019). In interviews with emergency room doctors and nurses, Zwaigenbaum et al. (2016) found that the participants perceived that a challenge of caring for some young patients with ASD was aggressiveness or limited verbal functioning. The participants explained that the emergency room is an unfamiliar setting with lots of noise and people, which can be difficult for people with sensory issues. Another challenge is that it takes time to deescalate situations, but the emergency room is a busy place so if a nurse needs to take extended time with one patient, they are removed from their other duties (Zwaigenbaum et al., 2016).

Young people with ASD visit the emergency room at higher rates than typically developing young people (Kouo et al., 2021). Authors in one study found that children with ASD were three times more likely to need extra staff for intravenous placement, five times as likely to experience difficulty with triage vitals (e.g., blood pressure, body temperature, oxygen saturation), and four times more likely to have delays in emergency room care (Kouo et al., 2021). Additionally, adolescents with ASD in the emergency room setting in another study were more likely to have a psychiatric hospitalization than adolescents with ADHD, and more likely to have to come back to the emergency room. (Kalb et al., 2019). Psychiatric hospitalization often leads to outpatient and inpatient psychiatric services, which are quite expensive for families of young people with ASD, costing $4,000 per week on average (Mandell et al., 2019).

In a non-emergency medical setting such as the pediatrician's or dentist's office, there are other considerations when providing care for young people with ASD. Because of the complexity of ASD, many families need longer pediatrician appointments; some pediatricians accommodate this by scheduling longer office visits, but other pediatricians in a study were either not able or unwilling to do so (Carbone et al., 2010). The communication difficulties inherent in ASD mean that the child's ability to understand the dentist's or pediatrician's directions may be limited as well as the child's ability to express pain, fears, or needs to the dentist or pediatrician (Logrieco et al., 2021; Stein et al., 2014). Stein et al. found that children with ASD exhibited greater behavioral and physiological distress during routine dental visits than typically developing children. Those with lower expressive communication skills exhibited more distress than those with higher levels of expressive communication. Similarly, there were greater levels of distress in children with ASD who had sensory processing difficulties (Stein et al., 2014).

Despite the challenges some young people with ASD face in a dental setting, children with ASD have similar rates of periodontal disease compared to the typically developing population (U.S. Department of Health and Human Services, 2008), but some children with ASD may have poor oral hygiene because they refuse the toothbrush (Charles, 2010). Other dental issues associated with children with ASD are clenching/grinding teeth, tongue thrusting, and self-injurious behaviors (Charles, 2010; Pathmashri & Kumar, 2018) such as chin or jaw hitting, picking at gums or lips, or eating non-food objects (Charles, 2010).

Training Needs

Because of the complexities of ASD, several researchers have recommended more training for medical providers and medical students regarding ASD (Austriaco et al., 2019; Kuhlthau et al., 2015; Morris et al., 2019; Nicholas et al., 2016; Rhoades et al., 2007; Zwaigenbaum et al., 2016). There is a need for training on general characteristics and care strategies for individuals with ASD, as well as screening, diagnosis, and advice for caregivers regarding ASD (Rhoades et al., 2007). Pediatricians should also learn more about evidence-based practices for treating patients with ASD and resources to share with caregivers (Carbone et al., 2013).

In focus groups with caregivers of children with ASD, the caregivers perceived that their child's pediatrician did not take their concerns seriously, did not have helpful resources or information about ASD to share, and were not family centered (Carbone et al., 2010). The caregivers explained that they tended to find out about services and supports via word of mouth or other resources, rather than from their child's doctor. Additionally, they did not feel listened to or that they were considered the experts about their own children (Carbone et al., 2010). Similarly, Carbone et al. (2013) found a discrepancy between caregivers' perceptions and pediatricians' perceptions about the doctor's ability to provide care to children with ASD. Caregivers in the study rated their pediatrician's ability to provide ASD-specific care as "not good" on 14 of 17 measures, whereas the pediatricians rated themselves "good" in 10 of 17 areas. For example, caregivers gave pediatricians a significantly lower rating than the pediatricians gave themselves regarding the ability to make timely referrals. One exception was that if the parents reported their care as "family-centered" they were more likely to consider the pediatrician's abilities regarding ASD as "good" (Carbone et al., 2013).

Although the pediatricians surveyed by Carbone et al. (2013) perceived themselves to be good at providing care to families of children with ASD, other studies of medical providers' perspectives have shown a need for more training regarding ASD. Medical providers in another study expressed interest in training and strategies for de-escalation of children with ASD (Nicholas et al., 2016). Austriaco et al. (2019) surveyed medical students and pediatric trainees about their knowledge and training regarding ASD. Both groups perceived they had low general knowledge about ASD and did not know much about sensory issues with ASD and did not feel they had been adequately prepared in their training programs to interact with children with ASD. Both groups expressed interest in further training, particularly through small group learning and interactions with patients with ASD (Austriaco et al., 2019).

Similarly, in a survey of dentists, Weil and Inglehart (2010) found that most participants did not feel they had been adequately prepared in their dental programs to provide dental care for patients with ASD. However, there was a significant correlation between dentists who perceived that their dental training prepared them well for patients with ASD and their comfort and knowledge treating patients with ASD. Also, those who perceived that their training prepared them well were more likely to say that they liked providing care to patients with ASD (Weil & Inglehart, 2010).

To address the need for training, Donnelly et al. (2020) implemented a half-day ASD training for hospital staff that addressed the symptoms of ASD and evidence-based practices for working with individuals with ASD. Following the training, participants perceived that their knowledge of ASD and confidence in their ability to support patients with ASD increased. Participants also increased their knowledge of evidence-based practices (Donnelly et al., 2020). In a more extensive training study, Mazurek et al. (2017) implemented a six-month pilot study with 12 clinics concerning ASD screening and identification of ASD, and medical and psychiatric management of comorbidities associated with ASD. The primary care providers received professional development credits for their participation. A post-test found significant improvements in self-efficacy and the use of ASD-specific resources, and an overall high satisfaction with the training (Mazurek et al.). While more research is needed in this area, these studies show that training can be effective at improving medical providers' knowledge and self-efficacy when treating patients with ASD.

Suggestions for Successful Interactions

Table 21.2 provides suggestions for caregivers of children with ASD to prepare for successful interactions with medical providers. These suggestions are centered around the use of evidence-based practices (EBPs) for teaching children with ASD (Steinbrenner et al., 2020). Another suggestion for caregivers from the dental literature was to avoid using sugary treats for behavioral rewards, particularly if the child dislikes tooth brushing (Charles, 2010).

To prepare for trips to the emergency room, Venkat et al. (2016) provided a form for caregivers to complete before the emergency. The form includes basic information and baseline characteristics about the child with ASD, such as the child's communication ability, social interaction, behavioral patterns, dietary patterns, other medical conditions, home medications and other therapies, and preferred comfort object (Venkat et al., 2016). Other suggested information included environmental factors that might agitate the child, the best way to communicate with the child, and medications that have worked for sedation or pain as well as medications that should be avoided (Venkat et al., 2016).

Table 21.2 Tips for Caregivers of Children with Autism to Prepare for Medical and Dental Visits

Evidence-Based Practice (EBP)	Description	How to Use EBP with Doctor or Dentist
Task Analysis	An activity or behavior is broken into small chunks so that the caregiver can teach the desired skill or behavior. Task analysis is often used in conjunction with video modeling.	A task analysis could describe the steps needed to walk into a medical office, check in for the appointment, and sit with quiet hands and feet in a waiting room.
Video Modeling	A desired behavior or skill is recorded on video and show to the child, to help the child learn how to engage in the behavior or skill.	Video modeling could be used to show the child what happens at a regular dental appointment (e.g, check in, wait, walk to exam room, sit in chair, dental hygienist says hi, dental hygienist begins brushing child's teeth, etc).
Social Narratives	A social situation is described in a narrative, often with pictures, and is used to portray desired behaviors or skills. It shows examples of the appropriate way to respond in a particular situation.	A social narrative could be written to show the child what to expect at a regular pediatrician appointment (e.g., weight, blood pressure, temperature, etc) and desired behaviors for the appointment.
Visual Supports	A visual display is shown to the child to support desired behavior or skills.	A series of pictures could portray a child at a pediatrician or dental appointment complying with the medical provider's requests.

Note. Description of EBPs based on the report conducted by Steinbrenner et al. (2020).

Table 21.3 provides suggestions to support positive interactions between medical providers and children with ASD. These suggestions are guided by the characteristics of ASD (e.g., deficits in social communication and social interaction; restricted, repetitive patterns of behavior; Centers for Disease Control and Prevention, 2020) and are drawn from the medical and dental literature.

Researchers provided several strategies for successful interactions between medical providers and children with ASD. A key recommendation in the medical and dental literature was to include caregivers in the process (Brown et al., 2014; Duker et al., 2019; McGonigle et al., 2014; Nicholas et al., 2016; Zwaigenbaum et al., 2016). Caregivers know their child best, including their preferences, dislikes, communication style, and calming strategies (Duker et al., 2019; Nicholas et al., 2016; Zwaigenbaum et al., 2016). Including caregivers was important for the

Table 21.3 Tips for Medical Providers Providing Care to Children with Autism

Characteristics of Autism	Tips for Medical Providers
Deficits in social communication and social interaction	Use concrete language such as, "Sit here," instead of, "Why don't you hop up on the table?" Use concrete descriptions/visuals to show patients with autism each tool and explain how it will be used. Create visual supports to show patients with autism the steps involved in a regular medical/dental visit. Create a social narrative for going to the dentist/going to the doctor that is available in the office waiting room.
Restricted, repetitive patterns of behavior	Praise/reinforce appropriate behavior. Reduce extra noise and bright lights when possible. Consider providing desensitization appointments to allow the child to become more comfortable before the regularly scheduled medical or dental. Doctors: Find out which behaviors are normal for the child and which behaviors are new—these new behaviors might tell you something about symptoms. When possible, keep visits with the same support staff in the same room. Ask caregivers if the child has a preferred toy or object for soothing during the appointment.

Note. Characteristics based on the diagnostic criteria for autism in the DSM-5. (CDC, 2020).

emergency room setting (McGonigle et al., 2014; Nicholas et al., 2016; Zwaigenbaum et al., 2016) and in the dental setting (Brown et al., 2014; Duker et al., 2019). Nicholas et al. (2016) suggested the development of a short screening tool that can be administered during emergency room registration. The caregivers can answer questions about their child's communication styles, specific needs, triggers, and strategies to work with the child (Nicholas et al., 2016). This helps the caregivers feel like valued members of the medical team (Nicholas et al., 2016).

Caregiver involvement is particularly helpful in emergency room settings. Emergency room staff should establish which behaviors are typical for the patient with ASD and which behaviors are new (Kong, 2015; McGonigle et al., 2014). The staff can ask the caregivers how the behaviors have changed and the antecedents for the new behaviors (McGonigle et al., 2014). These new behaviors may illuminate a medical issue that the patient cannot otherwise express, due to limited verbal functioning (Kong, 2015).

Another suggestion in the literature was to keep wait time short, when possible (Brown et al., 2014; Duker et al., 2019; Nicholas et al., 2016), as individuals with ASD may become increasingly anxious the longer they wait for an appointment. This can be difficult in an emergency room.

A parent in a qualitative study suggested a page system so that they would not have to wait in the emergency room but could be called on the phone when their child was ready to be seen (Nicholas et al., 2016). Emergency rooms can also provide alternate quiet spaces with art supplies, computers, and televisions (Nicholas et al., 2016) or just a quiet, private space (Zwaigenbaum et al., 2016). Similarly, dental researchers suggested maintaining a calm waiting room where children can play with their preferred toys (Brown et al., 2014).

Quiet and calm waiting rooms can also reduce the sensory issues associated with ASD. Patients with ASD may struggle because of the unfamiliar, bright, and loud setting of the emergency room (McGonigle et al., 2014). Some suggestions in the dental literature may apply to other medical settings as well. For example, researchers suggested providing sunglasses, dimming the lights, and allowing the use of noise-canceling headphones (Stein et al., 2014; U.S. Department of Health and Human Services, 2008). For dental visits, Stein et al. (2014) also suggested allowing patients with ASD to rinse more frequently and to use no-taste cleaning products such as pumice. To keep the patient and medical staff safe, the area around the chair should be kept clear (Pathmashri & Kumar, 2018; U.S. Department of Health and Human Services, 2008). Another suggestion in the dental literature was to provide one or more desensitization appointments (Duker et al., 2019; Stein et al., 2014; U.S. Department of Health and Human Services, 2008). In a desensitization appointment, the dentist allows the child to visit the office before the appointment so they can become familiar with the staff, office, and equipment. At the appointment, staff should have the child sit in the chair or the stool if they prefer. Dental staff would perform an initial exam with fingers, then use a toothbrush when the child is comfortable, because the toothbrush is a familiar sensation (U.S. Department of Health and Human Services, 2008).

Because individuals with ASD tend to dislike change, a recommendation from the dental literature is to use the same staff and the same room for each dental appointment (Pathmashri & Kumar, 2018; U.S. Department of Health and Human Services, 2008).

Because of the communication difficulties associated with ASD, children with ASD might not respond positively to strategies that usually work with neurotypical children such as coaxing, reassurance, or explanations (McGonigle et al., 2014). Researchers suggested providing clear, concrete directions rather than abstractions (Kong, 2015; McGonigle et al., 2014; Pathmashri & Kumar, 2018; Stein et al., 2014). For example, a doctor should tell a patient with ASD to get on the table instead of saying, "Why don't you hop up here and let me check you out?" (Kong, 2015, p. 2). Brown et al. (2014) recommended a calm, conversational style and to avoid talking for the sake of making conversation. Also, doctors should provide time for patients with ASD to respond, rather than overwhelming them with information and questions (Kong, 2015). Lastly, doctors and dentists should model what they are going to do before they do it (Brown et al., 2014; McGonigle et al., 2014). In the dental literature, this is described as a "tell, show, do" approach (Pathmashri & Kumar, 2018; U.S. Department of Health and Human Services, 2008). In this approach, dentists explain each procedure before beginning it, show the patient the instruments, and explain how they work (U.S. Department of Health and Human Services, 2008).

Another way to address communication issues in medical settings is through visual supports (Brown et al., 2014; Chebuhar et al., 2013; Kouo & Kouo, 2020; Stein et al., 2014). For example, Chebuhar et al. (2013) examined the effect of picture schedules for children with ASD in medical settings. Most of the medical staff and caregivers involved in the study perceived that the picture schedules decreased anxious and distressed behaviors in young patients with ASD (Chebuhar et al.). This may be more feasible in a non-emergency setting such as the pediatrician's or dentist's office. Another way to use visual supports is through social narratives (Brown et al., 2014; Stein et al., 2014). Social narratives are an evidence-based practice that uses short stories to describe target behaviors during individualized social situations (Steinbrenner et al., 2020). These narratives are written from the learners' perspective and provide information regarding the appropriate responses and the perspectives of others. When preparing to interact in medical settings social narratives can support the individual with ASD in preparing for the visit. For example, a caregiver can prepare a social narrative from the perspective of a child who is going to have their teeth cleaned. The narrative would visually depict the process the child will go through in preparing for the dental visit. Then describe in short sentences why they are going to the dentist, the process of arriving at the dental office, the act of sitting in the dental chair, and what tools will be used for the dental cleaning. Describing this process will allow for the individual with ASD to visually process and prepare for the dental visit.

A final recommendation for pediatricians is to prepare families for the transition to an adult primary care provider. Kuhlthau et al. (2015) interviewed healthcare providers about the strategies they use to transition their patients to adult providers. The providers gave families written medical summaries to give to the new providers and a list of adult providers accepting new patients (Kuhlthau et al., 2015).

It is imperative that medical professionals and first responders understand ASD. By developing the knowledge and awareness of the characteristics of ASD professionals will be better prepared to support and treat individuals with ASD. As the prevalence of ASD continues to rise, it is inevitable that first responders will respond to more non-emergency and emergency calls for service involving someone with ASD. Likewise, medical professionals will continue to see an increase in new and established patients with ASD. Having the skills and strategies to make environmental, communication, and behavioral adaptations will increase the quality of treatment provided to all individuals with ASD.

References

Austriaco, K., Aban, I., Willig, J., & Kong, M. (2019). Contemporary trainee knowledge of ASD: How prepared are our future providers? *Frontiers in Pediatrics, 7*(165), 1–8. https://doi.org/10.3389/fped.2019.00165

Brown, J., Brown, J., & Woodburn, J. (2014). Dental services for children with ASD spectrum disorder: Jeremy Brown and colleagues describe a pilot study to assess how parents perceive good practice and barriers to care. *Learning Disability Practice, 17*(3), 20–25. https://doi.org/10.7748/ldp2 014.03.17.3.20.e1527

Bureau or Justice Statistics. (2021). *Crime against persons with disabilities, 2009-2019 statistical tables.* https://bjs.ojp.gov/library/publications/crime-against-persons-disabilities-2009-2019-statistical-tables

Carbone, P. S., Behl, D. D., Azor, V., & Murphy, N. A. (2010). The medical home for children with autism spectrum disorders: Parent and pediatrician perspectives. *Journal of ASD and Developmental Disorders, 40*(3), 317–324. https://doi.org/10.1007/s10803-009-0874-5

Carbone, P. S., Murphy, N. A., Norlin, C., Azor, V., Sheng, X., & Young, P. C. (2013). Parent and pediatrician perspectives regarding the primary care of children with autism spectrum disorders. *Journal of ASD and Developmental Disorders, 43*(4), 964–972. https://doi.org/10.1007/s10803-012-1640-7

Centers for Disease Control and Prevention. (2020, June 29). *Diagnostic criteria.* Centers for Disease Control and Prevention. https://www.cdc.gov/ncb ddd/ASD/hcp-dsm.html

Center for Disease Control and Prevention. (2022). *Data & statistics on autism spectrum disorder.* www.cdc.gov/ncbddd/autism/data.html

Charles, J. M. (2010). Dental care in children with developmental disabilities: attention deficit disorder, intellectual disabilities, and ASD. *Journal of Dentistry for Children, 77*(2), 84–91.

Chebuhar, A., McCarthy, A. M., Bosch, J., & Baker, S. (2013). Using picture schedules in medical settings for patients with an autism spectrum disorder. *Journal of Pediatric Nursing, 28*(2), 125–134. https://doi.org/10.1016/ j.pedn.2012.05.004

Crane, L., Maras, K. L., Hawken, T., Mulcahy, S., & Memon, A. (2016). Experiences of autism spectrum disorder and policing in England and Wales: Surveying police and the autism community. *Journal of Autism & Developmental Disorders, 46,* 2028–2041. https://doi.org/10.1007/s10 803-016-2729-1

DePew, S., & Thistle, J. J. (2021). Supporting communication between individuals with disabilities and first responders: A preliminary case-based interview study. *Perspective of The ASHA Special Interest Groups, 7*, 115–122. https://doi.org/10.1044/2021_PERSP-21-00123

Diamond, L. L., & Hogue, L. B. (2021a). Preparing students with disabilities and police for successful interactions. *Intervention in School and Clinic, 57(1)*, 1–12. https://doi.org/10.1177/1053451221994804

Diamond, L. L., & Hogue, L. (2021b). *Individuals with disabilities and first responders*. Paper Presentation at the Northern Rocky Mountain Educational Research Association Annual Conference. Sun Valley, ID.

Diamond L. L., & Hogue L. B. (2022). Law enforcement officers: A call for training and awareness of disabilities. *Journal of Disability Policy Studies*. https://doi.org/10.1177/10442073221094803

Donnelly, L. J., Cervantes, P. E., Guo, F., Stein, C. R., Okparaeke, E., Kuriakose, S., Filton, B., Havens, J., & Horwitz, S. M. (2020). Changes in attitudes and knowledge after trainings in a clinical care pathway for autism spectrum disorder. *Journal of Autism and Developmental Disorders*. https://doi.org/10.1007/s10803-020-04775-y

Duker, L. I., Florindez, L. I., Como, D. H., Tran, C. F., Henwood, B. F., Polido, J. C., & Cermak, S. A. (2019). Strategies for success: A qualitative study of caregiver and dentist approaches to improving oral care for children with autism. *Pediatric Dentistry, 41(1)*, E4-E12.

Gardner, L., Campbell, J. M., & Westdal, J. (2019). Brief report: Descriptive analysis of law enforcement officers' experiences with and knowledge of autism. *Journal of Autism and Developmental Disorders, 49*, 1278–1283.

Gibbs, V., & Haas, K. (2020). Interactions between the police and the autistic community in Australia: Experiences and perspectives of autistic adults and parents/carers. *Journal of Autism and Developmental Disorders, 50*, 4513–4526. https://doi.org/10.1007/s10803-020-04510-7

Kalb, L. G., Stuart, E. A., & Vasa, R. A. (2019). Characteristics of psychiatric emergency department use among privately insured adolescents with autism spectrum disorder. *ASD, 23(3)*, 566–573. https://doi.org/10.1177/1362361317749951

Kelly, E., & Hassett-Walker, C. (2016). The training of New Jersey emergency service first responders in autism awareness. *Police Practice and Research, 17(6)*, 543–554. https://doi.org/10.1080/15614263.2015.1121390

Kong, M. Y. F. (2015). Diagnosis and history taking in children with autism spectrum disorder: Dealing with the challenges. *Frontiers in Pediatrics, 3*, 55–65. https://doi.org/10.3389/fped.2015.00055

Kouo, T. S., Bharadwaj, N. Kouo, J. L., Tackett, S., & Ryan, L. (2021). Assessing ease of delivering emergency care for patients with autism spectrum disorders. *Journal of Developmental & Behavioral Practices, 42(9)*, 704–710.

Kouo, J. L., & Kouo, T. S. (2021). A scoping review of targeted interventions and training to facilitate medical encounters for school-aged patients with an autism spectrum disorder. *Journal of Autism and Developmental Disorders, 51(8)*, 2829–2851. https://doi.org/10.1007/s10803-020-04716-9

Kuhlthau, K. A., Warfield, M. E., Hurson, J., Delahaye, J., & Crossman, M. K. (2015). Pediatric providers' perspectives on the transition to adult health care for youth with autismspectrum disorder: Current strategies and promising new directions. *Autism, 19*(3), 262–271. https://doi.org/10.1177/136236131 3518125

Logrieco, M. G. M., Ciuffreda, G. N., Sinjari, B., Spinelli, M., Rossi, R., D'Addazio, G., Lionetti, F., Caputi, S., & Fasolo, M. (2021). What happens at a dental surgery when the patient is a child with ASD spectrum disorder? An Italian study. *Journal of Autism and Developmental Disorders, 51*(6), 1939–1952. https://doi.org/10.1007/s10803-020-04684-0

Love, A. M. A., Railey, K. S., Phelps, M., Campbell, J. M., Cooley-Coook, H. A., & Taylor, L. (2020). Preliminary evidence for a training improving first responder knowledge and confidence to work with individuals with autism. *Journal of Intellectual Disabilities and Offending Behaviour, 11*(4), 211–219. https://doi.org/10.1108/JIDOB-04-2020-0007

Mandell, D. S., Candon, M. K., Xie, M., Marcus, S. C., Kennedy-Hendricks, A., Epstein, A. J., & Barry, C. L. (2019). Effect of outpatient service utilization on hospitalizations and emergency visits among youths with autism spectrum disorder. *Psychiatric Services, 70*(10), 888–893. https://doi.org/10.1176/appi. ps.201800290

Mazurek, M. O., Brown, R., Curran, A., & Sohl, K. (2017). ECHO ASD: A new model for training primary care providers in best-practice care for children with autism. *Clinical Pediatrics, 56*(3), 247–256. https://doi.org/101177/0009922816648288

McGonigle, J. J., Venkat, A., Beresford, C., Campbell, T. P., & Gabriels, R. L. (2014). Management of agitation in individuals with autism spectrum disorders in the emergency department. *Child and Adolescent Psychiatric Clinics of North America, 23*(1), 83–95. https://doi.org/10.1016/j.chc.2013.08.003

Modell, S. J., & Mak, S. (2008). A preliminary assessment of police officers' knowledge and perceptions of persons with disabilities. *Intellectual and Developmental Disabilities, 46*(3), 183–189.

Morris, R., Greenblatt, A., & Saini, M. (2019). Healthcare providers' experiences with autism: A scoping review. *Journal of ASD and Developmental Disorders, 49*(6), 2374–2388. https://doi.org/10.1007/s10803-019-03912-6

Myers, S. M., & Johnson, C. P. (2007). Management of children with autism spectrum disorders. *American Academy of Pediatrics, 120*(5), 1162–1182. https://doi.org/10.1542/peds.2007-2362

Nicholas, D. B., Zwaigenbaum, L., Muskat, B., Craig, W. R., Newton, A. S., Cohen-Silver, J., Sharon, R. F., Greenblatt, A., & Kilmer, C. (2016). Toward practice advancement in emergency care for children with autism spectrum disorder. *Pediatrics, 137*(2), S205-S211. https://doi.org/10.1542/peds.2015-2851S

Pathmashri, V. P., & Kumar, M. P. S. (2018). Dental management of children with autismspectrum disorders. *Drug Intervention Today, 10*(7), 1190–1194.

Perry, D. M., & Carter-Long, L. (2014, May 6). How misunderstanding disability leads to police violence. The Atlantic. https://www.theatlantic.com/health/arch ive/2014/05/misunderstanding-disability-leads-to-police-violence/361786/

Perry, D. M., & Carter-Long, L. (2016). The Ruderman white paper on media coverage of law enforcement use of force and disability. *Ruderman Family Foundation*.

Railey, K. S., Bowers-Campbell, J., Love, A. M., & Campbell, J. M. (2020). An exploration of law enforcement officers' training needs and interactions with individuals with autism spectrum disorder. *Journal of Autism and Developmental Disorders,* 50, 101–117. https://doi.org/10.1007/s10 803-019-04227-2

Rava, J., Shattuck, P., Rast, J., & Roux, A. (2017). The prevalence and correlates of involvement in the criminal justice system among youth on the autism spectrum. *Journal of Autism and Developmental Disorders,* 47, 340–346. https://doi.org/10.1007/s10803-016-2958-3

Rhoades, R. A., Scarpa, A., & Salley, B. (2007). The importance of physician knowledge of autism spectrum disorder: Results of a parent survey. *BMC Pediatrics,* 7(1), 37–47. https://doi.org/10.1186/1471-2431-7-37

Richdale, A. L. (1999). Sleep problems in ASD: Prevalence, cause, and intervention. *Developmental Medicine and Child Neurology,* 41(1), 60–66. https://doi.org/10.1017/S0012162299000122

Stein, L. I., Jane, C. J., Williams, M. E., Dawson, M. E., Polido, J. C., & Cermak, S. A. (2014). Physiological and behavioral stress and anxiety in children with autism spectrum disorders during routine oral care. *BioMed Research International,* 2014, 1–10. https://doi.org/10.1155/2014/694876

Steinbrenner, J. R., Hume, K., Odom, S. L., Morin, K. L., Nowell, S. W., Tomaszewski, B., Szendrey, S., McIntyre, N. S., Yucesoy-Ozkan, & Savage, M. N. (2020). *Evidence-based practices for children, youth, and young adults with* autism. National Clearinghouse on ASD Evidence and Practice Review Team. https://ncaep.fpg.unc.edu/sites/ncaep.fpg.unc.edu/files/imce/documents/EBP%20Report%202020.pdf

Tint, A., Palucka, A. M., Bradley, E., Weiss, J. A., & Lunsky, Y. (2017). Correlates of police involvement among adolescents and adults with autism spectrum disorder. *Journal of Autism and Developmental Disorders,* 47, 2639–2647. https://doi.org/10.1007/s10803-017-3182-5

Tint, A., Palucka, A. M., Bradley, E., Weiss, J. A., & Lunsky, Y. (2019). Emergency service experiences of adults with autism spectrum disorder without intellectual disability. *Autism,* 23(3), 792–795. https://doi.org/10.1177/136236131 8760294

U.S. Department of Health and Human Services. (2008). *Practical oral care for people with autism.* National Institutes of Health. https://www.nidcr.nih.gov/sites/default/files/2017-09/practical-oral-care-ASD.pdf

Venkat, A., Migyanka, J. M., Cramer, R., & McGonigle, J. J. (2016). An instrument to prepare for acute care of the individual with autism spectrum disorder in the emergency department. *Journal of Autism and Developmental Disorders,* 46(7), 2565–2569. https://doi.org/10.1007/s10803-016-2778-5

Viljoen, E., Bornman, J., Wiles, L., & Tönsing, K. M. (2017). Police officer disability sensitivity training: A systematic review. *The Police Journal,* 90(2), 143–159. https://doi.org/10.1177/0032258X16674021

Wachob, D., & Pesci, L. J. (2017). Brief report: Knowledge and confidence of emergency medical service personnel involving treatment of an individual with autism spectrum disorder. *Journal of Autism & Developmental Disorders,* 47, 887–891. https://doi.org/10.1007/s10803-016-2957-4

Wang, L. W., Tancredi, D. J., & Thomas, D. W. (2011). The prevalence of gastrointestinal problems in children across the United States with autism spectrum disorders from families with multiple affected members. *Journal*

of Developmental & Behavioral Pediatrics, 32(5), 351–360. https://doi.org/
10.1097/DBP.0b013e31821bd06a

Weil, T. N., & Inglehart, M. R. (2010). Dental education and dentists' attitudes
and behavior concerning patients with autism. *Journal of Dental Education,*
74(12),   1294–1307.   https://doi.org/10.1002/j.0022-0337.2010.74.12.
tb05005.x

Zwaigenbaum, L., Nicholas, D. B., Muskat, B., Kilmer, C., Newton, A. S., Craig,
W. R., Ratnapalan, S., Cohen-Silver, J., Greenblatt, A., Roberts, W., & Sharon,
R. (2016). Perspectives of health care providers regarding emergency depart-
ment care of children and youth with autism spectrum disorder. *Journal of
Autism and Developmental Disorders, 46*(5), 1725–1736. https://doi.org/s10
803-016-2703-y

Chapter 22

Teaching and Supporting Sexuality Education

Meaghan M. McCollow[1] and Peggy Schafer Whitby[2]
[1]Department of Educational Psychology, California State University East Bay
[2]Department of Curriculum and Instruction, University of Arkansas

Teaching and Supporting Sexuality Education

According to the World Health Organization, sexuality education is a human right (WHO, 2018). While the WHO includes individuals with disabilities, people with ASD/DD continue to be excluded from accessing comprehensive sexuality education that meets their individual needs. This exclusion seems to be rooted in the influence of eugenics and the historical treatment of disabled people in the United States (for a more comprehensive history, see: Graham Holmes & SIECUS, 2021; Wehmeyer, 2013). The effects, though, are the continuation of a belief in harmful stereotypes and myths about disability and sexuality. The myths include the ideas that people with disabilities are asexual or, conversely, hypersexual; people with disabilities are dependent on non-disabled people and are child-like; people with disabilities cannot or should not have children; people with disabilities should only be in relationships with other disabled people (Graham Holmes & SIECUS, 2021; McCollow et al., 2021). The belief in these myths results in youth with disabilities receiving little or no information about sex education, whether at home or school (Graham Holmes & SIECUS, 2021). As a human right, it is critical that learners with autism spectrum disorder and developmental disabilities (ASD/DD) are provided access to sexuality education. Without information and opportunities to safely explore their sexuality, these individuals are at a heightened risk for sexual abuse (Dion et al., 2013), sex trafficking (Reid, 2018), bullying (Gutmann Kahn & Lindstrom, 2015), cyber victimization (Normand & Sallafranque, 2015), suicide (Kirby et al., 2019; Marshal et al., 2011) and poor life outcomes (Gutmann Kahn & Lindstrom, 2015).

The taboo nature of sexuality, concerns of legal issues associated with delivering sexuality education, and cultural differences across families and supporting professionals can result in a delay in sexuality education or limited scope of content until problem sexualized behavior occurs. Providing comprehensive sexuality education is key to improving life

DOI: 10.4324/9781003255147-26

outcomes for individuals with ASD/DD. Teaching sexuality education to learners with ASD/DD is complex. For educators who support learners with ASD/DD, it is essential to work with parents in teaching sexuality education to their children, to work with IEP teams to develop individual sexuality education programs, and to enhance inclusion in general education sexuality education.

This chapter provides an overview of sexuality education through the lens of human rights, suggestions on how to teach sexuality education as it relates to individuals with ASD/DD, suggestions on how to collaborate to increase socio-sexual outcomes for individuals with ASD/DD, and a discussion on current issues in sexuality education for people with ASD/DD (i.e., sexual orientation and gender identity; social media; diversity and culture). The key points of this chapter are:

1. Sexuality education for people with ASD/DD is a disability rights issue.
2. Current issues regarding sexuality education include heteronormativity, technology, and intersectionality.
3. Teaching sexuality education to individuals with ASD/DD can mitigate problem sexualized behavior.
4. Collaboration is key to successful sexuality education and life outcomes.

PJ is 19-years-old and was diagnosed with autism spectrum disorder at a young age. PJ is currently a freshman in a college program and has moved away from home for the first time. PJ was adopted as a young baby. PJ is a bi-racial and has adoptive parents who are white. PJ has a younger brother who is the biological son of PJ's adoptive parents. PJ's family is upper middle class and deeply religious. PJ's family lives in a conservative area of the South. PJ has come out as gay and has requested others use the pronouns they/them/theirs as PJ is exploring their gender identity. PJ's family is deeply troubled by this announcement and are unsure if PJ is acting out, understands sexuality or gender identity, or what education should be provided.

Sexuality Education

In 2021, the Sexuality Information and Education Council of the United States (SIECUS) published a "call to action" for providing sexuality education to youth with disabilities. SIECUS states that for sexuality education, youth with disabilities should be included in general education classes and provided appropriate accommodations; should be represented in materials used; should be provided the opportunity to learn self-advocacy, bodily autonomy, and consent; and can benefit from role playing, interactive exercises, and concrete examples (Grahams Holmes & SIECUS, 2021).

The National Sex Education Standards (NSES) provide guidelines on core content and skills that are age-appropriate for K-12 students. The principles, values, and framework of the NSES are aligned with a rights-based approach to sexuality and disability. The principles and values of the standards include high expectations: functional knowledge and skills: trauma-informed, social, racial, and reproductive justice and equity: intersectionality: and language inclusivity (Initiative, 2020). The framework for the NSES approaches sex education from the social-learning theory, recognizing that learning occurs within social contexts (Initiative, 2020). The key concepts of the NSES theoretical framework are personalization, susceptibility, self-efficacy, social norms, and skills (Initiative, 2020). The NSES can be used as the core standards that can be used to teach sexuality education to all students. The standards are centered around the learner across the lifespan in order to build skills and expand knowledge.

The NSES helps IEP teams identify which skills need to be taught and at what age they should be taught. Many times, young children with ASD/DD will be missing important skills that should have been learned at a younger age. The IEP team should assess skills from the early age groups to determine which skills need to be taught or re-taught. Deciding what to teach is the hard part. Really. Members of the IEP team already possess and use specialized evidence-based teaching strategies for students with ASD/DD. These same teaching strategies should be applied when teaching sexuality education. Resources on evidence-based practices for teaching sexuality education include: Evidence-Based Practice for Children, Youth, and Young Adults with Autism Spectrum Disorder (Steinbrenner et al., 2020), found at https://ncaep. fpg.unc.edu/, and An Educators Guide to Evidence-Based Practice and Autism-Phase 2 (NAC, 2015), found at https://nationalautismcenter. org/resources/for-educators.

Individual Education Program teams should familiarize themselves with the National Sexuality Education Standards (NSES; Initiative, 2020) and plan for instruction in the same way academic instruction is planned. This may involve collaborating with other educators and colleagues within the school, considering accommodations for learners, checking that materials are representative of learners and the spectrum of sexuality and gender, providing opportunities for active learning such as role-plays, and ensuring self-advocacy and consent are included in the instruction. The NSES helps educators to make teaching decisions across the lifespan by understanding what an individual should know by certain ages and what a learner will need to know in the future.

During high school, it was reported that PJ made inappropriate comments to other boys in the bathroom. As a result, they were teased and called names by the other students. They spent most of their time on the internet trying to form relationships. Their family struggled with the behavior and were embarrassed by the reports of PJ's inappropriate comments to other boys. They punished PJ. As a result, PJ had to sneak on the internet to find information on their sexuality. PJ did this without guidance and accessed inappropriate illegal content. After legal involvement, PJ's team realized that an appropriate assessment of their knowledge and sexuality education was in order, along with parent education.

Addressing Problem Sexualized Behavior

When addressing problem sexualized behaviors, it is important to appropriately assess the behavior in the same way other challenging behavior is assessed. Utilizing tools such as the functional-assessment interview (FAI), functional assessment screening tool (FAST), questions about behavioral function (QABF), and observation of non-nude behaviors are tools already used to assess the function of behaviors. Additional assessment tools that can be used include the Test of Young Adult Social Skills Knowledge (TYASSK), Perceived Parental Reactions Scale (PPRS), Tools for the Assessment of Levels of Knowledge Sexuality, and Consent-Revised (TALK-SC-R), and the Socio-Sexual Knowledge and Attitudes Test-Revised (SSKAAT-R). While several of these assessment tools could be used outside of problem sexualized behavior to assess knowledge and skills related to knowledge about sexuality (e.g., TYASSK, TALK-SC-R, SSKAAT-R), these assessments can be used to better understand behaviors related to sexual offense or abuse. Table 22.1 provides a description of sexuality knowledge assessments. These assessments can be utilized to complete a functional behavior assessment (FBA) to set the foundation for developing an appropriate behavior intervention plan.

In many cases, the function of a problem sexualized behavior may be sensory related with pleasure being the sought-after input. As function is determined, a skill deficit analysis should be analyzed to determine what skills may be impacting the pleasure- seeking. For example, in a case where an individual is inappropriately fixating on minors, a question may be: Does the individual understand age? Is the person able to discriminate the concept and indicators of age across people and settings? Does the person understand the social and legal norms regarding minors and consent?

In other cases, the function of the behavior may have started as sensory seeking but is shaped into attention-seeking or escape-maintained

Table 22.1 Assessments for Sexuality Knowledge and for Addressing Problem
Sexualized Behaviors

Assessment	Description
Test of Young Adult Social Skills Knowledge (TYASSK)	Criterion-referenced assessment used to evaluate young adults' knowledge related to specific social skills (Laugeson, 2017)
Perceived Parental Reactions Scale (PPRS)	32-item measure of parental/caregiver reactions to sexual orientation disclosure (Willoughby et al., 2010). The original use was for parents of sons (e.g., males), but it has been used in other contexts as well.
Tools for the Assessment of Levels of Knowledge Sexuality and Consent-Revised (TALK-SC-R)	Pre/post assessment can be used during sex education-related training to determine an individual's baseline knowledge and identify gaps in knowledge (Hingsburger et al., 2014). There is a consent assessment included in the TALK-SC-R that provides information on a person's knowledge of consent-related skills.
Socio-Sexual Knowledge and Attitudes Test-Revised (SSKAAT-R)	The criterion-based measure of sexual knowledge and attitudes of IDD populations, particularly related to appropriate boundaries and behaviors (Griffiths & Lunsky, 2003)

behavior. It is important not to assume a function and to assess the environmental factors before developing a behavior plan. If the function is sensory seeking, work with the family to teach masturbation skills if needed and teach appropriate location. A person's bedroom should be emphasized as the place for self-stimulation as bathrooms are frequently shared, and some individuals with ASD may struggle with generalizing which bathrooms are appropriate. If the function of the behavior is not sensory but attention or escape, other interventions will need to be developed. Sometimes individuals with ASD learn that self-touch results in immediate attention or removal from a situation. Never teach school or public places as appropriate places to masturbate. This sets the individual up for great risk. Instead, assist the family in teaching self-stimulation skills at home.

As problematic sexualized behavior is assessed, it is important to keep the ethics of assessing the behavior at the center. In some cases, a behavior that looks deviant may just be different, which is not necessarily unacceptable. Examples of this may include issues of solo sex, same-gender relationships, gender differences, etc. Remember to work with the family in teaching their loved one and provide education to the family so that they feel supported and competent in addressing sexuality with their child. Given that certain skills build upon each other, or can be generalized to different settings, situations, and people, teachers should consider teaching to behavioral cusps.

Behavioral Cusps

One approach to teaching new skills is to utilize behavioral cusps or pivotal behaviors. A behavioral cusp is defined as:

> A behavior that has consequences beyond the change itself, some of which may be considered important.... What makes a behavior change a cusp is that it exposes the individual's repertoire to new environments, especially new reinforcers and punishers, new contingencies, new responses, new stimulus controls, and new communities of maintaining or destructive contingencies. When some or all of those events happen, the individual's repertoire expands; it encounters a differentially selective maintenance of the new as well as some old repertoires, and perhaps that leads to some further cusps.
>
> (Rosales-Ruiz & Baer, 1997, p. 534)

The advantage of a behavioral cusp is that by teaching one skill or set of skills, an individual may, after learning those skills, have access to many more skills. This is important when considering complex skills such as which social behaviors. An example of a behavioral cusp is reading. After learning how to read, one is able to access many more environments, engage with a variety of stimuli (e.g., books, magazines, websites, and menus), and can elicit new responses related to communication and writing.

Pivotal behaviors are related to behavioral cusps. Pivotal behaviors have been described as "a behavior that, once learned, produces corresponding modifications or covariations in other adaptive untrained behaviors," (Cooper et al., 2007, p. 59). Since pivotal behaviors (i.e., pivotal- response training) have been researched frequently within the area of social skills (e.g., Koegel & Frea, 1993; Ma et al., 2021; Ona et al., 2020), it is possible this is an area that can, and should, be further explored in the teaching of sexuality education. Pivotal response training (PRT) has been studied in classrooms, indicating its feasibility for use in school settings (Suhrheinrich et al., 2020).

To explore how pivotal behaviors might be identified and used to support teaching in sexuality education, we can begin by selecting an NSES and going through the instructional planning process (plan, teach, assess, re-teach). Indeed, the NSES are designed to lead to additional skills that build upon each other if early skills are taught. For example, in the grade K-2 standards, a core concept is "list medically accurate names for body parts, including the genitals" (AP.2.CC.1; Initiative, 2020, p. 18). As learners age, this knowledge and skill is built upon by specifying more specific body parts and variations humans may have to those body parts, how body parts respond and function, and the role of hormones and pleasure in human sexuality (Initiative, 2020). In this way, the skill of accurately naming body parts is built upon in age-appropriate ways across childhood, adolescence, and young adulthood. Accurately naming body parts becomes a pivotal skill in learning how body parts work and how human bodies respond to the sexual-response cycle. A further connection would be that having the skill of accurately naming body parts allows an individual to accurately describe cases of abuse and/or assault or describe areas of pain or injury, as an example. Table 22.2 provides examples of possible behavioral cusps.

Upon assessment, it is revealed that PJ did not understand that information on the internet was illegal. They were looking at young men and women who were near their age but were minors. PJ downloaded multiple files without looking at the files first. This resulted in very graphic material being stored on their computer. PJ did not understand that the pornography was not real and that modeling these behaviors at school does not result in relationship development and sexual relationships, but gets them in trouble and makes PJ appear weird to their peers, at the minimum, and can lead to arrest if they make these statements to underage adolescents. Given PJ's situation, all electronic devices need to be monitored, PJ needs to be provided intensive education, and a gradual release of technology supervision implemented, guided by a therapist.

Ethical Considerations

Educators who are teaching comprehensive sexuality education to individuals with ASD/DD should be aware of ethical considerations both in general and related to state and federal laws. If we approach sexuality education from a rights-based perspective, we are already upholding that our teaching and support will:

- Value the human rights of all individuals
- Be scientifically accurate
- Address the spectrum of gender identity and expression
- Provide a safe and healthy learning environment
- Utilize effective, participation-based instructional approaches
- Empower learners and promote self-advocacy

(Berglas et al., 2014)

To then address ethical considerations, educators will need to set aside their values and beliefs regarding sexuality and gender in order to make room for varied experiences, values, and beliefs. Beginning with reflecting

Table 22.2 Possible Behavioral Cusps Teaching Sexuality Education or People with Disabilities

Behavior/Skill	Possible Expansion of the Skill
Identify medically accurate names for body parts	Accurately describing body parts during medical appointments
	Identifying body parts and expected reactions during the sexual response cycle
	A more accurate description should abuse/assault be reported
	Access resources and supports related to abuse and/or assault
	Access resources and supports related to medical support such as gynecological checks, STI testing, and treatment
Identify uncomfortable or dangerous situations, such as bullying, teasing	Identify abuse and/or assault
	Identify safe vs. unsafe people and/or situations
	Identify boundaries with a variety of people in their lives
	Identify and utilize consent skills
	Access resources and supports related to abuse and/or assault
Define and discuss gender and gender-role stereotypes	Identify and describe the ways individuals express their gender
	Access medically accurate sources of information about gender, gender identity, and gender expression
	Identify how they want to express their gender and gender identity
	Access resources and supports, as needed, related to their gender and gender identity
Identify what reproduction is and describe what it is related to living things	Explain intercourse and human reproduction
	Explain pregnancy and contraception methods
	Explain and define STIs, including symptoms
	Access resources related to pregnancy, contraception, and STIs

on one's own beliefs and experiences related to sexuality and gender allows one to begin to explore their feelings about sexuality education. Withholding information is not an ethical practice. Acknowledging a need to find out more information and that the topic can be uncomfortable are both OK.

Ethical educators will begin by reflecting on and acknowledging their own biases, values, and beliefs related to sexuality and gender. They will also understand their scope of practice and begin seeking ways to expand their knowledge and skills related to sexuality education in order to provide better support. Ethical educators will also collaborate with other professionals in order to best meet the needs of the individuals supported. This includes collaborating with other professionals to seek the support they are uncomfortable providing, or unable to provide. Ethical educators put the needs of the individuals they support at the center.

There are boundaries to what educators can provide in terms of instruction related to sexuality education. Common sense and judgment should be used when considering appropriate instructional practices. For instance, there are boundaries to the use of common instructional practices such as modeling and video modeling. While there are well-made video modeling resources available (e.g., amaze.org), educators need to exercise judgment when considering creating other materials for use in instruction. Interventions should be developed and implemented by an IEP team. The IEP team works with the family to determine what should be taught and how the information will be taught. This provides multiple lenses' for problem-solving and provides support for families and special education teachers who may feel alone in addressing sexuality education.

Should an educator encounter a situation in which illegal activity is taking place, the educator needs to take the appropriate actions. In the United States, educators are mandated reporters who are required to report suspected child abuse and neglect, which includes sexual abuse and assault of minors. There are trained sexuality counselors who provide appropriate support to individuals with ASD/DD who are engaging in predatory and/or illegal sexual behaviors. These professionals should be sought in cases that go beyond the scope of knowledge and practice of educators.

Educators must follow district and state policies on teaching sexuality education. Each district and state will have its own guidelines and laws regarding sexuality education. SEICUS provides a state-by-state law and policy chart on sexuality education that can be found at https://siecus.org/siecus-updates-sex-ed-state-law-and-policy-chart/. Educators should familiarize themselves with their district and state laws, discuss the needs of the individuals with ASD with their administrator, and provide sexuality education through the IEP system. It is important that educators work with teams who help them make decisions so that they are not making decisions in isolation as sexuality education should be taught across environments to assure generalization of skills. Sexuality education needs to be taught across contexts and supported by people across settings. Collaboration among stakeholders and IEP team members should be facilitated. Many times, this includes the individual, family, special- and general- education teachers, related service providers, and sometimes siblings or peers. IEP team leaders should take great care in planning, implementing, and progress monitoring across settings and people.

Collaboration

Collaboration is important given how people learn and how behavior is supported by the environment. If behavior is increasing or stable, it is somehow being reinforced. Inconsistent implementation of a skill acquisition plan or a behavior reduction program can lead to no or slow progress. Behaviors can be inadvertently reinforced by stakeholders without their knowledge. The inadvertent reinforcement by one team member can result in a variable reinforcement schedule, thereby strengthening a behavior that the team may be trying to decrease. Fortunately, strategies can be taught to stakeholders to ensure successful interventions.

The first strategy is to educate all stakeholders on the need for the program and how their implementation of the program will help the individual. It is important for stakeholders to remember that problem behaviors may increase before they get better. Stakeholders need to remember that an appropriate replacement behavior must be taught in order to make the problem behavior irrelevant. For example, if a person is masturbating in public for sensory gratification, they must be taught when, where, and how to masturbate so they can meet their needs. If blocked from masturbating in public and given no appropriate opportunity to masturbate, the individual will most likely find another inappropriate place to masturbate. Stakeholders must understand the need for the program and why the behavioral intervention will help. If both the individual and stakeholders help develop the intervention, both will be more likely to implement the plan with fidelity.

Once stakeholders understand the intervention, they must be given the opportunity to commit to implementing the program, or an opportunity to say they are not comfortable and remove themselves from the team. Beliefs and values regarding sexuality and sexual behaviors differ across cultures. Each member of the IEP team should examine their own bias and knowledge of teaching sexuality, given the personal preferences and culture of the individual. It is better for a person to step forward at the planning stage of the intervention and say they are not comfortable implementing the intervention or are not knowledgeable about sexuality needs of the individual than to commit to implementing with fidelity and then not doing so.

Ongoing planning must be in place as the plan will need to be adapted as the individual develops new skills or data indicates the plan is not working. Using the data as a guide, the team will slowly adjust reinforcement, assess motivation, and change the intervention. First, the team should assess implementation fidelity and retrain if needed. Second, the team can assess whether reinforcement in the natural environment is being provided, or if the reinforcer continues to serve as a reinforcer or is strong enough to maintain the behavior. Last, the team can decide to change the intervention. When addressing sexuality, all decisions should be team based including the individual and family.

Current Issues

Much has been written about the myths/barriers regarding disability and sexuality (e.g., Baglieri & Shapiro, 2017; McCollow et al., 2021), and it is becoming clearer to practitioners that these myths can, and should, be dispelled. More current issues that must be addressed are heteronormativity, the use of technology, and intersectionality.

Heteronormativity

Heteronormativity is, broadly, the attitude or assumption that heterosexuality is the "norm" and natural expression of human sexuality (Warner, 1991). There is an assumption that individuals with ASD/DD are heterosexual. However, the broad spectrum of sexuality that all humans experience is represented within the ASD/DD population as well. Recently, the experiences of individuals with ASD/DD who identify as belonging to the LGBTQ+ community are emerging in the research literature (Narby, 2012), and findings suggest a high rate of gender variance among individuals with ASD, reporting that this population may be nearly eight times more likely to report gender variance than the neurotypical population (Janssen et al., 2016).

Assuming one is heterosexual and teaching from a heteronormative lens creates problems for individuals with ASD who identify with the LGBTQ+ community. These individuals are left without access to information needed to develop relationships and stay safe. The reported experiences of individuals with ASD/DD from the LGBTQ+ community include abuse, discrimination, lack of support, and lack of access to services (Dinwoodie et al., 2020). The lived experiences of individuals with ASD/DD who identify as LGBTQ+ need to be explored and shared as there is limited research providing a platform for these individuals.

Given the limited knowledge base regarding the experiences and needs of individuals who are ASD/DD and are part of the LGBTQ+ community, inclusive comprehensive sexuality education for all individuals becomes even more pertinent. Creating access to gender-affirming support services, providing language and terms to describe feelings and experiences that include a variety of lived experiences, and acknowledging that not all individuals experience sexuality and gender in the same way gives all individuals an opportunity to safely explore and understand their own identities. Table 22.3 provides an overview of terms related to sexuality and gender identity.

Technology

In today's society, technology plays an important role in social interactions, relationship development, and representation for those who may not have role models in their home communities. Teaching appropriate use of the internet and technology is imperative as the use of the internet poses risks for those who may not be able to discriminate between legal versus illegal activities. Without education, people with

Table 22.3 Terminology for Understanding Diversity in Sexuality/Gender

Term	Definition
Cisgender	"A term used to describe a person whose gender identity aligns with those typically associated with the sex assigned to them at birth" (HRC, nd)
Transgender	"An umbrella term for people whose gender identity and/ or expression is different from cultural expectations based on the sex they were assigned at birth. Being transgender does not imply any specific sexual orientation. Therefore, transgender people may identify as straight, gay, lesbian, bisexual, etc." (HRC, nd)
Sexual rights	"The fulfillment of sexual health is tied to the extent to which human rights are respected, protected, and fulfilled. Sexual rights embrace certain human rights that are already recognized in international and regional human rights documents and other consensus documents and in national laws" (WHO, 2018)
Gender expression	"External appearance of one's gender identity; frequently expressed through behavior, clothing, haircut, voice; may or may not conform to socially defined behavior or characteristics associated with being masculine or feminine" (HRC, nd)
Gender identity	"One's innermost concept of self as male, female, a blend of both, or neither. One's gender identity can be the same or different from their sex assigned at birth" (HRC, nd)
Non-binary	"An adjective describing a person who does not identify exclusively as a man or a woman. Non-binary people may identify as being both a man and a woman, somewhere between, or as falling completely outside these categories. While many also identify as transgender, not all non-binary people do" (HRC, nd)
Queer	"A term people often use to express fluid identities and orientations. Often used interchangeably with 'LGBTQ'" (HRC, nd)
Asexual	"The lack of a sexual attraction or desire for other people" (HRC, nd)
Bisexual	"A person emotionally, romantically or sexually attracted to more than one sex, gender or gender identity though not necessarily simultaneously, in the same way, or to the same degree" (HRC, nd)
Genderqueer	"Genderqueer people typically reject notions of static categories of gender and embrace fluidity of gender identity and often, though not always, sexual orientation. People who identify as 'genderqueer' may see themselves as both male and female, neither male or female or as falling completely outside these categories" (HRC, nd)
Lesbian	"A woman who is emotionally, romantically or sexually attracted to other women. Women and non-binary people may use this term to describe themselves" (HRC, nd)

Table 22.3 Cont.

Term	Definition
Gay	"A person who is emotionally, romantically or sexually attracted to members of the same gender. Men, women and non-binary people may use this term to describe themselves" (HRC, nd)
Pansexual	"Describes someone who has the potential for emotional, romantic, or sexual attraction to people of any gender though not necessarily simultaneously, in the same way, or to the same degree. Sometimes used interchangeably with bisexual." (HRC, nd)
Gender dysphoria	"Clinically significant distress caused when a person's assigned birth gender is not the same as the one with which they identify" (HRC, nd)
Intersex	"Intersex people are born with a variety of differences in their sex traits and reproductive anatomy. There is a wide variety of difference amount intersex variations, including differences in genitalia, chromosomes, gonads, internal sex organs, hormone production, hormone response, and/or secondary sex traits" (HRC, nd)
Outing	"Exposing someone's lesbian, gay, bisexual transgender or gender non-binary identity to others without their permission. Outing someone can have serious repercussions on employment, economic stability, personal safety or religious or family situations" (HRC, nd)
Sexual orientation	"An inherent or immutable enduring emotional, romantic or sexual attraction to other people … an individual's sexual orientation is independent of their gender identity" (HRC, nd)
Heteronormativity	The attitude or assumption that heterosexuality is the "norm" and natural expression of human sexuality (Warner, 1993)

ASD/DD can be vulnerable. Fortunately, safety skills can be taught, and discrimination skills can be built upon as behavioral cusps or pivotal skills. There are resources educators and parents can use to help teach social skills online and safety skills online. Table 22.4 provides a list of resources to assist parents and educators in teaching internet/social media use.

Intersectionality

It is critical to recognize that individuals do not exist within a vacuum. That is, individuals with disabilities, however those disabilities are present, have other identities as well. Youth with disabilities live within intersecting identities that include race, sexual orientation, gender identity and expression, and other cultural and religious backgrounds. "Sex education provides a vehicle to tackle not only myths around disability

Table 22.4 Resources for Teaching Internet Safety

Resource
Center on Transition https://centerontransition.org/asd/pdfs/FastFacts/InternetSafety.pdf
Federal Trade Commission (2016) www.consumer.ftc.gov/articles/pdf-0002-heads-up.pdf
Frank Porter Graham University of North Carolina https://csesa.fpg.unc.edu/sites/csesa.fpg.unc.edu/files/Internet%20Safety%20for%20   Adolescents%20with%20Autism.pdf (Clinard, 2016)
Pornography Literacy www.aboutsexpodcast.com/e/pornography-literacy-with-barb-gross/

facing [youth with disabilities] but also the white supremacy supported by and entwined with ablest structures of oppression" (Graham Holmes & SIECUS, 2021, p. 25). The only way to move forward toward inclusive comprehensive sexuality education is to recognize and include youth with disabilities, youth of color, and LGTBQ+ identities when designing and implementing sex-ed curriculum.

The need for comprehensive sexuality education that is inclusive of marginalized identities is critical. In a 2021 call to action, 10 organizations summarized the need and urgency for sex education that provides foundational information and knowledge to keep youth safe and healthy, particularly for youth who identify within the marginalized LGBTQ+ community (Advocates for Youth, et al., 2021). Without reliable, accurate, supportive information, youth within this intersection are more at risk for engaging in risk-taking behaviors. Inclusive comprehensive sex education that is supportive of LGBTQ+ youth includes "age-appropriate and medically accurate information; incorporate[s] positive examples of LGBTQ+ individuals, relationships and families; emphasize[s] the need for protection during sex for people of all identities; and dispell[s] common myths and stereotypes about behavior and identity" (Advocates for Youth et al., 2021, p. 1). However, this information is frequently unavailable to LGBTQ+ youth due to misunderstandings, a lack of information (on the part of educators and others), laws barring the information, or a heavy emphasis on heteronormativity resulting in ignoring other expressions of sexuality and gender identity.

It is important to understand that individuals from multiple marginalized populations experience more than an additive impact of the marginalization. These identities intersect. For example, a young man with a disability who identifies as Hispanic and as a gay man will have different experiences than a young man with a disability who identifies as White and a gay man, depending upon the culture of the family and social norms of the community in which he lives. Without representation and support within a community, individuals from multiple marginalized populations may struggle in different ways.

PJ continues to receive sexuality education and behavior support. They have a better understanding of developing relationships but are still at high risk for accessing inappropriate information on the internet. Their family has accepted that PJ is a young gay person and accept them. PJ will continue to need services as they navigate adulthood. These services and sexuality education should decrease

Table 22.5 Resources and Curricula for Teaching Sexuality Education

Resource	Description
Gratton, F.V. (2019). *Supporting transgender autistic youth and adults: A guide for professionals and families.* Jessica Kingsley Publishers.	Book providing guidance for professionals and families who support transgender autistic youth and adults
Elevatus Training www.elevatustraining.com	Training and curriculum for sexuality education for individuals with developmental disabilities
Intimate Relationship and Sexual Health: A Curriculum for Teaching Adolescents/Adults with High-Functioning Autism Spectrum Disorders and Other Social Challenges (Davies & Dubie, 2012)	Comprehensive curricula for teaching sexuality education for individuals with ASD.
LGBTQ+ and ASD Resources www.autismspeaks.org/lgbtq-information-and-resources	Resources on intersectionality between ASD and LGBTQ+
RespectAbility www.respectability.org/resources/sexual-education-resources/	Sexual Education resources for young adults with developmental disabilities
SexEd Mart https://sexedmart.com/	Products, toolboxes, activity kits, sequencing cards, etc. for teaching sexuality education
Sexuality Information and Education Council of the United States (SIECUS) http://siecus.org/	Provides guidelines and resources for comprehensive sexuality education; also published a Call to Action for Comprehensive Sex Education for Youth with Disabilities
State Regulations	SEICUS (2020) https://siecus.org/wp-content/uploads/2020/05/SIECUS-2020-Sex-Ed-State-Law-and-Policy-Chart_May-2020-3.pdf
Teaching Children with Down Syndrome about their Bodies, Boundaries, and Sexuality: A Guide for Parents and Professionals (Couwenhoven, 2007)	Basic curriculum for teaching hygiene, body, and safety. Limited content for relationship development.

PJ's risk for legal involvement and problem sexualized behavior as they support PJ's sexuality and relationship development.

Conclusion

Teaching sexuality education is a sensitive topic that many people feel uncomfortable addressing. The lack of comfort, along with a lack of knowledge, many times, results in no sexuality education, misinformed sexuality education, or reactive sexuality education. The IEP team is the ideal setting to collaborate, plan, and teach sexuality education. By listening to the family and individual, a team approach can be used to develop an individualized plan to provide appropriate sexual education to a student. Table 22.5 provides resources educators and others may find useful to teaching sexuality education.

Special education teachers have knowledge of evidence-based practices for teaching individuals with ASD, and these evidence-based practices can be used to teach sexuality. Teachers can utilize behavioral cusps or pivotal skills in teaching individuals with ASD, as many skills taught during early childhood can be generalized to sexual behaviors and relationship development. Collaboration as an IEP team the unique opportunity to address sexuality education as a comprehensive need for individuals with ASD.

References

Advocates for Youth, Answer, GLSEN, Black and Pink, Equality Federation, the Human Rights Campaign (HRC) Foundation, National LGBTQ Task Force, Planned Parenthood Federation of America (PPFA), the Sexuality Information and Education Council of the United States (SIECUS), Unite for Reproductive & Gender Equity (URGE). (2021). A call to action: LGBTQ+ youth need inclusive sex education.

Baglieri, S., & Shapiro, A. (2017). *Disability studies and the inclusive classroom: Critical practices for embracing diversity in education.* Routledge.

Berglas, N. F., Constantine, N. A., & Ozer, E. J. (2014). A rights-based approach to sexuality education: Conceptualization, clarification and challenges. *Perspectives on Sexual and Reproductive Health, 46*(2), 63–72.

Clinard, A. (2016). *Internet Safety for Teens with ASD (Autism at a Glance Brief).* The University of North Carolina, Frank Porter Graham Child Development Institute, CSESA Development Team.

Cooper, J. O., Heron, T. E., & Heward, W. L. (2007). *Applied behavior analysis (3rd Edition).* Hoboken, NJ: Pearson Education.

Couwenhoven, T. (2007). *Teaching children with down syndrome about their bodies, boundaries, and sexuality.* Bethesda, Maryland: Woodbine House.

Davies, C. & Dubie, M. (2012). *Intimate relationships and sexual health: A curriculum for teaching adolescents/adults with high-functioning autism spectrum disorders and other social challenges.* Shawnee Mission, Kansas: AAPC Publishing.

Dion, J., Paquette, G., Tremblay, K. N., Cyr, M., & Dionne, C. (2013). Sexual abuse of intellectually disabled youth: A review. *The Prevention Researcher*, *20*(3), 14–16.

Dinwoodie, R., Greenhill, B., & Cookson, A. (2020). 'Them two things are what collide together': Understanding the sexual identity experiences of lesbian, gay, bisexual and trans people labelled with intellectual disability. *Journal of Applied Research in Intellectual Disabilities*, *33*(1), 3–16.

Gratton, F. V. (2019). *Supporting transgender autistic youth and adults: A guide for professionals and families*. Jessica Kingsley Publishers.

Graham Holmes, L., & Sexuality Information and Education Council of the United States (CIRCUS): Sex Ed for Social Change. (2021). Comprehensive sex education for youth with disabilities: A call to action.

Griffiths, D., & Lunsky, Y. (2003). Sociosexual knowledge and attitudes assessment tool (SSKAAT-R). *Woodale, IL: Stoelting*.

Gutmann Kahn, L., & Lindstrom, L. (2015). "I just want to be myself": Adolescents with disabilities who identify as a sexual or gender minority. In *The educational forum* (Vol. 79, No. 4, pp. 362–376). Routledge.

Hingsburger, D., Beattie, K., Charbonneau, T., Hoath, J., Ioannou, S., King, S., & Woodhead, S. (2014). Tool for the assessment of levels of knowledge sexuality and consent (TALK-SC). *Vita Community Living Services and The Center for Behavioural Health Sciences: Toronto, ON*.

Human Rights Council (n.d.). *Glossary of Terms*. HRC. www.hrc.org/resources/glossary-of-terms?utm_source=GS.

Initiative, F. o. SE (2020). National sex education standards: Core content and skills, K-12. Future of Sex Education Initiative.

Janssen, A., Huang, H., & Duncan, C. (2016). Gender variance among youth with autism spectrum disorders: A retrospective chart review. *Transgender Health*, *1*(1), 63–68.

Kirby, A. V., Bakian, A. V., Zhang, Y., Bilder, D. A., Keeshin, B. R., & Coon, H. (2019). A 20-year study of suicide death in a statewide autism population. *Autism Research*, *12*(4), 658–666. https://doi.org/10.1002/aur.2076

Koegel, R. L., & Frea, W. D. (1993). Treatment of social behavior in autism through the modification of pivotal social skills. *Journal of Applied Behavior Analysis*, *26*(3), 369–377.

Laugeson, E. (2017). *PEERS® for young adults: Social skills training for adults with autism spectrum disorder and other social challenges*. Routledge.

Ma, Z., Travers, J. C., Martinez, J. R., Johnson, J. V., & Bross, L. A. (2021). A systematic review of intervention intensity in pivotal response training and scripting research. *Review Journal of Autism and Developmental Disorders*, 1–14.

Marshal, M. P., Dietz, L. J., Friedman, M. S., Stall, R., Smith, H. A., McGinley, J., Thoma, B. C., Murray, P. J., D'Augelli, A. R., & Brent, D. A. (2011). Suicidality and depression disparities between sexual minority and heterosexual youth: A meta-analytic review. *Journal of Adolescent Health*, *49*(2), 115–123.

McCollow, M. M., Heroux, J., & Kemper, T. (2021). Supporting the right to gender and sexuality diversity and disability. In E. A. Harkins, M. Fuller, & L. Stansberry (Eds.). *Diversity, autism, and developmental disabilities: Guidance for the culturally sustaining educator (Prism Series Vol. 13)*. Council for Exceptional Children.

Narby, C. N. (2012, January 3). *Double Rainbow: Navigating Autism, Gender, and Sexuality.* Bitch Media. www.bitchmedia.org/post/double-rainbow-nav igating-autism-gender-and-sexuality-feminism

National Autism Center. (2015). *National Standards Report* (S. M. Wilczynski, Ed.). Randolph, MA.

Normand, C. L., & Sallafranque-St-Louis, F. (2016). Cybervictimization of young people with an intellectual or developmental disability: Risks specific to sexual solicitation. *Journal of Applied Research in Intellectual Disabilities*, 29(2), 99–110.

Ona, H. N., Larsen, K., Nordheim, L. V., & Brurberg, K. G. (2020). Effects of pivotal response treatment (PRT) for children with autism spectrum disorders (ASD): A systematic review. *Review Journal of Autism and Developmental Disorders*, 7(1), 78–90.

Reid, J. A. (2018). Sex trafficking of girls with intellectual disabilities: An exploratory mixed methods study. *Sexual Abuse*, 30(2), 107–131.

Rosales-Ruiz, J., & Baer, D. M. (1997). Behavioral cusps: A developmental and pragmatic concept for behavior analysis. *Journal of Applied Behavior Analysis*, 30(3), 533–544.

Steinbrenner, J. R., Hume, K., Odom, S. L., Morin, K. L., Nowell, S. W., Tomaszewski, B., Szendrey, S., McIntyre, N. S., Yücesoy-Özkan, S., & Savage, M. N. (2020). *Evidence-based practices for children, youth, and young adults with autism.* The University of North Carolina at Chapel Hill, Frank Porter Graham Child Development Institute, National Clearinghouse on Autism Evidence and Practice Review Team.

Suhrheinrich, J., Rieth, S. R., Dickson, K. S., Roesch, S., & Stahmer, A. C. (2020). Classroom pivotal response teaching: Teacher training outcomes of a community efficacy trial. *Teacher Education and Special Education*, 43(3), 215–234.

Warner, M. (Ed.). (1993). *Fear of a queer planet: Queer politics and social theory* (Vol. 6). U of Minnesota Press.

Wehmeyer, M. L. (2013). The story of intellectual disability. *Baltimore, MD: Brookes.*

Willoughby, B. L., Doty, N. D., Braaten, E. B., & Malik, N. M. (2010). Perceived parental reactions scale. *Handbook of Sexuality-Related Measures*, 432–434.

World Health Organization. (2018, February 5). *Defining sexual health.* Sexual and reproductive health. www.who.int/reproductivehealth/topics/sexual_hea lth/sh_definitions/en/

Chapter 23

Neurodiversity and the Culture of Autism

Elizabeth A. Harkins Monaco,[1] Dylan Kapit,[2] and Gabrielle Agnew[3]
[1]College of Education, William Paterson University
[2]School of Education, University of Pittsburgh
[3]Graduate School of Biomedical Sciences, University of Texas Southwestern Medical Center

Introduction

This chapter aims to help scholars and practitioners actively engage with the views of autistic people and with the neurodiversity movement. First, we must address the concept of language in the autistic community. We use the term 'autistic individuals' because language is a critical tenant of the neurodiversity movement and the disability justice movement. The autistic community strongly advocates for the use of identity-first language, "autistic individual," when describing who they are versus the more traditional people-first approach, "individual with autism." Most people are taught to use person-first language but since we are prioritizing the wants and the needs of the autistic community, we are using their preferred terms and we recommend others do as well.

Case Study: Introduction

Autism is still viewed by many as a terrible, rare childhood disorder that affects predominantly white males. Due to this misinformation and lack of widespread knowledge regarding neurodiversity, clinicians are typically poorly trained to work with the autism population, if they are even trained at all. Consequently, females, people of color, and gender diverse individuals on the spectrum are often undiagnosed or misdiagnosed, which can easily lead to years of untreated mental and physical health concerns and untapped potential. It is not surprising that autistic people may learn to mistrust healthcare providers and have negative expectations regarding their care. Individuals with greater health literacy and resources may be able to better navigate the medical system and convey their

---

DOI: 10.4324/9781003255147-27

needs and concerns; however, even with literacy and resources, gaslighting and institutional betrayal is still common, particularly among diverse populations. Melissa's story is introduced in this chapter, and it examines the importance of intersectionality, of personal identity and history, the diagnostic process, and approach to care.

Literature Review

In the United States, we use the American Psychiatric Association's Diagnostic and Statistical Manual (DSM) as the standardized medical diagnostic criteria for autism. This manual is based on current trends in research conducted by leading 'experts'. We question the authenticity of the term 'experts' as much of the research is conducted by individuals who are not autistic and have not collaborated with autistic scholars to conduct their research, as evidenced by the divergency in the DSM's diagnostic criteria. We acknowledge that we may reference 'experts' that autistic individuals find controversial, and we would rather cite literature from autistic researchers, but the reality is that much of the research done on autism is not conducted by autistic people.

History of Autism

Autism has historically been defined through a deficit-first approach. First formally identified in 1943, autism was defined as a profound emotional disturbance that did not affect cognition in the DSM-I. The DSM-II (1953) defined autism as a childhood psychiatric condition that was based in schizophrenia and a result of cold parenting, based upon child psychiatrist Leo Kanner's (1949) concept that autistic children were raised in "emotional refrigerators" due to a lack of warmth from their primary caregivers, mostly the mothers.

> The DSM-III, published in 1980, established autism as its own separate diagnosis and described it as a "pervasive developmental disorder" distinct from schizophrenia. Prior versions of the manual left many aspects of the diagnostic process open to clinicians' observations and interpretations, but the DSM-III listed specific criteria required for a diagnosis. It defined three essential features of autism: a lack of interest in people, severe impairments in communication and bizarre responses to the environment, all developing in the first 30 months of life.
>
> (Zeldovich, 2018, paras 6–7)

The DSM-IV was originally published in 1994 and then revised in 2000. This marked the first time that autism was defined as a spectrum, and specifically listed categories, i.e., autistic disorder, pervasive developmental disorder not otherwise specified (PDD-NOS), Asperger's disorder, childhood disintegrative disorder, and Rett syndrome. Each of these categories was defined by a specific set of deficits alongside treatments to "fix" those deficits. Its goal was to promote the idea that autism was an inclusive diagnosis that allowed for a range of mild to severe deficits (Zeldovich, 2018). The labeling system also supported the research of the time that was trying to connect autism to specific genetics. In 2003 however, the Human Genome Project concluded that there wasn't an "autism gene," meaning there wasn't one gene that caused autistic traits in autistic people (Zeliadt, 2021). Another issue of the time was evidence of inconsistent diagnostic practices across the United States, with an unusual spike in diagnoses in the 2000s. Advocacy groups were blamed for significantly influencing the diagnostic process and the availability of services, so in 2013, the DSM tried to address these issues by reformatting its criteria again. The DSM-V combined the labels into the singular diagnosis of **autism spectrum disorder**. It also redefined its criteria as: 1) marked deficits in each of three areas of social communication and interaction and 2) marked deficits in at least two of four types of restricted, repetitive behaviors. It continued to offer guidelines to define the severity of these deficits (American Psychiatric Association, 2013).

Clearly, autism contains huge divergency in its diagnostic criteria. Some individuals do not have functional language and may experience developmental delays. Others identify with what was formerly called Asperger's, where individuals have average to above average IQ and no history of language delays. The Asperger's label stems from Dr. Hans Asperger, a doctor who is credited in 'discovering' these characteristics in children, but there is evidence to show that Asperger was associated with the Nazi regime and was granted career opportunities for his party affiliations.

> [He] publicly legitimized race hygiene policies including forced sterilizations and, on several occasions, actively cooperated with the child 'euthanasia' program. The language he employed to diagnose his patients was often remarkably harsh (even in comparison with assessments written by the staff at Vienna's notorious Spiegelgrund 'euthanasia' institution), belying the notion that he tried to protect the children under his care by embellishing their diagnoses.
>
> (Czech, 2018, para. 3)

The legacy of Asperger is incredibly problematic due to its distressing origins. *Note that Asperger syndrome is still used to classify autistic people in Europe.*

Autism has historically been defined by deficits such as "social communication difficulties, difficulties with cognitive empathy or theory of mind, the difficulties adjusting to unexpected change, a love of repetition or 'need for sameness', unusually narrow interests, and sensory hyper- and hyposensitivities" (Baron-Cohen, 2017, para. 3), but this kind of **deficit thinking** – thinking that places the responsibilities for addressing challenges and inequities onto autistic individuals (Davis & Museus, 2019) – undermines autistic people's success. We suggest that the strengths of an autism diagnosis are what's of value. "Autism is also associated with cognitive strengths, notably in domains such as excellent attention to detail, excellent memory for detail and a strong drive to detect patterns (or 'systemising')" (Baron-Cohen, 2017, para. 3).

Challenging the Concept of 'Disorder'

We acknowledge that autism is currently classified as Autism Spectrum Disorder (ASD) in the DSM-V, but we also acknowledge the various neurodivergencies in disability and therefore challenge the notion that autism is a disorder. 'Disorder' implies dysfunction, which means the concept of 'disorder' is stigmatizing and oppressive. This is not applied to other disabilities, like depression or ADHD. We argue that autism is better connected with the term 'disability'. "'Disability' should be used when the person experiences some of the following: thinks differently, processes their senses differently, moves differently, communicates and socializes differently, and needs help with daily living skills (ASAN, 2021). Disability indicates that everyone has areas of strength or difficulty; sometimes people can thrive in certain environments but that their [lack of] skills are disabling in other environments. Disability signals severity, without the stigma. For example, disability suggests that in autism-friendly environments, autistic people can function well or at higher levels than their non-autistic peers. We suggest that much of the time there is more evidence of disability in autism due to the need of support in one's environment, not because of one's inability to function (Lai, et al., 2013). To unpack these concepts more, we turn to Critical Disability Theory (CDT).

Critical Disability Theory (CDT): Disability as a Social Identity

Critical Disability Theory (CDT) is a framework that seeks to clarify the intersections of diversity and disability by distinguishing between the medical and societal understanding of disabilities. CDT rejects the view of disability as a medical condition which is the more traditional approach to defining disability and defining autism. The medical perspective uses biological, neurological, and hereditary impacts to define individuals by their disability's symptoms and emphasizes how to 'fix', 'improve', or 'cure' these symptoms. Thus, CDT rejects the very basis of the DSM's diagnostic process; instead, it emphasizes that much of disability is dependent upon how society supports – or doesn't support – disabled people. It points to the environments that fail to meet the needs of disabled people; it examines how societal expectations, norms, and settings impact how people can or cannot function in certain environments (Pearson, Hamilton, & Meadan, 2018).

> This interrelationship involves the individual's challenges, the individual's response to the challenges, and the social environments that the individual is a part of and has access to. All these factors help to create how the individual with disability sees themself, how society sees them, and how these two components interact to form societal norms.
>
> (Fuller et al., 2021, p. 7)

This connects with the **biopsychosocial model of disability** (World Health Organization, 2002), rooted in the **social theory of intersectionality,** which defines disability as a **social construct,** or social identity. The concept of intersectionality was first coined by Kimberlé Crenshaw (1989) who studied the intersection of Black females' racial identities (Black) and gender identities (female) and how those identities impacted their lived experiences (Crenshaw, 1989; Proctor, Williams, Scherr, & Li, 2017). Race and gender are two examples of social constructs that impact people's relationships and experiences; other examples include but are not limited to the following: socioeconomic class, sexual orientation, nationality, religion, [dis]ability, career, political orientation, language[s] spoken, parental status, family size, ethnicity, education, and values (Vance, 2021). Disability as a social construct is not **monolithic** meaning that individuals who identify as having disabilities may share that one commonality of disability, but also identify in many other ways. Abilities and disabilities vary across people, even people with the same disability, and therefore impact individuals differently. Disabled people also identify with other social constructs and groupings that may equally or increasingly impact their experiences beyond their disabilities.

Why Social Constructs Matter

Social constructs form patterns of overlapping social identities and ultimately people are often categorized by "how much one is similar to, or different from, others who occupy the same collective, or social identities" (Vance, 2021, para. 7). Therefore, social constructs create **social impact,** meaning that they impact how people think, perceive, interact, and feel and therefore, affect personal social connections and interactions. For example, a nonbinary autistic person who was assigned male at birth and identifies as Black and gay will have different social connections and experiences than their white, straight, male, non-autistic peers due to the intersection of their race, gender, sexuality, and disability (National Association of School Psychologists, 2017; Proctor, et al., 2017).

Case Study: Melissa

Melissa is an English-speaking 23-year-old African American cisgender female graduate student at a prestigious university. She presented to student health with frequent stomachaches, concentration difficulties, and constant worry. Melissa reported feeling stressed due to approaching final exams and a recent fight with her partner. She described her coursework this semester as particularly difficult, leading to feelings of anxiety and dread about attending classes. Melissa stated that she has one good friend in her cohort, but does not feel particularly close to her other classmates. "We're not necessarily interested in the same things, and I'm just too tired to hang out with them. Parties are just too loud and overwhelming." Melissa often feels so exhausted after class that she has no desire to socialize, leading to increased tension with her partner who often feels neglected. Melissa reported multiple daily crying spells for the past two weeks, in addition to difficulty getting out of bed in the morning.

Melissa grew up in a middle-class socioeconomic status two-parent household. She is the youngest of two daughters and described her childhood as "a roller coaster." From a young age, Melissa felt different from her peers and stated that she was socially awkward. However, she did not experience any physical or mental health symptoms until age 10, shortly before beginning middle school. While Melissa performed well academically, she continued to struggle socially. "It's still not easy for me today, but I make do." After speaking with a psychotherapist, she was diagnosed with social anxiety disorder and prescribed a selective serotonin reuptake inhibitor (SSRI) which somewhat alleviated her anxiety symptoms. The psychotherapist observed that Melissa answered questions succinctly, made little eye contact, frequently fidgeted with her hands, and swayed side to side in the swivel chair. Melissa later asked if she might have autism because of her sensitivity to loud noises or environments and social difficulties; however, the psycho-therapist dismissed this train of thought, stating, "You can't have autism because you can speak, make eye contact, and don't mind being touched. Anyway, autism is most common in males."

Concerned about her wellbeing, Melissa's family made the following suggestions: Melissa's grandmother encouraged her to pray and seek guidance from her pastor, and her older sister encouraged her to continue seeing the psychotherapist and ask about increasing SSRI dosage. Finally, Melissa's parents sug-gested carving out more time for self-care on the weekends. After taking everyone's advice, Melissa reported feeling slightly better but still felt disconnected from her peers and her partner. Ultimately, Melissa decided to take a leave of absence to recu-perate and re-think her future. "I'm not sure I'm cut out for academia after all."

Social impacts become problematic when people focus on and af-firm only the identities that they feel are the most personally rewarding, those that support their need to belong verses their fear or avoidance of being excluded. To reward the social intersections that lend themselves to this **sense of belonging**, people tend to create and reinforce societal disadvantages that support their preferred or dominant social identities. When people are unaware, ignorant, or unwilling to address this, others become or remain excluded and oppressed (Cooper, 2016; Crenshaw, 1989). This kind of oppression is often unconsciously distributed and therefore harder to correct (Vance, 2021). "For example, people without disabilities may not notice or recognize certain challenges people with disabilities face, which ultimately erase[s] the importance of the disabled person's needs and experiences – and in turn, their opportunities – in society" (Harkins Monaco, 2020, p. 72). Because people without dis-abilities aren't aware that they are missing these perspectives, there is an increased risk that these challenges won't be addressed.

Neurodiversity

The neurodiversity movement has grown over the past twenty years, due mostly to the advocacy efforts of the autistic community (Kras, 2009). Judy Singer, an autistic social scientist, first identified the **neurodiversity framework** in 1998. **Neurodiversity** defines neurodevelopmental con-ditions such as ADHD, learning disabilities (Baron-Cohen, 2017) and autism as diversity of the brain; it is "at the crossroads between sociology, critical psychology, critical medical humanities, disability studies, and critical autism studies" (Rosqvist et al., 2020, p. 2), and is "informed by insights developed within neuro-queer theory and crip theory" (p. 3), i.e., intersectional feminist theory and CDT. Neurodiversity goes beyond **neurotypical assumptions** held by the social majority, that define people according to symptoms and how to cure those symptoms (deficit thinking). Rather, it acknowledges that the autistic brain is not necessarily the majority brain (**neurotypical brain**), and that there actually is not a 'normal' brain because everyone's brains are different. For example, social interactions are perceived differently by many kinds of people because of the context or environment, not due to their levels of brain functioning. In this regard then, disability is a result of the interaction between an individual and an unaccommodating environment (Oliver, 1990; Leadbitter 2021).

Neurodiversity defines autism as a disability, but it simultaneously suggests that the variations in neurological development and functioning are natural and valuable, notably not pathological (Jaarsma & Welin, 2012; Kapp 2020; Leadbitter, 2021). It criticizes the lack of social and economic supports for people with differences (Rosqvist et al., 2020) by using intersectional social theory to connect autism to the multiplicity of social identities (Baron Cohen, 2017; Owren & Stenhammer, 2013). The **autistic theory of identity** then, defines autism as a social construct across identities, values, and experiences rooted in common values. The autistic theory of identity means different things to different neurodivergent people, pending on their lived experiences, self-awareness, and connections to community (Vance, 2021), just like any other social construct.

Neurodiversity "has brought about new ethical, theoretical and ideological debates within autism theory, research and practice" (Leadbitter, et al., 2021, abstract); it emphasizes collective strengths in cognitive diversity (Chapman, 2020; Kapp, 2020; Leadbitter, 2021) and fits within the intersections of the civil rights and disability rights movements (J.M. Hughes, 2016; J. A, Hughes, 2020). It recognizes and accepts that cognitive variance is a form of biodiversity and seeks to positively contribute to society (Chapman, 2020) by ending discriminatory policies and practices (Runswick-Cole, 2014; Leadbitter, 2021).

Case Study: Melissa and Neurodiversity

After a period of self-reflection and prayer, Melissa decided to seek a second opinion regarding her diagnosis. She figured that social anxiety did not fully explain her experiences, including feeling different from peers, difficulty with eye contact, social exhaustion, and sensory sensitivities. Melissa discovered neurodiversity while doing online research and wondered if she might be neurodiverse. She sought help from a mental health provider trained to work with and diagnose neurodiverse adults who confirmed that Melissa was, in fact, autistic.

Melissa was referred to a clinician experienced in working with the adult autism population for weekly psychotherapy at a local academic medical center. The clinician introduced Melissa to cognitive behavioral therapy (CBT) which is based on the idea that individuals' thoughts, feelings, and behaviors are all intertwined. To better tailor this model to Melissa's needs, spiritual beliefs and autism-specific situations (e.g., sensory overload) were also included. With this modified CBT, Melissa learned how these five components (thoughts, feelings, behaviors, spirituality, and autism-specific situations) influence each other, in addition to identifying patterns and learning how these patterns impacted her life. The clinician walked Melissa through completing a CBT thought record, in which Melissa dissected feelings of worthlessness around her academic performance: "I get so overwhelmed trying to keep up during class discussion and lectures that I get so anxious I don't participate. My professors and classmates think I'm lazy. Then, I get poorer grades and fear that I'm disappointing my family." In this case, sensory overload, potentially slower processing speeds, and misunderstandings by classmates and professors negatively impact Melissa's self-worth and esteem. Melissa and the clinician collaborated to create appropriate strengths-based coping mechanisms, including sharing her concerns with the professor, asking for notes or lecture slides before class, using fidget toys, mindfulness activities, talking to her friend, and/or excusing herself when starting to feel overwhelmed. Additionally, with the help of CBT thought logs, Melissa practiced questioning and looking for evidence against her automatic thoughts (e.g., "I'm a bad student" vs "I'm a hard-working student who deserves to be here, and simply needs more support to achieve my goals"; "I'm not smart enough for a job in academia" vs "I will continue to improve my areas of weakness and bring a new perspective to academia"). When she returned to class, Melissa received accommodations, including wearing noise-cancelling headphones, taking more frequent breaks during class, having a personal note-taker, and having more time to complete assignments. With the autism diagnosis, Melissa gained self-awareness and felt more prepared and empowered to complete her coursework and advocate for herself.

Another area of concern for Melissa was her interpersonal relationships with her grandmother and partner. Her grandmother was born and raised in Kenya before relocating to the US with her husband and children—including Melissa's mother. Many Kenyans, and people from various non-Western countries, believe autism has medical and non-biomedical causes, such as the presence of evil spirits, witchcraft, or curses (Gona, et al., 2015). Melissa thought her grandmother recently began treating her differently than her sister and cousins. "I feel more distanced from her. I know she loves me, but she doesn't spend as much time with me as she used to. She tells me all the time, 'I'll pray for you.'" Melissa attributed this to her grandmother's belief in evil spirits. As a result, Melissa feels sad and unlovable, and she fears that her partner—who is not yet aware that she is autistic—may react the same way. The clinician helped Melissa dissect her core belief of unlovability and reframe negative thoughts into positive thoughts (e.g., "I am unlovable because I'm autistic" vs "I have social and behavioral differences, but I am also kind, detail-oriented, and unique.") Melissa and the clinician created a gradual, step-by-step approach to build her confidence to discuss being on the spectrum with her grandmother and her partner. While her grandmother remained hopeful that she would be "cured of the evil spirits" through prayer, Melissa accepted that they would agree to disagree regarding the need for a cure and learned to appreciate the fact that her grandmother continues to pray for her. "That's her way of showing she loves me. In addition to taking my medication and taking care of myself, I find solace in prayer, too. Each week, I discuss the daily devotional with my clinician as part of our session, which I appreciate." Additionally, Melissa was able to better communicate her needs to her partner which improved their relationship.

Neurodiversity and Autism Research

The neurodiversity movement is also important because of the historical implications of autism research in the United States. Autism research has perpetuated problematic ideas about autism and has ultimately caused harm to the autistic community. As a starting point, most research on autism is done by non-autistic researchers who tend to pathologize autism; this is oppressive because 1) the researchers are typically not autistic and 2) their descriptions of the autistic people are biased (Ainslow,

2021). For example, autism is typically defined by negative behavioral characteristics that reduce or eliminate diagnostic traits and implicitly define being 'typical' as a goal, which is likely to cause harm to disabled people because it 1) may directly oppose their personal goals and 2) may be used to 'fix' traits that aren't causing harm to the individuals or people around them (Ne'eman, 2021). Another way research has inaccurately portrayed autistic people is when autistic people are described as amoral or incapable of comprehending morality. "There is a long history of neurotypical medical professionals attempting to portray autistic people as amoral or incapable of comprehending morality" (Ainslow, 2021, para. 1). These kinds of studies have elicited responses from the autistic community, including

> As an autistic adult, the framing of this paper concerns me enormously, both because of the obvious problem of the suspect, highly biased and pathologizing language used to describe autistic individuals in comparison to so-called "healthy controls", i.e. allistic individuals; as well as more broadly the implication that a consistent ethical stance is somehow indicative of pathology at all . . . The authors seem to have developed the premise "autistic morality is dysfunctional", then bent over backward to uphold this predetermined conclusion, despite all evidence to the contrary. I suspect a better frame through which to present the authors' data would be "Right temporoparietal junction underlies pervasive moral inconsistency in Neurotypical Spectrum Disorder"
>
> (Ainslow, 2021, para. 1)

If authors are aware of concerns, they may choose to work towards addressing them, but the reality is that non-autistic people are likely to reject these kinds of perspectives. When an autistic person thinks, lives, or experiences things differently than the non-autistic social majority, they are challenging non-autistic people's senses of self, which threatens the social hierarchies that benefit non-autistic people. Non-autistic people's **intersectional preferences** most likely benefit their neurotypical identities, therefore non-autistic people are likely to reject anything that would disrupt these preferred experiences (Vance, 2021).

It is important to discuss the impact of the neurodiversity movement on autism research (Leadbitter, 2021). For example, there is an increase in research of 1) the language used to describe autism and autistic people (see Kenny et al., 2016; Bury et al., 2020); 2) mental health and improved quality of life for autistic individuals (Autistica, 2015; National Autistic Taskforce, 2019; Leadbitter, 2021); and 3) person-centered mental health interventions (see Crane et al., 2019; Cassidy et al., 2020; Parr et al., 2020). There is also a call for further research on whether social difficulties result from deficits within individuals or as the neurodiversity movement suggests, communication breakdowns between individuals who have cognitive variances (Milton, 2012; Crompton et al., 2020).

Case Study: The biopsychosocial-spiritual approach to care

In Melissa's case, a biopsychosocial-spiritual approach to care is beneficial. Rather than focusing solely on problematic thoughts, the clinician incorporated features related to autism and spirituality, utilizing a holistic approach. An autistic life is defined by more than neurological differences; it also entails navigating a foreign, unintuitive, socially hierarchical, neurotypical world often encountering discrimination from one's home environment to academic and medical settings. Therefore, neurodivergent individuals cope in a variety of ways, including seeking social support, religion, and accommodations, as seen in the case study. As educators, healthcare providers, and other individuals in positions of power, it is our responsibility to cultivate a better understanding of the neurodiverse population and determine how to best serve this community. Autism is not a disease to be cured; it is a different way of experiencing the world.

Positionality Statement

It should be noted that Dylan Kapit (they/them), the author of this section of the chapter, is #actuallyautistic. Therefore, this section is written based on personal experiences in the education system and practices that would have been helpful for them in their educational experiences growing up. Additionally, Dylan asked other #actuallyautistic adults what they wish educators would have done for them in the K-12 classroom and incorporated some of those answers into this section. While these are recommendations and suggestions based on the experiences of #actuallyautistic learners, many autistic folks speak to the trauma and harm caused by educators who have not used some of these practices. As educators should always try to minimize the harm that is caused to their students, we strongly encourage trying to work some of these autistic adult recommended practices into your classroom.

Recommendations for Educators and Practitioners

When thinking about how to design a classroom that is validating for and affirming of neurodivergent students, there are several important things to keep in mind. First, please remember that we will reference both 'neurodivergent students' and 'autistic students' as many strategies are effective for students with neurdivergencies beyond autism. Second, remember that neurodiversity is a normal part of the human condition. No two people have brains that work the same way; therefore, no two people will learn the same way. Even in classrooms where students do not have documented disabilities and everyone is assumed to be neurotypical and otherwise abled, each student is going to need differentiated and individualized instruction. However, when dealing with students who are autistic, neurodivergent or otherwise disabled, educators will need to take more care to ensure that their classroom is set up in a way that is validating for and affirming of neurodivergence, and that it is welcoming to students whose brains exist in non-typical ways.

Some of the ways to make sure that a classroom is inclusive of autistic learners are easy and straightforward, and others take a little bit more work. If you are choosing to be an educator or practitioner who works with autistic students, you need to be prepared to do this type of work. Educators who do not put in the work are more likely to create long-lasting harm to autistic students.

Before we get into some autism affirming best practices, it is important to remind you that the education of autistic and otherwise neurodivergent learners has historically been decided by people who are neurotypical. Most administrators and educators serving autistic students are not neurodivergent themselves, which means that people making decisions about how to best educate autistic individuals are people who have never experienced what it is like to be neurodivergent. This leads to a huge disconnect between what gets written *as* best practice verses what *is* best practice according to autistic and otherwise neurodivergent people. One easy example of this is person first vs. identity first language – one is what is considered best practice by neurotypical educators and has been for many years, while the other is what is being requested by the neurodivergent community themselves. Our suggestion for educators who are interested in hearing about what neurodivergent people believe to be best practices are to go consult with neurodivergent adults about ways that their educators could have and should have supported them throughout their learning. Not all neurodivergent people have the same viewpoints. Therefore, it is that much more important to ask neurodivergent people their own preferences. By listening to autistic adults, we can better educate autistic youth. The more frequently that this happens, the more likely that what is considered best practices in education will shift.

Best Practices that Neurodivergent Adults Encourage Educators to Use in Their Classrooms

Many neurodivergent students engage in a behavior called stimming, which is shorthand for self-stimulatory behavior (Kapp et al., 2019).

There are many ways that neurodivergent folks stim, including but not limited to: tapping, flapping, rocking, humming, and other repetitive behaviors. This behavior is one that neurotypical educators often find distracting or that it makes it harder for them to teach, and therefore often work to eradicate in the classroom. Stimming is a coping skill for neurodivergent folks, a way to self-regulate, and is not a behavior that should be eradicated unless students are stimming in ways that are harmful to the student – hitting, biting, scratching, or kicking themselves. If a stim is hurting the student, then the behavior can be eradicated or restructured. If the stimming behavior is not hurting anyone, it does not need to be eradicated, even if it feels inconvenient to the educator or other students. Instead of trying to get rid of the behavior entirely, teachers should work to understand what is causing the student to stim (why is the student dysregulated) or structure the stimming in ways that make sense for both the student and the class-room environment.

Another common practice in classrooms with neurodivergent students is to try and force neurodivergent students to make eye contact when speaking, or practice something called "whole body listening" that involves eye contact. Autistic adults say that making eye contact with a speaker does not make them more likely to absorb what the speaker is saying and many neurodivergent self-advocates have written about how eye contact causes physical pain for them. The pressure for students to make eye contact often leads to students focusing so hard on eye contact that they are not able to listen as well as they would otherwise. Instead, a neurodivergent affirming educator must understand that students might not make eye contact, but that that does not mean that a student isn't paying attention. Asking students what paying attention looks like for them, how they listen best, or how they learn best can better help educators understand their neurodivergent students.

In addition to not wanting to make eye contact, many neurodivergent students do not sit still while listening or learn best in traditional body positions. A student might not be their most productive seated at their desk with their feet on the floor and their hands still on top of their desk. Many neurodivergent students need to be fidgeting in some way to pay attention. Having sensory toys or fidgets around might aid the student in being able to focus on a lesson. Some students might even learn best sitting on the floor or in another position, and this should be allowed if it is not interfering with the student's learning. Common examples of this might be that a student needs to stand while working, work with music on, wear noise canceling headphones, or a variety of other accommodations that will allow a student to work best in ways that do not involve traditional seating or expected classroom behaviors.

For many neurodivergent students, things in the classroom might be distracting that would not be distracting to someone who is neurotypical. Educators do not have to understand why something is bothering the student to help the student navigate the stimulation that is bothering them. There might be no explainable reason that something is interfering with their learning or distracting the student – it just is. If helping a student be less distracted by something does not get in the way of their learning, make the accommodation. Oftentimes it is as easy as offering them a new location like a quiet corner or noise canceling headphones.

It is also incredibly important that educators and practitioners who work with neurodivergent students do not privilege spoken language over other forms of communication. While many neurodivergent students do communicate with spoken language, many prefer other modes of communication. There are many forms of assistive technology that allow for students to communicate. Examples include apps on iPads or smartphones, text to speech which allows students to type out answers to questions and then have them read aloud, or traditional pen and paper to communicate ideas. When neurodivergent students become nonspeaking due to feelings of overstimulation, other forms of communication should also be valued as equal forms of contribution.

Additional Resources

Instead of offering research papers or other academic texts to learn about neurodivergence, we recommend that people follow #actuallyautistic and otherwise neurodivergent individuals on social media, such as Twitter and Instagram. Here are some of our favorites (Table 23.1):

Table 23.1 Social Media Accounts to Follow

Instagram	- @transteachertales
	- @autinelle
	- @fidgets.and.fries
	- @the.autisticats
	- @auteachofficial
	- @galaxibrain
	- @divergentlessons
	- @kidish.bambino
	- @autism_advocate_
Twitter	- @autistichoya
	- @autisticats
Websites by autistics for autistics:	- Autistic Women & Nonbinary Network (AWN) – https://awnnetwork.org

Note. This table illustrates only some recommended social media accounts; we are sure there are others to follow as well.

Conclusion

Autism is still considered a neurological disability (Vance, 2021), but we must acknowledge the need for increased reflection and conversation around how service provision should align with a neurodiversity framework (Leadbitter, et al., 2021). The historical exclusion of neurodivergent individuals from the academy means that much of published academic research about neurodivergence is written by people who are not neurodivergent, and therefore, sometimes end up writing about neurodivergence in a variety of problematic ways. Researchers who are not autistic must reframe their current practices to adopt "a balanced view of neurodiversity [that] recognizes . . . diversity brings fundamental collective advantages" (Leadbitter, 2021, para 5). Only when we bridge between the historical implications of autism and the current neurodiversity movement will we be able to reevaluate the practices that seek to suppress or eliminate disability-related traits (Ne'eman, 2021). The following recommendations in Table 23.2 will help.

Table 23.2 Recommendations for Educators

Do this	Not this
Seek out autistic voices	(Do not) only reference non-autistic researchers
Use identity first language	(Do not) Use people-first language
Try to understand what is causing the student to stim	(Do not) Try to eradicate stimming
Why is the student dysregulated?	
Structure the stimming in ways that make sense for both the student and the classroom environment	(Do not) Force traditional seating or expected classroom behaviors
Understand that students might not make eye contact	(Do not) Force eye contact
This doesn't mean that a student isn't paying attention	
Ask students	(Do not) Force expected classroom behaviors
1. what paying attention looks like for them	
2. how they listen best	
3. how they learn best	
Allow for fidgeting and movement	(Do not) Force traditional seating or expected classroom behaviors
Make any accommodation	(Do not) Only focus on why something is bothering the student
Offer a new location, a quiet corner, or noise canceling headphones	
Value all forms of communication	(Do not) Privilege spoken language over other forms of communication

Note. This table illustrates what to DO and what NOT to do.

Author note

We used identity-first (*autistic person*) language as largely preferred by the autistic community.

References

Ainslow, M. A. (2021). *RE: Right TPJ in moralality in people with Autism*. www.jneurosci.org/content/41/8/1699

American Psychiatric Association (2013). *Diagnostic and statistical manual of mental disorders.* 5th ed. American Psychiatric Association.

Autistic Self Advocacy Network (2021). About Autism. https://autisticadvocacy.org/about-asan/about-autism/

Autistica (2015). Your questions: Shaping future autism research. www.autistica.org.uk/downloads/files/Autism-Top-10-Your-Priorities-for-Autism-Research.pdf (retrieved November 10, 2021)

Bury, S. M., Jellett, R., Spoor, J. R., & Hedley, D. (2020). "It defines who I am" or "It's something I have": What language do [autistic] Australian adults [on the autism spectrum] prefer? *Journal of Autism and Developmental Disorders.* 10.1007/s10803-020-04425-3

Cassidy, S. A., Robertson, A., Townsend, E., O'Connor, R. C., & Rodgers, J. (2020). Advancing our understanding of self-harm, suicidal thoughts and behaviours in autism. *Journal of Autism and Developmental Disorders, 50*(10):3445–3449.

Chapman, R. (2020). Neurodiversity and the social ecology of mental functioning. *Perspectives on Psychological Science. 16*(6), 1360–1372.

Cooper, B. (2016). Intersectionality. In L. Disch & M. Hawkesworth (Eds.), *The Oxford handbook of feminist theory* (385–406). Oxford University Press.

Crane, L., Adams F., Harper, G., Welch, J., & Pellicano, E. (2019). Something needs to change': Mental health experiences of young autistic adults in England. *Autism 23*(2), 477–493.

Crenshaw, K. (1989). Demarginalizing the intersection of race and sex: A Black feminist critique of antidiscrimination doctrine, feminist theory, and antiracist politics. *University of Chicago Legal Forum, 8*(1), 139–167. https://chicagounbound.uchicago.edu/uclf/vol1989/iss1/8

Crompton, C. J., Sharp, M., Axbe, H., Fletcher-Watson, S., Flynn, E. G., Ropar, D. (2020). Neurotype-Matching, but not being autistic, influences self and observer ratings of interpersonal rapport. *Frontiers in Psychology, 11.*

Czech, H. (2018). Hans Asperger, National Socialism, and "race hygiene" in Nazi-era Vienna. *Molecular Autism 9,* 1–43. https://doi.org/10.1186/s13229-018-0208-6

Davis, L. P., & Museus, S. D. (2019). What is deficit thinking? An analysis of conceptualizations of deficit thinking and implications for scholarly research. *Currents, 1*(1). https://quod.lib.umich.edu/c/currents/17387731.0001.110?view=text;rgn=main

Fuller, M. C., Harkins Monaco, E. A., Stansberry Brusnahan, L. L., & Lindo, E. J. (2021). In Harkins Monaco, E.A., Fuller, M. C., & Stansberry Brusnahan, L. L. (Eds.), *Diversity, autism, and developmental disabilities: Guidance for the culturally sustaining educator.* (pp. 1–22). Council for Exceptional Children.

Gona, J. K., Newton, C. R., Rimba, K., Mapenzi, R., Kihara, M., Van de Vijver, F. J. R., & Abubakar, A. (2015). Parents' and professionals' perceptions on causes and treatment options for Autism Spectrum Disorders (ASD) in a multi-cultural context on the Kenyan Coast. *PloS One, 10*(8), e0132729. https://doi.org/10.1371/journal.pone.0132729

Harkins Monaco, E. A. (2020). Intersectionality in the college classroom. *Excellence in College Teaching, 31*(3), 71–92.

Hughes, J. A. (2020). Does the heterogeneity of autism undermine the neurodiversity paradigm? *Bioethics, 35*, 47–60.

Hughes, J. M. (2016). Increasing neurodiversity in disability and social justice advocacy groups. *Washington, DC: Autistic Self Advocacy Network.*

Jaarsma P., & Welin, S. (2012). Autism as a natural human variation: reflections on the claims of the neurodiversity movement. *Health Care Analysis. 20*(1), 20–30.

Kanner, L. (1949). Problems of nosology and psychodynamics of early infantile autism. *American Journal of Orthopsychiatry, 19*(3), 416–426. https://doi.org/10.1111/j.1939-0025.1949.tb05441.x

Kapp, S. K., Steward, R., Crane, L., Elliot, D., Elphick, C., Pellicaor, E., & Russell, G. (2019). 'People should be allowed to do what they like': Autistic adults' views and experiences of stimming. *Autism, 23*(7), 1783–1792. https://journals.sagepub.com/doi/pdf/10.1177/1362361319829628

Kapp, S. (2020). *Autistic community and the Neurodiversity Movement: Stories from the Frontline* (ed. S. Kapp). Springer Nature, 1–19.

Kenny, L., Hattersley, C., Molins, B., Buckley, C., Povey, C., & Pellicano E. (2016). Which terms should be used to describe autism? Perspectives from the UK autism community. *Autism, 20*(4), 442–62.

Kras J. F. (2009). The ransom notes affair: When the neurodiversity movement came of age. *Disability Studies Quarterly, 30*, 1065. 10.18061/dsq.v30i1.1065

Lai, M. C., Lombardo, M., Chakrabarti, B., & Baron-Cohen, S. (2013). Subgrouping the autism 'spectrum': Reflections on DSM-5. *PLoS Biology*, 11.

Leadbitter, K., Buckle, K. L., Ellis, C., & Dekker, M. (2021). Autistic self-advocacy and the neurodiversity movement: Implications for autism early intervention research and practice. *Frontiers in Psychology, 12,* 10.3389/fpsyg.2021.635690

Milton, D. E. (2012). On the ontological status of autism: the 'double empathy problem'. *Disability and Society. 27*, 883–887.

National Association of School Psychologists (2017). *Understanding intersectionality.* [Handout]. Bethesda, MD: Author.

National Autistic Taskforce (2019). An independent guide to quality care for autistic people. https://nationalautistictaskforce.org.uk/wp-content/uploads/RC791_NAT_Guide_to_Quality_Online.pdf (retrieved November 10, 2021).

Ne'eman, A. (2021). *When disability is defined by behavior, outcome measures should not promote "passing."* AMA Journal of Ethics, https://journalofethics.ama-assn.org/article/when-disability-defined-behavior-outcome-measures-should-not-promote-passing/2021-07

Oliver, M. (1990). *The Politics of disablement.* Palgrave.

Owren, T., & Stenhammer, T. (2013). Neurodiversity: Accepting autistic difference. *Leraning Disability Practice, 16*(4), 32–37. 10.7748/ldp2013.05.16.4.32.e681

Parr, J. R., Brice, S., Welsh, P., Ingham, B., Le Couteur, A., Evans, G., Monaco, A., Freeston, M., & Rodgers, J. (2020). Treating anxiety in autistic adults: Study protocol for the Personalised Anxiety Treatment-Autism (PAT-A©) pilot randomised controlled feasibility trial. *Trials, 21*(1), 265.

Pearson, J. N., Hamilton, M-B., & Meadan, H. (2018). "We saw our son blossom": A guide for fostering culturally responsive partnerships to support African American autistic children and their families. *Perspectives of the ASHA Special Interest Groups, 3,* 84–97.

Proctor, S. L., Williams, B., Scherr, T., & Li, K. (2017). Intersectionality and school psychology: Implications for practice. *National Association of School Psychologist (NASP).* Retrieved from www.nasponline.org/resources-and-publications/resources-and-podcasts/diversity/social-justice/intersectionality-and-school-psychology-implications-for-practice

Rosqvist, H. B., Chown, N. & Stenning, A. (eds). (2020). *Neurodiversity studies: A new critical paradigm.* Routlege: Taylor & Francis Group.

Runswick-Cole, K. (2014). 'Us' and 'them': the limits and possibilities of a 'politics of neurodiversity' in neoliberal times. *Disability and Society, 29,* 1117–1129.

Vance, T. 2021. The identity theory of autism: How autistic identity is experienced differently. https://neuroclastic.com/the-identity-theory-of-autism-how-autistic-identity-is-experienced-differently/?fbclid=IwAR1Xj1kr_DTHAE-OuriDyY_gatu7XuArvlHTdQ62g6fZUYPfbJpOZCXCWCI

World Health Organization (2002). Towards a common language for Functioning, Disability and Health (ICF). www.who.int/classifications/icf/icfbeginnersguide.pdf

Zeldovich, L. (2018). The evolution of 'autism' as a diagnosis, explained. *Spectrum.* www.spectrumnews.org/news/evolution-autism-diagnosis-explained/

Zeliadt, N. (2021). Autism genetics, explained. *Spectrum.* www.spectrumnews.org/news/autism-genetics-explained/

Index

Note: Page numbers in *italics* indicate figures, **bold** numbers indicate tables, on the corresponding pages

For Product Safety Concerns and Information please contact our EU
representative GPSR@taylorandfrancis.com
Taylor & Francis Verlag GmbH, Kaufingerstraße 24, 80331 München, Germany